MW00817083

WITH CONTRIBUTIONS BY:

Stephen I. Bistner, D.V.M.

Associate Professor of
  Comparative Ophthalmology
College of Veterinary Medicine
University of Minnesota
St. Paul, Minnesota
Diplomate, American College of
  Veterinary Ophthalmology

Lloyd E. Davis, D.V.M., Ph.D.

Professor of Clinical Pharmacology
Departments of Veterinary Clinical
  Medicine and Biosciences
College of Veterinary Medicine
University of Illinois
Urbana, Illinois
Fellow, American College of
  Veterinary Pharmacology and
  Therapeutics

Ralph A. Henderson, Jr., D.V.M., M.S.

Assistant Professor of Small Animal
  Surgery and Medicine
School of Veterinary Medicine
Auburn University
Auburn, Alabama
Diplomate, American College of
  Veterinary Surgeons

D. J. Krahwinkel, D.V.M., M.S.

Associate Professor of Surgery
Department of Urban Practice
College of Veterinary Medicine
University of Tennessee
Knoxville, Tennessee
Director of Surgical Services
Veterinary Teaching Hospital
Knoxville, Tennessee
Diplomate, American College of
  Veterinary Surgeons and
  American College of
  Anesthesiologists

SURGERY OF TRAUMATIZED SKIN:

Management and Reconstruction in the Dog and Cat

STEVEN F. SWAIM, D.V.M., M.S.

Associate Professor of Small Animal Surgery
Department of Small Animal Surgery and Medicine
Auburn University
School of Veterinary Medicine
Auburn, Alabama

W. B. SAUNDERS COMPANY
Philadelphia London Toronto

W. B. Saunders Company: West Washington Square
Philadelphia, Pa. 19105

1 St. Anne's Road
Eastbourne, East Sussex BN21 3UN, England

1 Goldthorne Avenue
Toronto, Canada M8Z 5T9, Canada

Library of Congress Cataloging in Publication Data

Swaim, Steven F

Surgery of traumatized skin.

1. Dogs—Surgery.   2. Cats—Surgery.   3. Skin—
   Surgery.   4. Skin—Wounds and injuries.   I. Title.
   [DNLM: 1. Dogs—Surgery.   2. Cats—Surgery.
   3. Skin—Surgery. SF991 S971s]

SF991.S93   636.7′08′97477   78–20729

ISBN 0–7216–8688–5

Surgery of Traumatized Skin: Management and
Reconstruction in the Dog and Cat   ISBN   0-7216-8688-5

© 1980 by W. B. Saunders Company.   Copyright under the International Copyright Union.   All rights reserved.   This book is protected by a copyright.   No part of it may be reproduced, stored in a retrieval system, or transmitted in any form or by any means, electronic, mechanical, photocopying, recording, or otherwise, without written permission from the publisher.   Made in the United States of America.   Press of the W. B. Saunders Company.   Library of Congress catalog card number 78-20729.

Last digit is the print number: 9   8   7   6   5   4   3   2

Proverbs 16:3

MEDICAL ILLUSTRATORS

Nadine K. Harper, B.S., M.S.

Medical Illustrator
Department of Learning Resources
School of Veterinary Medicine
Auburn University
Auburn, Alabama

Rhoda Pidgeon, B.F.A.

Medical Illustrator
Department of Learning Resources
School of Veterinary Medicine
Auburn University
Auburn, Alabama

George Batik, M.S.

Medical Illustrator
Biomedical Learning Resources Center
School of Health Sciences
University of Louisville
Louisville, Kentucky

Michael Schenk, M.S.

Medical Illustrator
University of Minnesota
School of Veterinary Medicine
St. Paul, Minnesota

Elizabeth Sue Tugwell, B.S.

Artist-Illustrator
Office of Communications
University of Tennessee
Knoxville, Tennessee

PREFACE

As stated by Peacock and Van Winkle, the skin is the largest organ of the body and also the most exposed organ. Thus, it is quite susceptible to both major and minor trauma. In addition to the defects caused by skin injury, skin defects also result from the surgical removal of pathologic conditions involving this organ (e.g., tumors, cysts, pyodermas). Regardless of the etiology, the end result is a skin defect which requires some form of reconstruction. It is the purpose of this text to provide the veterinary practitioner and the clinical veterinary student with information on the management and reconstruction of traumatized skin and skin defects, including some basic information on the anatomy and physiology of the skin, the etiology of skin trauma and defect and wound healing. It is not the purpose of this text to present information on reconstructive procedures designed to alter an animal's appearance to conform to man-made standards (e.g., ear trimming, tail docking, and the like).

When dealing with a case of skin trauma or defect, the practicing veterinarian should consider his patient and its owner and adhere to the philosophy that *the simplest, least time-consuming, and most economical means of management and reconstruction should be considered first.* The more involved techniques of skin reconstruction (e.g., multistaged surgeries, such as the use of bipedicle tube flaps) should be considered when the nature of the wound indicates their use and the pet owners are willing to invest the expense and undertake the care that will be involved in such procedures.

All forms of surgery involve both science and art; however, the art of surgery is of prime importance in plastic and reconstructive surgery. Though various reconstructive techniques have been described with regard to the shifting of local tissues and the use of various types of flaps to close skin defects, it is often necessary for the surgeon to call upon imagination to modify and combine some of the named procedures to provide an effective wound closure technique that will meet the demands of the situation.

Steven F. Swaim

Auburn, Alabama

ACKNOWLEDGMENTS

I am grateful to all individuals who have played a part in making this book a reality. The fine contributions of Drs. Bistner, Davis, Henderson, and Krahwinkel in their respective chapters is sincerely appreciated. I am grateful for Dr. B. F. Hoerlein's support and encouragement during the preparation of this book. In addition, the cooperation and interest of the numerous faculty members of the Department of Small Animal Surgery and Medicine have been a source of encouragement and are most appreciated.

A text such as this is not possible without adequate illustrations and photographs, and thanks go to Mrs. Nadine Harper, Mrs. Rhoda Pidgeon, Ms. Elizabeth Sue Tugwell, Mr. Michael Schenk, and Mr. George Batik for their outstanding medical illustration work. I am also grateful for the contributions of the several medical photographers whose work was used in the text.

As with illustrations, typists are a vital part of producing a book, and the typing support of Mrs. Karen Lynch, Ms. Zenobia Carter, Mrs. Kathy Delehoy, and Ms. Angela Bratcher are gratefully acknowledged.

I am most appreciative of the unselfish help and support given by members of the staff and veterinary students of Auburn University in the preparation of this book. I am especially appreciative for the help given by Dr. William C. Sammons, Dr. John C. Faircloth, Mr. Harley H. Sutton, Ms. Pamela Jones, Ms. Karen Huffman, Mrs. Deborah Schubert, Ms. A. Louise Henley, and the veterinary library staff.

Mr. Carroll Cann, Mr. Robert Reinhardt, Mr. Raymond Kersey, and the entire staff of W. B. Saunders Company have been most helpful in the preparation of this book. The author is grateful for their support and guidance in its preparation.

I am especially grateful for the loving encouragement and understanding of my wife Marjorie during the preparation of this book. In addition to this support, the unselfish contribution of her time for typing and proofreading were vital in its preparation. The words of encouragement and understanding from my sons Tom and Matt during the book's preparation were very meaningful to me.

Steven F. Swaim

Auburn, Alabama

CONTENTS

SECTION I – INTRODUCTION

Chapter 1
ANATOMY AND PHYSIOLOGY OF THE SKIN 3

Chapter 2
ETIOLOGY OF SKIN TRAUMA AND DEFECTS 40

Chapter 3
WOUND HEALING 70

SECTION II – MANAGEMENT OF TRAUMATIZED SKIN

Chapter 4
MANAGEMENT OF CONTAMINATED AND
INFECTED WOUNDS 119

Chapter 5
THERMAL BURNS 214
Lloyd E. Davis, D.V.M., Ph.D.

SECTION III – RECONSTRUCTION OF TRAUMATIZED SKIN

Chapter 6
GENERAL PRINCIPLES OF DELAYED WOUND
EXCISION AND CLOSURE 237

Chapter 7
MOVING LOCAL TISSUES TO CLOSE SURFACE
DEFECTS 297

Chapter 8
SKIN FLAPS 321

Chapter 9
Z-, V-Y, AND W-PLASTIES 395

Chapter 10
SKIN GRAFTS 423

Chapter 11
BLEPHAROPLASTY 477
Stephen Bistner, D.V.M.
George Batik, M.S., Medical Illustrator
Michael Schenk, M.S., Medical Illustrator

Chapter 12
RECONSTRUCTIVE EAR SURGERY.. 520
Trauma, Infection, Neoplasia, and Developmental Deformities
Ralph A. Henderson, D.V.M., M.S.

Chapter 13
CORRECTION OF SPECIFIC SKIN DISEASES........................ 550
D. J. Krahwinkel, Jr., D.V.M., M.S.

INDEX... 573

SECTION I

INTRODUCTION

ANATOMY AND PHYSIOLOGY OF THE SKIN

FUNCTION OF SKIN

A human physiology text published in 1872 aptly described the skin. "The skin is a tough, thin, close fitting garment for the protection of the tender flesh. Its perfect elasticity beautifully adapts it to every motion of the body. We shall learn hereafter that it is more than a mere covering, being an active organ, which does its part in the work of keeping in order the house in which we live. It oils itself to preserve its smoothness and delicacy, replaces itself as fast as it wears out, and is at once the perfection of use and beauty."[31] Points of this description are as applicable to animals as they are to humans. The functions of the skin are many.

PROTECTION OF UNDERLYING STRUCTURES

The skin protects the fluid body from its dry environment and from hypotonic or hypertonic fluid surroundings.[20] It also protects the body from physical,[9, 20, 22, 28] chemical,[9, 22, 28] and microbiological[9, 20, 22] trauma. The skin protects the body from invasion by macroorganisms and particulate foreign bodies.[9] The body is protected from external deficiencies of water and humidity[9] as well as overexposure to sunlight and other radiation.[9, 28] The skin also provides protection against the loss of internal fluids, chemicals (including electrolytes), and macromolecules.[9, 22]

TEMPERATURE REGULATION

The skin performs a thermoregulatory function,[9, 20, 22, 28, 33] with the hair coat,[9, 22] sweating,[9] and the regulation of the cutaneous blood supply controlling body temperature.[22]

As stated by Muller and Kirk, the dog and cat do not possess the extensive superficial arteriovenous shunts that are present in man and pigs for the dissemination of heat in hot weather. Ordinarily, 75 per cent of the heat loss is accomplished by radiation, conduction, and convection, with the efficiency of these mechanisms varying with the external temperature and humidity. The efficiency is further modified by the animal's vasomotor and pilomotor responses. As the environmental temperature rises, the aforementioned factors become quite ineffective in producing heat loss, and heat loss by vaporization from the skin and lungs predominates. Dogs and cats vaporize large volumes of water from their respiratory passages as a means of heat loss. The cat has an additional heat loss mechanism. A hot environment, or sympathetic stimulation, produces a copious flow of watery saliva from the submaxillary salivary gland. This saliva is spread on the hair for additional water vaporization and cooling.[22]

When the environmental temperature drops, the body attempts to preserve heat by vasoconstriction in the skin and erection of the hairs to improve the insulating qualities of the skin and coat.[22]

SENSORY PERCEPTION

The skin serves as a sense organ through nerve endings for touch, pressure, temperature, pain, and itching,[9, 20, 22] all of which help the animal relate to its environment.[28]

SECRETION AND EXCRETION

The presence and function of apocrine, merocrine, and sebaceous glands in the skin make it a secretory organ.[9, 22] There are also modified sebaceous glands of the eyelid, tail, circumanal area, and anal sacs. Secretions of the glands help in maintaining a buffered surface film with some antimicrobial and antifungal actions[9] in addition to keeping the skin supple and hydrated.[28] Glandular secretion is most developed in the mammary glands, which are a form of apocrine gland.[33] In some species the skin functions in a limited way as an excretory organ.[22]

SYNTHESIS AND STORAGE

Through solar radiation stimulation, the skin is able to produce vitamin D.[20, 22] As a storage organ the skin stores carbohydrates, electrolytes, fat, protein, water, and other materials.[9, 22, 28]

ADNEXAL PRODUCTION

The skin produces keratinized structures such as hair, vibrissae (tactile hairs), nails, and the horny layer of the epidermis (keratin).[9, 22]

BLOOD PRESSURE CONTROL

The skin helps to maintain normal blood pressure by means of peripheral vascular dynamics, which produce changes in the peripheral vascular bed that affect blood pressure.[9, 22]

PIGMENTATION

Melanin formation, vascularity, and keratinization all enter into the pigmentation process and help determine coat and skin color. Damage from solar radiation is prevented by skin pigmentation.[22]

RECOGNITION OF FOREIGN PROTEINS

The skin is capable of recognizing foreign proteins in the form of contact allergens, haptens, and venoms, and it can stimulate antibody production.[9]

INDICATOR

The presence of internal disease may be indicated by the skin.[22] An example of this is the rough, dry hair coat exhibited by cats suffering from a systemic disease.

SELF-MAINTENANCE AND REPAIR [9]

As stated earlier, one of the functions of the skin is to continually replace itself as it is worn out.[31] Surgery of the skin takes advantage of the skin's ability to repair itself. Whether it is the healing of a sutured wound or healing by second intention, the reparative processes of the skin are essential for success.

MOTION AND SHAPE

The flexibility, elasticity, and toughness of the skin are properties that allow motion and provide shape and form.[22] The skin is remarkably loose on the dorsal aspect of the neck and trunk, where it is possible to raise it in extensive folds.[30] These properties are useful to the surgeon in reconstruction of the skin. They allow the skin to be moved over defects from adjacent areas either by means of tension sutures or by means of skin flaps. The skin's toughness allows the placement of sutures to hold it in the new position.

SKIN AND HAIR IN GENERAL

Hair and skin are different on different parts of the body. Four general types of skin make up the canine integument: nasal, foot pad, scrotal, and hairy skin.[22] With regard to hairy skin, it is generally thicker on the back and on the extensor surfaces of the limbs than it is on the underside and flexor surfaces of the limbs.[33] More specifically, the skin is thickest over the dorsum and the neck and thinnest over the abdomen, sternum, axillary and

TABLE 1–1   EPIDERMAL AND DERMAL THICKNESSES[34]

Skin Type	Body Region
Thin epidermis, thin dermis	Pinna, axillary, and inguinal
Thin epidermis, thick dermis	Head, neck, shoulder, axillary, sternal, abdominal, back, tail, and prepuce
Thick epidermis, thin dermis	Lip and nasal septum
Thick epidermis, thick dermis	Digital pads

inguinal region, and the inner lining of the pinna.[22, 28, 34] Various combinations of thick and thin dermis and epidermis are found over the body (Table 1–1). A microscopic study of cat skin showed a decrease in thickness from dorsal to ventral on the trunk and from proximal to distal on the limbs.[32]

The type and density of hair coat will vary from one point to another on the body. In dogs, and cats especially, there is an inverse relationship between hair coat density and epidermal thickness;[22] the thickened epidermis on sparsely haired areas helps afford some of the protection given by the hair coat in areas of dense hair.

The skin, hair, and subcutis of a newborn puppy constitute 24 per cent of the body weight; however, at maturity these structures only represent 12 per cent of the body weight.[20, 22] As an animal ages, certain changes take place in the skin and hair. Senile changes in dog skin are similar to those in humans, except that there are no vascular changes and no senile elastosis or dermal basophilia.[3, 22] It is possible that the extra pigmentation and dense hair coat of dogs may protect them from some of the changes caused by light in aging human skin. Changes may not be due entirely to poor blood supply and nutrition; the accumulation of metabolites may play a part. With increasing age there is an increased incidence of carcinoma of the skin.[22] This could, of course, lead to the need for surgical removal and skin reconstruction in the aged animal.

Changes in senile dog skin vary with its location on the body but are mainly in the form of cellular atrophy, with a decrease in both size and numbers of cells. The atrophy affects the epidermis, appendages, and dermis. Follicular atrophy is exhibited by hair loss, which is generally bilateral in areas of wear. The apocrine glands do not regress in the dog but do contain yellow granules, which are not iron. In addition to these senile changes, the arrector pili muscles degenerate by becoming eosinophilic, fragmented, and vacuolated until they are absent in extreme old age. Hyperkeratosis of the hair follicles and epidermis, with the claws becoming malformed and brittle and the foot pads becoming hyperkeratotic, has also been noted.[3, 22]

Changes in the hair are also seen with aging in that a young adult dog will have profuse and abundant hair growth, whereas old dogs will have a thinner, shorter hair coat that may be gray[20] as a result of atrophy of pigment cells in the hair follicles.[22] The hairs also become more brittle[20] along with skin and subcuticular changes in the form of increased dermal pigmentation and loss of flexibility.[20, 22] Such changes are of interest to the surgeon in that the lack of flexibility of senile skin may have some bearing on the type of skin flap that can be used to correct a defect.

Opinions vary as to the effect of clipping and shaving on the rate of hair growth. It has been stated that clipping and shaving have no effect on hair growth or the stage of its growth cycle.[20] However, evidence has been obtained that shaving is closely followed by some degree of stimulation of hair growth. In this study it was found that two rates of growth occurred after clipping and shaving the hair: (1) an initial slow growth rate of about 0.04 mm. per day and (2) a second, more rapid growth rate of 0.18 mm. per day; it was also stated that further study was necessary to determine whether this was the normal growth pattern after clipping and shaving.[6] Even though generalizations may be misleading, normal or short hair coats usually take about 130 days to regrow after shaving, whereas long hair coats, such as that of the Afghan hound, may take up to 18 months.[22] Further studies are needed before we can accurately answer the client's question, "When will the hair grow back, doctor?"

EPIDERMIS

BASIC ANATOMY AND PHYSIOLOGY

The skin is made up of two main layers: the outer layer, called the epidermis, the superficial epithelial layer, or surface epithelium, and the subjacent layer, called the dermis or corium, which is composed of dense connective tissue[9, 18, 29] (Fig. 1–1). The epidermis has a high degree of elasticity[33] and is lacking in blood vessels, with its nourishment coming from tissue fluid that penetrates from the deeper layers[18] and from nearby capillaries in the dermis.[9] Generally, the canine epidermis is thinner than that

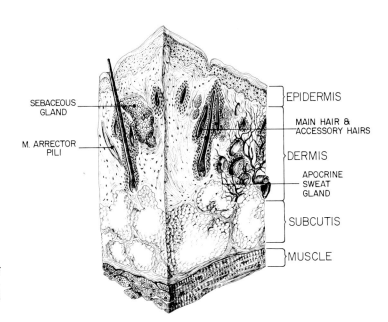

SEBACEOUS GLAND

M. ARRECTOR PILI

EPIDERMIS

MAIN HAIR & ACCESSORY HAIRS

DERMIS

APOCRINE SWEAT GLAND

SUBCUTIS

MUSCLE

Figure 1–1: Basic anatomy of the skin. (After Kral, F.: Noninfectious dermatoses in dogs and cats. Vet. Scope 2:8, 1957.)

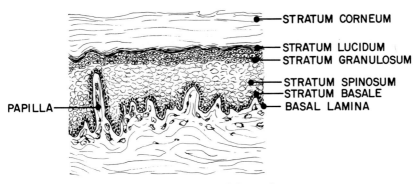

Figure 1–2: Layers of the epidermis.

of humans. It is less than 100 μ thick in all areas except the lips, digital pads, and nasal septum. In hairy regions its thickness is between 30 and 40 μ, with the thinnest epidermis being over the sternum.[20, 28] Epidermal papillae are found on the skin. These papillae measure from 0.33 to 0.35 mm. in diameter and project from 0.25 to 0.48 mm. above the skin. They are composed of epidermis, which is six to 12 cell layers thick, overlying a projection of the dermis that is composed of fine, closely packed connective tissue fibers.[19, 20]

The primary function of the epidermis is to produce a horny coat through the process of keratinization.[9] This is basically brought about by five cell layers in the epidermis (Fig. 1–2). However, the majority of the skin's epidermis is made up of three of the layers, the stratum basale, stratum spinosum, and stratum corneum, with the remaining two layers, the stratum granulosum and stratum lucidum, being evident in those areas where keratinization is retarded.[19, 20] The stratum basale constitutes the basal layer of the epidermis, and it is responsible for the production of the cells of the other layers of the epidermis with the resultant keratinization (Fig. 1–2). The mitotic frequency within these cells is greatest during sleep,[33] with fewer mitotic figures being present in the stratum basale of hairy skin than in the same layer in the foot pads and planum nasale.[20] This is in keeping with the epidermal thickness of these areas, since there is an inverse relationship between hair covering and dermal thickness.[22] Studies have shown the total epidermal cell renewal time in normal beagles to be 22 days. This is from the basal cell layer to the stratum granulosum.[2, 22] Clipping the hair has been found to decrease the cell renewal time to 15 days and to stimulate melanocytes so that increased melanin pigment was found in epidermal cells. The epidermis seems to respond to irritants such as inflammation, trauma, and metabolic changes by a shortened keratinocyte cycle and by increased melanin deposition. Clinically, this is seen as scaling and darkening of the skin.[22]

Basal Lamina

In animals the undersurface of the epidermis is smooth, undulating, and more or less parallel to the skin surface. In humans this dermoepidermal junction is thrown into distinct folds called rete ridges. These ridges are normally seen in the skin of the scrotum in small animals, whereas they are seen in other areas only as a result of pathological processes. At the dermoepidermal junction there is a chemical interface known as the basal lamina. This is not a membrane even though it has been called the basement membrane[22] (Fig. 1–2).

Basal Layer

The basal layer of the epidermis (stratum basale, stratum cylindricum) is the deepest layer of epidermis that lies in contact with the basal lamina. The cells in this layer are columnar cells with cytoplasmic processes that penetrate the basal lamina.[22, 33]

Most of these cells are keratinocytes that are constantly reproducing and pushing upward to replenish the epidermal cells above, which are eventually shed as dead horny cells.[22] Keratinocytes are particularly abundant in the skin of the foot pad and planum nasale.[28] The keratinocytes produce the dead fibrous protein keratin, which is the primary constituent of the outermost horny layer of skin. In dogs and cats there is soft keratin, which forms the outer layers of the hair epidermis, and hard keratin, which forms the outer layer of the claws.[22]

The melanocyte is the second type of cell in the basal layer. It produces melanin, which is responsible for hair color and for naturally occurring general and local skin pigmentation.[18, 22] Since these cells are located in the basal layer, most of the skin pigment is in this area; the horny layer is usually unpigmented. When exposed to sunlight, irritation, or inflammation, these cells produce an increased number of melanin granules. White skin and dark skin do not differ in the number of melanocytes that they contain; however, dark skin contains more melanin, which indicates greater activity of the melanocytes. Albinos have about the same number of melanocytes as normal animals, but they do not form melanin owing to a lack of tyrosinase (Fig. 1–2).[22]

Prickle Cell Layer

The prickle cell layer (spinous cell layer, stratum spinosum, stratum malpighii) is two to three cells thick in the hairy skin and is composed of cells that are daughter cells of the basal layer cells. In the foot pad and planum nasale, these cells appear to be connected by fine spines or intercellular bridges, which are tonofibrils radiating from desmosomes in the cell membrane.[20, 22] The function of these fibrils may be to reinforce the epithelium.[33] These cells fill the depressions between the dermal papillae[33] and are generally inactive mitotically unless the surface epidermal layers are stripped off.[22] However, these cells should be considered viable nucleated cells that actively synthesize keratin.[22] Owing to their viability, they are classified along with the basal layer as the stratum germinativum.[28, 33] In dark-skinned animals, melanin granules are present in and between the cells of this layer.[28] In white or light-colored animals, pigment is found mainly in this layer, but in black skin it is found in all layers of the epidermis as well as the papillary area of the dermis.[34] Dendritic cells located in the upper prickle cell layer are called Langerhans' cells. They resemble melanocytes but do not stain for melanin. These cells have an obscure function and significance and may be phagocytic (Fig. 1–2).[22]

Granular Cell Layer

The stratum granulosum is a layer of cells that is dying.[22] There are differing opinions as to the location and thickness of this layer. Some believe that it may not be present,[22] and others believe that it is present except on the face, head, and ears.[28, 34] It may be one cell layer thick on certain parts of the body,[22, 28, 34] or it may be up to five[33] or 15 layers thick.[28, 34] The cells are fusiform and finely serrated and show the first signs of keratinization in the form of shiny basophilic keratohyalin granules. These granules give a granular appearance to this layer. The nuclei of the cells shrink and undergo chromatolysis (Fig. 1–2).[33]

Clear Cell Layer

The clear cell layer (stratum lucidum) is absent in skin on hairy regions and is only present in the foot pads of the dog and cat.[22, 28, 34] It is a thin compact layer of nonnucleated dead cells[22] that have an acidophilic homogeneous appearance microscopically.[33] The keratohyalin granules are replaced by a specifically stainable substance (eleidin) that is allied with, but not essential to, keratinization.[33] The layer is fully keratinized (Fig. 1–2).[22]

Horny Layer

The horny layer (stratum corneum), which is relatively thicker in areas where the skin is subjected to constant pressure,[18] is present in all skin areas.[28] It is thinnest on the lip and thickest on the digital foot pads.[34] This layer is composed of cells that are usually flat but may, at times, be swollen and vesicular.[33] These cells have no nuclei and form fully keratinized, loose eosinophilic bands that run parallel to the skin surface.[28] These cells are dead and are constantly being shed as scales.[18, 22, 33] This is balanced by a proliferation of cells in the basal layer to maintain a constant epidermal thickness.[18, 22] The horny layer, along with the granular layer, forms the barrier zone that prevents the outward loss of fluid and other elements and the inward diffusion of chemicals, bacteria, and other noxious substances.[22] It contains less water than the other underlying epidermal cells, and it absorbs water when it is wet (Fig. 1–2).

The epidermis in hairy skin areas of cats is thin and consists of four distinct layers, with the stratum lucidum being absent. In the nonhairy skin of the cat, all five epidermal layers are present. The thickest epidermis is found on the metacarpal foot pad, the planum nasale, and the lip.[32]

DERMIS

BASIC ANATOMY AND PHYSIOLOGY

The dermis, or "true skin," is quite vascular and generally much thicker than the epidermis.[18] It is composed of fibers, ground substance, and cells[22] and is well supplied with blood vessels, lymphatic vessels, and nerves. In addition to these, it contains glands and their ducts, hair follicles, and smooth muscle fibers (Fig. 1–1).[18, 19, 22, 29] In hairy areas the dermis is divided into a distinct papillary layer and a reticular layer.[28] However, in one histological study on mongrel dogs, no distinct division was noted between the two layers.[34] The papillary layer is more superficial; its blunt conical prominences are called papillae and have within them vascular loops, nerves, or specific nerve endings.[18, 29] In hairy skin the papillae are small and poorly differentiated.[33] One study has shown *no* pegging of the epidermis in hairy areas of the skin. In place of this, the dermoepidermal junction is normally thrown into folds that parallel the surface contour of the skin.[19] However, in hairless or sparsely haired areas, the papillae are large and slender. Some papillae branch into more than one cone-shaped projection. These form compound papillae and are found in the foot pads of dogs.[33] Epidermal pegging is also present in the planum nasale and mucous membranes.[19] The reticular layer of the dermis is not sharply demarcated from the papillary layer. This is the deeper and heavier dermal layer where the fiber bundles interweave mainly in a horizontal plane.[33]

In areas of thick hairy skin, the dermis is relatively thicker than the epidermis, whereas in very thin skin, such as that of the scrotum, the thinness is due to a thin dermis.[22] The canine dermis is thickest over the scapular and sacral regions.[28] The main functions of the dermis are nutrition and physical support of the epidermis.[9]

The reticular layer of the deep dermis consists of a relatively loose network of coarse bundles of fibers. In most places there is no clear demarcation between it and the subcutis.[29] This presents a problem to the surgeon when trying to take a free full-thickness skin graft, since all subcuticular tissue should ideally be removed from the dermis on such a graft.

Ground Substance

The ground substance, which is composed of mucopolysaccharides in the form of hyaluronic acid and chondroitin-sulfuric acid, is the primary component of the dermis. It surrounds other structures of the dermis and fills the spaces, while allowing electrolytes, nutrients, and cells to traverse it freely in passing from the dermal vessels to the avascular epidermis. The ground substance decreases in amount as animals age.[22]

Fiber Content

The fibers of the dermis are collagenous, reticular, and elastic,[19, 22, 34] with the connective tissues being finer and denser under the epidermis than in deeper layers.[19] Collagenous fibers are the largest and most numerous type of fiber, constituting approximately 90 per cent of all the fibers. These fibers are generally in the form of thick bands composed of multiple protein fibrils.[22] However, the collagen fibers are of varying thickness and arrangement.[28, 34] In the papillary area of the dermis, small collagen bundles run parallel to the surface, with a few fibers going in every direction. Collagen bundles are wider in the deep or reticular area of the dermis. In areas where the skin is pliable, such as the axillary and flank region and the dorsum of the neck, collagen bundles are smaller and more loosely arranged. In areas of thick skin, such as the head region, digital pad, lip, nasal septum, and dorsal body surface, large collagenous bundles are arranged parallel to the surface.[34] The fact that androgens increase collagen production[22] may be of interest to the surgeon when planning a regimen in which good strong wound healing is desired.

The reticular fibers, also known as precollagen, are finely branched structures.[22] These fibers are present throughout the ground substance at birth and gradually decrease in number within four weeks. At this time they are concentrated around blood vessels, hair follicles, glands, and arrector pili muscles and beneath the basal cell layer of the epidermis.[28, 34] In all areas of the body the reticular fibers interdigitate between the basal cells of the epidermis and help form the epidermal basal layer. The fibers closely approximate collagen fibers with age.[22]

Elastic fibers are made up of single fine branches that have great elasticity.[22] These fibers are less abundant in the superficial dermis as compared with the deeper dermis;[28] however, a study has shown these fibers to be more numerous in the superficial area of the dermis in regions where the skin is more pliable, such as the axillary and flank region and the dorsum of the neck.[34] In general, elastic fibers in the papillary zone are finer and woven into a network, although single fibers have been found. In the deep or reticular layer of the dermis, elastic fibers are more numerous with fewer networks.[34]

The fiber content of the dermis plays a role in determining the presence and direction of tension lines in the skin. These lines have been mapped out in humans and dogs and are important to surgeons in that incisions made along these lines tend to heal more cosmetically than those made across tension lines. The significance of these lines will be discussed in more detail in Chapter 7.

Cellular Content

The major cell types in the dermis are (1) fibroblasts, (2) histiocytes, and (3) mast cells (Fig. 1–3).[22]

The fibroblasts produce tropocollagen fibrils, which are the precursors of collagen fibers. They are often found adjacent to the surface of collagen bundles[22] and are responsible for producing elastic[9] and reticular fibers.

The histiocytes are mature lymphoid-type cells. They possess phagocytic characteristics.[22]

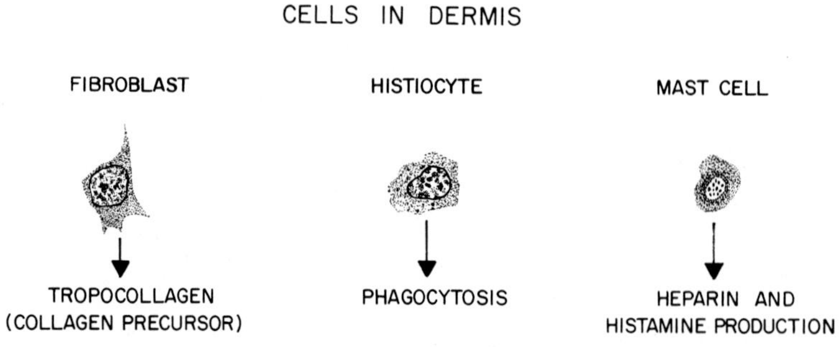

CELLS IN DERMIS

FIBROBLAST   HISTIOCYTE   MAST CELL

TROPOCOLLAGEN   PHAGOCYTOSIS   HEPARIN AND
(COLLAGEN PRECURSOR)   HISTAMINE PRODUCTION

Figure 1–3: Cells of the dermis and their primary function.

Mast cells or tissue basophils are responsible for the production of heparin and histamine,[9, 22] which are released in response to tissue injury. As reported by Muller and Kirk, the histamine causes vasodilation and wheals as a result of increased extravasation of fluids from capillaries into the extracellular fluid space. The heparin prevents the formation of microclots either intracellularly or in small lymphatic or blood vessels. This process increases the removal of extravasated blood either by lymphatics or by phagocytosis by means of connective tissue macrophages.[22]

Considerable pigmentation of the dermis has been noted in the senile dog, especially in the palpebral margins. This pigment presumably screens the dermis from the harmful effects of light. Elastosis of the dermis is not seen in senile dog skin as it is in humans. This is possibly due to the protection afforded the skin by the hair. The obliterative changes seen in the skin vessels of aged humans have not been seen in the skin of senile dogs.[3]

In cats the dermis is composed of stratum papillare and reticulare,[23] with the collagenous fibers being largest in the stratum reticulare and the elastic fibers being more abundant near the arrector pili muscles and in flexible skin.[32] In the more flexible areas of skin on the cat, the collagenous bundles are smaller and more loosely arranged. These areas are the dorsal neck, the scapular area, and the lateral upper forelimb.[32] As a general rule, the skin of the cat is more flexible and movable than that of the dog. This is of benefit to the veterinary surgeon in that local skin can usually be shifted to close some rather large defects on the cat.

SUBCUTIS

ANATOMY AND PHYSIOLOGY

The subcutis is composed of connective tissue, nerves, blood vessels, and lipocytes.[22] The connective tissue consists of loose collagenous trabeculae, which contain many elastic fibers that cross each other to form a meshwork. The spaces of the meshwork are further subdivided by smaller bundles. A homogeneous adhesive ground substance converts the fiber nets to thin membranes, between which are narrow tissue spaces. These spaces are often filled with adipose tissue,[33] which may serve several purposes. The fat can serve as (1) a cushion or shock absorber (as in the foot pads); (2) a filler; (3) a sheath for easily injured parts (e.g., nerves and vessels); and (4) an insulator to protect the body from excessive heat loss.[33] Canine females generally have a thicker fat layer than males.[28, 34] In areas where the skin is anchored tightly against underlying tissues, the subcutis and adipose tissue are absent or very thin. Such skin is found on the inner surface of the ear, the lips, the eyelids, the nose, the scrotum, and other areas.[33]

In spite of these favorable functions of subcuticular fat, it can present a problem to the surgeon when a free full-thickness skin graft is to be used to correct a skin defect. All subcuticular fat must be removed from the deep surface of the dermis so that it will not interfere with the penetration of capillaries from the wound bed into the dermis of the graft. On an obese animal in which the fat has invaded the deeper dermal areas, removal of this fat is perplexing in that the surgeon is uncertain how far to proceed with fat removal before damage is done to the bases of hair follicles. Such damage results in poor hair growth on the graft.

The degree to which the skin can be folded or displaced is dependent upon the development of the subcutis, i.e., the extensibility, length, and thickness of the fiber bundles that have already been mentioned.[33] This is important to the surgeon when attempting to close a skin defect by shifting local tissues. Skin that can be displaced easily as a result of the previously described subcutis development lends itself to this type of reconstruction more readily.

As reported by Nevrand and Schwartz, there are two distinct layers to the subcutis of a cat. The superficial part is the stratum adiposum subcutis, which contains fat, especially in the area of the hair shafts. The stratum fibrosum subcutis is the deeper layer. It is a connective tissue layer that is almost without fat and that contains the cutaneous muscle in the various body regions.[23]

HAIR FOLLICLES

BASIC ANATOMY

The basic unit of hair production is the hair follicle; each shaft of hair is produced in a sleeve of epithelium that is continuous with the surface epidermis.[20] Follicles have a sac-like fundus, a narrow neck, and a wider funnel-shaped opening. The follicle is made up of a peripheral connective tissue portion (follicle proper) and an inner epithelial part (root sheaths).[33] The connective tissue part of the follicle is that part of the follicle contributed by the dermis, while the epithelial part is contributed by the epidermis.[29, 33] The epithelial part is divided into outer and inner root sheaths,[20, 22, 33] with the outer root sheath being a continuation of the basal layer of the epidermis. The inner root sheath, which is firmly connected to the outer sheath, grows upward with the hair from the papilla as far as the opening of the sebaceous gland, where it disintegrates.[22, 33] The innermost

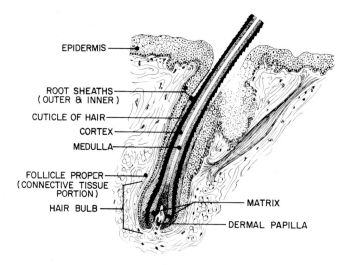

EPIDERMIS

ROOT SHEATHS
(OUTER & INNER)

CUTICLE OF HAIR

CORTEX

MEDULLA

FOLLICLE PROPER
(CONNECTIVE TISSUE
PORTION)

HAIR BULB

MATRIX

DERMAL PAPILLA

Figure 1–4:   Basic anatomy of a hair and its follicle.

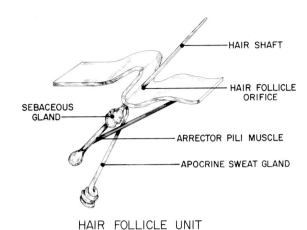

HAIR SHAFT

HAIR FOLLICLE
ORIFICE

SEBACEOUS
GLAND

ARRECTOR PILI MUSCLE

APOCRINE SWEAT GLAND

HAIR FOLLICLE UNIT

Figure 1–5: Simple hair follicle with its associated structures (arrector pili muscle, sebaceous gland, and apocrine gland) making up a hair follicle unit. (From Lovell, J. E., and Getty, R.: The hair follicle, epidermis, dermis, and skin glands of the dog. Am. J. Vet. Res. *18*:877, 1957.)

layer of the epithelial follicle is the cuticle of the sheath, which is a membrane similar in structure to the adjacent hair cuticle. The free edges of the cells of the cuticle are directed toward the papilla of the follicle so that they interdigitate with the free edges of the cells of the hair cuticle (Fig. 1–4).[33]

The hair follicle attains its greatest diameter at its base (the sac-like fundus previously mentioned), where it dilates in the shape of a bulb (hair bulb). This hair bulb is invaginated from the bottom by a dermal papilla containing blood vessels. The outer root sheath ends in a tapered edge at the neck of the papilla, while the inner root sheath and hair grow from a layer of nucleated cells (germinative epithelium, or hair matrix) covering the papilla (Fig. 1–4).[20, 22, 33]

Hair follicles can extend into the subcutaneous adipose tissue[19] and thus be damaged when harvesting a free full-thickness skin graft.

A hair follicle may also have associated with it an arrector pili muscle as well as apocrine and sebaceous glands that empty into it. These structures make up the hair follicle unit (Fig. 1–5).[22]

SINGLE AND COMPOUND FOLLICLES

At birth the hair follicles are simple or primary, with one hair per follicle. As the animal ages, accessory hairs develop in accessory or secondary follicles, which arise as buds from the original single follicle.[18, 19, 28] The result is a compound follicle in the adult animal[28] that appears from the surface as a single follicular orifice, with one coarse main or guard hair and a number of fine woolly hairs emerging from it.[28] The number of hairs emerging from the follicle may be from three to 15.[18-20, 22, 28, 33, 34] Hair shafts that share a common opening in the skin are enclosed in the same follicle down to the level of the sebaceous glands.[19, 20, 22, 33] At this point the hair shafts branch away from each other into their own individual hair follicle and bulb. The follicle and hair bulb of the cover or guard hair in the compound follicle are larger and penetrate deeper into the subcutaneous tissue than those of satellite or subsidiary hairs.[20, 22] Along with the satellite follicles and hairs, sebaceous glands and arrector pili muscles are formed to

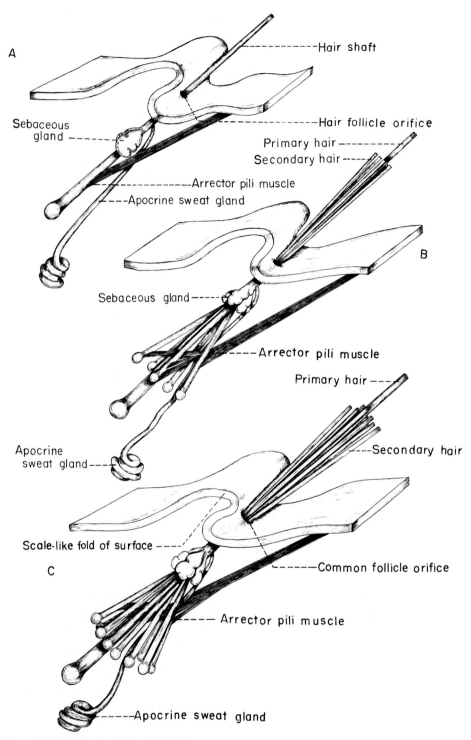

Figure 1–6:   Compound hair follicle during the 28th week of life. (From Lovell, J. E., and Getty, R.: The hair follicle, epidermis, dermis, and skin glands of the dog. Am. J. Vet. Res. *18:* 877, 1957.)

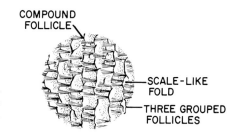

COMPOUND
FOLLICLE

SCALE-LIKE
FOLD

THREE GROUPED
FOLLICLES

Figure 1–7: A view of scale-like folds of the skin and arrangement of hair follicles. (After Lovell, J. E., and Getty, R.: The hair follicle, epidermis, dermis, and skin glands of the dog. Am. J. Vet. Res. *18*:878, 1957.)

accompany them.[19, 28] The hair follicles of the cat are like those of the dog. From 12 to 20 hairs diverge from a common follicle opening (Fig. 1–6).[32]

SKIN FOLDS

The skin surface is irregular owing to scale-like folds that form depressions into which the hair follicles invaginate.[13, 19, 20, 22] This scale-like pattern is most evident on the dorsum and less evident on the more thinly haired ventral surface of the dog.[13] These folds are also seen in cat skin (Figs. 1–6 and 1–7).[32]

HAIR GROUPS

Hair grouping is seen in canids. Hair bundles (compound follicles) may be single but are usually arranged in groups of two to four or more, with three-bundle groups being the most common. The groups are arranged in irregular rows. The guard hair of the centralmost bundle in a three-bundle group is coarser than the guard hairs of the other bundles of the group (Fig. 1–7).[13, 19, 20, 22, 30, 33, 34]

In the cat, hair bundle groups of two and three are more common on the dorsal aspect of the body, and groups of four and five are more common on the ventral aspect of the body and lower extremities.[32]

The primary follicle change that occurs with age is atrophy. This results in hair loss, with the number of hairs per follicle being reduced to zero in some cases.[3]

HAIR

BASIC ANATOMY

Hairs may be defined as epidermal structures that are flexible, elastic, horny threads; the free portion is called the hair shaft and the proximal portion is called the root. The root is almost always set obliquely in the skin, with the angle and direction varying with the species and body region. The root of the hair is attached to the underlying dermal papilla by means of its knob-like proximal end. The papilla causes the end of the bulb to be invaginated (Fig. 1–4).[29, 33] The angle and direction of hair growth are of importance to the surgeon when transferring a free graft or skin flap from one area of the body to another. When the graft or flap is in its recipient bed, the direction of hair growth should be the same as that of the surrounding hair.

The shaft of a hair is composed of medulla, cortex, and cuticle.[20, 22, 29, 33] The medulla in dog and cat hair is moderately wide[22] and gradually disappears toward the tip of the hair.[33] In the region of the root, the medulla is solid, but it contains air vacuoles in the shaft.[29, 33] These play a part in the graying of hair.[33]

The cortex is made up of tightly packed keratin cells[22, 29] that form the bulk of the hair.[20] These cells are fusiform, with the longitudinal axis parallel to the hair shaft. They are shorter, softer, and finally oval, with spheroid nuclei near the hair bulb. Hair color is determined by pigment in these cells.[29, 33]

The cuticle is a single layer of flat, cornified, nonnucleated cells that overlap like shingles, thus giving the hair a slightly serrated profile microscopically (Fig. 1–4).[20, 22, 29, 33]

HAIR TYPES

The type of hair as well as the direction of hair growth is important to the surgeon. Moving a graft or flap of skin from one area of the body to another may result in a different hair growth pattern than is present in the surrounding area.

Different means of classifying hair types have been used. One classification includes straight hair, bristle hair, and wavy bristle hair as protective types of hair and bristle wavy hair, large wavy hair, and fine wavy hair as components of the undercoat.[20] Another classification divides hair into three basic types: (1) tactile hairs (feelers, whiskers, vibrissae); (2) guard hairs (spines, bristles), which arise from the primary follicle of a compound follicle; and (3) fine, soft underhairs (wool, fur, or lanugo hairs), which arise from accessory or secondary follicles.[28]

The vibrissae are a special type of hair. They are large, stiff hairs with a rich sensory nerve supply and are embedded in vascular sinuses that are located between the outer and inner layers of the follicle;[28, 29] thus the name *sinus hairs*.[9, 33] These hairs are divided into five groups on the head of the animal: (1) mystacial on the muzzle, (2) submental on the mandible, (3) superciliary above the eye, (4) genal on the side of the face, and (5) interramal between the mandibles.[13, 20]

A third classification of hair type includes normal, long, and short hair coats.[11, 20, 22] The normal hair coat is like that seen on the German shepherd, Welsh corgi, and wild canids such as wolves and coyotes. The long hair coat is divided into two categories: (1) fine long hair as on the cocker spaniel, Pomeranian, and the chow), and (2) woolly or coarse long hair (as on the poodle, Bedlington terrier, and Kerry blue terrier). The short hair coat may be either coarse or fine, with the coarse coat being typified by the rottweiler and many of the terriers. There is a strong growth of primary hairs and a smaller growth of secondary hairs in this type of coat. The fine short-hair coat is seen in such breeds as boxers, dachshunds, and miniature pinschers. With this type of coat secondary hairs are numerous and well developed, and the primary hairs are reduced in size compared with the normal coat.[22]

There are two types of hair coats in cats: long hair or Persian, and short hair or "domestic," with short hair being the dominant gene. In domestic cats the secondary hairs considerably outnumber the primary hairs in all undifferentiated hairy regions.[22]

FUNCTION

The hair forms the first line of external defense by affording the animal protection against physical, chemical, and actinic trauma.[22, 28] It also performs sensory functions and plays a significant role in the thermoregulatory mechanism.[28] It insulates the skin from its external environment and aids in heat conservation.[22]

PIGMENT

A wide range of colors is possible in hair coats; however, microscopic examination has revealed only brown, black, and yellow pigment granules. The black-brown pigment is designated as "tyrosine-melanin" and is formed by enzyme oxidation of tyrosine to melanin. The yellow-red pigment is pheomelanin and is of unknown origin.[20, 22]

Hair color is produced by pigment cells in the bulb of the hair follicle. These cells place pigment granules in the cortical and medullary cells of the hair as they develop. Most of the granules remain in the cells, but some may remain between the cells, as in the medulla. The melanocytes of the follicles may produce pigment throughout the growth of the hair, or pigment deposition may vary. In a black hair, pigment deposition remains active throughout the growth period. However, in the agouti type of hair seen in the German shepherd and Norwegian elkhound, pigment deposition is not uniform, and the hair is white at its tip, black or dark brown at its thickest part, and lightly pigmented (yellow or red) at its proximal two-thirds.[20, 22] In the tabby cat, bands of pigment appear that indicate alternating periods of activity and quiescence of the melanocytes.[22]

In aging dogs there is a whitening of the hairs around the muzzle and elsewhere. This may be the result of some derangement in pigment production or an atrophy of pigment cells themselves. It has been suggested that hormonal imbalance produced by variable atrophy of the endocrine glands may play a part in the hair color change.[3] Another factor causing hair color change in dogs is the healing of skin, especially in dogs that have had inflammation of the skin. In light-colored areas, dark hairs will appear.[18] The author has also observed the opposite effect, with lighter hairs growing from a healed area on a dog with a dark coat.

In cats there is little relationship between skin and hair color. Hairy skin is devoid of pigment and the colors of the coat are concentrated in the hairs. In hairless areas of darker skin (e.g., lip, digital pads, and planum nasale), there are large amounts of pigment in the epidermis. Some specialized areas such as the scrotum, prepuce, anal sac, and teat also have some epidermal pigment.[32] The coat color of Siamese cats is temperature dependent, with the darker hair color being the result of a temperature-dependent enzyme that converts melanin precursors into melanin. The threshold temperature for pigment production varies in different parts of the body and varies with the sex. Higher temperatures result in lighter hair, while lower temperatures result in darker hair. This explains why newborn kittens and cats that are kept indoors or are in tropical climates are lighter in color. Inflammation and hyperemia result in a new growth of light hair, while senility (with poor circulation) and clipping to remove hair result in a darker new hair growth.[22] These are factors that should be taken into consideration and explained to the pet owner before undertaking any wound management or reconstructive procedure on a Siamese cat.

HAIR GROWTH PATTERN

Location

The density of hair coat varies in each individual; however, the coat is usually heavy and thick over the back and sides of the body, while the abdomen, inside of the ears and flanks, and underside of the tail are sparsely haired.[20, 22]

Direction

There are different implantation angles of the hair follicles on different dogs. The chow, Airedale, and Scottie have an implantation angle of 45 degrees, while other breeds, such as the long-haired dachshund, cocker spaniel, and Irish setter, have an implantation angle of less than 30 degrees. The majority of breeds that have been examined have an angle of between 30 and 40 degrees.[5] However, the long-haired dogs tend to have a higher implantation angle. In general, hairs slant caudally from the nose toward the tip of the tail.[20] The hair growth pattern has been described in terms of streams, convergent and divergent whirls (vortices), and lines where streams of different directions meet.[24, 29] These patterns are subject to variation. A study of gray foxes revealed a general hair slope pattern that is applicable to the dog as well, with some minor variations (Fig. 1–8).[13]

The areas of hair growth of different density on an animal's body and the direction of hair growth are important factors to consider when using skin flaps and skin grafts for reconstruction. Ideally, the hair on a flap or graft should be of the same density and slope as the surrounding hair for a com-

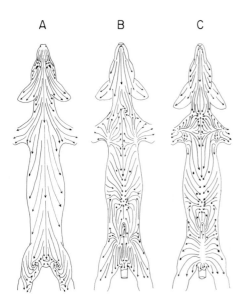

Figure 1–8: *A* and *B*, Direction of hair slope on the dorsal and ventral aspects of a gray fox. *C*, Hair slope pattern on the ventral aspect of a coyote. These patterns are applicable to the dog with some minor variations. (From Hildebrand, M.: The integument in canidae. J. Mammal. 33:420, 1952.)

pletely cosmetic effect. However, the surgeon may not be able to achieve the ideal in every case. Nevertheless, attempts should be made to have the same type of hair coat on a flap or graft as is on the skin surrounding the recipient area and to have the hair growing in the same direction as the surrounding hair. The tissue resemblance is not as good when skin is taken from a distant donor site as when it is taken from an adjacent donor site. An example of this is a pedicle flap taken from the thorax and transferred to the distal forelimb of a dog. Although the hair growth is in the same direction, the difference in hair density and length is more noticeable in the winter months when the dog develops its heavier winter coat.

Time

Several factors govern an animal's hair growth. These include the season, nutrition, temperature, and the general state of the animal's health. Internal conditions may be manifested by thinning or loss of hair, especially with hormonal disorders. There are various stimulating influences in animals that may provoke rapid hair growth. Hair growth in animals is more rapid in the winter than in the summer, resulting in a thicker, longer coat.[18] The times of heaviest shedding are the spring and the fall; however, shedding occurs throughout the year, with the hair growth pattern alternating between phases of rest and activity with neighboring follicles in the same phase.[6, 28] Other authors state that humans, guinea pigs, dogs, and cats have unsynchronized follicle growth, which results in hair replacement in a mosaic pattern. Adjacent hairs may be in any stage of the hair growth cycle.[22] No critical studies have been done on hair growth in dogs; however, some of the variations in hair growth that occur on individuals can be explained if there is a different rate of hair growth on different parts of the body, a different length of hair cycle on each body part, or a combination of both variables. This would explain why some breeds, such as the collie and chow, have long hair on the body and short hair on the face and feet. Likewise, a variation in the length of the hair growth cycle in different breeds could explain characteristic hair coats on dogs and differences in individual dogs.[22]

The hair growth cycle consists of three stages: (1) *anagen*, or the growing phase when the follicle is actively producing the hair; (2) *catagen*, or the transitional stage between the growth and resting periods, and (3) *telogen*, or the resting period when the hair is retained in the follicle as a dead or "club" hair, which is eventually shed.[20, 22] During anagen the hair is produced by mitosis in cells of the dermal papillae. In early catagen there is constriction of the hair bulb, with the hair above the stricture becoming the club hair. In late catagen the follicle below the club hair becomes thick and corrugated and pushes the hair outward. At the onset of telogen, the dermal papilla separates and an epithelial strand shortens to form a secondary germ. This brings the cycle to early anagen, when the secondary germ grows down around the dermal papilla and a new hair bulb is formed. The club hair is lost and the newly formed hair elongates as anagen progresses (Fig. 1–9).[22]

As previously mentioned, many factors affect the hair growth cycle. One of the most important factors is the photoperiod. As the daylight hours increase, the rate of shedding increases and the hair coat becomes coarser and less dense. This may be seen clinically in house dogs that are exposed to many hours of artificial light. These dogs shed yearlong. As the photoperiod

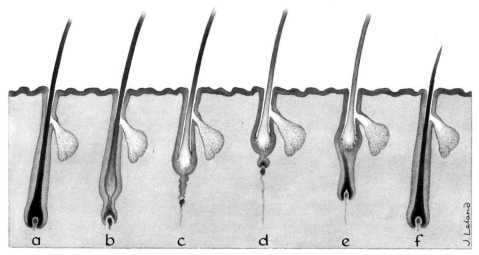

Figure 1–9: The hair cycle. *a*, Anagen. During anagen, the growing stage, hair is produced by mitosis in cells of the dermal papillae. *b*, Early catagen. In early catagen, the transitional stage, a constriction occurs at the hair bulb. The hair above this will become a club. *c*, Catagen. The distal follicle becomes thick and corrugated and pushes the hair outward. *d*, Telogen. This is the resting stage. The dermal papilla separates and an epithelial strand shortens to form a secondary germ. *e*, Early anagen. The secondary germ grows down to enclose the dermal papilla and a new hair bulb forms. The old club is lost. *f*, Anagen. The hair elongates as growth continues. (From Muller, G. H., and Kirk, R. W.: Small Animal Dermatology, ed. 2. Philadelphia, W. B. Saunders Co., 1976, p. 30.)

decreases, the coat is again shed and there is a stimulation of hair growth to produce a dense hair coat along with decreased sebum production, which results in a coat with improved insulating qualities.[22]

Poor health or generalized disease also affects hair growth by shortening the period of anagen, resulting in a large percentage of body hairs being in telogen at one time. These hairs are lost more easily, and the animal may shed excessively. In addition, disease states may cause faulty cuticle formation in which cuticle cells are pressed loosely against the cortex. As light strikes the hair shaft, it is reflected abnormally and the hair coat appears dull. Systemic illness or stress, such as pregnancy or parturition, may cause many hairs to enter telogen prematurely and simultaneously. These hairs are shed at the same time, and the altered hormone balance of parturition may also be a stimulus to end anagen.[22]

It is reasonable to assume that reconstructive procedures of the skin may alter the hair growth cycle. This would be particularly true with procedures that alter the blood supply to the skin (e.g., free full-thickness grafting). Damaged hair follicles caused by taking the graft may also account for the altered hair growth on free full-thickness grafts.

GLANDS

GENERAL INFORMATION

The glandular structures of the skin include the sebaceous glands and the apocrine and merocrine sweat glands. While sebaceous glands are more developed in the short- and rough-haired breeds, the sweat glands are more developed in the long- and fine-haired breeds.[30] In some areas of the body there are combinations of glands. One such area is the external ear canal, which has sebaceous and apocrine-type ceruminous glands, both of which are responsible for the cerumen of the ears.[9, 20, 25] These glands undergo hypertrophic proliferation and hypersecretion when the ear canal is inflamed.[25] Other areas of combination glands are in the anal sacs and tail gland area, where sebaceous and apocrine glands are present.[9, 20, 22, 25] In cats, sebaceous glands predominate in the anal sacs.[9]

The pH of dog skin is quite alkaline when compared with other species. Human skin has an acid pH that is detrimental to many organisms. It is not clear whether the pH of dog skin has an influence on skin disease.[22] However, the alkaline pH may provide a satisfactory environment to support some bacteria. For this reason it may be necessary to change dressings on dogs relatively often to help prevent problems with bacterial growth.

SEBACEOUS GLANDS

Sebaceous glands are simple alveolar holocrine glands that are present all over the skin in connection with hairs. However, a few are unassociated with hairs —those in the external ear canal, anus, glans penis, prepuce, labia, vulva, and tarsal glands of the eyelids.[22, 29, 33] In addition to being simple alveolar glands, these glands can also be of the branched alveolar or even tubular variety, with their size generally being in inverse ratio to the size of the hair.[29] The glands have been stated to be largest and most numerous in the lips, anus, and dorsal surface of the trunk and sternal area.[18, 20, 22, 25, 28-30, 33]

The glands appear as evaginations of the hair follicle and are connected to the upper part of the follicle by a short duct. The gland is composed of basal cells, which make up the peripheral germinative layer. These cells surround a central mass of large, foamy, lipid-filled cells (Fig. 1–10).[22] The secretion of the glands is called sebum and is made up of the products of these degenerated and disrupted cells.[18, 22, 33] It is an oily secretion containing cholesterol, cholesterol esters, squalene, waxes, and esterified fatty acids.[22] The emptying of this gland is by contraction of the arrector pili muscle.[18, 22, 33] The secretion tends to keep the skin and hair soft and pliable by forming an emulsion on the

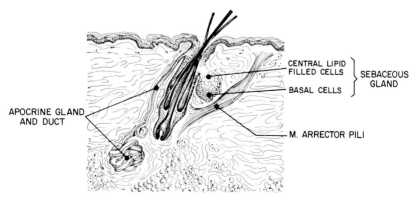

Figure 1–10: The relationship of a sebaceous gland, apocrine gland, and arrector pili muscle to a hair follicle.

skin and hair surface to retain moisture[18, 22, 33] and also by protecting them from excess moisture.[33]

These glands increase in size and activity up to maturity at about 7 months of age, when large amounts of sexual hormones are produced.[18, 28] Sebum production is continuous and is influenced by climate and environment.[18] The size of the glands often varies inversely with the diameter of the associated hair; the largest and most numerous glands are found in the eyelids, lips, sternal area, vulva, scrotum, anus, and the dorsal surface of the neck, trunk, and tail.[20, 22, 28] In the dog the glands are especially large at the mucocutaneous junctions[22, 23] and in the area of the tail gland.[22] Sebaceous glands may be multilobular, club shaped, and coiled.[22] Glands of individual follicles may bunch together or fuse,[20] or several glands may enter into a single opening of a hair follicle.[22]

Sebaceous glands are found only in hairy areas on the cat. The glands are largest on the dorsal tail and the lip and beneath the chin (submental organ).[32]

As an animal ages, there may be hyperplasia of the glands. The glands may also atrophy with age.[3]

TAIL GLANDS

The tail gland area on a dog is located on the dorsal surface of the tail not far from the sacrum (usually about 2 in. from the base of the tail). It is an oval or diamond-shaped area of skin in which the hair coat is composed of stiff, coarse hairs emerging from single follicles. There are numerous large sebaceous and apocrine glands that extend deep into the dermis and subcutaneous tissue in this area. As a result of the secretion from these glands, the skin has a yellow, waxy appearance.[19, 20, 22, 28]

CIRCUMANAL AND PERIANAL GLANDS

These glandular complexes are found in the area of the anal orifice. The circumanal glands are the superficial sebaceous glands the ducts of which empty into hair follicles[20] and onto the mucocutaneous anal surface.[9] Perianal glands (deep circumanal glands) make up the deeper, nonsebaceous part of the complex. They are composed of solid masses of large polygonal cells, and their ducts are believed to be solid, with no secretory activity.[20, 25] These glands are responsible for the formation of perianal adenomas in older male dogs.[9]

APOCRINE GLANDS

Dogs are capable of sweating and have two different types of sweat glands: (1) large, loosely coiled apocrine sweat glands that are distributed over the entire skin as an appendage of the hair follicles; and (2) small, densely coiled merocrine sweat glands that are present in the fatty fibrous tissue of the foot pads.[18, 25] The apocrine glands are more numerous in some areas. Greater numbers are found on the face and between the toes.[25, 28] The presence of both types of glands with their resultant secretions on the feet of dogs is an indication for frequent bandage changes. The combination of increased sweat secretion, an alkaline skin pH, and the presence of infection or wound drainage provides a favorable culture medium for bacteria and thus necessitates frequent dressing changes.

Specialized apocrine glands are also present in the external ear canal and in the eyelids in association with the cilia (glands of Moll).[22] The mammary glands are also apocrine in nature.[33]

One apocrine gland is associated with each follicle complex in the form of a coiled secretory tubule that extends deep into the dermis and subcutaneous tissue, generally parallel to the follicle. At the level of the sebaceous gland the lumen narrows to form the excretory duct. This extends up along the follicle complex and empties into the follicle above the opening of the sebaceous gland (Fig. 1–10).[20, 22, 28, 33]

The apocrine sweat glands do not appear to function under normal conditions,[33] as was shown in a study in which no spontaneous sweating was observed on the hairy skin of dogs even during excessive exercise.[1] However, the application of local heat and the injection of drugs (pilocarpine hydrochloride, acetylcholine, and adrenaline hydrochloride [Adrenalin Chloride]) to induce sweating has resulted in sweating from skin other than the foot pads.[1] Another study revealed general sweating on hairy skin following the infusion of adrenaline (Adrenalin) and noradrenaline. This suggested some control of the apocrine glands by circulating catecholamines.[16] It has also been found that sweat secretion occurs in localized patches, probably as a result of groups of glands alternating between periods of rest and secretion.[25] The sweat glands of the dog do not actively participate in the central thermoregulatory mechanism, but they serve mainly to protect the skin from an excess temperature rise[1, 20, 28] and apparently as a defense against the local elevation of skin temperature.[28]

In general, apocrine secretion is a proteinaceous, white, odorless, milky fluid that is slowly and continuously formed.[22] Even though there seem to be no morphological differences among apocrine glands, the biochemical properties of different glands vary. As an example, the apocrine secretion of the ceruminous glands of the ears differs from that of the anal sacs.[25]

The apocrine glands of the cat are glomoid or coiled in shape.[22, 32, 33] They have been reported by some to be in all general body areas and most prominently in the scrotum;[32] however, others have stated that these glands are poorly developed glands on the cat and can be found in only a few body areas (oral region, anus, lower jaw, and foot pads).[33]

MEROCRINE GLANDS

Merocrine sweat glands are found only in the foot pads of the dog and cat.[20, 22, 28, 32] These glands are small, tightly coiled, and tubular.[20, 28, 33] They are located deep in the dermis at its junction with the hypodermis[22] in the fat and fibrous tissue under the thick foot pad.[20] The excretory duct follows a tortuous path through the dermis and epidermis to a pore on the surface of the pad that is located in the crevices between the conical papillae of the foot pads (Fig. 1–11).[20, 22, 33]

Injections of epinephrine and acetylcholine induce secretion from these glands, as does the direct application of heat.[28] The secretion of these glands is watery;[20] however, they have no thermoregulatory function in the dog and cat.[22]

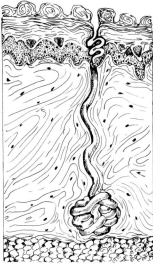

MEROCRINE GLAND
IN FOOT PAD

Figure 1–11: A merocrine gland and its duct located in the dermis and epidermis of a foot pad.

As mentioned earlier, secretion from these and the apocrine glands of the feet would tend to keep foot bandages moister than body bandages, making it necessary to change them more frequently.

ANAL SACS

Anal sacs are paired and lie on each side of the anal canal between the internal and external sphincter muscles. They are pockets of skin that open into the anal canal by a single duct. These pockets serve as a reservoir for the apocrine and sebaceous gland secretions.[20, 22]

MAMMARY GLANDS

The mammary glands are modified cutaneous glands[14, 21, 35] that are apocrine in nature.[33] The gross anatomy of these glands is important to the surgeon from the standpoint of their removal and the surgical correction of the resultant defect. Typically, the mammary glands are arranged in two bilaterally symmetrical rows that extend from the pectoral to the inguinal region, with five glands on each side of the midline for a total of ten glands. There may be as few as eight or as many as 12 glands, with four to six glands on each side of the midline. Occasionally there are more glands on one side than on the other.[14, 21, 27, 37] The glands have been designated as two pairs of pectoral glands, one pair of abdominal glands, and two pairs of inguinal glands.[27] A slightly different classification includes two pairs of thoracic glands (cranial and caudal), two pairs of abdominal glands (cranial and caudal), and one pair of inguinal glands (Fig. 1–12).[21, 37] Owing to the frequent variation in the number of glands, they have been numbered cranially to caudally from 1 through 5.[14, 27, 37]

The mammary glands are attached to the ventral belly wall in varying degrees. The cranialmost glands are closely adherent to the pectoral musculature, whereas the abdominal and inguinal glands are loose and pendulous, especially after lactation. The glandular tissue is located in a plane between the skin and cutaneous musculature. A discrete plane in the subcutaneous tissue of the lateral thorax and abdomen defines the lateral extent of mammary tissue. This line of demarcation is important when the surgeon is completely excising all glandular tissue, since small fragments of mammary tissue that are overlooked during surgical excision can lead to a recurrence of mammary neoplasia.[35]

The cranial and caudal thoracic mammary glands are innervated by the fourth through the seventh ventral cutaneous nerves of the thoracic nerves.

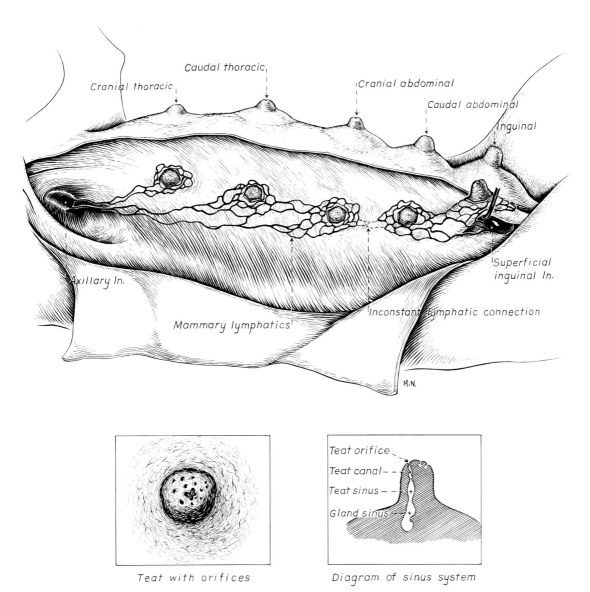

Figure 1–12: Topography of the mammary glands. (From Al Bagdadi, F., and Lovell, J.: The integument, Evans, H. E., and Christensen, G. C. (eds.): Miller's Anatomy of the Dog. Philadelphia, W. B. Saunders Co., 1979, p. 102.)

The abdominal and inguinal mammae are innervated by the inguinal nerve and the ventral superficial branches of the first three lumbar nerves. Additional innervation comes to the glands via sympathetic fibers accompanying the blood vessels.[21]

The mammary glands are quite vascular, with veins being more extensive than arteries. The thoracic mammae receive their arterial supply from the perforating sternal branches of the internal thoracic arteries, which penetrate the thoracic wall at the intercostal spaces. In addition to these, intercostal and lateral thoracic arteries may also contribute blood to the thoracic glands. At the caudal rib cage, the internal thoracic vessels divide, forming the cranial deep and the superficial epigastric arteries. These, along with the cranial and caudal branches of the caudal superficial epigastric artery, supply the abdominal and inguinal mammary glands.[14, 21, 37] Some of the caudal intercostal arteries also supply the cranial abdominal gland.[37] Segmental arteries from the abdominal wall and the circumflex iliac artery supply the lateral aspects of the glands, and labial vessels from the perineum enter glands in the area of the vulva.[35] Veins parallel the arteries to a large degree, with the cranial and caudal superficial epigastric veins being the major veins of the glands.[21, 37] There are numerous veins that cross the midline, and large superficial mammary veins are present on the ventral superficial abdomen over the mammary tissue.[35]

The lymphatic drainage of the mammae is important, since mammary neoplasias can metastasize more readily via this route than via the blood stream. Thus, the lymphatic drainage governs surgical removal of mammary glands in cases of mammary neoplasia.[21] Lymphatic drainage of the mammae is bilaterally symmetrical.[21, 27] Usually one to three main channels leave each gland and pass laterally and superficially to the nearest superficial lymph node.[21] When considered numerically from cranial to caudal regions, the first two glands drain directly by separate channels forward to the axillary lymph node.[14, 21, 27, 37] The third gland's drainage is inconsistent.[14, 21] In most instances it drains toward the axillary lymph node,[14, 21, 27, 37] but its lymphatics may join those of the fourth gland and drain toward the inguinal lymph node.[21, 37] When the gland drains cranially, it drains into the lymphatics of the second gland as well as by a separate channel to the axillary node.[14, 27, 37] Drainage of the fourth gland is into the lymphatic meshwork of the fifth gland as well as into the superficial inguinal lymph node by a direct channel. The fifth mammary gland drains into the superficial inguinal lymph node (Fig. 1–12).[14, 21, 27, 37] Occasionally, small lymphatics have been found to partially penetrate the superficial muscle layer beneath the mammary gland. However, lymphatics have not been observed to penetrate the abdominal or thoracic walls or to anastomose with lymphatics on the opposite side.[27]

The lymphatic drainage of the mammary glands would affect mammary neoplasia removal in the following ways:

1. For a tumor of the first mammary gland, resect only the tumor and affected gland,[14, 21] resect the first two mammary glands and the axillary lymph node,[35] or remove the first three glands[4, 10, 26, 37]
2. For a tumor of the second mammary gland, resect the tumor and the first two mammary glands on the affected side.[14, 21] The third gland of that side may also be removed,[10, 26, 27, 37] as may the axillary lymph node.[12]
3. For a tumor of the third mammary gland, resect the tumor and the first three mammary glands on the affected side.[10, 14, 21, 26, 27, 37] The relatively rare anastomosis of lymphatics between the third and fourth glands indicates

that it is occasionally advisable to remove all glands on the affected side[21, 27, 37] and the inguinal lymph node.[12]

4. For a tumor of the fourth mammary gland, resect the fourth and fifth glands[4] and the superficial inguinal lymph node.[10, 14, 21, 26, 27, 37] The third gland may also be removed.[12]

5. For a tumor of the fifth mammary gland, resect the fourth and fifth glands[4] and the superficial inguinal lymph node.[10, 12, 14, 21, 26, 27, 37]

Another approach to mastectomy has been the removal of the entire chain of mammary tissue in which the tumor or tumors are located.[12, 21] This is advocated because there is no way to specifically determine which glands contain neoplastic tissue, and if multiple neoplasms exist, the possibility of leaving tumors in the patient is increased if less than a total mastectomy is performed. There is also the possibility of lymphatic and vascular metastasis if partial unilateral mastectomy is performed.[35] Related to this is the potential lymphatic intercommunication among all glands.[12]

There is no evidence that any one of the procedures described for the removal of mammary tumors is any better than any other or may result in a significant increase in survival time. Until adequate studies can be devised to show the superiority of one technique over another, the extent of surgery is a matter of the surgeon's choice.[12]

It has been stated that it is not necessary to regularly remove the axillary lymph node in cases of neoplasia of the first three mammary glands.[14, 27] Metastasis of mammary neoplasms to the axillary or accessory axillary lymph nodes is infrequent in the bitch.[21] Others have advocated removing the superficial inguinal, popliteal, and axillary nodes only if they are visibly palpable or enlarged.[4]

MUSCLES

ARRECTOR PILI

The arrector pili muscle fibers originate from the outer root sheath of the hair follicle and join together in a common muscle.[20] The muscle extends from the lower one third of the follicle below and around the sebaceous gland, often by means of bifurcation, to the epidermis.[28, 33] The muscles are always found on the side of the hair follicle that forms an obtuse angle with the skin surface (Fig. 1–10).[33] In compound hair follicles the arrector pili muscles of the component follicles join together.[22] In the dog and cat these muscles are most developed in the dorsal midline along the neck, back, and tail,[20, 22, 28, 32] and their function is to elevate the hair and empty the sebaceous glands.[9, 18, 20, 22, 28, 29] These muscles are not present on tactile hairs and vibrissae.[22]

CUTANEOUS TRUNCI

The cutaneous trunci muscle is a thin leaf of musculature that covers almost the entire dorsal, lateral, and ventral walls of the abdomen and thorax. It originates in the gluteal area and runs cranially and ventrally to cover the dorsal and lateral abdominal and thoracic surfaces and ends in the axilla and on the caudal border of the deep pectoral muscle. It lies in the superficial fascia of the trunk.[21] This muscle is important in relation to the type of blood supply to the dog's skin, which will be pointed out in the following section on vasculature of the skin. When skin flaps are created on the trunk of a dog, this muscle is included in the flaps.

VASCULATURE

The skin of the dog, like that of humans, possesses a rich vascular system that, among other things, delivers nutrients to the skin and functions in thermoregulatory mechanisms.[28] "Detailed knowledge of the anatomy of the arterial circulation in the skin and subcutaneous tissue is of particular importance to the reconstructive surgeon who must form and transplant pedunculated flaps, the viability of which depend upon this vascularity."[7] Knowledge of the skin's vasculature is also important when dealing with free grafts, as will be pointed out in Chapter 10. Some parts of the skin are more vascular than others. As an example, some regions such as the subcutaneous fascia of the limbs carry larger and more prominent vessels, especially veins, than do other areas.[15]

The points of superficial emergence of the larger cutaneous arteries along the abdomen and thorax are quite suggestive of a segmental arrangement; however, the segmental arrangement is not as regular as in the case of nerves (Fig. 1–13). This is partly due to the extensive anastomosis between the vessels. Anastomosis between branches of different arteries and between adjacent branches of the same artery occurs in all areas to the degree that it is

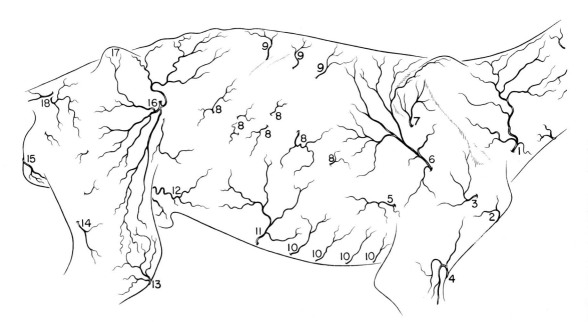

Figure 1–13: The superficial arteries of the trunk. *1,* Superficial cervical branch of omocervical. *2,* Cranial circumflex humeral. *3,* Caudal circumflex humeral. *4,* Proximal collateral radial. *5,* Lateral thoracic. *6,* Cutaneous branch of thoracodorsal. *7,* Cutaneous branch of subscapular. *8,* Distal lateral cutaneous branches of intercostals. *9,* Proximal lateral cutaneous branches of intercostals. *10,* Ventral cutaneous branches of internal thoracic. *11,* Cranial superficial epigastric. *12,* Caudal superficial epigastric. *13,* Medial genicular. *14,* Cutaneous branch of caudal femoral. *15,* Perineal. *16,* Deep circumflex iliac. *17,* Tuber coxae. *18,* Cutaneous branches of superficial lateral coccygeal. (From Evans, H. E.: The heart and arteries, in Evans, H. E., and Christensen, G. C. (eds.): Miller's Anatomy of the Dog. Philadelphia, W. B. Saunders Co., 1979, p. 713.)

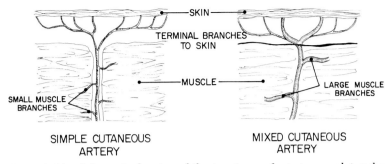

Figure 1–14: Schematic drawing of the two types of arteries supplying the skin of the dog.

difficult to say where any one vessel terminates. The sources of the arteries and their large primary branches in the subcutaneous fascia are generally constant in all dogs. The divisions and subdivisions of these arteries all run more or less parallel to the skin surface, with no constancy in the arrangement of the smaller vessels and no pattern common to all dogs.[15, 20]

Before it breaks down into plexuses, the vasculature of the skin is of two types. The *simple cutaneous arteries* reach the skin by running between muscle masses and giving small branches to the muscle tissue. The *mixed cutaneous arteries* pass through a more or less thick bed of muscle, supplying large muscular branches to it before terminating in the skin (Fig. 1–14).[15, 20, 22] Since these vessels pass through muscle masses, it is possible that the action of the muscle may influence the amount of blood flow through the arteries. In addition, the muscular blood supply may be increased at the expense of the skin. However, the extensive plexuses and anastomoses of vessels that supply the skin would assure adequate skin blood supply in the event of temporary flow reduction in the mixed cutaneous vessels.[15] Studies have shown 23 mixed cutaneous arteries and 16 simple cutaneous arteries located over the body of a dog. The previous material refers to arteries; however, it should be remembered that veins generally run parallel to the arteries.[15, 20]

Others have stated that the vasculature of loose-skinned animals, including the dog and cat, is composed of direct cutaneous vessels that run longitudinally under the skin in close association with the panniculus carnosus (cutaneous trunci) muscle.[8] If such is the case, this would be a definite indication for including this muscle in any skin flaps that are prepared on the trunk of a dog or cat.

Regardless of whether the arteries supplying the skin are simple cutaneous or mixed cutaneous arteries, both types are involved in the formation of the three vascular plexuses: (1) the subcutaneous (deep) plexus, (2) the cutaneous (middle or intermediate) plexus, and (3) the superficial (subepidermal or subpapillary) plexus.[15, 20, 22, 33] These all lie parallel to the surface of the skin.[20] The *subcutaneous plexus* is made up of the terminal branches of the two types of cutaneous arteries (i.e., simple and mixed) and lies in the superficial subcutaneous fat and areolar tissue deep to the dermis (hypodermis area). Where the cutaneous trunci muscle is present, the vessels lie both superficial and deep to the muscle and have some branches within the muscle.[15, 20, 22] The *cutaneous plexus* is derived from the subcutaneous plexus and lies in the dermis at the level of the skin glands and hair follicles. Branches from this plexus course superficially to form the third plexus as well as supply blood for the hair follicles, the ducts of tubular glands, and the arrector pili muscles.[15, 20, 22] The *superficial plexus* is located in the outer layers of the dermis. In those areas of the body where dermal papillae are well developed, this plexus supplies capillary loops in the papillae. Conversely, in areas of poor papillary development the loops are correspondingly few. Where the papillary body is absent, the plexus is a flattened capillary meshwork. Since the papillary body is absent or poorly developed in densely haired areas, its development in the dog is poor or absent owing to the dog's hair coat. It thus follows that capillary loops projecting into the papillae from the superficial plexus are not prominent in the dog (Fig. 1–15).[15, 20, 22]

The extensive microscopic plexuses of skin vessels appear to insure a continuous and complete blood supply to the skin, even in instances in which there is temporary blockage of the main vessels coming from the deeper layers. These plexuses in the subcutaneous fascia vary in the size of the areas enclosed by their macroscopic meshworks; however, they are especially prevalent over bony prominences (e.g., point of the elbow). In these areas the distance between vessels of the plexuses is small. Similar plexuses are present over large muscle masses (e.g., triceps brachii and biceps femoris), but the distance between vessels of the plexuses is greater.[15, 20] The vascular plexuses are not as rich in areas where the skin is relatively thin (e.g., the ventral aspect of the head, neck, and thorax; the medial aspect of the thigh and axillary region; and the lateral aspect of the thorax and abdomen).[15]

The vascular plexuses are important in gauging depth when cutting split-thickness skin grafts. A thin split-thickness graft will leave a donor site with many small surface bleeders (e.g., bleeding from the superficial plexus), whereas a thick split-thickness graft will leave a donor site with fewer but larger bleeders (e.g., bleeding from the cutaneous plexus).

LYMPHATICS

Lymphatics of the skin arise from capillary nets that lie in the superficial (papillary) area of the dermis or surround the follicles and glands. The vessels that arise from these nets drain into a subcutaneous lymphatic plexus.[18, 20, 33] Their main function is to transport the capillary transudate.[18] In the first few days after placement, a skin graft is maintained by plasmatic imbibition; during this time severed lymphatics and blood vessels in the graft absorb fluids and hemic elements from the graft bed. This gives the graft an edematous appearance. This will be discussed in more detail in Chapter 10.

NERVES

Nerves of the skin serve as sensory receptors and also control the sweat glands and arrector pili muscles.[18] The nerves of the skin lie in the subcuticular area and are continued by a nerve plexus that extends through the dermis to the epidermis. Nerve branches arising from this plexus innervate the epidermis, glands, muscles, and hair follicles. In addition, some branches terminate in special nerve endings.[20, 33] The sensory nerve fibers of this plexus have been divided into three types of terminal receptors: (1) the dermal nerve network, (2) the hair follicle network, and (3) specialized end-organs (Fig. 1–16).[22, 36]

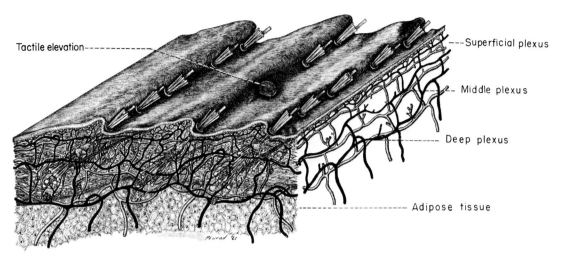

Figure 1–15: Schematic section of the skin of the dog showing epidermal papilla and blood vessels (*veins in black*). (From Al Bagdadi, F., and Lovell, J.: The integument, in Evans, H. E., and Christensen, G. C. (eds.): Miller's Anatomy of the Dog. Philadelphia, W. B. Saunders Co., 1979, p. 97.)

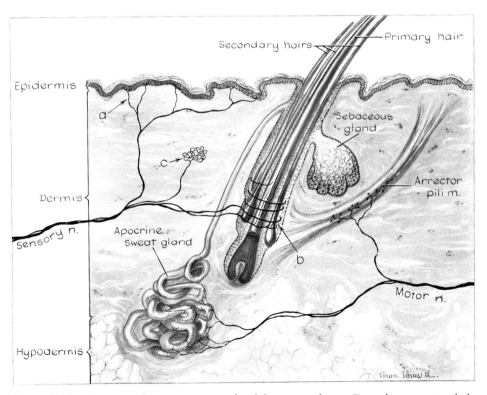

Figure 1–16: Sensory and motor nerve supply of the canine skin. *a*, Dermal nerve network. *b*, Hair follicle network. *c*, Specialized end-organs. (From Muller, G. H., and Kirk, R. W.: Small Animal Dermatology, ed. 2. Philadelphia, W. B. Saunders Co., 1976, p. 36.)

The nerve fibers form cells of the dorsal root ganglia come together in the skin to form fine dermal networks. These fibers become finer as they approach their termination and end as terminal twigs in the skin and mucous membranes. The density of dermal networks in the skin varies inversely with the hair coverage of the area. In hairy skin they are sparse, while in hairless skin they are extensive. The dermal networks function in pain perception and temperature variation.[22]

In hairy skin, sensory nerve fibers form a double network around each primary hair that is known as the hair follicle network. In mammals this network is the principal organ for perception, especially for touch.[22] Every hair has a nerve ending associated with it. The nerve penetrates the follicle below the sebaceous gland duct and divides to arrange itself parallel to the long axis of the hair.[20] The mechanism of touch perception is more refined in the sinus or tactile hairs where engorgement of the vascular sinus surrounding the base of the hair follicle enhances sensory acuity.[20, 22]

In addition to the dermal and follicle networks, the hairless skin also contains many encapsulated nerve endings that make up the specialized receptors. These special end-organs are primarily found at the mucocutaneous junctions and in the foot pads. The end-organs are similar to the hair follicle network except that the final axon filaments are rolled into an encapsulated coil or ball instead of being associated with the hair follicle.[22]

The skin is also supplied with adrenergic sympathetic motor nerves to blood vessels, arrector pili muscles, and myoepithelial cells around the apocrine sweat glands. There do not appear to be any other motor fibers to apocrine or sebaceous glands themselves or to hairs or other epidermal appendages (tactile hair excepted).[22] A study has demonstrated the existence of this sympathetic innervation, which is probably of adrenergic nature, to the apocrine glands in the dog's hairy skin.[16] Likewise, stimulation of the sympathetic trunk results in cutaneous vasoconstriction, and norepinephrine appears to be the stimulating, mediating substance of the adrenergic fibers. Parasympathetic (cholinergic) vasodilator fibers are not known to occur in the skin as they do in the salivary glands and the penis (Fig. 1–16).[28]

The sensory innervation to the skin is important to the reconstructive surgeon when dealing with skin grafts and skin flaps in that these structures are reinnervated after they are placed in their new location. Reinnervation of grafts and flaps and the possible problems associated with it are discussed in Chapters 8 and 10.

SPECIAL SKIN AREAS

FOOT PAD

On the flexor surface of the carpus and digits of the forelimb are hairless, cushion-like pads. The carpal pad is located medial and distal to the accessory carpal bone. The metacarpal pad is the largest in the area and is situated behind the distal ends of the metacarpal bones and the greater part of the proximal phalanges. The pad is composed of two unequal lateral lobes, making it heart shaped, with the apex distally located. The metapodiophalangeal joints rest on this pad when the paw supports weight. The digital pads are smaller and oval and support the second digital joints.

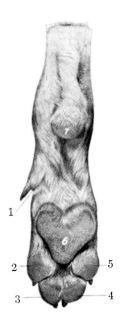
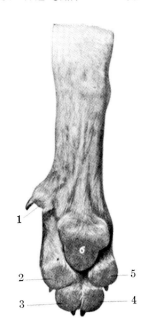

Figure 1–17: *A*, Pads of the right fore-paw of the dog: *1* through *5*, digital pads; *6*, Metacarpal pads; *7*, carpal pad. *B*, Pads of the right hind paw of the dog: *1* through *5*, digital pads; *6*, metatarsal pad. (From Sisson, S.: Common integument, in Getty, R. (ed.): Sisson and Grossman's The Anatomy of Domestic Animals, ed. 5. Vol. 2, Philadelphia, W. B. Saunders Co., 1975, p. 1782.)

The foot pad arrangement on the pelvic limb is like that on the thoracic limb with regard to the digital and metatarsal pads. The main difference is the lack of a tarsal foot pad (Fig. 1–17).[30]

The foot pads are modified to absorb shock and to resist abrasion.[22] When they are lost or damaged as a result of trauma to the distal limb, the veterinary surgeon is faced with the problem of repairing or replacing the pads.

The outer portion of the foot pad is tough, thick, and heavily pigmented. The surface may be rough as the result of being covered with numerous conical papillae that are keratinized and readily visible to the naked eye. However, friction may wear these papillae to a rounded shape or smooth.[19, 20, 22, 30] The epidermis of the foot pad is composed of all five of the previously described layers, with the most marked feature being the stratum corneum. The stratum corneum consists of a thick layer of keratinized, non-nucleated material that is thicker than all other cell layers combined;[19, 20] it is arranged in a jagged, saw-toothed or papillary manner.[22]

In the dermis the collagen tissue is fine and fibrillar in the upper portions and becomes denser in the deep parts of the dermis.[22] In addition to reticular fibers, the dermis contains collagenous and elastic fibers along with fibroblasts, blood vessels, and nerves.[19] The merocrine sweat glands of the foot pads are numerous in the lower dermis and nearby adipose tissue, with their ducts passing through the dermis to enter the epidermis at the depths of the epidermal pegs. At this point the epithelium of the duct joins the stratum basale of the epidermis. The lumen of the duct then follows a tortuous path through the epidermal cells to the surface.[19, 20, 22] Just below the epidermis the connective tissue of the dermis is dense and papillate, forming conical connective tissue cores for the epidermal conical papillae.[19]

The hypodermis is composed of abundant adipose tissue that is partitioned by reticular collagenous and elastic fibers (Fig. 1–18).[19, 20, 22] Many elastic fibers are present in the deep layers of the subcutis, as are the merocrine sweat glands and lamellar corpuscles.[19] The hypodermis is tightly ad-

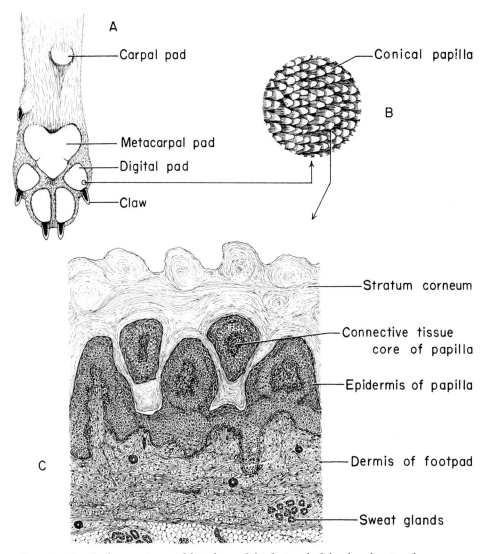

Figure 1–18: Surface contour and histology of the foot pad of the dog showing the gross appearance of foot pads (*A*), a view of the conical papillae arrangement on the surface of the digital pad (*B*), and a histological section of a foot pad (*C*). (From Lovell, J. E., and Getty, R.: The hair follicle, epidermis, dermis, and skin glands of the dog. Am. J. Vet. Res. *18*:876, 1957.)

herent to the overlying skin and connected by trabeculae to the underlying bones and tendons.[30]

SCROTUM

The scrotal skin in general is thin; however, it has a relatively thick epidermis and a particularly thin dermis. The stratum corneum of the epidermis is quite thin, and the basal layer of the epidermis contains large numbers of melanin pigment granules. In the dermis there are numerous smooth muscle fibers and capillaries. Other features of scrotal skin include prominent epidermal ridges and a sparse hair coat.[22]

NASAL SKIN

Nasal skin is pigmented, tough, and moist. The surface of the planum nasale appears irregular owing to numerous shallow grooves that divide the surface into polygonal plaque-like areas. There are only three layers in the epidermis: the stratum basale, the stratum spinosum, and the stratum corneum.[19, 20, 22] The cells of the stratum spinosum do not undergo typical kera-

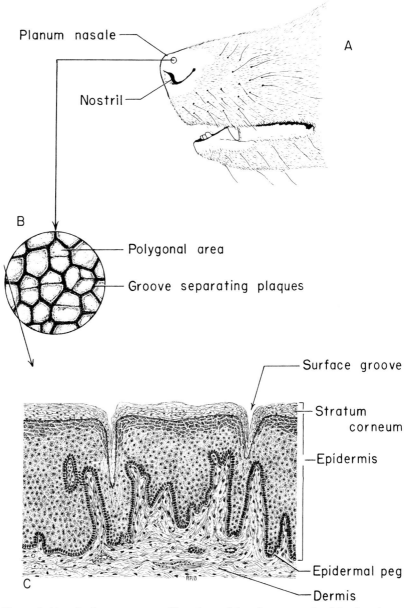

Planum nasale

Nostril

A

B

Polygonal area

Groove separating plaques

Surface groove

Stratum corneum

Epidermis

Epidermal peg

Dermis

C

Figure 1–19: Surface contour and histology of the planum nasale of the dog showing (A) the gross appearance of nasal skin, (B) a view of polygonal plaque-like areas of the planum nasale, and (C) a histological section of the planum nasale. (From Lovell, J. E., and Getty, R.: The hair follicle, epidermis, dermis, and skin glands of the dog. Am. J. Vet. Res. 18:874, 1957.)

tinization as they reach the surface of the skin; instead they remain as thin, atypical, nucleated stratum corneum that is four to eight cell layers thick.[19, 20] Another feature of nasal skin is the lack of hair and glandular structures within it.[19, 20, 22] The dermis of the planum nasale is composed of reticular, elastic, and collagenous fibers, together with fibroblasts, blood vessels, and nerves (Fig. 1–19).[19, 20]

REFERENCES

1. Aoki, T., and Woda, M.: Functional activity of the sweat glands in the hairy skin of the dog. Science 114:123, 1951.
2. Baker, B. B., Maibach, H. I., Park, R. D., et al.: Epidermal cell renewal in the dog. Am. J. Vet. Res. 34:93, 1973.
3. Baker, K. P.: Senile changes in dog skin. J. Small Anim. Pract. 8:49, 1967.
4. Bostock, D. E., and Owen, L. N.: Neoplasia in the Cat, Dog, and Horse. Chicago, Year Book Medical Publishers, Inc., 1975.
5. Brunsch, A.: Vergleichende Untersuchungen am Haarkleid von Wildcaniden und Haushunden. Z. Tierzuchtung Zuchtungs Biol. 67:205, 1956.
6. Comben, N.: Observation on the mode of growth of the hair of the dog. Br. Vet. J. 107:231, 1951.
7. Conway, H., Stark, R. B., and Nieto-Cano, G.: The arterial vascularization of pedicles. Plast. Reconstr. Surg. 12:348, 1953.
8. Daniel, R. K., and Williams, B. H.: The free transfer of skin flaps by microvascular anastomoses: An experimental study and reappraisal. Plast. Reconstr. Surg. 52:16, 1973.
9. Doering, G. G., and Jensen, H. E.: Clinical Dermatology of Small Animals: A Stereoscopic Presentation. St. Louis, The C. V. Mosby Co., 1973.
10. Fidler, I. J., Abt, D. A., and Brodey, R. S.: The biological behavior of canine mammary neoplasms. J. Am. Vet. Med. Assoc. 151:1311, 1967.
11. Gair, R.: Die Wuchstormen des Haarkleides bei Haustieren nach Untersuchungen beim Hunde. Z. Tierzuchtung Zuchtungs Biol. 11:57, 1928.
12. Harvey, H. J.: General principles of veterinary oncologic surgery. J. Am. Anim. Hosp. Assoc. 12:335, 1976.
13. Hildebrand, M.: The integument in canidae. J. Mammal. 33:419, 1952.
14. Hoffer, R. E.: Skin and adnexa, in Archibald, J. (ed.): Canine Surgery, ed. 2. Santa Barbara, Calif., American Veterinary Publications, Inc. 1974.
15. Hughes, H. V., and Dransfield, J. W.: The blood supply to the skin of the dog. Br. Vet. J. 115:199, 1959.
16. Iwabuchi, T.: General sweating on the hairy skin of the dog and its mechanism. J. Invest. Dermatol. 49:61, 1967.
17. Jenkinson, D. M., and Blackburn, P. S.: The distribution of nerves, monoamine oxidase and cholinesterase in the skin of the cat and dog. Res. Vet. Sci. 9:521, 1968.
18. Kral, F.: Compendium of Veterinary Dermatology. New York, Chas. Pfizer and Co., 1960.
19. Lovell, J. E., and Getty, R.: The hair follicle, epidermis, dermis, and skin glands of the dog. Am. J. Vet. Res. 18:873, 1957.
20. Lovell, J. E., and Getty, R.: The integument, in Miller, M. E., Christensen, G. C., and Evans, H. E. (eds.): Anatomy of the Dog. Philadelphia, W. B. Saunders Co., 1964.
21. Miller, M. E., Christensen, G. C., and Evans, H. E.: Anatomy of the Dog. Philadelphia, W. B. Saunders Co. 1964, and Evans, H. E., and Christensen, G. C.: Miller's Anatomy of the Dog, ed. 2, 1979.
22. Muller, G. H., and Kirk, R. W.: Small Animal Dermatology, ed. 2. Philadelphia, W. B. Saunders Co., 1976.
23. Nevrand, V. K., and Schwartz, R.: Light microscopic studies of feline skin, epidermis, corium, and subcutis. D.T.W. 76:521, 1969.
24. Niedoba, T.: Untersuchungen über die Haarrichtung der Haussaugetiere. Anat. Anz. 50:178 and 204, 1917.
25. Nielsen, S. W.: Glands of the canine skin — morphology and distribution. Am. J. Vet. Res. 14:448, 1953.
26. Owen, L. N.: Mammary neoplasia in the dog and cat: III. Prognosis and treatment of mammary tumors in the bitch. J. Small Anim. Pract. 7:703, 1966.
27. Schlotthauer, C. F.: Neoplasms in the mammary glands in dogs: Their pathology and surgical treatment. J. Am. Vet. Med. Assoc. 96:632, 1940.
28. Schwartzman, R. M., and Orkin, M.: A Comparative Study of Skin Diseases of Dog and Man. Springfield, Ill., Charles C Thomas, Publisher, 1962.
29. Sisson, S.: Common integument, in Getty, R. (ed.): Sisson and Grossman's The Anatomy of Domestic Animals, ed. 5. Philadelphia, W. B. Saunders Co., 1975, vol. 1.

30. Sisson, S.: Common integument, in Getty, R. (ed.): Sisson and Grossman's The Anatomy of Domestic Animals, ed. 5. Philadelphia, W. B. Saunders Co., 1975, vol. 2.

31. Steele, J. D.: Fourteen Weeks in Human Physiology. New York, American Book Company, 1872.

32. Strickland, J. H., and Calhoun, M. L.: The integumentary system of the cat. Am. J. Vet. Res. 24:1018, 1963.

33. Trautmann, A., and Fiebiger, J. F.: The Fundamentals of the Histology of Domestic Animals. Ithaca, NY, Comstock Publishing Associates, 1957.

34. Webb, A. J., and Calhoun, M. L.: The microscopic anatomy of the skin of mongrel dogs. Am. J. Vet. Res. 15:274, 1954.

35. Wilson, G. P., and Fowler, E. H.: The mammary glands: Mammary tumors, in Bojrab, M. J. (ed.): Current Techniques in Small Animal Surgery I. Philadelphia, Lea & Febiger, 1975.

36. Winkelmann, R. K.: Similarities of cutaneous nerve end organs in cutaneous innervation: A Brown University symposium, in Montagna, W. (ed.): Advances in Biology of the Skin. London, Pergamon Press, Inc., 1960, vol. 1.

37. Withrow, S.: Mammary tumors in the dog. Sci. Proc. Am. Anim. Hosp. Assoc. 2:118, 1975.

2

ETIOLOGY OF SKIN TRAUMA AND DEFECTS

GENERAL

Instances of traumatic injury are often encountered by the practicing veterinarian, and such injury can affect all tissues of the body. Since the skin is the outer covering of the body, it is especially subject to external traumatic injury. The frequency with which the small animal practitioner encounters traumatic injury may be related to the leash laws and their enforcement within the community. However, there are other sources of skin trauma and skin defects.

A study conducted at the University of Pennsylvania Veterinary Hospital from 1971 to 1972 revealed that of 1000 trauma cases, 87.1 per cent involved dogs and 12.9 per cent involved cats, with a predominance of males over females. The average age was 1.9 years for the dogs and 1.3 years for the cats. The sources of injury were divided into nine etiological categories: motor vehicle, animal interaction, sharp object, fall from height, crush, weapon (guns and knives), burn (thermal, electrical, and chemical), abuse, and unknown cause.[36] Many of these sources can induce skin trauma or defects or both. In the study it was found that burns and weapons caused the greatest number of severe injuries, while sharp objects and abuse caused the least severe injuries. It was also found that dogs sustained significantly more injuries to the extremities and fewer injuries to the head than did cats.[36]

Sixteen of the more frequently encountered sources of skin trauma or defect will be covered in this chapter. Those sources include:

1. Simple lacerations
2. Degloving injuries
3. Bite wounds
4. Snakebites
5. Insect bites and stings
6. Skin tumors
7. Mammary tumors
8. Gunshot wounds
9. Radiation injury
10. Decubital ulcers
11. Application of casts, bandages, and splints
12. Burns
13. Perivascular injections
14. Bacterial and fungal infections

15. Granulomas
16. Weather trauma

Miscellaneous sources of trauma will be discussed briefly at the end of this chapter, and other specific conditions that can be considered forms of skin trauma will be covered in Chapter 13.

SIMPLE LACERATIONS

One of the simplest forms of skin trauma that is often encountered in dogs and cats is the simple laceration. It may be long or short, superficial or deep. Any sharp object may inflict such a wound. As a rule, uncomplicated superficial lacerations produce little damage to surrounding and underlying tissues and lend themselves to primary closure rather nicely. The defect in the skin may appear large as a result of tension-line traction on the wound edges. However, if no skin has been lost, the wound should close without difficulty.

Uncomplicated deep lacerations can result in the separation of underlying tissues (i.e., muscles, tendons, nerves, and blood vessels). As with superficial lacerations, little damage occurs to adjacent underlying tissues. Naturally, these tissues require some form of repair prior to closure of the skin laceration.

Many times lacerations are contaminated with hair, dirt, and other types of debris. In addition to these, added trauma to adjacent fissues may result if the laceration is combined with other forms of trauma such as crushing injury and degloving injury. Management of this type of injury is more involved than that associated with the simple skin laceration.

DEGLOVING INJURIES

A degloving injury is the extensive loss of skin from a limb as a result of wringer or roller injury. In humans the usual cause is either catching the limb in power-driven rollers or running over the limb with a tire and scraping the skin against the tire or the road.[12, 39] Both of these cause a sudden, severe, shearing strain on the skin.[39] The latter source of injury is all too common in animals and familiar to the veterinary practitioner.

With this injury the skin is either anatomically or physiologically flayed. The skin is actually torn off with anatomical flaying (Figs. 2–1 and 2–2). In physiological flaying the skin surface is intact; however, there is complete disruption at the deep fascial level, with undermining. The vascular network of the skin is damaged more or less severely at this time by the sudden, extreme tension caused by the shearing strain. This damage is usually severe enough to result in ischemic necrosis of the skin and superficial fascia (Fig. 2–1).[39]

In humans, degloving injuries can occur on the palmar or the dorsal surface of the hand. The skin on the dorsal surface is laxer but less well attached deeply. It gives more with the shearing strain than does palmar skin, but it does not withstand the strain as well. The result is that it degloves more readily than the palmar surface, with the cleavage plane being between the skin and the superficial fascia.[38] In the author's experience, a

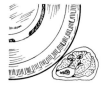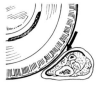

"PHYSIOLOGICAL   "ANATOMICAL
DEGLOVING"   DEGLOVING"

Figure 2–1: Physiological and anatomical degloving injury produced by a car tire. (From McGregor, I. A.: Fundamental Techniques of Plastic Surgery, ed. 6. Edinburgh, Churchill Livingstone, 1975, p. 167.)

similar situation occurs in dogs in that there seem to be more degloving injuries on the dorsum of the feet than on the volar or plantar (pad) surfaces.

A pure degloving injury damages the skin selectively without injuring the deeper structures such as the nerves, tendons and bone. However, many degloving injuries are a combination of degloving and crushing in which bone damage and varying degrees of deeper soft tissue damage are present along with the skin injury.[38]

The primary pathology of a degloving injury occurs in the blood vessels supplying the skin as a result of the tremendous stretching. There may be epidermal damage; however, this is usually in addition to vascular damage. In a pure degloving injury, the epidermis is still viable, and it is probable that the dermal capillaries are still intact but are without a supportive blood supply for maintenance.[38] The survival time of such a degloved flap of skin is a matter of hours at normal temperatures but could be prolonged by cooling the skin.[38]

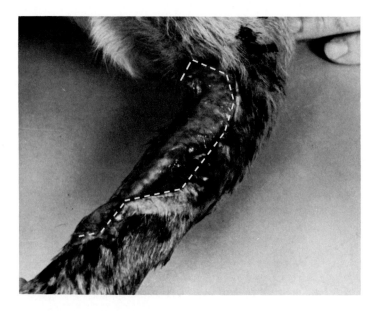

Figure 2–2: Anatomical degloving of a dog's forelimb. See color plate I–A, p. 568.

Of the skin injuries seen by veterinarians, the degloving injury can be one of the most perplexing and leaves the surgeon with two problems. The first problem is to differentiate between the viable and nonviable tissue and to excise or eliminate the nonviable tissue. This will be discussed further in Chapter 4. The second problem is to reconstruct the remaining skin defect with either local or distant skin.

BITE WOUNDS

In areas where leash laws are nonexistent or are poorly enforced, dog fight victims may account for a significant portion of the practitioner's case load. Dog bite wounds can range from almost insignificant wounds to extremely difficult and challenging injuries.[42]

What appears to be a simple wound at first may turn out to be an extremely complex wound when thoroughly examined. The skin is freely movable in most areas of the body, and the canine tooth will often only make a puncture wound. However, with the slashing action of a biting dog, the tooth moves through the underlying subcutaneous and muscular tissues. Although the skin slides with the movement of the tooth, the deeper tissues that do not slide are torn via the small puncture wound.[42] The dynamics of such an injury become evident when one considers what a carnivore does when it catches its prey — it shakes the prey violently. A puncture-type wound may be compared to an iceberg in that only a small part of the damage is seen on the surface, with much more significant underlying damage (Fig. 2–3).

The problem of wound infection is inherent in animal bite wounds, despite the cliché "clean as a hound's tooth."[9] Not only do bacteria come from the attacker's mouth but also from the victim's skin and, in many cases, from soil organisms. There may be a large amount of torn, devitalized tissue beneath the skin, with much dead space in which serum can accumulate and allow bacteria to proliferate.[42] Such areas may present a problem in that the skin puncture wound will heal, but the underlying bacteria in the pabulum will proliferate until a large area of abscessed necrotic tissue and its overlying skin slough, leaving a large open area for the surgeon to deal with.

A study of bite wounds in humans has shown that cat bite wounds are more likely to become infected than dog bite wounds. In this study the cat bite wounds were small puncture wounds, with small punctate abscesses

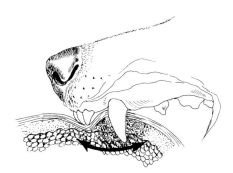

Figure 2–3: Dynamics of a dog bite wound. A skin puncture wound results in more extensive damage to underlying tissues as the tooth moves through these tissues.

being common; only one half of the infected wounds caused lymphangitis and lymphadenitis. Positive cultures from the infected wounds revealed *Staphylococcus aureus, Staphylococcus albus,* and *Streptococcus pyogenes.* The infections were sensitive to ampicillin, cloxacillin sodium, and a combination of penicillin and cloxacillin sodium.[16] If left untreated, cat bite wounds can develop into serious infections, including the abscesses and sloughs previously mentioned.

In the author's experience, some of the most severe dog fight injuries have occurred when three or more large dogs have been penned together and one dog was attacked by the others. Massive skin loss and underlying soft tissue trauma have resulted, since the victim had no place to retreat.

Dog and cat bite injuries may result in the direct loss of skin or a secondary loss of skin as the result of infection and slough of tissue.

SNAKEBITES

Another source of skin defect is snakebite and the effect of venom on the local tissues (Fig. 2–4). Of the pit vipers, the true rattlesnakes of the genera *Crotalus* are the most dangerous owing to their size and venom capacity.[1, 48–50] The majority of human deaths from snakebites are caused by rattlesnake bites.[9] Among rattlesnakes, the eastern diamondback has the reputation of being quite dangerous,[1, 34, 48–50] with few dogs or small animals surviving its bite[1, 48, 50] or that of its fellow, the western diamondback.[1, 50] Also considered to be dangerous among the pit vipers is the water moccasin (cottonmouth).[1, 9, 34, 48, 49] The copperhead and pygmy, or ground rattler, are not as dangerous as the aforementioned snakes.[1, 9, 48–50] The toxin of the pit vipers is primarily a hematoxin, whereas that of the coral snake is primarily a neurotoxin.[23, 47, 48, 50]

Snake venoms are primarily proteinaceous and are composed of enzymes and toxins. The enzymes that have been identified in snake venoms include hyaluronidase, L-amino-oxidase, various proteases, phospholi-

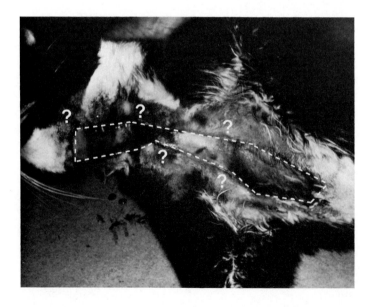

Figure 2–4: Necrotizing effect of snake venom on the cranioventral skin of a cat. The skin is of questionable viability(?). See color plate I–B, p. 568.

pases, phosphatases, phosphatidases, and coagulases.[1, 23, 50] Numerous hemolysins and neurotoxins have also been identified.[23] Pit viper venoms are primarily active in causing hemolysis and tissue necrosis.[23, 50] These actions are produced by the various enzymes in the venoms. The phosphatidases act on the heart and circulation and cause hemolysis, while the proteolytic enzymes destroy local tissues and capillaries. "Spreading factors," which include hyaluronidase, enhance the spread of the venom within the tissues.[1, 49, 50]

In addition to the changes caused by the components of the venom, changes are produced by bradykinin, adenylic compounds, and histamine released by the tissues.[1, 35, 50] Lysolecithin, which is formed in the tissues by the venom, may cause hemolysis.[1] Based on the known actions of the various components of pit viper venoms, it can be seen that they have the potential for causing severe soft tissue damage, including damage to the skin.

The severity of a snakebite and the amount of soft tissue destruction will vary with several factors. An animal's age, weight, general health, general body condition, and composition (fat or lean) are factors that will affect snakebite severity. The presence of a thick hair coat or subcutaneous fat layer that could absorb the venom or impede its absorption as well as the location and nature of the bite (a glancing scratch as opposed to a deep wound) have a bearing on the severity of the bite.[23, 48] However, it has been stated that a large rattlesnake with fangs as long as 1 in. or more usually deposits venom in the subcutaneous tissue and only rarely as deep as the muscles.[1, 50] The majority of snakebites in animals occur on the head, face, shoulder, neck, chest, and forelegs.[48]

Factors related to the snake also determine the gravity of a snakebite, such as the size and species of snake, its general health, and the virulence of its venom. In addition to these, the time since the snake's last feeding, the length and strength of its fangs, and the amount of venom injected contribute to the severity of a snakebite.[23, 48] The eventual result of a snakebite may also be influenced by the presence of pathogenic bacteria either within the snake's mouth or on the victim's skin.[23] Infection with such bacteria can complicate the soft tissue destruction associated with envenomation.

A snakebite wound can be considered a contaminated, venom-laden, necrotic, and anaerobic puncture wound that provides an excellent milieu for bacterial growth. Serious local complications are often present in the form of gangrene, infection, and tissue slough.[1, 50] Immediately following envenomation, an animal may show excruciating local pain, edema, discoloration and erythema of the area, and serum or lymphatic transudation from the fang punctures.[1, 23, 35] These local signs progress in the form of swelling that extends proximally and distally from the bite.[23] Destruction of the capillary endothelium results in serum and blood loss into the tissues in the form of petechiae, ecchymoses, and finally hemolytic effusions.[23, 50] The hemolysis mentioned earlier also takes place.[35, 50] Anemia and local tissue slough almost invariably result from severe envenomation.[1, 50] Even with an incision and suction over the venom injection sites, wide local sloughs of the soft tissue may occur. This was shown in a study in which venom from an eastern diamondback rattlesnake and a water moccasin was injected into dogs. Of the injected venom, 53.6 per cent could be recovered after 15 minutes of suction and the treatment was lifesaving; however, wide local sloughs of soft tissue still occurred.[57]

The subcutaneous injection of rattlesnake venom in monkeys showed it to be a powerful tissue irritant that causes necrosis and actual dissolution of blood vessels, with subsequent extravasation of erythrocytes and serum into the tissues. The most outstanding lesion was a marked hemorrhagic edema at the site of injection that spread widely throughout the adjacent subcutaneous tissues. The skin over the lumbar injection site was dark red, and this appearance extended into the anterior abdominal wall. However, an autopsy revealed intense hemorrhagic edema that was much more extensive than was indicated by the discoloration of the overlying epidermis. This was accompanied by marked thickening of the subcutaneous connective and adipose tissue and regional hemorrhagic lymphadenitis.[19]

An unrelated study in which snake venom was injected into dogs revealed findings similar to those found in monkeys. Lymph and serum collected at the injection site, and the venom was mixed with these fluids. There was slow dispersion throughout the surrounding area, causing much tissue destruction and hemolysis.[34]

The local tissue destruction associated with a snakebite may consist of an area where the skin has sloughed away, leaving the immediate underlying musculature, vessels, and nerves plainly visible. The musculature is usually dark red or nearly black and edematous, and there may be necrosis of the lymph nodes that drain the area.[34]

Bacterial contamination further complicates tissue destruction by snake venom. Numerous types of microorganisms may be present in snakes' mouths as well as on the skin of the bite victim. These may result in serious wound-borne infections accompanying snakebites, since the organisms have a very suitable atmosphere for growth in the moist, warm environment surrounding the bite.[23, 35] Enteric and coliform bacteria have been identified as the predominant bacteria in snakes' mouths and venom,[47, 48] with the more commonly found organisms being *Proteus vulgaris, Escherichia coli, Corynebacterium,* diphtheroid sp., *Paracolobactrum* sp., and *Streptococcus* sp.[47] In addition, clostridial organisms, including those that cause gas gangrene and tetanus, may be found in snakes' mouths.[23, 48, 57] Because of the presence of these organisms, the use of broad-spectrum antibiotics[35, 48] and gas gangrene and tetanus antitoxins[48] has been advocated in treating snakebites.

INSECT BITES AND STINGS

Some of the biting arthropods may cause quite severe local tissue destruction, with or without severe systemic symptoms (Fig. 2–5). Certain insects will leave a part of the stinging apparatus in the tissues of the victim after injecting their venom. When venom sacs are retained in the tissues, more local absorption and tissue destruction can occur. In the case of ticks, the biting mouth parts may be left within the tissues and this may produce a granuloma.[9]

Spiders

There are only four species of spiders in North America capable of producing clinical signs that justify medical management. These spiders are

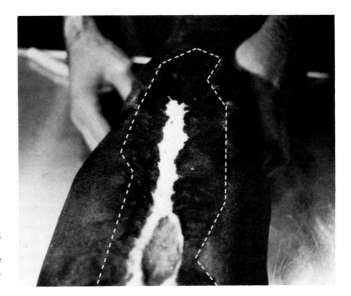

Figure 2–5: A wide scar on a dog's back (*dotted lines*) resulting from the open healing of an extensive tissue slough caused by an insect bite or sting. See color plate I–C, p. 568.

(1) the black widow spider, (2) the red-legged widow spider, (3) the brown recluse spider, and (4) the common brown spider. The two widow spiders produce venoms that are neurotoxic, inducing signs that may last several days. The bites of the two brown spiders produce more chronic effects.[23] The brown recluse spider deposits a toxin that produces both a local reaction and a systemic reaction.[9, 15, 20] Initially, the bite of the brown recluse seems minimal; however, the victim begins to experience severe pain shortly thereafter at the area of the bite. This develops into a small area of necrosis that spreads gradually, increasing daily. Without excision the necrotic skin will slough.[9] In animals the bite area typically ulcerates, leaving a necrotic center.[23] This ulcer may be from one to many centimeters in diameter, with a healing time directly proportional to its size.[15, 20] In humans, small ulcers usually heal in about three weeks;[20] however, the veterinary literature has stated that several months may be needed for an indolent ulcer to heal.[23]

In humans, one prescribed treatment is excision of the involved skin soon after a diagnosis of brown spider bite has been established. If excision is delayed until later, a skin graft is usually needed 5 to 10 days after excision.[9]

When dealing with animals, it would be difficult to establish an early diagnosis of brown spider bite unless the biting incident was actually observed; consequently, late excision would be the rule. It is not uncommon to have to excise the chronic lesion and place a skin graft in the defect.[15, 23] However, it has been reported that such grafts in humans may take poorly or may not be successful.[15, 20]

Bees and Wasps

Bee and wasp venoms are both neurotoxic and hemolytic. In the normal individual, the reaction to a bee or wasp sting includes acute pain, erythema, local induration, edema, and later pruritus.[23] Wasp and hornet stings may be more severe than bee stings from the standpoint of infection.

Since wasps and hornets are scavengers, they are likely to transmit infection with their venom, which may develop as a cellulitis some hours or days after the sting. The responsible organisms may include the anaerobic bacteria that produce gas gangrene.[20] Therefore, the potential for tissue destruction and loss is present with the sting of a wasp or a hornet.

SKIN TUMORS

Skin tumors are included as a source of skin trauma or defect, since one or both may result from such a pathological condition. An ulcerated mastocytoma or any other ulcerated skin tumor can be examples of trauma. Removal of skin tumors (whether large or small, traumatized or not) leaves a skin defect that the surgeon must close. The postsurgical skin defect may be the result of removing the skin tumor itself or a tumor involving skin secondarily[39] (Fig. 2–6). An example of the latter would be the removal of mammary gland tumors.

Various figures have been stated for the incidence of skin tumors in dogs and cats. Depending upon the source of data, it has been reported that from 20 per cent to 50 per cent of all canine tumors and from 15 per cent to 47 per cent of all feline tumors are skin tumors.[6, 8, 10, 11, 30, 31, 41, 52]

When dealing with malignant skin tumors, the surgeon should separate, in his mind at least, the excision of the tumor and the defect repair. This is done so that the tumor will be treated according to its nature and extent without regard for the potential problems to be encountered with repair.[39, 52]

General guidelines have been established for the marginal extensions to be used when excising skin tumors. In the veterinary literature, wide skin margins (0.5 to 1.5 cm.) have been advocated for tumor removal.[27, 31, 61] One report stated that a margin of 0.5 to 1.0 cm. is adequate, with a 1.0-cm. margin yielding an almost certain cure, since most lesions extend less than 6 mm. from the visible margins.[2] The following would be a guide for the

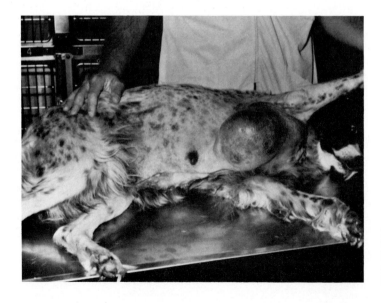

Figure 2–6: A large tumor, the removal of which will leave an extensive skin defect requiring some form of reconstructive surgery.

excision of tumors: (1) nodular lesions, a 0.5- to 1.0-cm. margin; (2) ulcerative-invasive lesions, at least a 1.0- to 1.5-cm. margin; and (3) morphea-like or fibrosing lesions, at least a 1.0- to 1.5-cm. margin.[44]

Generally, the more exophytic the lesion, the less deeply it invades the tissues. A nodular exophytic lesion usually requires complete removal of the dermis only, unless dissection reveals the lesion to extend more deeply. The fibrosing or morphea-like lesion will probably require removal of the first anatomical mesodermal barrier (i.e., fascia, periosteum, perichondrium, or subcutaneous tissue when present). Deeper dissection is usually not necessary unless further invasion can be demonstrated.[44]

The margins of resection for a squamous cell carcinoma are more standardized; they should include at least 1 cm. of clinically normal tissue in all planes.[44]

In addition to conventional surgical removal, other techniques have been described for skin tumor removal. These include electrosurgery (surgical diathermy — desiccation and coagulation) or cutting.[11] Cryosurgery may also be used for tumor removal.

Skin tumors on certain areas of the body may present unique problems to the surgeon. Squamous cell carcinomas and malignant melanomas are important neoplasias of the digits. Squamous cell carcinomas in the digital region often invade the adjacent phalanges, causing marked osteolysis that is readily visualized on radiographs. Unless there is inoperable metastasis, early diagnosis should be followed by digital amputation.[8]

In cats (especially white cats), squamous cell carcinomas commonly occur in the head region, particularly in the tips of the pinnae and the eyelids.[8] Following removal of such tumors, some form of blepharoplasty or otoplasty would be needed for defect closure.

Histiocytomas have been found frequently in the skin of the head, particularly in the pinnae.[8] As with squamous cell carcinomas of this area, some form of otoplasty would be indicated for reconstruction.

Ceruminous gland tumors are among the most common skin tumors of cats. They arise from the wax-secreting glands of the external auditory canal and are usually malignant. They appear as a solitary, rapidly growing, dome-shaped, fleshy mass that protrudes into the ear canal. Owing to the inaccessible nature of the site and the invasiveness of the tumor, total excision is difficult and local recurrence is usual. However, cures can be affected in early cases by radical excision. This type of tumor may respond well to cryosurgery.[5, 6] Again, some type of reconstructive otoplasty is indicated with this type of tumor.

Hepatoid or perianal adenomas in male dogs arise from the hepatoid cells in the subcutaneous tissues around the anal ring, lateral to the prepuce, and on the dorsal and ventral surfaces of the root of the tail. The most common site of this neoplasia is the perianal region, especially in males. After wide surgical excision, the prognosis is good; however, owing to the nature of the site, complete removal is not always feasible, especially with large tumors.[5, 6] About 35 per cent of the adenomas around the anal ring recur after surgical removal.[6]

Three to five intralesional injections of 10 to 20 mg. each of a long-acting preparation of diethylstilbestrol every two to three weeks will usually induce dramatic shrinkage. This type of treatment is valuable in reducing the size of large tumors prior to surgery but cannot be relied upon as the sole therapeutic regimen.[5, 6, 41] By reducing the size of the tumor, the extent of postexcisional reconstructive surgery can be reduced. Castration may reduce the size of many large tumors prior to excision[6] and may be effective in preventing recurrence following tumor removal.[41]

The surgical removal of even large subcutaneous lipomas is often easy. In some dogs strict dieting for several months has reduced the size of such tumors so that surgical excision has been easier.[6] This should be kept in mind when dealing with an extremely large lipoma, the removal of which might result in a large skin defect.

Reconstruction of an area following tumor removal will require a knowledge of skin tensions and the principles of reconstructive surgery. The surgeon has at his disposal the use of three basic techniques for reconstruction: (1) shifting local tissue, (2) using a pedicle flap, and (3) using a free skin graft. One of these will be chosen as a means of skin closure. Free skin grafts may have the advantage of not obscuring the field in case of tumor recurrence in the underlying tissues. Flaps would be indicated when tumor excision leaves a surface that cannot take a free skin graft, e.g., cortical bone or tendon.[39] Shifting of local tissues could also be used in the latter instance.

Mast Cell Tumors

The mast cell tumor has been identified as the most important and most clinically significant skin tumor in the dog.[4, 5, 8]

The mastocytomas are important to the surgeon, since they constitute a large portion of the skin tumors and since inadequate removal or follow-up therapy or both could result in increased chances for metastasis or recurrence of the tumor at the surgical site.

Mastocytomas can occur anywhere in the skin, with little predilection for any other organ. They can be single or multiple and vary from slowly growing, soft, and flabby tumors to rapidly growing, firm, multinodular masses (Figs. 2–7 and 2–8). The latter can invade the skin and cause ulceration and local irritation.[6] Owing to the varying forms, mastocytomas can present the surgeon with a reconstructive challenge following removal.

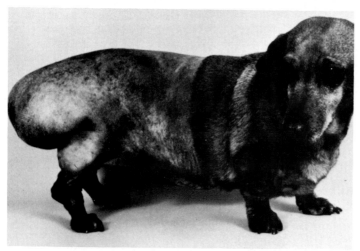

Figure 2–7: Slow-growing, ill-defined mastocytoma.

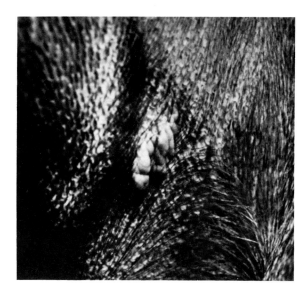

Figure 2–8: Small, firm, multinodular masto-cytoma. (Courtesy of M. D. Wiggins.)

These tumors have been histologically graded from 1 to 3, with grade 1 being a poorly differentiated tumor, grade 2, an intermediately differentiated tumor, and grade 3, a well-differentiated tumor.[4] This is important for prognosis following surgical removal[29] in that the cure rate of dogs with grade 3 tumors has been found to be greater than that of dogs with the other two grades of tumor.[4] Following the removal of slowly growing, well-differentiated mastocytomas, more than 80 per cent of the dogs are cured.[6] Dogs that survive longer than 30 weeks postoperatively appear to be cured.[4] Less well-differentiated tumors tend to recur locally and to metastasize to regional lymph nodes and thus have a guarded prognosis. Over 70 per cent of the dogs with poorly differentiated tumors have to be killed because of regrowth following surgical excision.[6] Many tumors that were well developed before surgical removal recur and are more anaplastic than the original tumors.[41]

Based on clinical grounds alone, it has been stated that if a mast cell tumor has been present for more than 28 weeks before removal, the prognosis should be favorable, since 83 per cent of the animals with such a history survived more than 30 weeks after surgery.[4]

In all fairness to the animal and its owner, the surgeon should take into consideration the previously mentioned characteristics and prognostic factors associated with mastocytomas and discuss these with the animal owner prior to surgical intervention.

The surgical approach to mastocytomas should be wide excision of the primary cutaneous tumor.[5, 31, 32, 41] Regional lymph node removal,[5, 41] radiation therapy,[5, 6, 31, 32, 41] and corticosteroid therapy[31, 41] have also been advocated as part of the treatment. Chemotherapy in the form of a vinblastine, cyclophosphamide, and prednisolone combination has been reported.[41] Radiation therapy is especially recommended when dealing with the intermediately or poorly differentiated tumors.[5] If the tumor is a single, primary, mature, well-granulated mastocytoma, additional therapy may not be needed. However, this decision should be based on histopathological interpretation and should consider (1) the degree of malignancy of neoplastic cells; (2) the gross physical characteristics of the tumor (nodular or diffuse); (3)

the condition of regional lymph nodes; and (4) the presence or absence of uninvolved tissue at the periphery of the tumor in histological sections.[32]

Other nonneoplastic tumor-like lesions of the skin require surgical removal and consequently reconstruction of the skin. Such lesions include calcinosis circumscripta, cysts, and granulomas.[6]

MAMMARY TUMORS

Mammary gland tumors are another type of pathological entity that is frequently encountered by the practitioner. These tumors are considered from the standpoint of the skin defect that is created when they are removed. This defect can become rather large in some cases of extensive tumor involvement and when one or both mammary chains are removed. These tumors reportedly account for 25 per cent[6] to 52 per cent[5] of all neoplasms in female dogs and less than 3 per cent of those in male dogs.[5] Various histological types of neoplasms have been observed in dogs, but a large portion of them are mixed tumors.[5, 6, 55] It has been stated that about 70 per cent of the bitches with mammary neoplasia will have mixed tumors, but 50 per cent of these have coexisting malignant neoplasms of a different type.[60]

In bitches the inguinal mammary glands are involved in neoplastic transformation three to four times more often than the more cranially located glands.[5, 6, 8] However, it has been reported that careful patient evaluation reveals frequent tumor occurrence throughout the mammary chain, especially in the area of the cranial superficial epigastric vessels.[60] Tumors that do occur in the inguinal glands provide an advantage for the surgeon in that the skin in this area (the lateral abdominal and flank area) may be more abundant and therefore more suitable for closure of the defects created by removal of the glands.

Mammary tumors are quite rare in male cats but account for about 22 per cent of the total tumors in female cats.[5] From 80 per cent to 95 per cent of the mammary tumors in cats are diagnosed as adenocarcinomas.[5, 6, 8] Clinically, feline tumors grow rapidly, are multinodular and locally invasive, tend to ulcerate, and often metastasize. They do not show a predilection for the caudal mammary glands: all four mammary glands are more or less equally affected.[5, 8] Generally, feline mammary tumors have a more malignant behavior pattern and a worse prognosis.[5]

Mammary gland tumors have various clinical characteristics and the surgeon should be aware of these. One study has divided mammary gland tumors into three groups, depending upon their growth characteristics: group I, tumor growth is slow and often persists for many months or years without harming the host; group II, growth is slow at first, often for months or years, then there is a sudden growth spurt and the tumor becomes invasive and metastatic; and group III, from the time of first detection growth is quite rapid and the tumors appear malignant soon after their onset.[8] Most benign mammary gland tumors grow slowly and are usually sharply demarcated from the surrounding tissue. They are freely movable without infiltration and are occasionally pedunculated, and the covering skin over the tumor can be moved.[43] Some benign mixed mammary tumors tend to be very slow growing but may increase in size in the immediate postestrus period, with incomplete regression during anestrus.[6] The statement that benign tumors tend to be firmer than malignant ones is not reliable in the case of mammary tumors. Well-encapsulated nonadherent tumors may still be malignant.[43]

The surgeon should suspect malignancy and consider a poor prognosis when a tumor shows infiltration, fixation to the skin or deeper tissues (including the regional lymph nodes), a rapid growth rate, ulceration, palpable enlargements in the lymphatics between the gland and lymph node, hemorrhaging, and radiographic evidence of lung metastasis.[31, 43] However, with large benign mixed mammary tumors, the tumor may become ulcerated as a result of trauma.[6] Edema of the pelvic limb or forelimb may be indicative of metastasis to the inguinal or axillary lymph nodes, respectively; however, axillary node involvement is rare. Either of these signs warrants a poor prognosis. Edema of the mammary gland itself may be due to lymphatic blockage or an inflammatory response.[43] Size has been used to determine whether surgical treatment of a mammary tumor is necessary. It should be remembered that widespread metastasis may be present even though the size of the mass appears to be static. Regardless of its size, a tumor of the mammary glands should be considered malignant.[60]

Thoracic radiographs to check for pulmonary metastasis are advisable.[43, 60] These should be done whether an animal shows signs of respiratory involvement or not. There is usually little value in excising the primary tumor when lung metastasis has occurred. However, the presence of lung metastasis is not an immediate indication for euthanasia, since the growth of such metastasis is quite variable.[43] The preoperative work-up should include a physical examination and pertinent laboratory determinations.

The surgical removal of mammary tumors and glands should be done early, while the tumor is still small and localized, for the best results as well as safety and convenience. However, good results frequently follow surgical removal of large or multiple tumors, and one should not advise against surgery unless the lesion is undoubtedly inoperable. Tumors might be considered inoperable if there is extensive local involvement or demonstrable metastasis of the neoplasm. A patient that is in poor physical condition may be considered a poor surgical risk and inoperable.[55]

The surgical removal of mammary gland tumors and related glands and lymph nodes has been discussed from an anatomical standpoint in Chapter 1. Factors related to the actual surgical procedure will be discussed at this point. Owing to the lack of controlled comparisons between the various methods of mammary tumor removal, it is difficult to be certain which procedure is most effective. It seems likely, by analogy with the results obtained in human treatment, that wide excision to include normal tissue is essential if local recurrence is to be prevented. However, wide removal of adjacent glands and regional lymph nodes may not be necessary unless they are clinically involved. If there is evidence of involvement of the superficial lymph nodes, the deep lymph nodes, or the lungs, the prognosis must be guarded regardless of the procedure used.[5] As a general rule, mastectomy is done unilaterally at one time,[60, 61] since the amount of trauma caused by bilateral excision is great and the wound closure and healing may present some difficult problems. The most involved chain should be removed first and the patient should be allowed to recover sufficiently before the contralateral chain is excised.[60] It has also been reported that all of the caudal glands may be removed at one time in cases of bilateral involvement; however, this may not be possible in some animals because of extensive skin loss, and a second operation may be necessary.[43] Bilateral mammary gland removal may be considered but *only* if the surgeon, through preoperative planning, has been able to ascertain that sufficient skin *will* be available for closure of the defect after tumor removal. One technique that helps supply skin for closure of such a defect is to leave a "V"-shaped, cranially based flap of skin between the cranialmost mammary glands. This facilitates closure of the thoracic skin defect left by bilateral mammary gland excision. The defect closes in the shape of a "Y" (Fig. 2–9).[28] Leaving a bilateral mastectomy wound partially open in cases in which there is insufficient skin for closure can be justified if the tumors are bilateral, rapidly growing, and invasive. The area may be closed at a later time or may be left to heal as an open wound.[28]

The incisions for mammary gland removal may be straight or elliptical, and they should be sharp and wide.[31, 55, 62] The incision should conform to the size and shape of the mass and will vary with the number of glands to be removed. The surgeon should give consideration to the closure of the defect before the incision is made.[31] For total unilateral mastectomy, an elliptical incision may be made from the cranial pectoral region to the lateral vulvar region. The lateral incision is lateral to the definable glandular tissue, and the medial incision follows the ventral midline except near the cranial and caudal aspects of the incision.[60]

Dissection of the tumors may be carried out from the cranial to the caudal regions using blunt dissection of the chain from the abdominal musculature through the connective tissue layers.[55, 60, 62] Scissors, a scalpel blade, or a cautery may be used for dissection, with scissors probably being the most commonly used instrument.[55] At the cranial aspect of the chain, the glands are closely attached to the pectoral fascia and extend to varying degrees into the axilla, where dissection is tedious. While in this area, the axilla should be explored and the axillary lymph node should be removed, if indicated. As the thoracicoabdominal area is approached, the glands are more loosely attached and excision becomes easier.[60] If there appears to be any involvement of the fascia of exposed muscle, either by direct spread or via lymphatics, this tissue should be removed. Wound irrigation with a saline solution containing penicillin has been advocated for removing cellular debris, fat particles, and bacteria.[43] Gentle manipulation of tumors during their removal will help avoid tumor emboli.[62]

The ligation of large vessels supplying the mammary tissue is important from the standpoint of good hemostasis and prevention of tumor em-

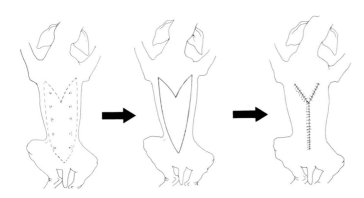

Figure 2–9: A technique for simultaneous removal of both mammary chains. The cranially based "V"-shaped flap left in the thoracic area aids in the relief of tension in this area as the wound is closed in a "Y"-shape.

boli problems.[43] As vessels are located they should be clamped or ligated before being severed.[31, 62] Other small bleeders are clamped and ligated as necessary for hemostasis. In the inguinal area, the caudal superficial epigastric vessels should be identified, transfixed, and ligated.[31, 60, 62] This is followed by removal of the inguinal lymph node, further careful removal of perivulvar glandular tissue, and adequate hemostasis in the area.[60]

At the time of wound closure, the wound edges should be examined for any glandular tissue that may have been overlooked.[60] Undermining of the wound edges should be done with discretion, if at all, since dead space, seroma, decreased blood supply to the skin edges, and necrosis could result from this procedure.[60, 62] However, some undermining may be necessary to achieve closure without undue tension.[31]

Subcuticular sutures have been advocated for closing dead space and preventing seromas and hematomas in the defect left by the mammary gland removal. These sutures are followed by skin sutures for final wound closure.[43, 55, 62] The use of interrupted horizontal mattress sutures to serve as tension sutures along the wound edge and simple interrupted sutures to appose the skin edges has been advocated. However, an occasional seroma may develop in the inguinal area because of the difficulty in eliminating the dead tissue space in this area during skin closure.[60] The application of a pressure bandage over the surgical site for 24 hours following surgery has been described for holding the skin in close apposition to the underlying muscles.[55] However, a pressure bandage in the area can impair venous drainage from the pelvic limbs and can further complicate the edema that may already be present as a result of removing the inguinal lymph nodes.[28] A technique that lends itself well to closure of the defects caused by mammary tumor removal is the "walking" suture technique, which is described in Chapter 7.

Ovariohysterectomy is recommended with mastectomy, not to stop the neoplasia, but because ovarian cysts or tumors, metritis, and pseudocyesis are common.[60] The resultant mammary atrophy in the remaining glands will allow identification of other tumors and easier surgical removal of the second chain.[31, 60]

An early aggressive approach should be taken with feline mammary gland tumors. Since all mammary gland nodules in the cat should be considered malignant until proved otherwise, a wide unilateral radical mastectomy and lymphadenectomy are the procedures of choice. Since the underlying tissues can be invaded by malignant cells, a partial or full-thickness resection of these tissues may be performed as needed. Copious flushing of the wound helps remove exfoliated cells. When there are tumors in both mammary chains, a bilateral mastectomy is performed, with the mastectomy of the second chain of glands being performed after the skin has healed adequately in the first incision.[27] Simultaneous bilateral mastectomy may be considered if, as previously mentioned, the surgeon has been able to ascertain, through preoperative planning, that there will be sufficient skin available to close the large defect.

GUNSHOT WOUNDS

Gunshot injuries occur in dogs and cats, and in many instances the owner is unaware of the trauma owing to the small pellets with which the animals are shot.[33] There are, of course, other instances in which a large wound is quite obvious as the result of a higher velocity or closer range gunshot. Gunshot injuries in males seem to predominate over those in females.[33]

Gunshot wounds are caused by one of three firearms: (1) pistols and civilian firearms, (2) shotguns and (3) military or high powered hunting rifles.[17, 40] Air rifles and pellet guns would be included in the first category of weapons. Pistols and civilian firearms produce less destruction than the high-powered or military rifles, which create severe soft tissue damage. The tissue damage done by a shotgun blast is dependent upon the pellet size and the range at which the gun was fired.

There are two types of high-velocity bullets, each of which produces a different type of wound. The jacketed or military type of bullet generally produces a cylindrical wound tract, the size of which does not increase appreciably as the missile progresses through the tissue. The missile itself is barely deformed as it passes through the tissue. In contrast to this is the expanding bullet that is used for game hunting in all areas of North America. When performing as it should, this bullet expands to several times its original caliber and thereby creates a very wide wound tract. The wound is in the form of a large cone rather than a cylinder (Fig. 2–10).[14, 37] Wound ballistics studies in which 150-grain .30 caliber bullets traveling at 2900 ft./sec. were fired through the thoraces of anesthetized dogs revealed different wounding capacities, depending upon whether the bullet was jacketed or expanding. When a jacketed bullet was used, the wound of entrance was 0.75 cm. in diameter, the wound of exit was 2.0 cm. in diameter, and the wound volume was 23.5 cu. cm. An expanding missile produced a wound of entrance of 0.75 cm. in diameter, a wound of exit of 12.5 cm. in diameter, and a wound volume of 917 cu. cm.[14] These figures show that an expanding missile has the capacity to produce not only a large amount of tissue damage within a wound but also a sizable skin wound at the point of exit. High-velocity bullet wounds in which the bullet has been tumbling as it passed through the tissue also have a larger volume of tissue damage if the missile had traveled straight through the tissue.[17]

Several factors govern the wounding characteristics of a missile: mass, shape, aerodynamic and hydrodynamic stability, deformation and breakup, and velocity.[17] Two of these factors, velocity and mass, can be placed in a formula to determine the energy related to a missile. This formula is:

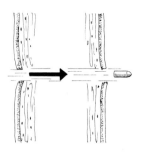

JACKETED
BULLET

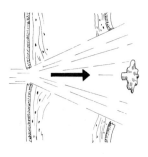

EXPANDING
BULLET

Figure 2-10: The difference between wound patterns of jacketed and expanding bullets. A jacketed bullet makes small wounds of entry and exit and a cylindrical wound tract. An expanding bullet makes a small wound of entry, a large wound of exit, and a large cone-shaped wound tract.

$$\text{Kinetic energy} = \frac{\text{Mass} \times \text{velocity}^2}{2}$$

The velocity of a missile is the primary factor in determining its wounding capacity. Doubling the mass doubles the kinetic energy, but doubling the velocity quadruples the kinetic energy.[14, 17, 25, 37, 63]

The wounding capacity of a low-velocity missile, such as that of pistols and civilian weapons, is less than that of the military or high-powered rifle, which has a higher velocity missile. The low-velocity missiles have been considered to have a velocity of less than 1000 ft. per/sec.,[25] and their action in soft tissue has been likened to that of a rod being plunged through soft snow where the snow piles up in front of the rod and is pushed ahead. When the rod is withdrawn, a hole is left the diameter of which is little more than that of the rod. Thus, damage to tissues by a low-velocity missile is the result of their immediate displacement by the moving projectile.[26] The result is generally only a laceration and crushing of tissue, with minimal cavitation and the area of damage confined to the permanent cavity perimeter.[25, 37]

More involved dynamics accompany high-velocity missile injuries, thus producing more tissue damage. Two of the factors involved are (1) the creation of a temporary cavity as the energy of the missile is transmitted radially to the tissues so that tissue cells adjacent to the wound tract become secondary missiles that move outward at tremendous speeds;[3, 14, 22, 37, 63] and (2) the creation of shock waves, which are pulses of high pressure (well over 1000 lbs./sq. in.) that pass through the tissues with the speed of sound in water or tissue (about 4800 ft./sec.).[22, 26]

Not only the energy of a missile but the physical properties of the tissues themselves govern the extent of tissue damage. In general, the higher the specific gravity (sp. gr.) of a tissue, the more the damage from missile passage.[14, 37] In one study, extreme wound severity was produced in bone (rib, sp. gr. of 1.11) when it was struck by a high-velocity missile, whereas lung tissue (sp. gr. of 0.4 to 0.5) was at the other end of the scale, with only minimal wound severity. Muscle, liver, skin, and fat were intermediate in severity between bone and lung. Muscle (sp. gr. of 1.02 to 1.04) and liver (sp. gr. of 1.01 to 1.02) were similar in wound characteristics, with marked wound severity. Skin (sp. gr. of 1.09) sustained a marked wound severity also.[14] It is known that elastic tissues, such as fascia and skin, and spongy tissues, such as lung, show little devitalization when struck by high-velocity missiles. However, other soft, bulky, homogeneous, solid tissues, such as muscle bellies, liver, and spleen, are violently damaged by high-velocity missiles.[63]

Since this text deals primarily with trauma and reconstruction of the skin, the effects of high-velocity missiles on the skin are of primary interest. It is important to remember that the wound of exit is not necessarily larger than the wound of entrance. As has been pointed out in the discussion on jacketed and expanding missiles, the size of the skin wound will vary with the stability, shape, and cohesiveness of the missile. It will also be governed by the amount of foreign material and bone carried into and out of the body. Other facts to bear in mind are that skin wounds do not necessarily reveal the caliber of the missile that created them and entrance and exit wounds do not indicate the extent of tissue destruction within a wound.[63]

Skin has been found to be more resistant to penetration by a missile than other tissues.[22] There can be disintegration of a large mass of tissue under the

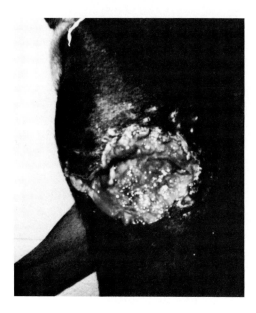

Figure 2–11: Close-range shotgun injury with avulsion of the skin and underlying muscle. See color plate I–D, p. 568.

skin despite small entrance and exit holes in the skin itself. The temporary cavity expansion is the cause of the severe disintegration of the inner tissues. The small skin holes of entry and exit are attributable to the greater structural resistance of skin to expansion and to the skin's elasticity. This elasticity allows it to return to nearly the original size despite the temporary stretch it undergoes.[26] Skin tends to have a confining effect on underlying tissue damage. This has been demonstrated in studies in which high-velocity steel balls are fired into the limbs of dead rabbits. In skinned limbs, a larger crater was formed in the flesh at the site of entry, with greater destruction of tissue than was noted when the same injury was inflicted on a limb covered with skin.[3] It has been observed that with ordinary high-velocity missile injuries, only a thin margin of skin (1 to 2 mm. in width) immediately surrounding the point of perforation needs to be excised.[63] However, it should be remembered that the design (jacketed or expanding) of a high-velocity missile can alter the amount of skin damage.

Shotgun injuries vary greatly in the amount of tissue destruction, depending on the weapon, load, distance, and pattern of shot.[40] At close range shotguns are capable of avulsing skin and muscle over a wide area, which may require skin reconstruction (Fig. 2–11). In addition, there may be massive swelling as well as nerve and blood vessel damage from the multiple foreign bodies. Treatment of these wounds requires careful appraisal of each case.[40] At the other extreme are shotgun injuries from long ranges or with light loads that cause little tissue damage.[33, 40] These injuries seldom need débridement.[40] However, they can be troublesome if a shot enters the eye or if infection ensues.[33]

Traumatic open wounds produced by gunshots are contaminated at the time of production as microorganisms are carried to the depths of the wound by the wounding agent or are sucked into the wound depths by the negative pressure wave associated with tissue cavitation. The conditions present at the time of wounding and the method of wound production have a bearing on the number and type of organisms present in the wound. The organisms multiply, produce toxic products, overcome body defenses, and produce local and systemic body reactions. The greater the tissue destruction, the more ideal is the pabulum for bacterial growth. In such instances it is difficult for the body to mobilize its local defenses to kill these bacteria.[63] Bacterial contamination of a gunshot wound has the potential for causing significant tissue destruction if not managed properly. The loss of this tissue, including skin, could leave the surgeon with a formidable reconstructive surgery job.

RADIATION INJURY

Radiation injury to the skin in the form of acute radiodermatitis may leave the practitioner with an integumentary defect that needs reconstruction. Acute radiodermatitis has been classified into four degrees: (1) A first-degree reaction (threshold erythema) is characterized by reddening of the skin surface. (2) A second-degree reaction (dry desquamation) produces a loss of the superficial layers of the epidermis. (3) A third-degree reaction (moist desquamation) is characterized by exudation with loss of the basal layer of the epidermis. (4) A fourth-degree reaction (necrosis) is irreversible ulceration with dermal destruction (Fig. 2–12).[45] It has been found that a dose of 610 rad. produces erythema, of 1220 rad. causes dry desquamation, of 1830 rad. results in moist desquamation, and between 2440 and 3660 rad. causes acute ulceration and necrosis. Of the ulcers caused by the higher radiation doses, those produced by a dose of 2440 rad. were smaller and most of them healed by the eighth postoperative week. The ulcers produced by a dose of 3660 rad. were larger and had not healed after 50 postoperative days. It is possible to predict acute or chronic radiodermatitis by noting the erythema after radiation. The more severe the erythema and the shorter the time interval after irradiation for its appearance, the more severe the maximum acute reaction.[45, 46]

The nonhealing ulcers that result from higher doses of radiation are the result of vascular changes and dermal scarring, causing avascular areas in the irradiated skin. Vessels at the periphery of irradiated skin are large, tortuous, and dilated, probably as the result of narrowing of their lumens in the irradiated

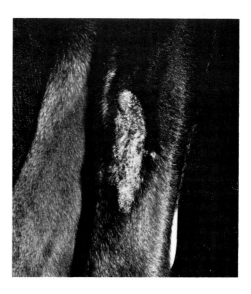

Figure 2–12: Radiation skin injury on the forelimb with ulceration and dermal destruction. (Courtesy of J. E. Bartels.)

area. The connective tissue proliferation in the radiated dermis may also limit revascularization and vessel size by external interference and pressure.[46]

The avascularity of radiation-damaged skin affects the surgical approach to the skin in two ways. First, the area must be deeply excised beyond the damaged zone. If this is not done, the granulation tissue formed may be of poor quality and the chances of a free skin graft taking are poor. Second, the suture-holding properties of therapy-damaged skin are poor and the tissues heal slowly.[39]

When a radiation ulcer does heal, it is by epithelialization, with new epithelium extending into the ulcer from the periphery, and in some instances epithelial islands will erupt in the center of an ulcer.[45]

Before reconstructing the site of an ulcer that has resulted from irradiating a neoplasm, a biopsy should be performed to exclude malignancy, since this would influence the extent and depth of excision. It should be remembered that a malignant ulcer developing in an area of radiation damage is seldom clinically typical and may appear as radionecrosis until a biopsy specimen reveals the true state of the condition. When a recurring postradiation tumor is excised, the entire area of therapy change should be considered potentially neoplastic, since this is the area of the original neoplasm.[39]

When evaluating the pathological effects of radiation and deciding on the type of repair, it must be decided which tissues have borne the brunt of the damage. The mobility of the skin is a good indicator of whether the deeper structures are involved. If only the skin is involved, excision and replacement with a graft are usually satisfactory. However, if there is an indication that deeper structures are involved, excision of the ulcer should be as radical as is technically feasible both in depth and in clearing away radiation-damaged skin at the margins. If bone is involved, sequestrectomy may be done at the time of wound débridement. A blood-carrying flap may be necessary to repair an area of more extensive damage.[39]

DECUBITAL ULCERS

Decubital ulcers develop most commonly in patients that have been recumbent for long periods, including paraplegics, tetraplegics, and orthopedic cases that have multiple fractures (Fig. 2–13). In general, decubital ulcers result from compression of soft tissues between a bony prominence and the surface on which the patient has been resting. The problem is made worse in paralyzed patients that feel no discomfort when left in one position too long.[24, 58]

Factors that predispose skin to the development of decubital ulcers include the following: (1) lessening of the padding between the skin and the bone as a result of disease, atrophy, or loss of fat from debility; (2) loss of tissue elasticity; (3) malnutrition (hypoproteinemia, anemia, vitamin deficiencies); (4) maceration of the skin; (5) chafing of the skin; (6) burns and scalds of the skin; (7) skin friction; (8) circulatory and lymphatic stasis; (9) urinary and fecal incontinence; and (10) inadequate nursing care and poor skin hygiene.[21, 24, 53, 54, 58, 59]

When one or a combination of these factors is present and pressure is placed directly on blood vessels, ischemia results.[21, 24, 58] The tissue ischemia leads to tissue acidosis, increased capillary permeability, extravasation, and vascular thrombosis.[7, 54, 56] An increase in intensity or duration of pressure or

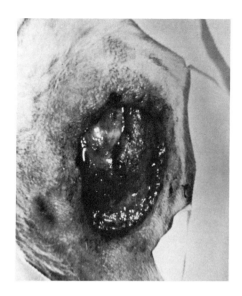

Figure 2–13:   Large decubital ulcer over the scapula.

both will cause interference with cellular metabolism and may result in epithelial, adipose, connective, and muscle tissue necrosis in the involved area.[18] When the necrotic tissue sloughs or is debrided, an ulcer remains.[21, 24, 58]

When ischemia is not prolonged, relief of pressure causes reactive hyperemia, which flushes out harmful metabolites and restores the tissue. Ischemia lasting from six to 12 hours damages skin, and continuous ischemia lasting from 24 to 48 hours or even less results in skin necrosis.[21, 58]

The pathogenesis of skin breakdown has been divided into four stages in humans. Stage 1 is hyperemia that is observed within 30 minutes or less after pressure starts. The hyperemia will disappear within one hour after pressure relief. Stage 2 is ischemia that develops after two to six hours of continuous pressure. The redness associated with ischemia takes at least 36 hours to disappear after pressure relief. Stage 3 is necrosis that occurs unless pressure is released within six hours. Stage 4 is ulceration that occurs within two weeks as the necrotic area becomes ulcerated and infected. Muscle and bone may be involved in this stage of skin breakdown.[18] It is reasonable to assume that similar processes take place in animals.

It has been shown that patients with spinal cord injuries possess an abnormal vascular reflex owing to a disturbance in the sympathetic chain, and dermal trauma in such patients may have a neurogenic basis.[54]

Secondary infection may develop in a decubital ulcer. For example, if drainage of the ulcer is insufficient, systemic infection may result, or if necrosis penetrates more deeply, the underlying bone may become exposed and infected.[24, 58] In human paraplegics, decubital ulcers tend to have an "iceberg" quality, with extensive undermining and osteitis of the underlying bone and possibly suppurative arthritis.[39] Undermining of the skin beyond the ulcer edges is not uncommon in dogs and should be considered during surgical excision and débridement. Of importance to the surgeon is the fact that healing of anesthetized tissues in paraplegics is poor. A wound may fail to heal in such a patient following surgery.[39]

When dealing with a patient that has been or will be in a prolonged recumbent position, as a preventive measure it is wise to check the pressure

① TUBER ISCHII

② TROCHANTER MAJOR

③ TUBER COXA

④ ACROMION OF SCAPULA

⑤ LATERAL EPICONDYLE OF HUMERUS

⑥ LATERAL CONDYLE OF TIBIA

⑦ SIDES OF FIFTH DIGITS

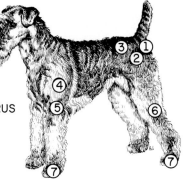

Figure 2–14: Areas to watch for decubital ulcers. (From Swaim, S. F., and Votau, K.: Prevention and treatment of decubital ulcers in the dog. Vet. Med. Small Anim. Clin. *70*:1073, 1975.)

points often for impending decubital problems. The areas to check are the skin over the tuber ischii, trochanter major, tuber coxae, acromion of the scapula, lateral epicondyle of the humerus, lateral epicondyle of the tibia, and lateral aspects of the fifth digits (Fig. 2–14).[58] An impending decubital ulcer may not be noticed as readily in animals as in humans because of the animal's hair coat. This is especially true in long-haired animals. Prevention of decubital ulcers is the best way to circumvent the problems associated with them.

CAST AND BANDAGE APPLICATION

The overzealous application of casts and bandages may result in restricted blood supply to an area and avascular necrosis of tissues. In such instances, skin as well as other structures may be involved in the necrosis. This type of damage is similar to that associated with decubital ulcers. Pressure bandages are necessary in some cases; however, these should be applied with care. Bandage, splint, or cast application is an art that requires a fine touch. The bandage, splint, or cast should be tight enough to accomplish its purpose and yet not so tight that it interferes with the circulation in the area, which could lead to severe soft tissue damage and slough. An animal that licks and chews at a bandage may just be that kind of animal; however, it is possible that the animal is indicating that the bandage is too tight.

Bandages, casts, and splints should be applied and observed carefully, and bandaged areas should be unbandaged and observed if there is any indication of a problem. When avascular pressure necrosis is encountered, some form of reconstructive surgery (skin flap or graft) is often needed, and in some instances amputation of a part or parts (e.g., digits) may be necessary.

THERMAL BURNS

Thermal injuries in animals are not frequent; however, when they do occur, they can be quite devastating from the standpoint not only of skin damage but also of their effect on other tissues and organs. The effect of thermal burns on the skin and other tissues as well as their treatment will be covered in detail in Chapter 5.

Most animals have enough intelligence or lack of intelligence to avoid fire and hot objects; consequently, practically all cases of burns in animals occur either because the animal cannot escape or there is no warning of potential harm. An example of the first instance would be a building in which the animal is housed (private home, stables, kennel, or veterinary hospital) catching fire (Fig. 2–15).[13] Burns caused when an animal was confined in a defective dryer[13] or when an anesthetized dog was laid on an electric heating pad are also examples of animals being unable to escape. Burns resulting from lack of forewarning occur when a dog chews on an electrical cord or is placed in extremely hot bath water. The satisfaction of a sadistic tendency in certain members of our society is another source of thermal injury to animals.[13]

PERIVASCULAR INJECTION OF IRRITANTS

The perivascular injection of irritating medicants is another source of skin trauma and defect. Pentobarbital sodium and the substituted phenyl arsenoxides, which are used to treat heartworms, are examples of such medicants. They may cause a severe local tissue reaction and end in a sloughing of the skin in the area. Unfortunately, such reactions are usually on the limbs where there is not an abundance of surrounding skin for repair of the defect. In these cases the surgeon may have to resort to the use of skin flaps from the animal's torso or free skin grafts to repair the defect.

BACTERIAL AND FUNGAL INFECTIONS

Resident skin bacteria include *Staphylococcus epidermidis* (coagulase negative), *Corynebacterium* spp. (lipophilic), and *Pityrosporon* spp. The transient organisms on the skin, which include *Escherichia coli, Pseudomonas, Enterobacter, Streptococcus,* and *Clostridium,*[41] do not multiply or become

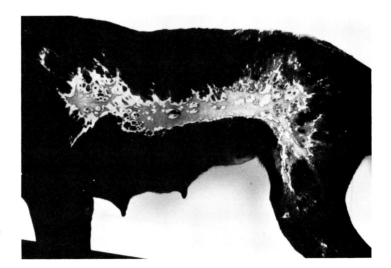

Figure 2–15: Large burn injury. See color plate I–E, p. 570.

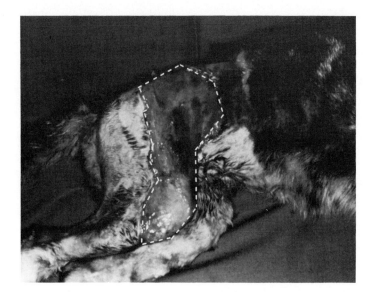

Figure 2–16: Skin slough (*dotted lines*) resulting from a large undetected subcutaneous abscess on a cat. See color plate I–F, p. 568.

significant unless they become involved in pathological processes as secondary invaders.

The number of resident skin bacteria tends to vary with individuals — some have many organisms, others have few. The number of bacteria per individual may remain constant unless the bacteria are disturbed by antibacterial therapy or changes in climate. Oily skin and moist intertriginous areas of the skin tend to have higher bacterial counts. The skin flora seems to increase in warm, wet weather as opposed to cold, dry weather.[41]

Bacteria are normally present on the skin and are thus a potential source of skin loss when they invade injured skin and underlying structures. In humans, antibiotics have made fulminating cellulitis uncommon, but it may still occur as a result of an uncontrolled *Streptococcus pyogenes* infection or a progressive bacterial synergistic gangrene.[39] Antibiotics have also helped to control the severe skin infections that are seen in veterinary medicine; however, massive skin infection and skin loss are still encountered as a result of bacterial infection. An example of such an infection is the extensive and undetected subcutaneous abscess formation on a cat that results in the slough of a large area of skin (Fig. 2–16). Other types of skin infection may also result in skin loss, either from the infection itself or from the surgical removal of the infected area.

Some infections can cause skin loss of such magnitude that reconstruction by grafting is necessary. Once the infection has been controlled, two conditions must be present before reconstruction by grafting can take place: (1) the granulation tissue must be healthy, with evidence of marginal healing, and (2) the bacterial flora must be innocuous.[39] The quantitative evaluation of bacteria in a wound is discussed in Chapter 4.

Several forms of bacterial skin infection require surgical exicison of the affected skin as part of the therapy, and reconstruction of the area generally accompanies such an excision. These skin conditions usually fall into the classification of pyodermas. Interdigital pyoderma requires excision of the cystic as well as the inflamed skin for good results.[31] Pyoderma of the lip, facial, tail, and vulvar folds requires surgical removal of the infected skin folds and reconstruction of the area. Pyoderma of the calluses on the elbow, hock, and sternum also requires surgical removal and reconstruction of the area. In addition to the pyodermas, surgical drainage of the external ear canal by one of the resection techniques or ablation of the external ear canal may be necessary for the correction of refractory ear infections.[41] Another source of skin trauma and defect in which bacterial infection plays a role is the perianal fistula. The surgical techniques for correction of many of these conditions will be covered in other chapters.

Not only do some bacterial infections of the skin require surgical correction, but some mycotic infections also require such treatment. Cutaneous blastomycosis and histoplasmosis may appear as slowly growing, suppurative granulomas of the skin and subcutaneous tissues. The lesions may ulcerate deeply and be covered by a yellowish-gray exudate from tortuous subcutaneous fistulas. The subcutaneous tissue involvement of these conditions may result in the skin's being fixed to the underlying fascia. Since it is difficult to ascertain the true extent of the infection, surgical excision should be wide and may be difficult. If there is evidence of involvement of the lymph nodes, lungs, or bones, surgery may not be indicated. Cutaneous cryptococcosis is a public health hazard and euthanasia should be considered.[31] Mycetoma infections and phaeohyphomycosis are other cutaneous mycoses that require surgical excision.[41]

Cutaneous nocardiosis is another example of a cutaneous infection that may require excision of a granulating mass. However, if the mass is too large or is located in an area where total excision is impossible, drainage should be attempted to reduce the size of the mass before surgical excision.[31]

GRANULOMAS

There are several types of cutaneous granulomas that may require surgery. An acral or lick granuloma appears as a thickened, firm, oval plaque on the cranial surface of the lower foreleg or hind leg and is caused by a dog's continual licking (Fig. 2–17).[41] Lick granulomas have also been reported in the palmar, carpal, and metacarpal regions and they sometimes occur in the lateral,

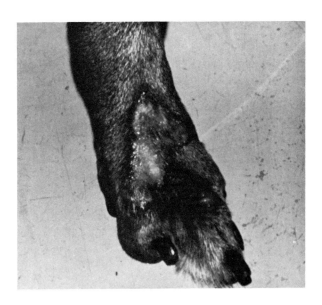

Figure 2–17: Lick granuloma. (Courtesy of M. D. Wiggins.)

tarsal, or metatarsal regions. Large breeds of dogs are primarily affected.[31] Among other treatments, surgical excision with primary closure and excision with repair of the defect by a skin graft have been reported.[31, 41]

Eosinophilic granulomas and pressure point granulomas have also been treated by surgical excision.[41] Various treatments of lick granulomas are discussed in more detail in Chapter 13.

Secretion granulomas have been described in dogs. They are caused by normal products of skin, such as sweat, sebum, hair, or keratin, that have been displaced or inserted into the dermis by rupture of a cutaneous cyst or disintegrating hair follicle. Surgical removal of the central core of such a lesion usually results in its healing.[31]

WEATHER TRAUMA

Feline solar dermatitis affects the white ears of cats and is the result of repeated sun exposure (Fig. 2–18). The condition may advance to a squamous cell carcinoma. With this dermatitis, amputation of the ear tips may be required for cosmetic purposes. When a squamous cell carcinoma develops, amputation of the affected portion of the pinna or radical amputation of the pinna may be necessary.[41] These techniques will be discussed in Chapter 12.

Frostbite resulting from exposure to severe cold weather may damage the ear tips of cats and erect-eared dogs. Other areas that may be affected are the scrotum of dogs and places where the hair covering is sparse and peripheral circulation is poor. In severe cases in which necrosis of the tissue occurs, amputation should be performed; however, amputation of affected tissue should not be performed too early, since more tissue may be viable than is actually expected.[41]

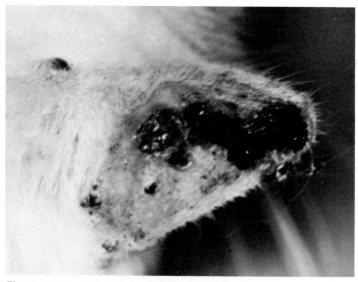

Figure 2–18: Feline solar dermatitis of the ear that has progressed to a neoplastic condition. (Courtesy of J. R. August.)

MISCELLANEOUS SOURCES OF SKIN TRAUMA OR DEFECT

Ear fissures develop on the distal edge of the pinna as a result of scratching or "flapping" the ears. These start as small wounds but enlarge with further trauma, since the skin's healing process is constantly interrupted. Fissures are triangular tears in the ear margin that may range in size from 2 or 3 mm. to 3 cm.[41] The surgical correction of these fissures is covered in Chapter 12.

Intercutaneous cornifying epitheliomas, calcinosis cutis, and epidermal cysts are also treated by surgical excision.[41] Other skin cysts that require surgical excision are dermoid, follicular, retention, and pilonidal cysts.[31]

REFERENCES

1. Snake Venom Poisoning: Its Pathogenesis and Clinical Management. Fort Dodge, Iowa, Fort Dodge Laboratories, 1976.
2. Beirne, G. A., and Beirne, C. G.: Observations on the critical margin for the complete excision of carcinoma of the skin. Arch. Dermatol. 80:344, 1959.
3. Black, A. N., Burns, B. D., and Zuckerman, S.: An experimental study of the wounding mechanism of high-velocity missiles, in Winfield, S. P. (ed.): War Medicine: A Symposium. New York, F. Hubner and Co., Inc., 1942, p. 68.
4. Bostock, D. E.: The prognosis following surgical removal of mastocytomas in dogs. J. Small Anim. Pract. 14:27, 1973.
5. Bostock, D. E.: Neoplasia of the skin and mammary glands in dogs and cats, in Kirk, R. W. (ed.): Current Veterinary Therapy VI. Philadelphia, W. B. Saunders Co., 1977, p. 493.
6. Bostock, D. E., and Owen, L. N.: Neoplasia in the Cat, Dog, and Horse. Chicago, Year Book Medical Publishers, 1975.
7. Braver, S. D.: Surgical treatment of decubitus ulcers in paraplegic patients. Ohio State Med. J. 64:582, 1968.
8. Brody, R. S.: Canine and feline neoplasia. Adv. Vet. Sci. Comp. Med. 14:309, 1970.
9. Committee on Trauma, American College of Surgeons: Early Care of the Injured Patient. Philadelphia, W. B. Saunders Co., 1972.
10. Conroy, J. D.: Tumors of the skin, in Kirk, R. W. (ed.): Current Veterinary Therapy IV. Philadelphia, W. B. Saunders Co., 1971, p. 304.
11. Conroy, J. D.: Neoplasms of the skin and subcutis, in Kirk, R. W. (ed.): Current Veterinary Therapy V. Philadelphia, W. B. Saunders Co., 1974, p. 444.
12. Converse, J. M., and Brauer, R. O.: Transplantation of skin, in Converse, J. M. (ed.): Reconstructive Plastic Surgery: Principles and Procedures in Correction, Reconstruction, and Transplantation. Philadelphia, W. B. Saunders Co., 1964, vol. 1.
13. Davis, L. E.: Thermal burns in the dog. Vet. Scope 8:2, 1963.
14. DeMuth, W. E.: Bullet velocity and design as determinants of wounding capability: An experimental study. J. Trauma 6:222, 1966.
15. Dillaha, C. J., Jansen, G. T., Honeycutt, W. M., et al.: North American loxoscelism: Necrotic bite of the brown recluse spider. J.A.M.A. 188:33, 1964.
16. Douglas, L. G.: Bite wounds. Am. Fam. Physician 11:93, 1975.
17. Dziemian, A. J., Mendelson, J. A., and Lindsey, D.: Comparison of the wounding characteristics of some commonly encountered bullets. J. Trauma 1:341, 1961.
18. Enis, J. E., and Sarmiento, A.: The pathophysiology and management of pressure sores. Orthop. Rev. 2:25, 1973.
19. Fidler, H. K., Glasgow, R. D., and Carmichael, E. B.: Pathological changes produced by the subcutaneous injection of rattlesnake (Crotalus) venom into Macaca mulatta monkeys. Am. J. Pathol. 16:355, 1940.
20. Frazier, C. A.: Diagnosis and treatment of insect bites. Clin. Symp. 20:75, 1968.
21. Freeman, B. S.: Treatment of bedsores in paraplegic patients. Surgery 21:668, 1947.
22. French, R. W., and Callender, G. R.: Ballistic characteristics of wounding agents. Wound Ballistics, p. 91, 1962.
23. Frye, F. L.: Bites and stings of venomous animals, in Kirk, R. W. (ed.): Current Veterinary Therapy VI. Philadelphia, W. B. Saunders Co., 1977, p. 166.
24. Griffith, B. H.: Pressure sores, in Ruge, D. (ed.): Spinal Cord Injuries. Springfield, Ill., Charles C Thomas, Publisher, 1969, p. 135.

25. Hampton, O. P.: The indications for debridement of gunshot (bullet) wounds of the extremities in civilian practice. J. Trauma *1*:368, 1961.

26. Harvey, E. N.: Studies on ballistics, in Andrus, E. C., Carden, G. A., Winternitz, M. C., et al. (eds.): Advances in Military Medicine. Boston, Little, Brown and Co., 1948, p. 191.

27. Harvey, H. J.: General principles of veterinary oncologic surgery. J. Am. Anim. Hosp. Assoc. *12*:335, 1976.

28. Henderson, R. A.: Personal communication, 1977. School of Veterinary Medicine, Dept. of Small Animal Surgery and Medicine, Auburn University, Auburn, AL 36830.

29. Hess, P. W.: Canine mast cell tumors. Am. Anim. Hosp. Assoc. Sci. Proc. *2*:126, 1975.

30. Hess, P. W.: Canine and feline skin tumors. Am. Anim. Hosp. Assoc. Sci. Proc. *2*:130, 1975.

31. Hoffer, R. E.: Skin and adnexa, in Archibald, J. A. (ed.): Canine Surgery, ed. 2. Santa Barbara, Calif., American Veterinary Publications, Inc., 1974, p. 107.

32. Hottendorf, G. H., and Nielsen, S. W.: Canine mastocytoma — a review of clinical aspects. J. Am. Vet. Med. Assoc. *154*:917, 1969.

33. Keep, J. W.: Gunshot injuries to urban dogs and cats. Aust. Vet. J. *46*:330, 1970.

34. Knapp, W. A., and Flowers, H. H.: Treatment of poisonous snakebite in the dog with cortisone acetate. Vet. Med. *51*:475, 1956.

35. Knowles, R. P., Snyder, C. C., Glenn, J. L., et al.: Bites of venomous snakes, in Kirk, R. W. (ed.): Current Veterinary Therapy IV. Philadelphia, W. B. Saunders Co., 1971, p. 111.

36. Kolata, R. J., Kraut, N. H., and Johnston, D. E.: Patterns of trauma in urban dogs and cats: A study of 1,000 cases. J. Am. Vet. Med. Assoc. *164*:499, 1974.

37. Lipowitz, A. J.: Management of gunshot wounds of the soft tissues and extremities. J. Am. Anim. Hosp. Assoc. *12*:813, 1976.

38. McGregor, I. A.: Degloving injuries. J. Br. Soc. Surg. Hand 2:130, 1970.

39. McGregor, I. A.: Fundamental Techniques of Plastic Surgery, ed. 6. Edinburgh, Churchill Livingstone, 1975.

40. Morgan, M. M., Spencer, A. D., and Hershey, F. B.: Debridement of civilian gunshot wounds of soft tissue. J. Trauma *1*:354, 1961.

41. Muller, G. H., and Kirk, R. W.: Small Animal Dermatology, ed. 2. Philadelphia, W. B. Saunders Co., 1976.

42. Neal, T. M., and Key, J. C.: Principles of treatment of dog bite wounds. J. Am. Anim. Hosp. Assoc. *12*:657, 1976.

43. Owen, L. N.: Mammary neoplasia in the dog and cat: III. Prognosis and treatment of mammary tumors in the bitch. J. Small Anim. Pract. 7:703, 1966.

44. Palletta, F. X.: Tumors of the skin: A plastic surgeon's viewpoint, in Converse, J. M. (ed.): Reconstructive Plastic Surgery: Principles and Procedures in Correction, Reconstruction, and Transplantation, ed. 2. Philadelphia, W. B. Saunders Co., 1977, vol. 5, p. 2817.

45. Park, R. D., O'Brien, T. R., Baker, B. B., et al.: Acute radiodermatitis in the beagle dog: Gross observations after single-dose exposure with x-irradiation. J. Am. Vet. Rad. Soc. *14*:49, 1973.

46. Park, R. D., O'Brien, T. R., Baker, B. B., et al.: Single dose x-irradiation of canine skin. J. Am. Vet. Rad. Soc. *15*:108, 1974.

47. Parrish, H. M., MacLaurin, A., and Tuttle, R. L.: North American pit vipers: Bacterial flora of the mouths and venom glands. Va. Med. Monthly *83*:383, 1956.

48. Parrish, H. M., and Scatterday, J. E.: A survey of poisonous snakebites among domestic animals in Florida. Vet. Med. *52*:135, 1957.

49. Parrish, H. M., Scatterday, J. E., and Moore, W.: The use of antihistamine (phenergan) in experimental snake venom poisoning in dogs. J. Am. Vet. Med. Assoc. *129*:522, 1956.

50. Parrish, H. M., Scatterday, J. E., and Pollard, C. B.: The clinical management of snake venom poisoning in domestic animals. J. Am. Vet. Med. Assoc. *130*:548, 1957.

51. Priester, W. A.: Skin tumors in domestic animals: Data from 12 United States and Canadian colleges of veterinary medicine. J. Natl. Cancer Inst. *50*:457, 1973.

52. Ross, G. E.: Skin tumors, in Kirk, R. W. (ed.): Current Veterinary Therapy III. Philadelphia, W. B. Saunders Co., 1968, p. 305.

53. Sather, M. R., Weber, C. E., and George, J.: Pressure sores and the spinal cord injury patient. Drug Intelligence Clin. Pharm. *11*:154, 1977.

54. Saunders, D. E., and Jaison, A. R.: The management of decubital ulcers. Del. Med. J. *38*:129, 1966.

55. Schlotthauer, C. F.: Neoplasms in the mammary glands in dogs: Their pathology and surgical treatment. J. Am. Vet. Med. Assoc. *96*:632, 1940.

56. Settel, E.: Decubitus ulcer. Med. Times 97:220, 1969.

57. Snyder, C. C., Knowles, R. P., Pickens, J. E., et al.: Pathogenesis and treatment of poisonous snake bites. J. Am. Vet. Med. Assoc. *151*:1635, 1967.

58. Swaim, S. F., and Votau, K.: Prevention and treatment of decubital ulcers in the dog. Vet. Med. Small Anim. Clin. 65:1069, 1975.

59. Torelli, M.: Topical hyperbaric oxygen for decubitus ulcers. Am. J. Nursing 73:494, 1973.

60. Wilson, G. P., and Fowler, E. H.: The mammary glands: Mammary tumors, in Bojrab, M. J. (ed.): Current Techniques in Small Animal Surgery I. Philadelphia, Lea & Febiger, 1975, p. 269.
61. Withrow, S.: Surgical management of cancer. Am. Anim. Hosp. Assoc. Sci. Proc. 2:93, 1975.
62. Withrow, S.: Mammary tumors in the dog. Am. Anim. Hosp. Assoc. Sci. Proc. 2:118, 1975.
63. Ziperman, H. H.: The management of soft tissue missile wounds in war and peace. J. Trauma 1:361, 1961.

3

WOUND HEALING

"I dressed the wound, and God healed it."

Paré

INTRODUCTION

Volumes have been written on the subject of wound healing, including all levels (i.e., from the macroscopic to the molecular level) and the various factors affecting the process. However, the purpose of this chapter is to present only the *basics* of wound healing as they relate to the skin and *some* of the factors that affect the wound healing process. It is hoped that this chapter will give the practitioner a working knowledge of wound healing. For the student, the author particularly recommends the works of Bryant,[11] Johnston,[34–36] Madden,[46] Peacock,[54, 55] and Peacock and Van Winkle.[56]

TYPES OF WOUNDS

There are many types of wounds of the skin, and the reader is referred to Chapter 2 for more in-depth information. Each type has certain anatomical, physiological, pathological, and microbiological factors associated with it. Although all of these factors have a bearing on the wound healing process, the basics of the process remain the same.

STAGES OF HEALING

The classifications of the stages of wound healing have varied with the individual who conducted the study. In this text, the classification used by Johnston[34] will basically be followed. This classification breaks the process of healing into (1) the inflammatory stage, (2) the débridement stage, (3) the repair stage, and (4) the maturation stage. In general, these processes occur on a temporal basis, and treating each stage separately will facilitate discussion. However, it is important to remember that the wound healing process is a continuum, with overlapping of the various stages. The stage of repair overlaps in time with that of inflammation; scar maturation may begin while collagen production continues; epithelialization of the surface may begin well ahead of the repair stage; and contraction may be in progress during the repair stage. Some of the processes of healing may continue for years after the physical integrity of the wounded tissue has been reestablished.[11, 35, 36, 55]

GENERAL PATTERN OF WOUND HEALING

Simple tissues, such as fat and connective tissue, regenerate rapidly and completely after injury. However, skin is a highly complex organ containing multiple structures that are derived from several germ layers. In mammals, the complex organs and appendages have lost the ability to regenerate, and damaged tissue is replaced by fibrous scar tissue that is covered by remodeled epithelium. In general, skin restores its surface continuity by epithelialization, synthesis of dense connective tissue, and contraction.[34]

The general pattern of wound healing in an incised wound begins with the reestablishment of epidermal continuity over the wound. The repair (fibroplastic) process of wound healing then starts in the area of subcutaneous tissue, which has a dense population of fibroblasts by about the fifth to the eighth day of healing. The active connective tissue proliferation that occurs in this area expands upward into the wound. Connective tissue also proliferates downward from the papillary layer of the dermis. The reticular layer of the dermis takes little part in producing connective tissue to fill the intradermal area, and the collagen that is eventually deposited in this area originates primarily in the connective tissue that has extended into the intradermal space from the subcutaneous tissues.[4, 43, 53, 64] As a result of this process, the center of the healing wound may remain somewhat inverted until the underlying connective tissue synthesis pushes the epithelium up into an everted position.[55] In general, wound healing occurs from the bottom and progresses upward (Fig. 3–1).

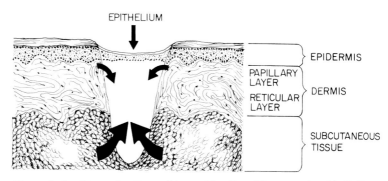

Figure 3–1: General pattern of wound healing. The wound epithelializes, with most of the connective tissue proliferating from the subcuticular areas upward into the wound (*large arrows*). A smaller amount of connective tissue proliferates from the papillary layer of the dermis into the wound (*small arrows*). The reticular layer of the dermis takes little part in producing connective tissue to fill the intradermal area.

INFLAMMATORY STAGE

IMMEDIATE REACTIONS

Skin Retraction and Vessel Reaction

After a full-thickness skin loss, the normal elasticity of the skin and the external tension produced in some areas by muscle pull enlarge the defect according to the amount and direction of force that is exerted. As a result, the shape of a skin defect may have little relation to the size and shape of the skin segment that has been removed.[55]

Immediately following injury there is vasoconstriction of small vessels in the area, with actual vascular occlusion at the wound site that tends to limit hemorrhage (Fig. 3–2). However, vasoconstriction usually lasts only five to ten minutes and is followed by active vasodilatation.[11, 34, 56] Lymphatics, which are more friable than blood vessels, are usually damaged more severely than the vasculature. The leakage of fluid from venules provides fibrinogen and other clotting elements. Thus, fibrin plugs quickly form in damaged lymphatics and effectively stop lymphatic drainage from the injured area. As a result, the inflammatory reaction is localized to the immediate area surrounding the injury.[11, 55, 56] If lymphatic obstruction is prevented or if there is dissolution of the clots in the lymphatics, such as occurs in streptococcal infection through the action of fibrinolysin, there can be a rapid spread of inflammation and infection.[11]

Blood Clot and Scab Formation

Blood flows into the gap created by the cutting instrument and clots. This unites the wound edges. In the presence of enzymes that are released

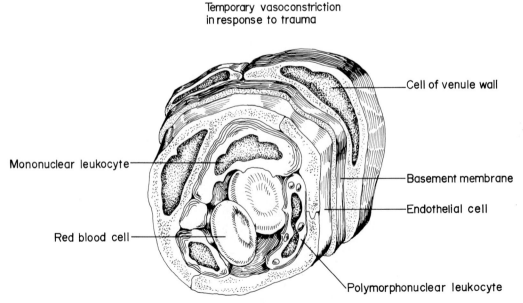

Temporary vasoconstriction in response to trauma

Cell of venule wall

Mononuclear leukocyte

Basement membrane

Endothelial cell

Red blood cell

Polymorphonuclear leukocyte

Figure 3–2: The immediate vascular response to injury is vasoconstriction.

from the blood and tissue cells, fibrinogen molecules from the blood link up to form interconnected fibrin strands. This fibrin acts as a hemostatic barrier and as a framework for the elements of repair.[34-36, 56]

Ideally, there should be only enough blood clotting to hold the tissues together, fill the dead space, and act as a framework for further healing. If there is excess blood in the area, pain, ischemia (caused by pressure on the surrounding tissues), necrosis, and delayed healing may result. The excess blood must be clotted, organized, degenerated, and absorbed before healing can continue. In the meantime, it can serve as a bacterial and a nutritional medium for cells that can later produce an inordinately large scar.[68]

In normal circumstances the clot contracts and dehydrates, and fibrin and other proteins on the surface dehydrate to form the scab.[4, 34-36, 55, 56] A scab provides limited protection from external contamination, maintenance of internal homeostasis, and a surface beneath which cell migration and movement of the wound edges can take place.[34-36, 55] Scabs are dark in color and hard when they contain blood pigment or yellow and pliable when blood pigment is not present in the wound fluids.[74] Although scabs protect a wound during healing, it has been demonstrated that their presence is not a prerequisite to healing. Granulation tissue can form and epithelial migration can occur in the absence of a scab.[72] This fact becomes obvious when the practitioner considers the healing of large open wounds by second intention.

LATER REACTIONS

In general, the inflammatory stage of healing is a vascular and a cellular response that serves to dispose of microorganisms, foreign material, and devitalized tissue. It also initiates the mechanisms responsible for wound repair.[11, 34] After an initial vasoconstriction of small vessels (Fig. 3–2), the later reactions of the inflammatory stage of healing ensue; these may be summarized as follows:

1. There is an increase in blood flow in the area, with vasodilatation.
2. Capillary and venule permeability increase as the endothelial cells of the vessels swell and "round up," creating gaps between the cells. This permeability may be initially caused by the action of histamine in the injured tissues; however, serotonins, kinins, prostaglandins, proteolytic enzymes, chemotactic agents, and macromolecular mediators have also been suggested as causes of vessel permeability.
3. Plasma-like fluid escapes from the vessels into the tissues. This occurs before any cells leave the affected vessels and may occur in the presence[11, 34] or absence[56] of gaps in the vessel walls. The fluid's presence in the tissues tends to dilute toxic substances and to aid in the movement of cells that enter the area from affected blood vessels. The fluid contains enzymes, proteins, antibodies, and complement.
4. Within 30 minutes after injury, the leukocytes become "sticky" and adhere to the endothelium of the local venules. The platelets and erythrocytes also become sticky but not to the same extent as the leukocytes. The erythrocytes may form rouleaux.
5. The leukocytes escape from the affected vessels. By diapedesis and active movement they force their way through the basement mem-

Active vasodilatation with increased
venule permeability in response
to histamine and other substances

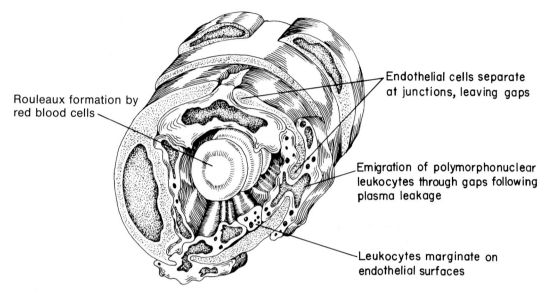

Rouleaux formation by
red blood cells

Endothelial cells separate
at junctions, leaving gaps

Emigration of polymorphonuclear
leukocytes through gaps following
plasma leakage

Leukocytes marginate on
endothelial surfaces

Figure 3–3:   The delayed vascular response to injury is vasodilatation.

brane of the vessels. After they are out of the vessels, the leukocytes travel by active movement and concentrate at the site of injury (Fig. 3–3).[11, 34, 41, 46, 55, 56, 64, 67, 68] The duration and intensity of this process are dependent on the amount of local tissue damage.[46]

DÉBRIDEMENT STAGE

The débridement stage of wound healing begins about six hours after wounding.[34-36] It has been stated that the neutrophil is the first leukocyte to enter a wound after about six hours, followed by the monocyte at 12 hours.[4, 34-36, 44] However, another theory seems to be more accepted. It states that neutrophils and monocytes migrate toward the wound at the same time and are in the same proportion as occurs in the blood stream (Fig. 3–4). This being the case, the polymorphonuclear cells would predominate, but these cells are short-lived compared with the mononuclear cells. When the neutrophils die, the mononuclear cells remain. Thus, in older wounds the mononuclear cells predominate.[11, 46, 56]

Neutrophils are necessary to clean up infected wounds, since healing will not progress until infection is controlled. In the absence of infection, healing could progress without neutrophils.[56] The activities of neutrophils can be summarized as follows:

1. They ingest organisms by phagocytosis.
2. The neutrophils degenerate and die. When their outer membrane ruptures, enzymes and ingested debris are released. The enzymes attack extracellular debris and facilitate the further breakdown of necrotic debris by monocytes.[11, 34-36, 46]

Monocytes are essential for wound healing.[56] Their activities include the following:

1. They become macrophages when they enter the wound.
2. Macrophages phagocytize dead and necrotic tissue and debris. This material is then partially digested. Some of the material ingested is that which has not been solubilized by the neutrophils (Fig. 3–5).
3. In addition to transforming into macrophages during states of chronic inflammation, the monocytes may also coalesce to form multinucleate giant cells. The mononuclear cells may also evolve into epithelioid cells and histiocytes.

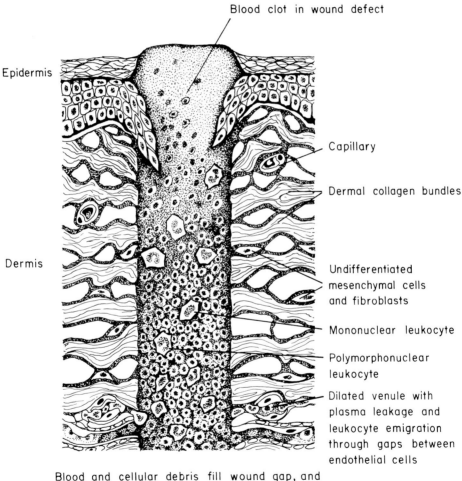

Blood clot in wound defect

Epidermis

Capillary

Dermal collagen bundles

Dermis

Undifferentiated mesenchymal cells and fibroblasts

Mononuclear leukocyte

Polymorphonuclear leukocyte

Dilated venule with plasma leakage and leukocyte emigration through gaps between endothelial cells

Blood and cellular debris fill wound gap, and the clot unites the wound edges. Epithelial cells begin migrating across the defect. Increased venule permeability permits the escape of serum, plasma, proteins, and leukocytes that enter the wound. Mature fibroblasts form from undifferentiated mesenchymal cells.

Figure 3–4: The débridement stage of wound healing. It has also been considered to be part of the inflammatory phase.[11]

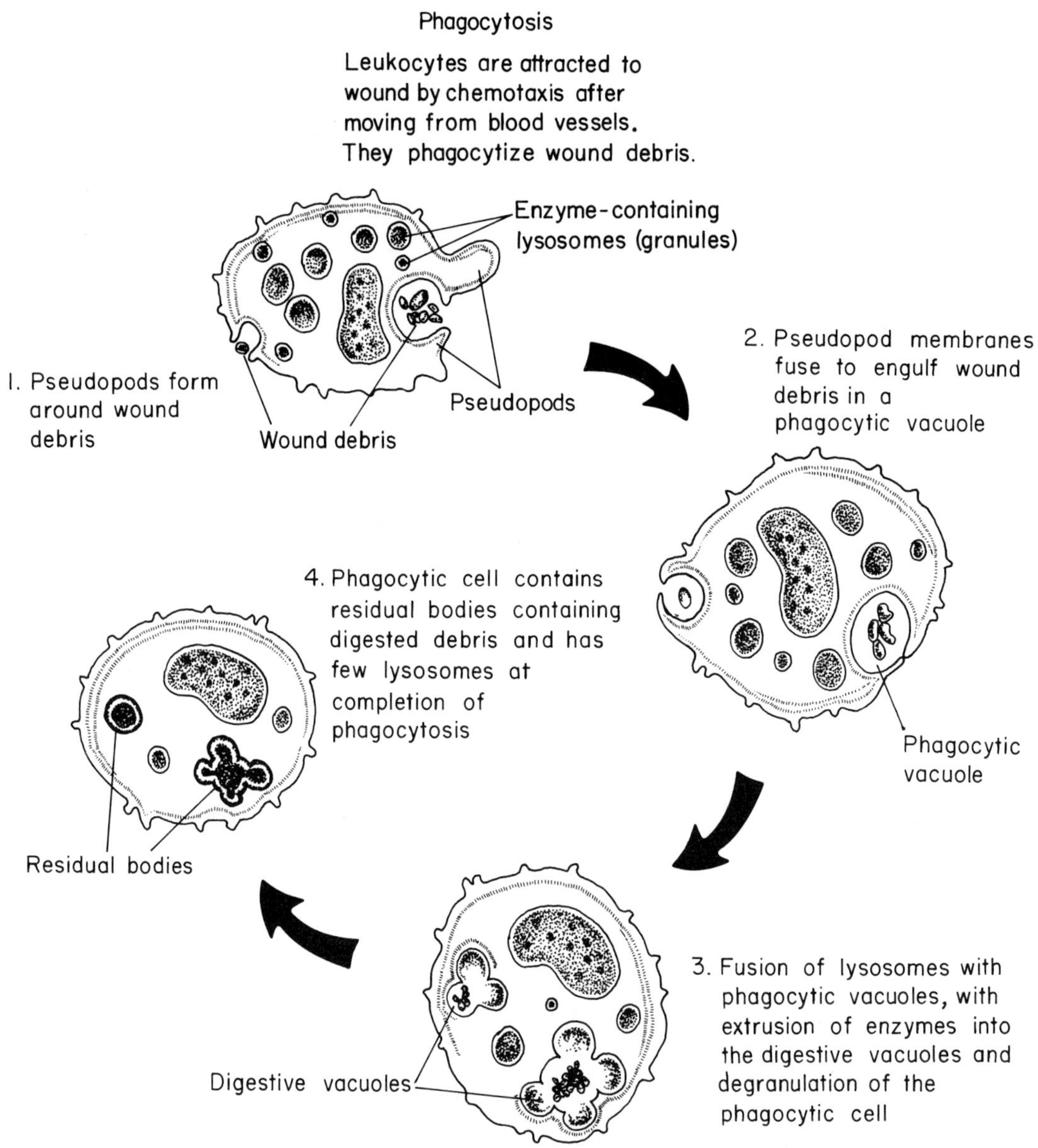

Phagocytosis

Leukocytes are attracted to
wound by chemotaxis after
moving from blood vessels.
They phagocytize wound debris.

1. Pseudopods form
around wound
debris

Enzyme-containing
lysosomes (granules)

Pseudopods

Wound debris

2. Pseudopod membranes
fuse to engulf wound
debris in a
phagocytic vacuole

Phagocytic
vacuole

4. Phagocytic cell contains
residual bodies containing
digested debris and has
few lysosomes at
completion of
phagocytosis

Residual bodies

Digestive vacuoles

3. Fusion of lysosomes with
phagocytic vacuoles, with
extrusion of enzymes into
the digestive vacuoles and
degranulation of the
phagocytic cell

Figure 3–5: Process of phagocytosis.

4.   Macrophages also serve to attract fibroblasts into a wound and perhaps influence them to undergo maturation and maximal collagen
synthesis.[11, 34-36, 56]

There may also be some large and small lymphocytes present in the
wound, which are perhaps indicative of some immunological response to
foreign materials.[11]

The fluid that has escaped from the vessels, combined with the migrating
leukocytes and dead tissue, makes up the inflammatory exudate that accumulates in the injured area. As the polymorphonuclear cells die and lyse, the
exudate takes on the character of pus. It should be realized that pus can accumulate even in the absence of bacterial invasion. Even though it may be

sterile, pus can still impair wound healing. The protease and collagenase associated with this exudate solubilize connective tissue. As a result, pus can interfere with the epithelialization and fibroplasia, which occur simultaneously with inflammation. Therefore, a minimal amount of pus is desirable so that wound healing can proceed unhindered.[11, 34, 56] It can be seen that adequate drainage of an infected wound is extremely important for the removal of exudate and the progression of healing.

REPAIR STAGE

BASICS OF REPAIR

The repair processes start almost immediately after injury and proceed as fast as necrotic tissue, blood clots, and other barriers are removed from the wound. The three processes that have been described in the repair stage of healing are (1) fibroblast proliferation, (2) capillary infiltration, and (3) epithelial proliferation and migration.[34] These processes, along with that of wound contraction, will be described in this section.

In uncomplicated simple wounds, the debris has usually been removed by the third to the fifth day, when fibroblast proliferation and capillary infiltration start in the wound area.[34] In an open wound this is recognized as the proliferation of granulation tissue.

FIBROBLASTS AND ELASTIC FIBERS

Fibroblasts: Origin and Movement

Although there have been other theories on the origin of fibroblasts in a wound, the currently accepted theory is that these cells originate from undifferentiated mesenchymal cells in nearby connective tissue (i.e., subcutaneous tissue and fat). These resting cells and fibrocytes are primarily associated with the adventitia of the small blood vessels in the area. They differentiate into fibroblasts, move into the wound area, multiply, and start their synthetic activity.[4, 11, 34-36, 46, 54, 56]

Fibroblasts move into a wound by advancing along fibers within the fibrin clot that formed early in the wound healing process (Fig. 3–6).[11, 44, 56] They have also been reported to move along capillaries that are growing into the wound.[44] Fibroblasts move and cease moving by contact guidance and contact inhibition, respectively, They move by forming a cytoplasmic extension called a ruffled membrane, which extends out from the cell and adheres to the solid substrate (i.e., fiber or capillary). The body of the cell then loosens from the substrate, and the cell streams in the direction of the ruffled membrane. When the cell encounters another fibroblast, movement ceases and the cells stick together — contact inhibition. If a free edge is still present on the cell, a new ruffled membrane will form, cell adhesion will be broken, and the cell will move off in another direction.[1, 46, 56, 64]

The times reported for the appearance of fibroblasts in the wound have ranged from 12 hours to six days.[4, 34, 41, 53, 56, 64] However, fibroblasts usually appear about the third day. These cells are active and multiply from 14 to 21 days.[56]

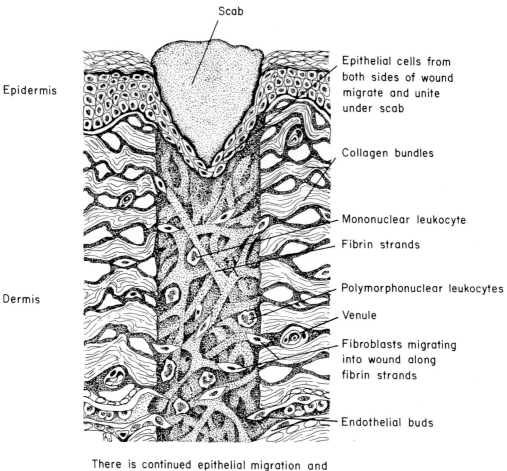

Scab

Epidermis

Epithelial cells from
both sides of wound
migrate and unite
under scab

Collagen bundles

Mononuclear leukocyte

Fibrin strands

Polymorphonuclear leukocytes

Venule

Dermis

Fibroblasts migrating
into wound along
fibrin strands

Endothelial buds

There is continued epithelial migration and
proliferation. Mononuclear leukocytes persist
after polymorphonuclear leukocytes and remove
remaining debris. Fibroblasts migrate into
the wound along fibrin strands, and capillaries
invade the area by budding. This tissue appears
as granulation tissue in the open wound.

Figure 3–6: Early repair stage of wound healing. It has also been classified as the migratory phase.[11]

Orientation of Wound Fibers

During the first three to four days following an incision-type wound, the fibrin strands of the clot within the wound are oriented vertically. As a result of this, fibroblasts growing along these fibers have a similar arrangement, as do the interweaving definitive new collagen fibers that they produce. The newly formed capillaries that are growing into the area also have a vertical arrangement. After the sixth day the intraincisional fibroblasts, fibrils, and capillaries gradually change in orientation until they lie parallel to the surface across the incision (Fig. 3–7).[34-36, 53, 64] There are two reasons for the early vertical orientation of the wound content.

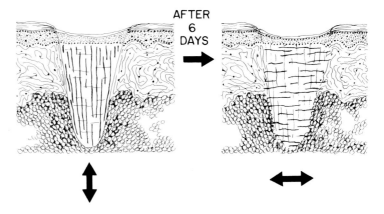

Figure 3–7: Orientation of wound fibers. In the early stages of wound repair, fibrin strands, fibroblasts, new collagen fibers, and new capillaries have a vertical arrangement. As wound healing progresses, the structures become horizontally arranged.

1. The wound closure materials (sutures or tapes) that are holding the wound edges in apposition exert pressure and thereby diminish the space available within the incision. As a result, newly formed connective tissue is squeezed into a vertical position.[53]

2. As mentioned earlier, the general wound healing pattern is such that the fibroplastic (repair) stage of healing progresses from the subcutaneous tissues up into the wound and also from the papillary region of the dermis down into the wound. Consequently, fibroblasts enter the wound area in a vertical plane, both upward and downward (Fig. 3–1).[53] Tension on the wound fibers seems to be the factor that governs the reorientation of the fibers from a vertical to a parallel arrangement.[56]

In a skin defect in which there has been a loss of tissue, the natural elasticity of the skin places tension on the fibrin clot that is adherent to the wound margins. This orients the fibrous components toward the wound margins. As the ingrowing fibroblasts enter the wound, they are guided by the fibrous elements, the position and orientation of which are such that they bring cells toward the center of the defect.[56, 64]

Products of Fibroblasts and Wound Strength

After fibroblasts have entered a wound, they begin to secrete protein-polysaccharides and various glycoproteins that constitute the wound's ground substance. The ground substance is an amorphous milieu composed of water, ions, and complex protein-polysaccharide polymers. It reaches its point of greatest development in about three to five days and is essential for effective collagen deposition. The mucopolysaccharides of this substance surround the fibroblasts and influence the aggregation and orientation of collagen.[4, 11, 34-36, 46]

It is generally believed that collagen synthesis by the fibroblasts begins on the fourth or fifth day. Collagen is synthesized by the fibroblasts from hydroxyproline and hydroxylysine. As these substances are synthesized, tropocollagen molecules are extruded into the extracellular space. These molecules aggregate to form young collagen fibrils close to the cell membrane. As these fibrils continue to bond together, collagen fibers are formed, and the collagen becomes increasingly less soluble. The collagen bundles are small at first but enlarge gradually to produce a dense collagenous scar that binds the edges of severed tissues together. As the collagen content of the wound increases, the glycoprotein and mucopolysaccharide contents decrease (Fig. 3–8).[11, 34-36, 41, 46, 53, 54, 56]

There are several factors that control and eventually lead to the cessation of collagen production.[34] As a sufficient amount of collagen is produced, the number of fibroblasts in the wound decreases. The decrease in fibroblasts marks the end of the repair (fibroplastic) stage of wound healing and the beginning of the maturation stage.[11] With the diminished number of synthesizing fibroblasts, the total collagen synthesis decreases and eventually balances the rate of collagen destruction.[56] Besides the decrease in fibroblasts, proliferating epithelial cells liberate collagenase, which is im-

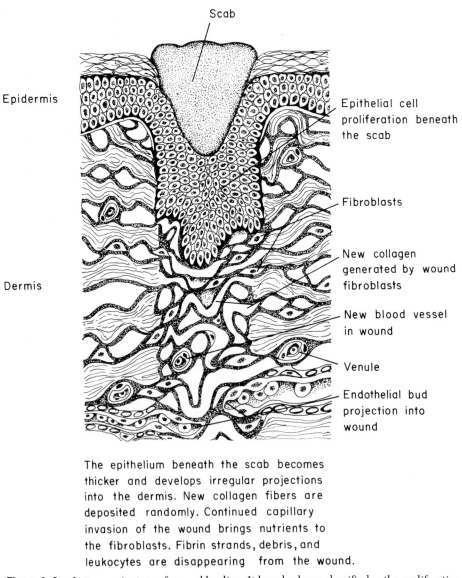

The epithelium beneath the scab becomes thicker and develops irregular projections into the dermis. New collagen fibers are deposited randomly. Continued capillary invasion of the wound brings nutrients to the fibroblasts. Fibrin strands, debris, and leukocytes are disappearing from the wound.

Figure 3–8:   Later repair stage of wound healing. It has also been classified as the proliferative phase.[11]

portant in controlling the collagen content of the wound. Fibroblasts that come into contact with the new epithelium also secrete collagenase.[34, 56] Though several time periods have been stated for the duration of the repair stage, some of the recent literature states that it lasts from two to four weeks, depending upon the nature of the wound.[34, 56] However, it should be mentioned again that the wound healing processes may overlap, with the fibroplastic stage extending into the maturation stage and vice versa.

It is generally accepted that there is an early rise in wound tensile strength as collagen is produced by the fibroblasts. This is followed by a slower gain in wound strength that takes place over a long period; this gain is initially due to increased collagen deposition and later to the maturation and remodeling of the collagen that is present in the wound. The reported times at which the various gains in wound strength occur vary, depending upon the source. The hydroxyproline content of a wound has been used as an indication of collagen concentration and thus of wound strength progression, and a review of this will give a basic view of the progression in wound strength. As stated in Johnston's review of wound healing, hydroxyproline in a wound increases rapidly beginning on the fourth day, with the highest rate occurring between the fifth and the 12th day. A lesser rate of increase takes place between the 12th and the 21st day, and a markedly lower rate occurs from the 21st to the 60th day.[34] There is an imperceptible gain in wound strength for at least two years;[35, 36, 44, 55] however, the strength of scar tissue never reaches that of normal skin or fascia.[35, 36] A study on wound healing in rats has shown that at the end of one year, the skin of a healed wound is only 80 per cent as strong as comparable unwounded skin.[40]

Elastic Fibers

In addition to collagen, the second major fibrous component of connective tissue is elastin. This fibrous protein is not readily replaced when removed, and it plays almost no role in wound repair.[56] In studies on pig wounds, fairly long segments of very fine, wavy, apparently new elastic fibrils that were aligned parallel to the surface first became apparent in wound healing tissue at 15 days. These remained in this form throughout the healing process.[53] The sparseness of elastic fibers within scar tissue explains its lack of elasticity.

CAPILLARY INFILTRATION

Oxygen Gradients

Oxygen is necessary for cell migration, cell multiplication, and protein synthesis. Fibroblasts synthesizing collagen require additional oxygen for the hydroxylation of proline and lysine to form hydroxyproline and hydroxylysine.[56]

Following the infliction of a wound, there exists a marked gradient of oxygen within the wound. The center of the wound is the most deficient of oxygen,[32, 34-36, 61] with the oxygen tension being as low as 5 mm. of mercury.[32] This gradient may be partially responsible for the branching and ingrowth of new blood vessels from the wound periphery into the wound.[34-36, 61] The disappearance of the hypoxic gradient within the wound after new blood vessels have grown completely across the wound lends support to this theory.[61]

The activity of fibroblasts is dependent upon the oxygen supply within a wound. Measurements of oxygen tension in the vicinity of the leading fibroblasts that are migrating into a wound suggest that the oxygen supply is always at the lower limit for migration; however, this tension is too low for replication and protein synthesis. Fibroblasts replicate best at oxygen tensions between 15 and 30 mm. of mercury, and collagen synthesis increases as arterial oxygen tension increases. A fibroblast can synthesize collagen only within about 60 μ (micrometers) from an intact capillary. It can be seen that fibroblastic replication and synthetic activity depend upon the rate at which new capillaries grow into the wound.[32, 56]

Granulation Tissue

A bright red granular tissue begins to appear in an open wound from three to six days after injury. This is the result of the proliferation of capillary loops. These loops originate from the endothelium of the cut capillaries in the wound and grow into the wound immediately behind the fibroblasts at a rate of 0.4 to 1.0 mm./day. In a small wound, this occurs beneath the scab (Fig. 3–6). In a large open wound, the development of granulation tissue can be seen. The capillary loops or "knuckles" give the wound a granular appearance. Each "granule" is composed of a raised capillary that is capped by fibroblasts, macrophages, and other wandering cells, with fibroblasts predominating. There are considerable anastomoses between these new vessels and with preexisting vessels within the wound tissue. In its healthy state, granulation tissue is red, firm, flat, and nonexuberant after it grows to cover the entire wound (Fig. 3–9). Initially, the

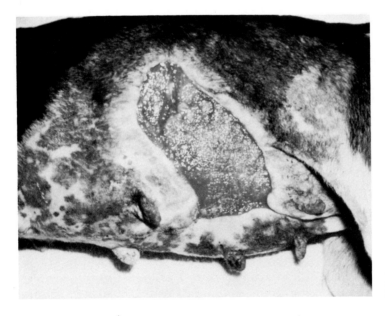

Figure 3–9: A bed of firm, flat, healthy granulation tissue.

capillaries of granulation tissue are quite fragile and easily damaged; as the granulation tissue develops, the simple blood channels differentiate progressively into arterioles, capillaries, and venules.[4, 11, 34-36, 55, 56, 64, 67, 68]

The endothelial cells of the new capillaries that are growing into a wound contain a plasminogen activator. The result of the action of this compound is fibrinolysis and breakdown of the original fibrin network that is present in the wound. This fibrin is replaced by collagen.[11, 34, 46, 56]

In essentially the same manner, though lagging a little behind the development of blood vessels, a system of lymphatic vessels is produced in the wound. These develop as the result of the migratory and mitotic activity of initially solid sprouts of lymphatic endothelial cells that arise from preexisting lymphatics.[64]

Granulation tissue is important in healing open wounds for several reasons:

1. This tissue is extremely resistant to infection.
2. The epithelium is able to migrate across its surface.
3. It is quite likely that the mechanism of wound contraction is centered in the granulation tissue.
4. It supplies cells (fibroblasts) that will produce collagen for wound healing.[34, 68]

Exuberant granulation tissue usually does not impair wound healing in the dog or cat. Although the excess granulation tissue may form, wound healing may progress in spite of its presence. In one study 20 per cent of the dogs exhibited an overproduction of granulation tissue in metatarsal wounds. However, the excess tissue was removed as the epithelium grew over the wound surface.[74] When excess granulation tissue does occur, it is because collagen fiber deposition has exceeded new capillary formation, and this may result in a mound of new tissue with a dusky, unhealthy appearance; this tissue is called proud flesh.[56]

EPITHELIALIZATION

General Information

Epithelial proliferation and migration are the first clear-cut signs of rebuilding.[34, 36] These can take place before connective tissue regeneration and the other events of wound healing occur.[56] As described by Johnston[34] and Peacock and Van Winkle,[56] there is a mobilization of the marginal basal cells as they lose their firm attachment to the underlying dermis. These cells enlarge, flatten, and extend outward and downward over the incised dermis. Excess cells migrate out over the defect to replace the epithelial cell deficit (Fig. 3–10). As a point of interest, the occurrence of mitosis in epidermal epithelium has a diurnal rhythm, being greatest during rest and inactivity and least during wakefulness and activity.[56]

In an incised wound, epithelial proliferation and migration can cover the wound in 12 to 24 hours.[35, 36, 55] However, in an open wound that fully penetrates the dermis, a layer of granulation tissue must form before the wound can epithelialize.[4, 68] There is usually a latent period of four or five days before epithelium starts to migrate from the wound margins across the developing granulation tissue in the bed.[64] Epithelial migration is rapid at

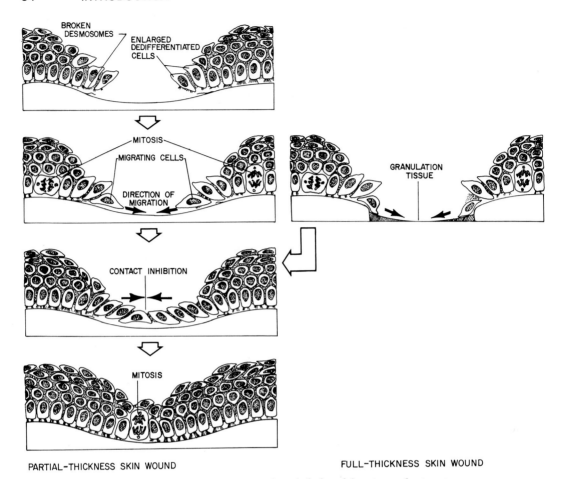

Figure 3–10: Basic processes of epithelial proliferation and migration.

first, but as the line of cells from the wound margin extends, the epithelium dwindles to a monolayer and progress becomes slower. Days or even weeks may pass before epithelialization is complete.[35, 36] In some large wounds, epithelialization may not be sufficient to cover the wound, or the epithelium may be so delicate in the center of the wound that it is continually knocked off, leaving exposed granulation tissue.

"Chalone"

There is evidence that a water-soluble and heat-labile substance known as chalone helps to control epithelial mitosis. Extracts of the epidermis and hypodermis contain this substance, which has an inhibitory effect on mitosis in these tissues. To be effective, chalone appears to require epinephrine. In a wound, the concentration and production of chalone would fall, and there would exist a decreasing concentration gradient from normal tissue to the wound defect, where it could presumably be zero. This would account for the narrow zone of increased mitotic activity at the wound edges. Chalone seems to be tissue-specific but not species-specific.[34, 56]

Epidermal Changes at Wound Edges

In preparation for epithelial migration over an open wound in the dog, an intense epidermal reaction occurs at and up to 5 mm. back from the wound's edge. The number of epidermal cell layers in the region increases until about the eighth day, at which time over 50 layers frequently are present, and in some cases over 90 cell layers are produced. The walls of regional hair follicles increase in thickness, and these cells add considerably to the number of cells capable of migration. Thus, a reservoir of cells is readied for migration across the wound surface.[76]

The cells that migrate are primarily from a newly developed stratum spinosum layer that is usually not present in normal canine epidermis but that is produced during the epidermal hyperactivity. A layer of cells derived from the stratum corneum accompanies these cells as they migrate over the wound. This layer of cells frequently moves in advance of other migrating cells, and in some regions its cells are the only ones to move into the lesion during the early stages. This layer is continuous with the normal stratum corneum and extends into the wound as a single or double column of cells.[76]

Hair Follicle Contribution

The walls of the hair follicles that are physically damaged during wound infliction react within 24 hours and show cellular hypertrophy and an increase in the rate of mitotic division. These cells form in the spinous layer of the follicle and are capable of migration. Transected follicles from all parts of the wound perimeter contribute to the number of epithelial cells that are capable of migration. However, in the portion of the wound that lies in the direction of hair flow, migrating cells from the ends of cut follicles give rise to a special feature. New epithelium can first be seen growing on the wound surface in the portion of the wound lying in the direction of hair flow. This is explained as follows. Within two or three days of wound infliction, the cut skin edge in the region of the wound that is situated in the direction of hair flow becomes oblique and assumes an obtuse angle to the wound. The result is that the cut lower parts of the hair follicles lie from 1 to 2 mm. closer to the wound center than does the epidermal edge itself. After four to five days the migratory epithelial cells, which are derived from the ends of the cut follicles, are the most advanced of the migrating cells. Coalition of these cells with each other and with cells from the cut epidermal edge results in the early formation of an epithelial crescent on this edge of the wound (Fig. 3–11).[75]

Figure 3–11: Hair follicle contribution to wound epithelialization. The edge of the wound that is situated in the direction of hair flow becomes oblique (forms an obtuse angle) with the wound. The cut lower parts of the hair follicles lie 1 to 2 mm. closer to the wound center than does the epidermal edge. Epithelialization occurs from the ends of the cut follicles and from the epidermal edge.

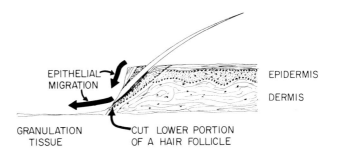

The thickness of follicle walls and the size of the individual cells begin to return to normal after about the 12th day. Once a well-formed sheet of advancing epithelium has been established by the eighth to the 12th day, the cells derived from the hair follicles no longer participate in epithelial migration.[75]

In dogs the sebaceous glands do not contribute to the healing of the wound; however, they do regenerate. After injury some degeneration of the glandular cells takes place in the first four to six days. The basement membrane then reforms, and new glands develop. They are usually smaller than normal but possess an almost normal shape and structure.[75]

Contact Guidance and Inhibition

As with fibroblasts, epithelial migration occurs by contact guidance and inhibition, and the reader is referred to this section for the basics of these phenomena. Although most cells maintain some attachment to like cells during contact guidance, it has been reported that a number of epithelial cells move independently and pass into the center of the wound. These cells arise from both the tip and the lower surface of the advancing epithelial shelf, and they may be important in determining the plane of and the direction taken by the migrating epithelium.[76]

If a scab is present, the migrating epithelium moves under the scab until it contacts the underlying granulation tissue bed. The migrating cells produce a proteolytic enzyme (collagenase) that dissolves the base of the scab so that it can be shed (Fig. 3–6).[4, 34, 46, 54-56]

In contact inhibition, cells stop moving when they are surrounded by like cells on all sides. This usually occurs when epithelial cells progressing from all sides of the wound meet in the center of the wound. However, there are instances in which epithelial cells stop moving even though they are not surrounded on all sides.[18] Examples of this are open wounds that have healed to an extent by contraction and epithelialization, with the centers of the wounds remaining as open granulation tissue.

As reported in Russell and Billingham's[64] review on the repair process, several factors may stop epithelial proliferation and migration. Infection may stop and even cause regression of epithelial migration. Repeated dressing changes can mechanically remove delicate regenerating epithelium. An inadequate oxygen supply will stop cell division and movement. Extreme hypothermia will also inhibit epithelialization.

As epithelial cells advance over a wound, a number of cells from directly behind the leading edge move downward into the underlying tissues. These usually survive only a short time. However, if migrating epithelium comes in contact with an area of infection from which the exudate has detached, these cells persist and form finger-like projections that grow into the wound tissues. One of these projections undermines the injured area, and its cells become a new tip of the migrating epithelial sheet. Within a short time, the connective tissue pushes the epithelium up to the original surface plane of the wound.[76]

Changes in Epithelium After Wound Coverage

As previously mentioned, the cells that cause epithelialization in dogs' wounds are those of the newly developed stratum spinosum. They roll over the basal cells at the wound edge and out onto the wound surface, where they assume the form of basal cells. In large excised wounds, all stages of epithelial repair may be seen at the same time. At the edge of the migrating epithelium, a single layer of flattened cells is moving across the wound. Farther back some cells are undergoing mitosis. Beyond these cells, upward migration is occurring to produce stratification of the new epithelium. Where several layers of cells cover the wound, differentiation and keratinization occur, and at the original wound edge there is hyperplastic thickening of the original epithelium.[34, 56] Winstanley has reported this same phenomenon.[76]

Prominent downgrowths develop on the lower surface of the newly formed epithelium by about the tenth to the 12th day after wounding. These invade the underlying connective tissue, giving rise to "pseudorete pegs" or "epithelial spurs" that reach their maximum size and extent between the 18th and the 21st day (Fig. 3–8).[53, 56, 64, 76] In dogs these spurs regress until the 36th day, when the lower border of the regenerated epidermis is relatively smooth.[76] In addition to regressing, the spurs have been reported to separate from the epithelium and form internally keratinizing epithelial "pearls," "nests," or "islands" that usually degenerate and disappear (Fig. 3–12).[11, 43, 56] The resulting smooth undersurface of the new epithelium provides a weak junction between connective tissue and epithelium;[56] thus, this new epidermis is easily traumatized and knocked off a healing wound.

It was long thought that specialized epithelial structures of the skin (i.e., hair follicles and sebaceous glands) did not regenerate if they were totally destroyed. However, research on wound healing in rabbits has shown that these appendages can be regenerated by differentiation of migrated epidermal epithelium. This adnexal neogenesis occurs after surface epithelialization is completed by the downgrowth of projections of new epithelium. These epithelial buds mature into hair follicles and their associated sebaceous glands.[7, 8, 34, 37, 54, 56, 64]

Winstanley observed short white hairs at the periphery of healed open wounds in dogs. He theorized that these grew from preexisting follicles that were displaced or had migrated into the wound.[74]

Macroscopic Appearance of Epithelialized Wounds and Surrounding Tissues

In Winstanley's study on dogs, epithelium first appeared in a crescent shape in the sector of an open wound that lay in the direction of hair flow. The reason for this has already been discussed. Within one to three days of its appearance, new epithelium was visible around the entire wound circumference. Epithelialization then progressed centripetally to cover the wound.[74]

Winstanley also observed that a crescentic area of alopecia developed along the side of an open wound that lay in the direction of hair flow. Conversely, hair grew more quickly and tended to be thicker than the surrounding hairs along the side of the wound that lay against the direction of hair flow. The alopecia on one side of the wound was due to damage to the bulbs of the follicles, while the increased hair growth on the opposite side of the wound was due to the rapid growth of hairs of a larger diameter from follicles that had only had their tops cut off, leaving their bulbs in situ (Fig. 3–13).[74, 75]

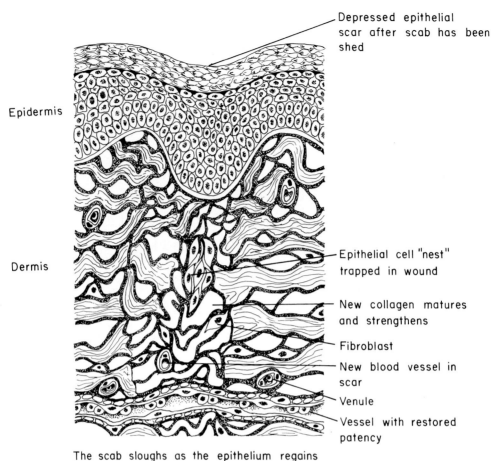

Depressed epithelial scar after scab has been shed

Epidermis

Dermis

Epithelial cell "nest" trapped in wound

New collagen matures and strengthens

Fibroblast

New blood vessel in scar

Venule

Vessel with restored patency

The scab sloughs as the epithelium regains normal stratification. New collagen increases in quantity and remodels in form to become more organized. Wound strength increases but does not reach that of uninjured skin. Fibroblasts disappear, and the vascular network is restored.

Figure 3-12: Maturation stage of wound healing.

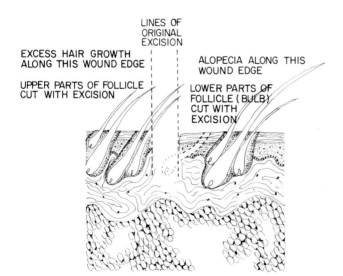

LINES OF ORIGINAL EXCISION

EXCESS HAIR GROWTH ALONG THIS WOUND EDGE

UPPER PARTS OF FOLLICLE CUT WITH EXCISION

ALOPECIA ALONG THIS WOUND EDGE

LOWER PARTS OF FOLLICLE (BULB) CUT WITH EXCISION

Figure 3-13: The alopecia along the side of a wound that lies in the direction of hair flow and the excess hair growth along the side of a wound that lies against the direction of hair flow are due to the way the follicles are cut.

The phenomenon of a thick crop of hair sprouts along wound margins has been explained by the epidermal hyperactivity that occurs along the margins of healing wounds, even in simple incision-type wounds. This regrowth of hair occurs considerably earlier than it appears over areas that have been shaved for surgery.[64]

The pigmentation of new epithelium over wounds has been stated to occur only in areas of dark skin on dogs. It is first seen on the 18th day, and the pigmented areas are small and restricted to the peripheral regions.[74]

Epithelialization of Incised and Sutured Wounds

The epithelium on each side of an incision reacts within 24 hours of injury by thickening and beginning to migrate across the intra-incisional clot that lies beneath the scab (Fig. 3–4). Usually within 48 hours the two new advancing epithelial sheets unite across the incision (Fig. 3–6). These sheets tend to invert at the point of union. In instances in which the epithelial sheets have migrated down the wall of the wound before uniting, the epidermal cells may invade defects in these walls and grow into suture tracts that are held gaping by horizontal suture tension. After the second postoperative day, the new epithelium over the wound thickens, and in most cases some further downgrowth of epithelium occurs, forming epithelial spurs (Fig. 3–8). As the epithelium thickens, its cells become more columnar and mitotic activity is increased. The epithelium becomes layered and acquires some of the structural features of adjacent uninjured epidermis. As keratin is produced in the uppermost epithelial cells of a wound, the overlying scab is loosened and dislodged; this usually occurs by the fifth day (Fig. 3–12).[34-36, 43, 46, 53]

In sutured wounds, epithelium can migrate down suture tracts. When the epithelium in the tracts thickens and keratinizes, it can produce a marked foreign-body reaction and sterile abscesses (Fig. 3–14).[34, 46, 55, 56] Thus, early suture removal can help prevent epithelialization of suture tracts and the problems associated with it.

In a study using pigs, Ordman and Gillman stated several possibilities for the healing pattern of incised adnexal structures (e.g., hair follicles and sweat glands). In general, new epithelium grows from the severed ends of these structures. This new tissue growth may (A) grow across an incision to rejoin the other part of the severed adnexa; (B) grow up the cut surface of the dermis to unite with the downgrowing spur or spurs of surface epithelium; (C) grow laterally or downward within the incision to join deep-lying in-

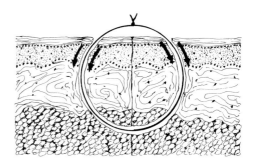

Figure 3–14: Epithelial migration along suture tracts. When epithelium in tracts thickens and keratinizes, it can produce a foreign-body reaction and sterile abscesses.

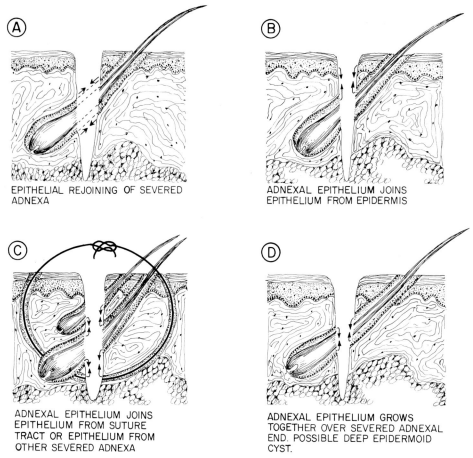

Figure 3–15: Possibilities for the healing of severed adnexa. See text for an explanation of parts A through D.

jured adnexal or perisutural epithelium; or (D) become sealed off when the epithelium grows together at the line of severance. The result may be a deep-lying microscopic epidermoid cyst (Fig. 3–15).[53]

Epidermal Abrasions

The margins of an abraded area are usually superficial and may involve only the outer epidermal layers. The center of the wound may extend deep to the basement membrane of the dermis. The defect is initially filled with a blood clot and necrotic debris that dehydrate to form a scab.[11]

A traumatic epidermal abrasion is quite similar to a split-thickness skin graft donor site or to intentional cosmetic dermabrasion. Although surface epithelium has been removed, transected adnexa remain. With proper protection from invasive infection, epidermal cells can regenerate from the epithelial lining of these foci and may appear as numerous islands of new epithelium on the wound surface. The cells of these islands migrate outward to reepithelialize the exposed dermal surface.[11, 56]

WOUND CONTRACTION

General Information

Wound contraction is the reduction in size of an open wound as the result of centripetal movement of the whole-thickness skin that surrounds the lesion. While granulation tissue is being formed and epithelialization is occurring, the granulation tissue contracts, pulling the skin margins inward so that the area to be covered by epithelialization is reduced. This contraction was once attributed to the contraction of collagen fibers but has since been found to be caused by other factors. No new skin is formed, but the size of the wound is reduced by the movement of surrounding full-thickness skin toward the wound's center.[4, 34-36, 46, 56, 72]

In areas on animals where skin is loosely attached to underlying structures, wound closure can virtually be completed by wound contraction, leaving minimal scar tissue. There are areas, however, where contraction cannot reach the ideal conclusion and a wider scar is left.[34-36] To determine how much a wound will contract, the wound edges should be grasped with forceps, and gentle traction should be applied in an attempt to coapt the edges. Any deformity or defect that is produced by this maneuver (e.g., joint flexion or distortion of the surrounding structures) will probably remain if the wound heals by contraction.[14, 54-56]

Wound contraction and wound epithelialization are two different processes that are independent of each other. Wound contraction proceeds beneath the newly formed epithelium, which is gradually obliterated as the full-thickness skin margins move toward each other.[34-36, 46, 56, 64]

Various times have been stated as to when wound contraction begins. In dogs there seems to be a lag period of five to nine days before significant contraction is visible.[34] It has been stated that in laboratory situations, wound contraction takes place between three and 47 days, with wide clinical variation.[14]

Previous Theories on Wound Contraction

Several theories have been proposed to explain the mechanism of wound contraction. They have generally received names corresponding to their proposed modes of action. Following are some of these theories.

Push Theory. This theory states that increased pressure caused by inflammatory edema in the surrounding unwounded skin pushes the wound margins inward. There is no convincing evidence to support this theory.[36, 45, 72]

Growth and Push Theory. This theory maintains that the wound margins may grow and push themselves inward by pushing on the surrounding skin. This proposal is not valid, since experimental evidence shows that growth has not occurred; rather, contraction has resulted in tension of the surrounding skin.[36, 72]

Sphincter Theory. This theory states that contractile material at the wound edge may act as a sphincter to reduce the wound size. Experimental evidence has negated this theory.[36, 45, 72]

Picture Frame Theory. According to this theory, active cells (fibroblasts) within the wound margin migrate inward, pulling on the material within the margins of the defect. Although no studies have disproved this theory, none have conclusively proven it either.[34-36, 45, 56, 64, 72]

Pull Theory.   This theory states that material within the granulation tissue of the defect contracts, thus pulling the margins of the defect inward. It has been shown that granulation tissue contains fibroblasts that develop characteristics typical of smooth muscle, including contractile ability. These cells have cell-to-cell and cell-to-stroma attachments. Stromal attachments include those to the wound bed and those to the panniculus and the dermis at the wound edge. When tested pharmacologically in vitro and in vivo, the behavior of these cells was found to be similar to that of smooth muscle cells. These cells are called myofibroblasts and will be discussed in the next section. Thus, the weight of experimental evidence favors this theory.[11, 21-23, 34-36, 45, 46, 49, 56, 72]

In Russell and Billingham's review of the mammalian repair process, two factors of interest that might relate to wound contraction were mentioned. Florey stated in this review that in rodents, spasm of the panniculus muscle, which is intimately attached to the skin, may play a role in initially bringing the wound edges together.[64] Billingham and Russell stated that excision of the panniculus muscle along with the dermis resulted in slower wound contraction.[7] They also mentioned that desiccation of the exudate in a wound might play some role in wound contraction; however, this has been disputed.[64]

Myofibroblasts and Wound Contraction

As previously stated, there are fibroblasts within an open wound that have modulated into contractile cells, which are responsible for wound contraction. These cells have the following properties in common with smooth muscle cells:
1.   They contain a cytoplasmic fibrillar system.
2.   Their nuclei show complicated folds and indentations that indicate cellular contraction.
3.   They have surface differentiations that adapt them for cell-to-cell and cell-to-stroma attachments.
4.   The cells demonstrate immunofluorescent labeling of their cytoplasm with human antismooth muscle serum.
5.   Strips of granulation tissue, when tested pharmacologically in vitro, behave similarly to smooth muscle. The granulation tissue contracts when exposed to smooth muscle stimulants and relaxes when exposed to smooth muscle inhibitors.[21-23, 54, 56]

In addition to their smooth muscle properties, myofibroblasts are capable of producing collagen.[56]

Reaction of Surrounding Skin to Contraction

Skin is not homogeneous; it contains cells, a fibrous network of collagen and elastin, and an amorphous ground substance composed of protein-polysaccharides, glycoproteins, globular proteins, salts, and water. Its heterogeneous composition, along with the physical arrangement of its components, is responsible for its mechanical properties. Skin has tension and extensibility. Tension is probably related to the content and direction of dermal elastic fibers. The extensibility of skin is the amount that it will stretch before it breaks. Two parameters determine extensibility: elastic stretch, which is dependent on elastic fibers and not collagen, and nonelastic stretch or plastic flow. Age and location are factors that affect both the tension and the extensibility of skin.[56]

As a wound contracts, the surrounding skin is stretched, thinned, and subjected to tension. It also has an increased water content. However, this state does not persist. Gradually, new collagen is laid down in the dermis so that tension is relieved. Thus, the dermis regains its degree of thickness. In addition, new epithelial cells are produced in areas under tension until the skin is restored to full thickness. The procedure is called intussusceptive growth.[6, 34, 56]

Cessation of Wound Contraction

The following are the three basic reasons for cessation of wound contraction:

A. When the wound edges meet, contact inhibition of the cells sets in to stop further movement.

B. If the tension in the surrounding skin equals or exceeds the force of contraction, further centripetal movement will cease and backward movement may occur. This may occur before the wound edges meet and is particularly a problem in areas where the skin is immobile.

C. In some wounds, contraction stops before the wound edges meet and while there is still some laxity in the surrounding skin. In these wounds the granulation tissue is paler and smoother and is probably composed primarily of collagen and ground substance. Thus, there is a lack of myofibroblasts[11, 34, 46, 56] (Fig. 3–16).

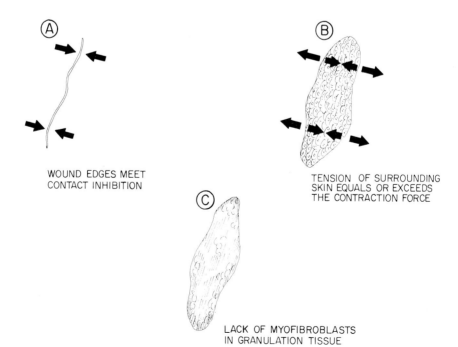

WOUND EDGES MEET
CONTACT INHIBITION

TENSION OF SURROUNDING
SKIN EQUALS OR EXCEEDS
THE CONTRACTION FORCE

LACK OF MYOFIBROBLASTS
IN GRANULATION TISSUE

Figure 3–16: Cessation of contraction. See text for explanation of parts *A* through *C*.

When the force of contraction and the tension of the surrounding skin reach equilibrium before the skin edges meet, a defect remains, and collagen may continue to be laid down in the defect. This area will begin to increase in size. This expansion of the scar in unclosed wounds is a late phenomenon. The extent of scar expansion is related in part to growth: it is greatest in young, growing animals and least in adult animals in which the growth rate is minimal.[56]

Wound Shape and Its Effect on Contraction

It has been found that various-shaped wounds heal in different patterns and at different rates in animals.

Rectangular Wounds.   On the torso of an animal the cranial and caudal edges of a rectangular wound contract faster than the other edges. Owing to mutual interference at the corners, the corners tend to remain stationary. The resulting scar has been described as two "V's" pointing toward each other with the points connected by a thin line or as a four-pointed star[34, 45, 56, 72] (Fig. 3–17). In studies of wound contraction in rabbits, Russell and Billingham found that rectangular wounds that were covered with Vaseline gauze decreased in size by about 7 per cent on each day during all but the first three and last five days of a 45-day healing period. The initial wound size played no significant part in the contraction rate.[34-36, 64]

Square Wounds.   Square wounds heal in a pattern similar to that of rectangular wounds, with the result being a stellate scar.[45, 46] These wounds also contract faster in a craniocaudal direction than in a lateral direction (Fig. 3–18).[56]

Triangular Wounds.   Triangular wounds contract to form a thin-bladed, three-pointed stellate scar (Fig. 3–19).[64]

Circular Wounds.   Circular wounds have been found to contract in a crumpled, unpredictable pattern, with a reduction of almost 40 per cent in perimeter. The movement of the skin across the wound is impeded and contraction is about 30 per cent slower than that of rectangular, square, or triangular wounds[34-36, 56, 64] (Fig. 3–20A and B). This may have some practical application in the creation of colostomies. If the skin is cut in the shape of a square or an ellipse, the process of contraction may constrict the stoma and result in obstruction, whereas a carefully designed circular skin wound will not contract to constrict the stoma.[56] However, in the interest of cosmetics, contraction of a circular wound can be undesirable.

Benefits of Wound Contraction

Wound contraction is an important factor in the healing of open wounds in animals and in humans. In humans the ill effects of wound contraction equal, if not exceed, the beneficial effects; however, in animals the beneficial effects of wound contraction predominate.[34, 36]

Wound contraction is a naturally occurring phenomenon that greatly facilitates the management of large skin defects. In animals in the wild, contraction is the primary process by which surface wounds heal.[14] Once contraction has started, it will continue to completion; however, this does not always close the skin defect. On the torso, closure can be almost complete, with

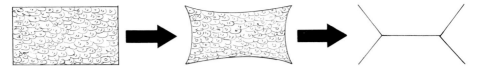

Figure 3-17:   Contraction pattern of a rectangular wound.

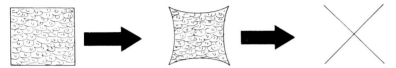

Figure 3-18:   Contraction pattern of a square wound.

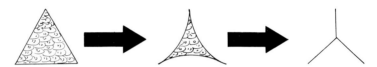

Figure 3-19:   Contraction pattern of a triangular wound.

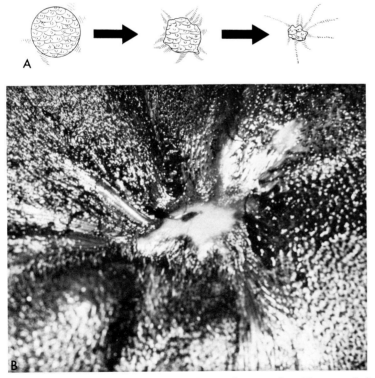

Figure 3-20:   *A*, Contraction pattern of a circular wound. *B*, The crumpled appearance of a scar that resulted from the open healing of a large circular wound over a dog's shoulder. See color plate I–G, p. 568.

a minimal amount of scarring. In other areas on the body, contraction stops before the wound is closed.[34]

The beneficial effects of wound contraction in animals are due to the large areas of mobile skin overlying the well-developed layer of cutaneous striated muscle, the panniculus carnosus. This muscle and the tenuous attachment of the skin to underlying structures permit wound contraction to occur to its fullest extent without interfering with the mechanical function of underlying structures. In humans the cutaneous striated muscle is vestigial, and the skin is more closely attached to underlying structures (i.e., immobile fasciae, major musculature, or bone). Thus, contraction may exert a force on these underlying structures, with resultant deformity.[4, 6, 56, 72]

Disadvantages of Wound Contraction

Deformity and loss of function as a result of wound contraction are usually not a problem in animals;[14] however, the following are some instances in which skin contraction or lack of contraction can cause problems:

1. Wounds near the flexor surface of a joint, when allowed to heal by contraction, may form a web of tight skin or scar tissue across the flexor surface that limits joint extension (Fig. 3–21).[14, 34]
2. When allowed to heal by contraction, wounds near a body opening may cause stenosis. Stenosis of the anus following cryosurgical treatment of perianal fistulae is an example.[34]
3. Wounds on the limbs, where there is insufficient mobility of surrounding tissue to allow complete healing by contraction, may be a problem. Epithelialization may cover these wounds, but this may take a long time, and the epithelium is easily traumatized and abraded from the wound owing to its loose attachment to underlying tissue. Some areas may not even epithelialize (Fig. 3–22).[10, 34, 41, 46]
4. Wounds in which skin shortening has occurred present a problem. The surface has a satisfactory covering with no gross deformity; however,

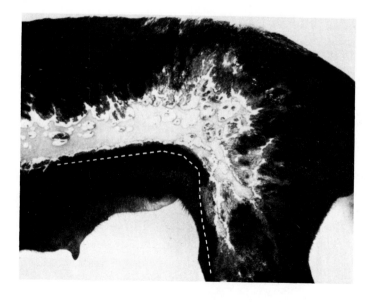

Figure 3–21: A web of tight skin across the flexor surface of the hip (*dotted line*) that resulted from the open healing of a burn lesion. Because of the inability to extend the joint, the dog walked sideways. See color plate I–H, p. 568.

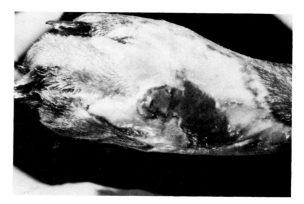

Figure 3–22: Insufficient skin to contract over a wound resulted in epithelialization with very delicate epithelial tissue that was easily abraded. The center of the wound did not epithelialize. See color plate II–A, p. 569.

the skin is so tight that it does not permit the normal functions of flexion and extension. The patient cannot bend in the skin envelope. The condition worsens if the patient gains weight, since the dense scar will not distend for new fat (Fig. 3–23).[10]

Effect of Skin Grafts and Flaps on Contraction

Contraction of a wound can be minimized or prevented by replacing skin immediately with thick skin grafts or pedicle flaps. However, once contraction has started, free grafts and pedicle flaps are much less effective in stopping contraction. The thickness of the dermis in a graft has a bearing on the cessation of contraction; thin grafts with less dermis have much less effect on contraction.[46, 54, 56] It has been stated that full-thickness grafts in animals will completely inhibit wound contraction.[7]

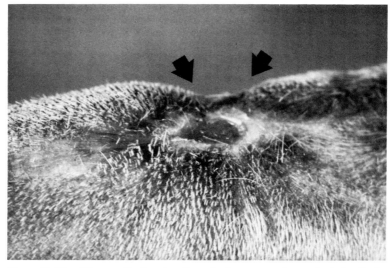

Figure 3–23: The result of contraction of a large wound on a dog's forelimb. The wound healed; however, the skin was quite tight in one area (arrows). The dog could walk normally, but the area of constricted skin on the forelimb limited extension during running, and the dog carried the leg.

MATURATION STAGE

EARLY WOUND STRENGTH

During the lag phase of four to six days, there is not an appreciable gain in wound strength. However, even within the first 24 hours a properly coapted wound has an effective strength. The fibrin in the clot seems to contribute to this strength. Within the first five days, epithelialization has occurred and the adhesive forces existing in the epithelial cells add to the early strength of the wound. The ingrowth of capillaries into the ground substance of the wound is another major factor contributing to wound strength. Also adding to early wound strength is the coagulation of protein in the wound. During this early stage of wound healing, the biological machinery for collagen synthesis is being mobilized and established so that it can add to later wound strength (Fig. 3–6).[34-36, 46, 53, 55, 56, 64]

LATE WOUND STRENGTH

Maturation and Remodeling of Collagen

The deposition of collagen in a wound has already been discussed in the section on wound repair. Collagen accumulates rapidly during the first three weeks of healing (Fig. 3–8). After this, the collagen content stabilizes, and there is no further increase in the amount of collagen in the wound. At this point there seems to be a balance between the deposition and the dissolution of collagen. Various tissue collagenases participate in the dissolution of collagen by removing nonfunctional and unnecessary collagen fibers. Functionally oriented fibers are preserved. Despite the dissolution of some collagen and the disappearance of fibroblasts with a resultant reduction in collagen synthesis, wound strength increases during a period of maturation and remodeling. As discussed earlier, this maturation and remodeling take place over a period of time (sometimes for years), and the rate of gain in wound strength becomes gradually less as time advances. The gain in wound strength is due to increased intermolecular and intramolecular cross-linkage of collagen fibers and a change in the physical weave of the collagen fibers. The purposefully oriented collagen fibrils increase slightly in thickness and compactness and tend to become grouped into bundles that present a whorled appearance. The junction between preexisting collagen bundles in the wound edges and newly formed bundles becomes progressively more difficult to define as the fibers of the two intermingle (Fig. 3–12). Though the strength of skin and fascia increases with time in a wound, it still remains 15 to 20 per cent weaker than that of surrounding normal tissue.[4, 11, 34–36, 44, 46, 47, 53, 55, 56] There is increasing evidence that even old scar tissue is in a state of dynamic equilibrium and that some collagen is constantly being synthesized and removed. This dynamic activity seems to be confined to a zone of approximately 15 mm. around the wound.[56]

Initially, the scar tissue of a healed wound is quite vascular and cellular, but as the scar matures and contracts, the vessels and cells become sparser. Macroscopically, a scar appears raised and pink at first, but as maturation occurs and the number of vessels and cells decreases, the scar takes on a white, flattened appearance.[4, 43, 44, 68] Although strong, scars are inelastic because of their denser than normal collagen content and their sparsity of elastic fibers.[46, 56]

Strength in Sutured or Tape-Closed Wounds

It has been reported that wounds on rats that were closed by tape had 90 per cent of the tensile strength of unwounded skin when evaluated five months after surgery. Sutured wounds in the same study were only 70 per cent as strong as unwounded skin; however, the sutured wounds were more pliable than those closed by tape. Both types of wound closure eventually had the same ability to resist rupture.[20]

Widened Scars and Their Prevention

Lacerations or incisions across the skin tension lines tend to cause a relatively greater spreading of the wound compared with those parallel to the skin tension lines.[41] If skin sutures are removed before the wound edges are stabilized by collagen, the scar tends to widen to approximately the width that the skin edges were separated before the skin sutures were inserted (Fig. 3-24).[34, 56] Scar widening is more marked in wounds that are across skin tension lines than in wounds that are parallel to skin tension lines or within skin creases.[46] The widened scars are usually not a problem in veterinary surgery; however, in some reconstructive procedures they are significant.[34] On shorthaired dogs or on areas of the body where the hair is naturally short, a widened scar may be objectionable.

To help prevent widened scars, a subcuticular suture of nonabsorbable material may be placed in the dermis and left permanently or for at least 30 to 40 days. A more common technique is to place a row of fine, long-lasting sutures deep in the dermis to accurately coapt the skin. This is followed by placing another row of fine sutures to coapt the epidermis. The latter sutures are

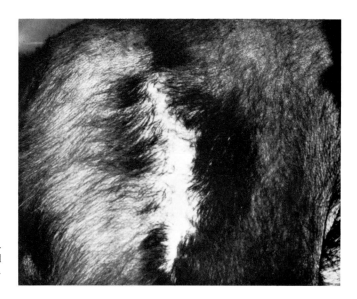

Figure 3-24: A widened scar resulted from tension on a healed wound after the skin sutures were removed. See color plate II-B, p. 569.

removed by five to six days, and the deeper dermal sutures hold the wound together until the collagen production has occurred.[34] A disadvantage of absorbable buried sutures is that they cannot maintain the physical integrity of the healing area for the time required for active remodeling of the collagen.[54] The reader is referred to Chapters 6 and 9 for further information on the prevention and correction of widened scars.

The placement of sutures close to the skin's edge is generally accepted as a means of preventing the "ladder-type" suture marks in a scar. However, there is an argument in favor of the wide placement of skin sutures. It has been found that normal wound collagen is lysed for a distance of approximately 5 mm. back from the wound edge. This area then becomes weaker, and if collagen synthesis does not take place, sutures that are placed in this region are likely to pull through the skin. The problem with wide suture placement is the tendency to tie the sutures too tightly and thus to strangulate tissue.[2]

FACTORS AFFECTING WOUND HEALING

AGE AND OBESITY

Wounds tend to heal more slowly in aged individuals owing to decreased fibroplasia and cell proliferation, nutritional factors, and an increased susceptibility to infection. Although young individuals heal rapidly, sutures may not hold well in the dermis and subcuticular areas because of tissue friability.[4, 41] Tissues in obese animals are usually friable and do not hold sutures well.[4]

ANABOLIC STEROIDS

Anabolic steroids allegedly increase the rate of healing, especially in fractures. These substances stimulate general protein synthesis in the body and therefore might be expected to stimulate wound repair.[56] A study of gingival healing in rats produced some evidence that oxandrolone* given orally to rats one day before and continually during the healing process increased the rate of healing in tooth extraction sites as compared with those in untreated control animals.[71] Synthetic anabolic steroids have been reported to antagonize the effects of steroids,[15] and therefore it has been suggested that they be used with caution.[56]

ANEMIA AND BLOOD SUPPLY

Chronic anemia[5, 36] and hypovolemic anemia[31, 32] have been found to be detrimental to wound healing; however, normovolemic anemia does not seem to affect wound healing.[31, 32, 56] The effect of hypovolemic anemia on wound healing seems to be related to hypoxia of the wound.[31]

An adequate arterial, venous, and microcirculatory supply to a wound is necessary to furnish oxygen and nutrients for healing. Injury to regional blood vessels, pressure by old or new scar tissue, the tight application of casts,

---

*Anavar is supplied by Searle Laboratories, Chicago, IL 60680.

bandages, or splints, and the tying of sutures too tightly can all interfere with blood supply and thus slow healing.[36, 41, 56] In addition, severe trauma may cause microvascular coagulation or sludging and thus interfere with wound oxygenation and nutrition.[56] It has been stated that adequate tissue perfusion seems to be more important than the oxygen-carrying capacity of the blood for adequate healing. Hemorrhage or anemia alone may not alter the oxygen tension of tissues; hypovolemia, vasoconstriction, and increased blood viscosity can profoundly affect local oxygen tension.[46]

ANTIBIOTICS

It has been found that wounds bandaged with neomycin are not slowed in their healing process.[28] In regard to systemic antibiotics, a study on rats showed that intravenously administered chloramphenicol inhibited the healing of skin defects.[12] However, massive doses of penicillin did not affect the tensile strength of healing skin incisions.[57] The reader is referred to Chapter 4 for more information on the use of systemic and topical antibiotics in contaminated and infected wounds.

ANTI-INFLAMMATORY DRUGS

Phenylbutazone, Indomethacin, and Aspirin

Phenylbutazone, indomethacin, and aspirin have been found to have an effect on wound healing.[24, 36, 46, 56] It has been theorized that phenylbutazone acts by decreasing capillary permeability and thus causes a delay in wound healing.[36] It is probable that the anti-inflammatory action of aspirin and indomethacin is mediated by their action on prostaglandins.[56] However, it should be remembered that in ordinary therapeutic doses, aspirin and phenylbutazone have no effects on the course or quality of wound healing.[46, 56]

In a study performed on horses, it was found that oxyphenbutazone,† when given in a loading dose of 12 mg./kg. (two days) and a maintenance dose of 6 mg./kg. (five days), significantly reduced the inflammatory response of tissue in artificially created surgical incisions and also resulted in a reduced amount of granulation tissue formation.[24]

Steroids

Steroids and steroid-related factors, including ACTH, cortisone, and stress,[56] have been reported to have a retardant effect on wound healing. Although ACTH and adrenocortical hormones are released at the time of stress to insure an animal's survival, it is unlikely that physiological levels of these hormones adversely affect wound healing.[4]

Steroids have been reported to affect the processes of wound healing in the following ways:

1. Inhibition of the processes associated with inflammation. There is a decrease in edema, fibrin deposition, capillary dilatation, and the

---

†Tandearil is supplied by Geigy Pharmaceuticals, Ardsley, NY 10502.

accumulation and activity of inflammatory cells.[16, 35] Cortisone increases the integrity of the lysosome, and it is the release of lysosomal enzymes that plays a prominent part in the inflammatory process.[16, 46, 56]

2. Suppression of fibroplasia. Cortisone and ACTH appear to retard the production of all mesenchymal cellular elements of repair. There is a reduction in both mucopolysaccharide and collagen synthesis.[16, 17, 36, 44, 46, 56] Chronic stress may also produce this effect.[56] In addition, cortisone may increase collagenolytic activity.[54]

3. Depression of capillary proliferation.[16, 36, 46] Both systemic and topical adrenocortical steroids inhibit the formation of granulation tissue.[56]

4. Inhibition of epidermal regeneration.[16, 46, 56] Some, however, have reported no noticeable impairment of epithelialization in wounds as a result of steroids or their analogs, even though the number of dermal elements is markedly reduced.[36]

5. Retardation of wound contraction.[56, 64]

6. Decrease in wound tensile strength.[16]

If they are administered after inflammation is established, steroids retard healing to a much lesser degree.[17] Cortisone in moderate to high doses after the third day following injury does not inhibit wound strength and apparently does not inhibit collagen synthesis.[16]

Chronic stress or the repeated administration of high doses of steroids, particularly if they are given just prior to or at the time of injury, may have an inhibitory effect on wound healing. However, it has been stated that an appreciable amount of corticosteroids given at the time of surgery usually does not affect the wound healing process significantly. Steroids given in doses that do affect wound healing usually slightly retard the healing rate; however, complete healing eventually occurs. All processes of healing take place, but at a slower rate.[46, 56] It should be remembered that in the presence of mild starvation and protein depletion, the effect of cortisone is greatly enhanced so that relatively low doses have a marked inhibitory effect on fibroplasia.[56] Acute stress and a low or a single dose of cortisone have no effect on healing.[54, 56]

Vitamin A and Steroids

Both topical and systemic vitamin A have been used successfully in humans to accelerate the healing of wounds whose progress has been retarded by cortisone.[31] As previously mentioned, the anti-inflammatory activity of steroids occurs at the lysosomal level. Steroids tend to stabilize lysosomal membranes, thus preventing the release of lysosomal enzymes that are necessary for the inflammatory process.[16, 46, 56] Vitamin A acts as an antagonist against the anti-inflammatory effects of cortisone at the lysosomal level by acting as a lysosomal labilizer.[16, 56] Synthetic vitamin A as an acid, alcohol, or ester can reverse the effects of steroids.[16]

The antagonism of vitamin A against steroids affects both inflammation[16, 56] and tensile strength.[16] Vitamin A acid accelerates the local accumulation of collagen in a wound.[27] Ehrlich and associates reported that the number of cells, capillaries, and collagen fibers is depressed in the wounds of glucocorticoid-treated rats; however, when vitamin A was given concurrently with glucocorticoids, there was a restoration of the inflammatory process and increased collagen deposition. In addition, vitamin A alone was found to stimulate fibroblasts and the accumulation of collagen.[17]

Since vitamin A may antagonize other effects of cortisone, caution has been advocated for its use in patients who are receiving cortisone to suppress inflammation.[16, 31]

BANDAGING

Bandaging has been found to be beneficial to wound healing from several standpoints, some of which are discussed in Chapter 4. In animals, occlusive dressings have been reported to speed the healing process.[77] With regard to epithelialization, bandaging seems to benefit migration rather than mitosis. Mitosis of epidermal cells occurs at the same rate in bandaged and air-exposed wounds. However, epithelium in humans has been found to cover superficial skin incisions that are bandaged with a nonadherent dressing by 24 hours after injury whereas similar incisions left unbandaged did not epithelialize until 72 hours.[63] This slower epithelial migration in the open wounds was probably related to the desiccation of both the epidermal cells and the wound edges. The increased drying of the wound and thicker crust forced the epithelial cells to cleave their way at a deeper level.[18, 63] It has been stated that epithelial cell movement occurs more rapidly if two surfaces are present rather than one. The cover provided by an artificial material or a natural dressing (i.e., a scab) provides more protection for the movement of epithelial cells.[54] Thus, epithelialization should occur smoothly between a moist wound bed and an overlying nonadherent dressing. Adherent dressings are detrimental to epithelialization, since they allow the growth of epithelial cells into the interstices of the dressing, and these cells are removed when dressings are changed. This does not seem to be a problem with nonadherent dressings.

CARTILAGE

The topical application of cartilage or cartilage extracts to wounds has been found to be beneficial to wound healing.[46, 58, 59, 62] The cartilage can be applied as (1) a powder,[46, 58, 59] (2) cartilage pellets implanted subcutaneously at a distance from the wound,[59] (3) saline extracts of cartilage injected at a distance from the wound,[46, 59] and (4) whole bovine ear cartilage sutured over the wound.[62] Histological studies suggest an increase in fibroblast density and collagen formation during the early phases of repair. Cartilage powder implanted within polyvinyl sponges stimulates collagen production.[46]

In Roberts' work, bovine ears from Brahman cattle were obtained from an abattoir. The skin was removed from the outer surface of the ear, leaving the skin on the inner surface. The ears were washed with surgical soap, placed in normal saline solution to which penicillin and streptomycin had been added as a preservative, and then frozen. The material was thawed and used as needed. When tested on fresh surgical wounds of dogs, the ear cartilage was nonirritating. When applied to the open wounds of horses, the whole bovine ear cartilage was found to be nonirritating, and its ability to stimulate healing was comparable to that of cadaver skin.[62] Further studies on the application of allograft or xenograft whole ear cartilage to the open wounds of dogs would be of interest.

Prudden and colleagues, in a review of how cartilage accelerates wound healing, proposed several theories; however, the topic is still speculative.[59]

DENERVATION

Denervated areas of skin on animals develop spontaneous ulcers even though contraction, epithelialization, and the rate of gain in tensile strength in such wounds are normal. Denervated skin appears to be more susceptible to trauma and pressure as the result of a lessened defense against mechanical injury. The author has noted this especially on the limbs of animals in which peripheral nerves have been irreparably damaged. Although the animal is able to compensate for motor paralysis either naturally or as a result of some surgical procedure (e.g., joint arthrodesis), the skin of the limb seems to be more subject to breakdown than it would be on a normal animal. This increased susceptibility is also evident in the extensive necrosis and ulceration of the skin and underlying tissues in paraplegics, which can be caused by minimal ischemia or pressure. Collagenase activity has been measured in these necrotic wounds and has been found to be quite high. The reason for such increased collagenase production in denervated dermis is unknown. Serum inhibitors generally prevent the manifestation of this activity; however, even during short periods of ischemia, the tissues are deprived of the serum inhibitors and the high level of the enzyme can exert its full effect.[56]

DEHYDRATION AND EDEMA

It has been demonstrated that dehydration delays healing; however, moderate edema has little or no effect on the gain in tensile strength. Marked edema has a slight and temporary inhibiting effect on wound healing, which may be more mechanical than biochemical in nature.[56]

In a study on rabbits, bilateral incisions were made on the feet of the pelvic limbs. In one limb, edema was induced by inflating a pneumatic cuff around the limb for 48 hours. The result was a diminution of tensile strength in the edematous wound, which was most marked by seven days. By two weeks the two sides were essentially the same with regard to tensile strength. Histological examination of the wounds revealed lymphatic dilatation and excessive fibrin deposition in the edematous limb; however, epithelialization, fibroplasia, and collagen deposition were not visibly impaired. The application of an external pressure device to the edematous limbs markedly inhibited edema formation, but prevention of the swelling did not materially improve the wound's tensile strength. Thus, edema per se does not seem to inhibit wound healing, but the factors that initiate edema do. A careful technique and avoidance of constrictive bandages have been advocated. If edema develops despite precautionary measures, skin sutures should remain in place for at least nine days.[50]

FOREIGN BODIES

If a foreign body causes irritation or infection, the wound will usually not heal until the foreign material is extruded or removed. This is an example of "tissue intelligence," which is designed to prevent the formation of deep and spreading infection. As long as a draining tract remains open to the surface, the foreign body does little harm. When the tract closes, there is danger of a deep-seated abscess.[36] The subject of foreign bodies in wounds is discussed in more detail in Chapter 4.

GENERAL CONDITION OF THE PATIENT

The general health of the patient will affect wound healing. Nutritional deficiencies, dehydration, endocrine imbalances, and cardiac, renal, or liver disease can complicate and delay wound healing. For this reason, elective surgery should be delayed until an attempt has been made to correct such deficiencies.[4] When nonelective surgery is undertaken on a debilitated animal, all attempts should be made to correct deficiencies during the postoperative healing time.

HORMONES

The hormone that is of most importance in wound healing is insulin. Diabetes mellitus can cause a delay in wound healing because of the occurrence of small artery occlusion, susceptibility to infection, and tissue deficiency in wound healing capacity.[41] The role of insulin in the treatment of contaminated and infected wounds is covered in Chapter 4.

HYPOPROTEINEMIA

Adequate protein levels are necessary for proper wound healing. A protein intake of 1 gm./kg. (0.454 gm./lb.) of body weight per day is necessary for normal functioning in animals. A minimum of 2.2 gm./kg./day (1 gm./lb./day) should be given to insure a positive nitrogen balance. In addition to this, dextrose should be given at the rate of 4.4 gm./kg./day (2 gm./lb./day) for energy and as a protein-sparing measure to allow protein to be used for tissue repair and synthesis.[52]

Protein deficiency has a deleterious effect on wound healing. The repair stage of healing is lengthened, with collagen deposition starting on the seventh or eighth day and progressing more slowly than normal. The number and activity of fibroblasts are reduced, mature collagen develops more slowly, the tensile wound strength is reduced, and wounds tend to disrupt more readily.[4, 41, 44, 52, 56, 64] Protein starvation has been reported to result in the failure of collagen to form in granulation tissue.[44]

It has been stated that the decreased rate of wound healing is not well correlated to plasma protein levels, and it would seem that the lag phase is not prolonged; rather fibroplasia is diminished. However, if the serum protein level goes below 2 gm./dl., there is inhibition of healing.[56] A report in the veterinary literature states that the normal plasma protein level ranges from 7.0 to 7.5 gm./dl. When this level falls to 6.0 gm./dl., wound healing is slowed. At levels below 5.5 gm./dl., a 70 per cent incidence of wound disruption has been reported. Albumin accounts for 85 per cent of the colloidal osmotic pressure of plasma; therefore, it is the most important plasma fraction in wound healing.[52]

A high-protein diet is indicated in animals that are undergoing wound healing. Experiments have shown that maximum wound strength was reached two days earlier in animals receiving a high-protein diet than in those receiving a low-protein diet. In addition, high levels of protein prevent tissue edema and promote increased fibroplasia to the point that wound strengths are three times greater than those at low levels of protein on the fifth postoperative day.[52] A high-protein diet does not shorten the lag period, but it does increase the rate of gain of tensile strength during the fibroplastic stage. An animal can synthesize fat from carbohydrates and carbohydrates from protein, but it cannot produce protein from any foods other than protein or its digestive products, peptides, and amino acids. For administering protein supplementation in large quantities, the oral route should be used.[52]

Supplementation of the diet with methionine and cystine will overcome the effects of protein depletion.[4, 32, 41, 44, 46, 55, 56, 64] The feeding of DL-methionine to protein-depleted animals has been shown to restore the lag phase to its normal duration and to increase the rate of fibroplasia. This suggests that the effects of protein deficiency are caused by the lack of a single specific amino acid. This amino acid appears to be necessary for the fibroblasts to synthesize mucopolysaccharides and collagen and thus complete the fibroplastic stage of healing. Later work has shown that methionine is converted to cystine, and this amino acid is the critical one for wound healing in protein-deficient animals. Although the explanation is unknown, it is theorized that cystine is a necessary component of one of the cellular enzymes involved in collagen synthesis.[56]

INFECTION

Bacteria interfere with wound healing by directly invading the injury site and by causing a chronic infection elsewhere in the body or a systemic infection. Local bacterial contaminations may lead to infections in the form of ulcers, abscesses, fistulae, or sinuses. A clostridial infection can result in gangrene.[4]

Infection can delay wound healing in several ways. Mechanical separation of the wound surfaces by exudate is a primary deterrent to healing.[4] Bacteria produce toxins that have been classified as enzymes with specific actions that retard wound healing. The necrotizing enzymes that produce tissue destruction include

1. Hyaluronidase, which favors the spread of infection.
2. Collagenases, which destroy and inhibit the production of collagen.
3. Fibrinolysins, which destroy developing fibrin and thereby impair the basic process of wound healing in its first phase.
4. Coagulases, which produce thrombosis of vessels that supply an area of infection and thereby inhibit or impair blood supply.
5. Hemolysins, which destroy hemoglobin.[3, 4]

There are other enzymes that impair the oxygen-carrying capacity of hemoglobin by causing the production of methemoglobin and sulfmethemoglobin. Other proteinases that have a broader target than fibrin and collagen are also produced by bacteria.[3]

Contaminated wounds can progress to infected wounds. This occurs when there is a large amount of necrotic tissue, when there are certain types of foreign bodies in the wound or its vicinity, or when something interferes with local tissue defenses, such as occurs in burns or in patients receiving immunosuppressive drugs. In the presence of any of these factors, small quantities of microorganisms may multiply before adequate tissue defense mechanisms are brought into action. When the organisms reach a concentration of 10^6/gm. of tissue, the wound is considered infected. The lower the initial concentration of organisms, the longer it takes to reach this point of infection. During this time local defense mechanisms have the opportunity to mobilize and work on the microorganisms.[56] The amount of devitalized tissue within a wound can play a significant role in the development of wound infection. Necrotic material in a wound must be removed before the final stages of healing can take place.[36] If there is a large quantity of devitalized tissue in a wound, the destructive phase (débridement stage) of healing will be prolonged, thereby delaying the proliferative phase (repair stage). During this time the necrotic tissue and its associated fluids afford a favorable environment for the proliferation of the bacteria that are present in wounds.[36] It can be seen that not only the number of bacteria but also the wound environment has a bearing on whether the wound becomes infected.

For more information on contaminated and infected wounds, the reader is referred to Chapter 4.

MOVEMENT

Movement of one portion of a wound with respect to another can rupture new capillary sprouts, disrupt organizing groups of reparative cells, and disturb the growth pattern of new fibers along with other undesirable results. Frequent mechanical disturbances near a wound surface as well as repeated hot poultices may bring about the deposition of excessive collagen fibers.[64] As mentioned in the section on bandaging in Chapter 4, there are two schools of thought on the immobilization of wounds. One group advocates the early mobilization of an injured part to help stimulate circulation to the wound and thus enhance healing. The other group supports immobilization of the injured area to prevent the aforementioned problems associated with wound movement. The author recommends a combination of the two methods: immobilize the wound surfaces against each other as much as possible with sutures, and then bandage, cast, or splint the affected limb or part so that the immediate wound area is immobilized and yet the whole part remains mobile for exercise.

NEOPLASIA

A combination of systemic and local factors associated with neoplasia affects the success of surgery. There is often a debilitating effect of generalized neoplasia that can either directly or indirectly affect many body systems.[4] As an example, if the surgeon encounters a nonhealing wound on a cat, it would be wise to check the animal for feline leukemia.

Wounds and incisions made in neoplastic tissue heal by proliferation of neoplastic cells. Healing of surgical wounds may be delayed or may fail to occur in the presence of a malignancy.[4] In light of this, it would be advisable to perform a biopsy on a nonhealing wound.

OXYGEN

Oxygen is essential for carbohydrate and protein metabolism, both of which are important in the wound itself.[32] With regard to protein metabolism, oxygen is necessary to provide energy for protein synthesis and to get newly synthesized collagen out of the cell.[32, 70] The amount of oxygen that is available for protein synthesis is dependent upon the partial pressure of oxygen in the blood, the capillary blood flow, and the diffusion of oxygen from the nearest functioning blood vessels to the healing wound edge.[70] Collagen synthesis is directly related to the supply of oxygen carried by the blood to the wound.[4, 70]

In a study on rats, it was found that an increase in Po_2 in inspired air resulted in an increase in wound tensile strength at one week.[70] Rats kept in an atmosphere of 10 per cent oxygen had reduced wound tensile strength, and the wound tensile strength of animals kept in an atmosphere of 40 per cent oxygen was increased when compared at one week with that of animals kept in an atmosphere of 20 per cent oxygen. The addition of oxygen accelerated healing only slightly; therefore, oxygen therapy for cleanly incised and closed wounds was not advocated. However, in patients with decreased oxygen delivery, extensive wounds, respiratory failure, and poor local perfusion, oxygen therapy could be beneficial.[70]

Increased Pco_2 in the atmosphere and in the wound has been found to be detrimental to healing and counteracts the accelerating effect of increased oxygen. It was theorized that in the healing wound, normal carbon dioxide accumulation is sufficient to provide conditions for maximal dilatation of small vessels and that an increased supply of carbon dioxide produces metabolic changes that impair healing.[70] Other theories on the effect of CO_2 on wound healing are stated in Chapter 4.

RADIATION AND CYTOTOXIC DRUGS

Acute ionizing radiation and other cytotoxic agents influence the wound healing rate.[46] In general, ionizing radiation is deleterious to wound healing. High doses of radiation, especially during the first three days of wound healing, significantly delay the rate of gain of wound strength.[46] Russell and Billingham have summarized the deleterious effects of irradiation as follows:

1. The formation of fibroblasts is depressed, and many of the fibroblasts that are produced are abnormal in appearance.
2. Collagen fibers become increasingly sparse at higher radiation doses.
3. At over 1000 rad., capillary regeneration becomes increasingly impaired.[64]

Most cytotoxic drugs interfere with cell proliferation in some way, and this affects wound healing. Any agent that prevents the proliferation of local fibroblasts or epithelial cells will prevent or delay healing.[46, 56] However, systemically administered mechlorethamine hydrochloride (nitrogen mustard), thiotepa, fluorouracil, chloroquine mustard, and other antimetabolites rarely reach high enough levels in the tissues to influence cell division in wounds.[46, 56] The long-term local application of mechlorethamine, thiotepa, and especially fluorouracil can completely prevent healing.[46] Cyclophosphamide, which also has an anti-inflammatory action, has been found to adversely affect wound healing. This adverse effect seems to be proportional to the debilitation of the experimental animals. Thus, it is questionable whether the adverse effect on wounds can be attributed directly to the drug.[56]

SECONDARY WOUND HEALING

There are two types of secondary wound healing. One type involves the healing of a second wound that has been made at some time after the primary wound. The second type is the secondary healing of a wound that has disrupted and been repaired.

In a study on rabbits, dorsal midline wounds were made five, nine, and 12 days after primary ventral midline wounds had been created. When wound tensile strengths were tested at five, nine, and 12 days after infliction of the secondary wounds and compared with those of the control wounds, it was found that those secondary wounds that were created nine and 12 days after primary wounding exhibited a significant increase in tensile strength. By the time of the second wounding at nine or 12 days, the primary wound was well into the collagen-producing stage of wound healing. These results suggest a secondary phenomenon that occurs when secondary wounds are created during the collagen-producing phase of the primary wound's healing. It is conjectured that a substance or substances are produced by the primary wound and are distributed systemically to enhance secondary wound healing, or perhaps a systemic reaction to the primary wound enhances secondary wound healing.[30]

Primary wounds that disrupt seem to heal more rapidly when resutured than those wounds that do not disrupt. It has been shown that resutured wounds show a significantly greater tensile strength on the third day after resuturing. This seems to be due to an immediate onset of fibroplasia in the wound, without the usual four- to six-day lag period. The sole difference between the healing of primary and secondary wounds is the lack of an initial lag phase in the latter type of wound. Disruption of the wound does not destroy macrophages or fibroblasts that are present. As a result, when the disrupted wound is resutured, the healing process that was already underway in the original wound takes up where it left off. No time period (lag phase) is required to activate and mobilize cells for healing in the disrupted wound as in healing of a primary wound.[56]

Madden and Smith have reported that disruption and resuturing of a wound at seven days did not alter the established rate of new collagen synthesis.[48] However, it has been suggested that there is more organization and cross-linking of existing collagen in secondary wounds, and therefore the gain in strength is rapid.[55, 56]

It is interesting to note that the excision of a strip of tissue ranging in size from 7 mm. to 1 cm. from around the edge of a disrupted wound will abolish the secondary wound healing phenomenon. This indicates that this type of secondary wound healing phenomenon is purely local.[55, 56]

SEROMAS AND HEMATOMAS

Collections of blood within or around a wound can delay healing by mechanically parting the tissues, thereby providing an excellent medium for bacterial growth. In addition, a large hematoma can exert sufficient pressure to interfere with the blood supply to adjacent tissues.[4, 36] Hematomas that are slow to be absorbed and that have not been therapeutically evacuated can result in rigid-walled cavities containing encapsulated fluid that encourages the growth of organisms.[36] Hematomas prolong the early stages of wound healing.

Seromas occur when dead space has not been obliterated in wound closure, when transected tissues are rich in lymphatics, when there is considerable movement in the wound, and when large amounts of surgical gut or other foreign material are in the wound.[36] The mechanical separation of the tissues and the potential for bacterial growth provided by the serosanguineous fluid can be significant deterrents to wound healing. For more information on hematomas and seromas and their prevention, the reader is referred to Chapter 4.

TEMPERATURE

It is believed that within physiological limits the effect of temperature on wound healing is related to an increase or a decrease in the blood supply to the wound.[36] As stated by Madden[46] and Peacock and Van Winkle,[56] wounds gain tensile strength faster at higher room temperatures than at lower room temperatures. Studies on rabbits have shown that warm environments favor healing, whereas cold or alternating cold and warm environments delay wound healing.[56] Wounds have been reported to heal faster at an ambient temperature of 30°C than at a normal room temperature of 18°C to 20°C. Lower environmental temperatures ranging from 12°C to 20°C decrease the tensile strength of wounds by about 20 per cent.[56] Reflex local vasoconstriction seems to be the factor involved in decreased wound healing at lower temperatures. The inhibiting effect of lower temperatures on wound healing can be eliminated by denervating the skin in the area.[46, 56] Bandaging a wound affects local wound temperature and thereby affects healing. For more information on this subject, the reader is referred to Chapter 4.

ADDITIONAL TRAUMA

Excessive trauma will prolong the first stages of healing, decrease the rate of gain of tensile strength, increase the possibility of infection, and result in excessive scar tissue that may affect the wound's appearance and decrease function. Rough handling of tissue, even in the absence of infection, can result in local edema and serum production. This may lead to a febrile reaction and can provide an ideal environment for bacterial proliferation.[4]

Prolonged exposure of the tissues during surgery is a form of additional wound trauma that can delay healing. Drying of tissue occurs as the result of exposure to the air and to the heat produced by the surgical lights. If solutions other than isomolar solutions are used to keep tissues moist, the cells may lyse, resulting in further cellular trauma. In addition, the possibility of bacterial contamination is increased when tissues are exposed for prolonged periods.[4]

The surgeon should exercise care to avoid causing trauma and contusion of the tissues by the instruments used in wound repair. Débridement should be done gently, carefully, completely, and with thorough and repeated flushing of the wound.[41]

VITAMINS

Several vitamins have an effect on wound healing. These effects are beneficial in some cases and detrimental in others. A discussion of some of the vitamins and their effects follows.

Vitamin A.   Vitamin A is essential for epithelial health.[41] It will overcome the membrane-stabilizing effect of vitamin E so that the wound healing rate will return to normal.[56] In a similar manner, it acts as an antagonist against the anti-inflammatory effects of cortisone.[16, 56] For more information on the effects of vitamin A on wound healing, the reader is referred to the section on anti-inflammatory drugs in this chapter.

Vitamin B Complex.   The vitamin B complex is necessary for cellular and enzymatic functions as well as carbohydrate metabolism.[32, 41]

Vitamin E.   Like steroids, vitamin E stabilizes membranes. It has been shown that high doses of vitamin E significantly retard wound healing and collagen production. As mentioned previously, vitamin A will reverse this adverse effect of vitamin E.[56]

Vitamin K.   Vitamin K is essential for blood clot formation, which is an integral part of wound healing.[41]

Vitamin C.   It has been stated that vitamin C is necessary for epithelial regeneration and the formation of blood vessel walls.[41] It is generally recognized that the primary function of vitamin C in wound healing is in the synthesis of collagen. A deficiency of vitamin C will cause a delay in wound healing. Although the building blocks may be present, if vitamin C is absent, complete collagen synthesis will not occur. If vitamin C is administered, collagen production can commence.[44] Vitamin C, along with ferrous iron, copper, α-ketoglutarate, and molecular oxygen, plays an important part in the hydroxylation of proline and lysine for the synthesis of collagen. The hydroxylation occurs after the amino acids have been synthesized into almost complete collagen molecules in the rough endoplasmic reticulum of the fibroblast. Without vitamin C, the hydroxyl groups are not added to proline and lysine. The collagen molecules remain incomplete and they may not be secreted by the fibroblast. Hydroxyproline and hydroxylysine are important in the cross-linking of peptide chains into the triple helix formation of collagen.[31, 36, 54, 56]

It is generally accepted that dogs and cats are among the animals that do not require an exogenous source of vitamin C. In one study on dogs it was shown that the mean plasma concentration of vitamin C was 0.88 mg/dl. of plasma, while the mean concentration in the buffy coat was 42.98 mg./10^8 cells. There was a significant day-to-day variation for both values.[13] In humans, minimal stores or a minimal dietary intake or both of ascorbic acid are sufficient for adequate wound healing, and it has been stated that a vitamin C deficiency must be quite severe before wound healing is impaired.[68] Some embryonic tissue culture studies of collagen formation have led to the conclusion that the synthesis of "normal" or "metabolic" collagen may not require ascorbic acid, but the requirement for rapid synthesis, as in wounds, may necessitate this vitamin.[56] Statements by others support these conclusions in that experimental studies have indicated that collagen synthesis can proceed at low rates in ascorbic acid–deficient animals. However, when circumstances require rapid collagen synthesis, ascorbic acid deficiency has a marked effect on collagen production. Supplying relatively small amounts of vitamin C restores normal healing, and an ascorbic acid saturation is not necessary.[46]

It is known in humans that the body loses ascorbic acid following major surgery and other stresses, such as burns and bacterial infections.[38, 68] Because of this, an adequate vitamin C supplementation might be advisable after wounding and before and after surgery.[68] There is the *possibility* that the vital levels of ascorbic acid in dogs and cats may also decrease following trauma, and this could be an indication for vitamin C supplementation in these species. Further research on vitamin C levels and its requirements in dogs and cats is needed.

ZINC

Zinc has been recognized as an essential element for all animals. The requirements for it are minute—20 to 100 parts per million; however, even slight to moderate deficiencies can retard growth, lower feed efficiency (the amount of body weight gained in relation to the weight of food taken in), and inhibit general well-being.[60] Zinc levels are subject to change, depending upon certain stress and traumatic conditions. A study has shown the mean serum zinc values to be 0.885 μg./ml. in male dogs and 0.957 μg./ml. in female dogs. Certain stress factors, such as hepatic disorders, hysterectomy, hypothyroidism, and infections, resulted in decreased serum zinc levels in the dogs.[19] In support of this latter statement, other studies have demonstrated that after trauma, surgical or otherwise, the amount of zinc in the blood and tissues may fall to low levels.[56] In one study, urinary zinc losses were determined in clinical patients during therapeutic weight reduction for obesity, after major surgery, and following severe burns. In all three groups of patients, accumulative zincuria was observed, with the magnitude being in proportion to the severity and duration of the metabolic insult and injury. There was an accompanying measurable reduction of zinc levels in serum, erythrocytes, and skin. In burned patients the average urinary loss of zinc per day was twofold or threefold greater than that of healthy patients. It was significantly greater after severe burns than after major surgical procedures.[26]

Zinc-deficient animals heal poorly, with characteristic epithelial defects and decreased wound tensile strength.[31, 36, 46, 60, 65, 66, 73] However, results vary as to the effect of zinc sulfate on wounds. When used topically to treat chronic leg ulcerations, zinc sulfate reportedly did not increase healing.[25] However, when zinc sulfate was administered orally, beneficial results were reported in the treatment of chronic ulcers[9, 33] and experimental burns.[39] Henzel and associates reported that supplemental zinc given to 16 zinc-deficient patients with impaired wound healing resulted in improved clinical wound healing along with a concomitant measurable increase in zinc concentration in the epithelium and granulation tissue of wounds.[26]

Zinc seems to be locally active at the tissue repair site, with a preferential accumulation of zinc within the healing wound after the administration of exogenous zinc to both zinc-sufficient and zinc-deficient animals. Peak concentrations are reached within 24 to 48 hours after injury.[26] Zinc transport to a wound site seems to be due to metabolic and electrochemical activity at the wound site.[42] Although zinc migrates rapidly into healing tissues, the effects of zinc deficiency or supplementation on healing are not evident for 12 to 15 days. However, results may be seen within three days in rapidly healing tissues such as the gingiva.[36, 60]

Reports indicate that zinc regulates DNA synthesis via zinc-dependent enzymes, i.e., DNA polymerase and reverse transcriptase. The decreased rate of wound healing in zinc-deficient animals has been attributed to decreased DNA activity in the skin. Because this decreased activity is related to the decreased function or amount of the two aforementioned enzymes, epithelial and fibroblast proliferation does not occur.[29, 56, 69]

The status of a patient with regard to zinc may be a governing factor in determining whether supplemental zinc will benefit wound healing. Following a study on rats, Sanstead and colleagues stated that zinc supplementation given to animals with normal zinc levels did not improve the rate of closure or tensile strength of wounds.[65] Others have supported this finding and have stated that uncomplicated surgical procedures rarely depress zinc levels markedly or for more than a few days.[56] Nadjafi reported that zinc sulfate produced no beneficial effect on the granulation tissue of standardized wounds of healthy dwarf pigs receiving a routine ration, nor was there an accumulation of zinc in the healing dermis.[51]

It has been reported that supplementing zinc in zinc-sufficient patients is not harmful, but it has no effect on delayed healing from other causes.[60] Others have stated that high levels of zinc could interfere with collagen cross-linking. This occurs when there is an antagonism between zinc and copper in the synthesis of lysyl oxidase, an enzyme necessary in collagen cross-linking. Excess zinc may displace the copper from the enzyme, thus interfering with the activity of lysyl oxidase. Zinc may also be detrimental to wound healing by stabilizing lysosomal enzymes and cell membranes. High levels of zinc can immobilize macrophages and decrease or inhibit phagocytosis.[56] Based on the latter statements, it would seem that the indiscriminant administration of high doses of zinc to wounded animals could cause a decrease in wound healing. At the other end of the scale, a lack of supplementation could result in poor wound healing in a zinc-deficient animal. There is a need for further research in the field of zinc deficiency and supplementation in dogs and cats as it relates to wound healing.

REFERENCES

1. Abercrombie, M.: The directed movements of fibroblasts: A discussion. Proceedings of the Zoological Society of Calcutta: The Mookerjee Memorial Volume., 1957, pp. 129–1400.
2. Adamsons, R. J., Musco, F., and Enquist, I. F.: The chemical dimensions of a healing incision. Surg. Gynecol. Obstet. 123:515, 1966.
3. Altemeier, W. A.: Wound Healing in Surgery: Proceedings of a Panel Discussion. Somerville, N. J., Ethicon Inc., 1970, p. 5.
4. Archibald, J., and Blakely, C. L.: Basic procedures and preoperative considerations, in Archibald, J. (ed.): Canine Surgery, ed. 2. Santa Barbara, Calif., American Veterinary Publications, Inc., 1974, pp. 22–24.
5. Bains, J. W., Crawford, D. T., and Ketcham, A. S.: Effect of chronic anemia on wound tensile strength: Correlation with blood volume, total red blood cell volume, and proteins. Ann. Surg. 164:243, 1966.
6. Billingham, R. E., and Medawar, P. B.: Contracture and intussusceptive growth in healing of extensive wounds in mammalian skin. J. Anat. 89:114, 1955.
7. Billingham, R. E., and Russell, P. S.: Studies on wound healing, with special reference to contracture in experimental wounds in rabbit's skin. Ann. Surg. 144:961, 1956.
8. Billingham, R. E., and Russell, P. S.: Incomplete wound contraction and the phenomenon of hair neogenesis in rabbit's skin. Nature 177:791, 1956.

9. Brewer, R. D., Leal, J. F., and Mihaldzic, N.: Preliminary observation of the effect of oral zinc sulfate on the healing of decubital ulcers. Proc. Annu. Clin. Spinal Cord Inj. Conf. *15*:93, 1966.

10. Brown, J. B., and McDowell, F.: Epithelial healing and the transplantation of skin. Ann. Surg. *115*:1166, 1942.

11. Bryant, W. M.: Wound healing. Clin. Symp. *29*:2, 1977.

12. Caulfield, J. B., and Burke, J. E.: Inhibition of wound healing by chloramphenicol. Arch. Pathol. *92*:119, 1971.

13. Crilly, J. C., Pugh, D. M., and Coffe, D. J.: Plasma and buffy coat vitamin C concentration in the dog. Folia Vet. Lat. *6*:289, 1976.

14. Dingwall, J. S.: Wound contraction. J. Am. Anim. Hosp. Assoc. *12*:668, 1976.

15. Ehrlich, H. P., and Hunt, T. K.: The effects of cortisone and anabolic steroids on the tensile strength of healing wounds. Ann. Surg. *170*:203, 1970.

16. Ehrlich, H. P., and Hunt, T. K.: Effects of cortisone and vitamin A on wound healing. Ann. Surg. *167*:324, 1968.

17. Ehrlich, H. P., Tarver, H., and Hunt, T. K.: Effects of vitamin A and glucocorticoids upon inflammation and collagen synthesis. Ann. Surg. *177*:222, 1973.

18. Epstein, E. H. Jr.: Wound healing, in Epstein, E., and Epstein, E. Jr. (eds.): Skin Surgery, ed. 4. Springfield, Ill., Charles C Thomas, Publisher, 1977.

19. Fisher, G. L.: Effects of disease on serum copper and zinc values in the beagle. Am. J. Vet. Res. *38*:935, 1977.

20. Forrester, J. C.: Wound Healing in Surgery: Proceedings of a Panel Discussion. Somerville, N. J., Ethicon, Inc., 1970, p. 5.

21. Gabbiani, G., Hirschel, B. J., Ryan, G. B., et al.: Granulation tissue as a contractile organ: A study of structure and function. J. Exp. Med. *135*:719, 1972.

22. Gabbiani, G., and Majno, G.: Dupuytren's contracture: Fibroblast contraction? Am. J. Pathol. *66*:131, 1972.

23. Gabbiani, G., Ryan, G. B., and Majno, G.: Presence of modified fibroblasts in granulation tissue and their possible role in wound contraction. Experientia *27*:549, 1971.

24. Gorman, H. A., Wolff, W. A., Frost, W. W., et al.: Effect of oxyphenylbutazone on surgical wounds of horses. J. Am. Vet. Med. Assoc. *152*:487, 1968.

25. Greaves, M. W., and Ive, F. A.: Double-blind trial of zinc sulfate in the treatment of chronic leg ulceration. Br. J. Dermatol. *87*:632, 1972.

26. Henzel, J. H., DeWeese, M. S., and Lichti, E. L.: Zinc concentrations within healing wounds: Significance of postoperative zincuria on availability and requirements during tissue repair. Arch. Surg. *100*:349, 1970.

27. Herman, J. B., and Woodward, S. L.: An experimental study of wound healing accelerators. Am. Surg. *38*:26, 1972.

28. Hinman, C. D., and Maibach, H. I.: Effect of air exposure and occlusion on experimental human skin wounds. Nature *200*:377, 1963.

29. Hsu, T. H., and Hsu, J. M.: Zinc deficiency and epithelial wound repair: An autoradiographic study of ^{3}H-thymidine incorporation (36415). Proc. Soc. Exp. Biol. Med. *140*:157, 1972.

30. Hugo, N. E., Epstein, L., Cone, A., et al.: The effect of primary wounding on the tensile strength of secondary wounds. Surg. Gynecol. Obstet. *131*:516, 1970.

31. Hunt, T. K.: Recent advances in wound healing. Surg. Annu. 2:1, 1970.

32. Hunt, T. K.: Wound healing in surgery: Proceedings of a Panel Discussion. Somerville, N. J., Ethicon, Inc., 1970, pp. 11–13.

33. Husain, S. L.: Oral zinc sulphate in leg ulcers. Lancet *1*:1069, 1969.

34. Johnston, D. E.: The processes in wound healing. J. Am. Anim. Hosp. Assoc. *13*:186, 1977.

35. Johnston, D. E.: Wound healing and reconstructive surgery. Am. Anim. Hosp. Assoc. Sci. Proc. 2:383, 1975.

36. Johnston, D. E.: Wound healing. Arch. Am. Coll. Vet. Surg. 3:30, 1974.

37. Joseph, J., and Townsend, F. J.: Experimental surgery — the healing of defects in immobile skin in rabbits. Br. J. Surg. *48*:557, 1961.

38. King, C. G.: Present knowledge of ascorbic acid (vitamin C). Nutr. Rev. *26*:33, 1968.

39. Leeds, E. B.: The role of zinc sulfate in wound healing. Arch. Am. Coll. Vet. Surg. *4*:2, 1975.

40. Levenson, S. M., Geever, E. F., Crowley, L. V., et al.: The healing of rat skin wounds. Ann. Surg. *161*:293, 1965.

41. Lewis, J. R.: The Surgery of Scars. New York, McGraw-Hill Book Co., 1963.

42. Lichti, E. L., Turner, M., Henzel, J. H., et al.: Wound fluid zinc levels during tissue repair: Sequential determination by means of surgically implanted Teflon cylinder. Am. J. Surg. *121*:665, 1971.

43. Lindsay, W. K., and Birch, J. R.: Thin skin healing. Can. J. Surg. 7:297, 1964.

44. Longacre, J. J.: Scar Tissue: Its Use and Abuse. Springfield, Ill., Charles C Thomas, Publisher, 1972.

45. Luccioli, G. M., Robertson, H. R., and Kahn, D. S.: The pattern of contraction during the healing of excised skin wounds in the rabbit. Can. J. Surg. 6:499, 1963.

46. Madden, J. W.: Wound healing: Biologic and clinical features, in Sabiston, D. C. (ed.):

Davis-Christopher: Textbook of Surgery, ed. 11. Philadelphia, W. B. Saunders Co., 1977.

47. Madden, J. W., and Peacock, E. E.: Studies on the biology of collagen during wound healing: III. Dynamic metabolism of scar collagen and remodeling of dermal wounds. Ann. Surg. *174*:511, 1971.

48. Madden, J. W., and Smith, H. C.: The rate of collagen synthesis and deposition in dehisced and resutured wounds. Surg. Gynecol. Obstet. *130*:487, 1970.

49. Majno, G., Gabbiani, G., Hirschel, B. J., et al.: Contraction of granulation tissue in vitro: Similarity to smooth muscle. Science *173*:548, 1971.

50. Myers, M. B., Cherry, G., Heimburger, S., et al.: The effect of edema and external pressure on wound healing. Arch. Surg. *94*:218, 1967.

51. Nadjafi, A. S.: Study of wound healing under application of zinc sulfate. Aerztl. Forsch. *26*:245, 1972.

52. Noffsinger, G. R., McMurray, B. L., and Jones, T. J.: Proteins in wound healing. J. Am. Vet. Med. Assoc. *131*:481, 1957.

53. Ordman, L. J., and Gillman, T.: Studies in the healing of cutaneous wounds. Arch. Surg. *93*:857, 1966.

54. Peacock, E. E.: Repair and regeneration, in Converse, J. M. (ed.): Reconstructive Plastic Surgery: Principles and Procedures in Correction, Reconstruction, and Transplantation, ed. 2. Philadelphia, W. B. Saunders Co., 1977, vol 1.

55. Peacock, E. E.: Wound healing and wound care, in Schwartz, S. I. (ed.): Principles of Surgery. New York, McGraw-Hill Book Co., 1969.

56. Peacock, E. E., and Van Winkle, W.: Wound Repair, ed. 2. Philadelphia, W. B. Saunders Co., 1976.

57. Pohl, R., and Hunt, T. K.: Penicillin G and wound healing. Arch. Surg. *101*:610, 1970.

58. Prudden, J. F., and Allen, J.: The clinical acceleration of healing with a cartilage preparation. J.A.M.A. *192*:352, 1965.

59. Prudden, J. F., Wolarsky, E. R., and Balassa, L.: The acceleration of healing. Surg. Gynecol. Obstet. *128*:1321, 1969.

60. Pullen, F. W., Pories, W. J., and Strain, W. H.: Delayed healing: The rationale for zinc therapy. Laryngoscope *81*:1638, 1971.

61. ReMensnyder, J. P., and Majno, G.: Oxygen gradients in healing wounds. Am. J. Pathol. *52*:301, 1968.

62. Roberts, D.: The use of bovine ear cartilage in speeding open-wound healing in the horse. Vet. Med. Small Anim. Clin. *61*:961, 1966.

63. Rovee, D. T., Kurowsky, C. A., Labun, J., et al.: Effect of local wound environment on epidermal healing, in Maibach, H. I., and Rovee, D. T. (eds.): Epidermal Wound Healing. Chicago, Year Book Medical Publishers, 1972, p. 159.

64. Russell, P. S., and Billingham, R. E.: Some aspects of the repair process in mammals. Prog. Surg. *2*:1, 1962.

65. Sanstead, H. H., Lanier, V. C., Shephard, G. H., et al.: Zinc and wound healing: Effects of zinc deficiency and zinc supplementation. Am. J. Clin. Nutr. *23*:514, 1970.

66. Sanstead, H. H., and Shephard, G. H.: The effect of zinc deficiency on tensile strength of healing surgical incisions in the integument of the rat. Proc. Soc. Exp. Biol. Med. *128*:687, 1968.

67. Schilling, J. A.: Wound Healing in Surgery: Proceedings of a Panel Discussion. Somerville, N.J., Ethicon, Inc., 1970, pp. 15–17.

68. Schwartz, P. L.: Ascorbic acid in wound healing: A review. J. Am. Diet. Assoc. *56*:497, 1970.

69. Stephan, J. D., and Hsu, J. M.: Effect of zinc deficiency and wounding on DNA synthesis in rat skin. J. Nutr. *103*:548, 1973.

70. Stephens, F. O., and Hunt, T. K.: Effect of changes in inspired oxygen and carbon dioxide tensions on wound tensile strength: An experimental study. Ann. Surg. *173*:515, 1971.

71. Tennenbaum, R., and Shklar, G.: Anabolic steroid effect on wound healing. Oral Surg. *30*:824, 1970.

72. Van Winkle, W.: Wound contraction. Surg. Gynecol. Obstet. *125*:131, 1967.

73. Winn, R. T.: A literature review of wound healing and the effects of zinc on wound healing. S.W. Vet. *28*:221, 1975.

74. Winstanley, E. W.: The macroscopical appearance of the healing full-thickness excised skin wound in the thoracic and metatarsal regions in the dog. J. Small Anim. Pract. *16*:143, 1975.

75. Winstanley, E. W.: The reaction of hair follicles in the vicinity of full-thickness excised skin wounds in the dog. J. Small Anim. Pract. *16*:661, 1975.

76. Winstanley, E. W.: The epithelial reaction in the healing of excised cutaneous wounds in the dog. J. Comp. Pathol. *85*:61, 1975.

77. Winter, G. D.: Epidermal regeneration studied in the domestic pig, in Maibach, H. I., and Rovee, D. T. (eds.): Epidermal Wound Healing. Chicago, Year Book Medical Publishers, 1972, p. 71.

SECTION II

MANAGEMENT OF TRAUMATIZED SKIN

4

MANAGEMENT OF CONTAMINATED AND INFECTED WOUNDS

Surgery of the skin cannot be discussed without considering the management of contaminated and infected wounds. All too often the structures underlying the skin are damaged by the agents that cause skin trauma and defect. In addition, many of the agents set the stage for wound contamination and subsequent infection. The author realizes that all practitioners have their own way and their preferred medications for treating wounds. The purpose of this chapter is to discuss some of the basic aspects of the management of contaminated and infected wounds.

TISSUE SUSCEPTIBILITY TO TRAUMA

The tolerance to destructive force varies with the type of tissue. Owing to its elasticity and vasculature, the skin can tolerate considerable insult.[66] However, it does have its limits and may be badly damaged if the destructive force is severe enough.

Subcutaneous tissue tolerates trauma poorly, and, when it is injured, the damaged tissue must be thoroughly excised. Muscle, which is quite vulnerable, is extensively damaged by injury. Tendons, fasciae, and nerves are more resistant to trauma.[66]

CLASSIFICATION OF WOUNDS

The early time period following the infliction of a wound is called the golden period. The period is variable in length. Times ranging from four to 12 hours have been stated in the literature,[22, 33, 66, 78, 79, 127, 154] and one study revealed the mean time to be 5.17 hours.[127] The length of the golden period is generally considered to extend for six hours after the time of injury. During this time wounds may be decontaminated by washing and débridement. After this period bacteria invade beyond the wound margins.[78] Three hours after injury is regarded as a critical time, since it has been found that bacterial numbers are approaching the dangerous level of greater than 10^5 bacteria per gram of tissue.[127] The effectiveness of prophylactic antibiotics in surgical wounds has been shown to be no more than three hours; therefore, the shorter the time between the contamination of a traumatic or a surgical wound and the administration of antibiotics, the more effective the antibotics are in preventing infection.[79]

Wounds have been categorized into three classes, depending on the progression of infection.[33] A class 1 wound is from zero to six hours old, during which time little bacterial multiplication has occurred. The period for a class 2 wound extends from six to 12 hours after injury, during which time organisms have started to divide but are not yet invasive. From 12 hours on the wound is considered a class 3 wound and is usually infected.

The time division in wound classification is arbitrary and will be modified by the nature of the wound, its blood supply, and the circumstances under which the wound was sustained.[33] A biologically oriented surgeon realizes almost intuitively that the length of time a wound has been open is not nearly so important as an accurate assessment of the natural defenses in the area, the known or suspected strength and type of inoculum introduced, and the treatment the patient has received during the interim between injury and definitive care. Discrimination between contamination (which can be converted to surgical cleanliness) and infection (which cannot be completely removed) is valuable. Mechanical wound closure is contraindicated in a wound that is red, warm, painful, or swollen following bacterial invasion, regardless of the length of time since wound infliction.[117]

FACTORS RELATED TO WOUND INFECTION

Many factors influence the magnitude of infection, including the type of microorganisms, tissue conditions, soil-related factors, the presence of wound fluids and cells, and other general conditions.

BACTERIA

The degree of contamination is an important determinant in the development of wound infection.[127] Not only is the number of bacteria important, but their virulence must also be considered.[78, 163] An algebraic equation has been stated that demonstrates the relationship between the number of bacteria, the type of bacteria, and the host's resistance:[78]

$$\frac{\text{dose of bacteria} \times \text{virulence}}{\text{host's resistance}} = \text{infection}$$

Although it would be impossible to place actual numbers in the equation, the algebraic principles hold true. An increase in either the dose or the virulence of bacteria increases the chance of infection, whereas an increase in the host's resistance decreases that chance.

The bacteria in a wound come from the soiling of a wound during injury and from in-hospital contamination.[4, 137] Soiling at injury may result from microorganisms and debris on the animal's skin and hair and from the same factors in the environment. In-hospital sources of bacteria include the human respiratory tract, the skin of the patient and the personnel who are treating the wound, and air or instrument contamination from nearby infected wounds.

Within the hospital the secondary contamination of wounds by pyogenic organisms often occurs before definitive treatment has begun. This argues for early wound protection and the use of the aseptic technique by the personnel who are treating the wounds.[4] These matters will be discussed in more detail later in the chapter.

Many different types of bacteria, either singly or in combinations, contaminate wounds.[4] Different bacteria and the problems associated with their growth in wounds will be discussed at various points throughout this chapter. Contaminating organisms exist in a commensal state within their host without causing infection or harm. This is true as long as they remain as contaminants. Although many contaminants are potential pathogens, they cannot be said to be pathogenic until they actually cause an infection. The same type or species of microorganisms may be either a contaminant or a pathogen and may change from one state to the other. Whether this conversion occurs is a result of what happens to the host's tissue in response to their presence.[17]

It is generally accepted that the critical level of bacteria within a wound is 10^5 bacteria per gram of tissue or milliliter of fluid. Beyond this level infection occurs, and the bacterial count must be at this level or below before a delayed wound closure or a graft will be successful.[127, 130] The types of obligate aerobes and facultative species contaminating a wound play a lesser role in the development of infection than does the quantity of bacteria.[37] Exceptions to the statement that more than 10^5 bacteria per gram of tissue produce infection are β-hemolytic streptococci and possibly some species of *Proteus*.[130]

Plasma does not have the bactericidal effect on streptococcal growth that it has on other bacteria. Many gram-positive organisms, including streptococci, produce a kinase which, when acted upon by plasminogen, produces the proteolytic enzyme plasmin. The plasmin inactivates complement, which is primarily active against gram-negative organisms, leaving gram-positive organisms unaffected. However, the streptococcal M proteins are an exception, with the plasma bactericidal properties against the streptococci being contained in the complement. In summary, streptococci produce kinase, which is acted upon by plasminogen to produce plasmin. Plasmin, in turn, inactivates the complement, which is the plasma factor that is bactericidal for streptococci. Because of the poor inhibitory effect of plasma against β-hemolytic streptococci, a lower inoculum of this organism is sufficient to cause infection.[130] It is stated by Davis in Chapter 5 that domestic animals do not have large quantities of plasminogen; therefore, a quantitative study on the effects of streptococcal infection in domestic animals would be of interest.

When considering bacterial infection in general, there are numerous substances that enter into the wound infection process. When bacteria colonize and invade a wound, their reaction with the tissue results in the production of a number of toxic substances that have profound local and systemic effects. There are necrotizing enzymes that cause tissue destruction. Spreading factors, such as hyaluronidase, favor the dissemination of infection. Collagenases destroy collagen and inhibit its production. Fibrinolysins destroy fibrin as it develops, thus impairing wound healing in its first phase. Coagulases cause thrombosis of the nutrient vessels supplying an area of infection and inhibit or impair the blood supply. Hemolysins destroy hemoglobin. There are enzymes that impair the oxygen-carrying capacity of hemoglobin by causing the formation of methemoglobin and sulfmethemoglobin. There are other proteinases that have a broader target than fibrin or collagen.[3] It is obvious that these bacterial products would have a deleterious effect on tissues.

The synergistic or cumulative activity of the bacteria that are present in a wound can also determine the nature and severity of an infection.[78] However, one study has shown that in infections caused by a combination of *Staphylococcus aureus* and *Staphylococcus albus* or *Staphylococcus aureus* and *Pseudomonas aeruginosa*, there does not appear to be synergism, infection enhancement, or inhibition between either of the organism pairs as occurs when the organisms are grown singly.[69]

The results of bacterial cultures are necessary for the proper treatment of accidental wounds.[123] Initially, a gram-stained smear of the infected wound should be taken. The wound should also be cultured, and antibiotic susceptibility tests should be performed on pure cultures of each potential pathogen that is isolated from the wound.[76] The question arises as to what antibiotic(s) should be used in cases of suspected infection until the culture results are available. Jennings has suggested three possible regimens: (1) cephalothin and kanamycin or gentamicin, (2) gentamicin and carbenicillin, or (3) cephalothin and carbenicillin.[76]

Repeated cultures will assist in the evaluation of therapy.[76] The author has found this to be a wise course of action. Early culture and susceptibility tests will yield information about the bacteria in the wound that are from "outside" sources. The same tests performed a few days later may reveal a different wound flora composed of antibiotic-resistant secondary contaminants from the hospital environment and possibly the original contaminating organisms that have become resistant to antibiotics.

A clinician's own senses may also aid in determining the type of bacteria in a wound. The odor and appearance of a wound and of its bandage may suggest *Pseudomonas* organisms. The blue-green pigment pyocyanin is indicative of a *Pseudomonas* infection. The more pathogenic forms of *Pseudomonas* are associated with pyoverdin or fluorescein. Burn wounds that are infected with the more pathogenic species of *Pseudomonas* have been observed to fluoresce under a Wood's light, and this fluorescence has been used to diagnose the infection while the bacterial density is less than that which is likely to produce invasive sepsis.[156]

CONDITION OF TISSUES

The presence of bacteria in a wound does not make infection a certainty. Evidence indicates that the physiological state of the tissue within the wound before and after contamination is more important than the presence of bacteria.[17, 78, 110] As stated by Pasteur in the last moments of his life, "The germ is nothing, it is the terrain in which it grows which is everything."[17]

A locally effective blood supply is a very important natural defense mechanism against infection, and damage to the blood supply of tissues greatly favors the development of infection by preventing local body defenses from becoming active at the wound.[17, 37, 57, 110, 117, 133, 163] In addition, the local release of vasoconstrictor substances in the damaged tissue results in poor perfusion and predisposes the wound to infection.[46] With the poor blood supply, the humoral and cellular defense mechanisms of the host have a decreased ability to combat the bacterial contaminants in the necrotic tissue. As a result, the necrotic tissue provides the nutrients for the infecting microorganisms, which multiply and reach high concentrations.[57] Wounds produced by sharp instruments (e.g., glass and knives) are much more resistant to infection and may heal without complication unless they are subjected to greater than 10^5 bacteria per gram of tissue. Wounds that are associated with more soft-tissue trauma may develop infections even when the bacterial count is considerably less than 10^5 bacteria per gram of tissue.[37] It can be seen that healing will be enhanced by adequately excising devitalized wounds with a sharp instrument, thereby exposing viable tissue with a good blood supply.

Surgeons have tended to follow an earlier premise of Pasteur and have concerned themselves more with the nature and control of bacteria than with the management and control of the tissues into which they have been introduced. Thus, a dependence on bacteriostatic and bactericidal agents rather than on the body's natural defense mechanisms has developed. Even though antibiotic therapy has probably decreased the incidence and severity of wound infections, some infections have developed because of an overdependence on these products.[17]

INFECTION-PRODUCING FACTORS IN SOIL

A study has shown that factors associated with the soil itself can contribute to wound infection. These are called infection-producing factors (IPFs). They reside predominantly in the clay (inorganic) or the organic soil fractions or both. The IPFs in the organic and clay fractions of soil can be characterized by their large surface area and high cation exchange capacity. These physical properties of the IPFs insure an active chemical exchange between the wound and the IPFs, which accounts for their deleterious effect.[133] Infection-producing factors also affect leukocytes and thus markedly inhibit the phagocytosis of bacteria. In addition, they inactivate the antibacterial action of natural serum antibodies.[37] It was found that a wound containing as few as 100 bacteria became infected as the result of adding 5 mg. of soil with its associated IPFs,[133] thus illustrating the deleterious effect of soil on wounds.

In the study it was found that of the colloidal clay minerals (montmorillonite, illite, and kaolinite), montmorillonite clay enhanced infection the most. Other inorganic soil components (sand and silt) did not potentiate infection nearly as much as clay. In fact, sand did not impair the tissue's ability to resist infection at all.[133]

The clinical significance of this information is prognostic. For example, a veterinarian can expect a lesser degree of infection in a wound that is contaminated predominantly with sand than in one that is heavily contaminated with clay.

WOUND FLUID, LYMPH, AND LEUKOCYTES

Even though it is generally accepted that a collection of fluid in a wound is an ideal culture medium that increases the risk of infection, there appear to be reasons to question this concept. As reported by Hohn and associates, investigators have demonstrated a potent heat-labile bactericidal activity in blood and serum. Others have shown that this antibacterial effect was due in part to a serum protein of high molecular weight that is related to the properdin systems. Still others have attributed this antibacterial effect to a natural or a specific antibody in the presence of complement. Gram-negative bacilli were the organisms most susceptible to these antibody-complement or properdin-mediated bactericidal systems. In addition to these heat-labile factors, blood sera from various mammals are capable of heat-stable antimicrobial activity against a variety of bacteria, and the active substances have been called β-lysins. Investigators have found these to be primarily effective against gram-positive organisms, with gram-negative bacteria and fungi being relatively resistant to the β-lysins.[64]

A study has examined and compared the survival rate of bacteria and of fungi in both human blood serum and wound fluid. Data from this study revealed that wound fluid is not an "ideal culture medium" and that human cell-free wound fluids contain proteins that kill or inhibit the growth of bacteria in vitro. These proteins appeared to be active against *Escherichia coli* and *Staphylococcus aureus*. The wound fluids showed either a bacteriostatic or a weak bactericidal activity against *Staphylococcus aureus* and the most striking antibacterial activity against *Escherichia coli*. The strain used in the study was rapidly killed by wound fluid. This was attributed to both heat-labile and heat-stable antibacterial substances in the fluid. The effect of the blood sera on the two organisms was not as marked.[64]

As reported by Hohn and colleagues, Martinez has found that human thoracic duct lymph contains multiple factors with different killing specificities for different types of bacteria. These antibacterial factors in cell-free lymph are complement-dependent and similar to those of β-lysin. After bacteria invade tissues, they are not bathed by blood serum but by the interstitial lymph fluid that is present at the portal of entry.[64]

In addition to the aforementioned antibacterial factors, leukocytes in wounds have been found to have bactericidal capacities.[64]

The antibacterial properties of fluid, lymph, and leukocytes in a wound are undoubtedly beneficial in helping to avert wound infection; however, it would still be advisable to prevent the accumulation of wound fluids within the dead spaces of a wound.

OTHER FACTORS

There are numerous other factors that predispose a wound to infection, including the following: (1) poor blood supply to the wound (see section on condition of tissues); (2) tissue injury (see section on condition of tissues); (3) contamination (see section on bacteria); (4) dead space and fluid accumulation;[17, 37] (5) foreign bodies;[17, 37] (6) dehydration;[78] (7) shock;[78] (8) malnutrition and hypoproteinemia;[46, 78] (9) exhaustion;[78] (10) uncontrolled diabetes;[78] (11) anemia;[46, 78] (12) systemic steroid therapy;[46] (13) irradiation and cytotoxic drugs;[46] (14) tension on the tissues;[17] (15) a poor surgical technique, including failure to remove devitalized tissue and inadequate hemostasis, which provides a pabulum for bacterial growth.[46, 163] The longer any of these factors that predispose the wound to infection is present, the greater are the chances of infection.[17] Some of these factors are discussed further in Chapter 3.

Factors that increase a wound's resistance to infection include the following:

1.   Correction of any of the previously stated problems is beneficial.
2.   Early ambulation has been advocated to enhance wound healing,[76]

since confinement usually results in catabolic rather than anabolic metabolism.[46]

3. Time can also work in favor of wound healing. A study has shown that during healing, wounds that were closed primarily or by delayed closure became increasingly resistant to infection. Likewise, the susceptibility of an open wound to infection decreased progressively during healing.[38]

EARLY WOUND MANAGEMENT

By the time many wounds are seen by the surgeon, they are often needlessly contaminated by an overzealous first aid attempt. The sight of blood arouses the overwhelming urge to "do something." Considerable restraint is required to do nothing more than apply a dressing at the scene of the accident.[66] Antiseptics, ointments, and powders should not be applied to wounds because of the possibility of further contamination and chemical injury to the tissues. Ointments increase the difficulty of final washing and débridement of the wound.[78] The early topical spraying of large, contaminated crush wounds with tetracycline or neomycin plus bacitracin has been advocated. This is not a substitute for débridement, but it helps to retard bacterial growth until débridement can be accomplished.[77, 100, 101] A degloving injury on the forelimb of a dog into which had been poured dehorning powder is an extreme and actual example of added chemical injury. The caustic effect of the powder only complicated an already severe injury.

The application of tourniquets is falling into disfavor except in the case of snakebite. The harm that results from improper tourniquet application outweighs the advantage. If venous flow is stopped without the occlusion of arterial flow, bleeding from an open wound on an extremity may become more profuse until the tourniquet is released. In addition, a tourniquet that is applied too tightly may cause irreparable damage to the underlying neurovascular structures.[77] During times of intermittent tourniquet release, blood loss may be extensive and underestimated.[33]

Ideally, there should be minimal interference with a wound before definitive treatment is undertaken. A large occlusive dressing of dry gauze or an improvised bandage of clean linen that is held firmly in place will help to protect the wound, prevent further contamination, and stop all but the most torrential hemorrhage. Continued bleeding is usually due to the failure to pack a cavity into which an artery is spurting.[37, 77]

When dealing with open wounds, the veterinarian should instruct his clients on how to care for the wound prior to bringing the animal to the clinic. This insures that further trauma is not inflicted on the tissues prior to definitive care.

WOUND PROTECTION AND PREPARATION OF THE SURROUNDING AREA

Protection of the wound is essential while preparing the surrounding area. The most popular technique for protecting the wound is to pack it with moistened sterile gauze sponges.[8, 13, 22, 66, 82, 95] Other protective measures include temporary closure of the wound with towel forceps,[8] Michel wound clips,[8, 32] Allis' forceps,[8] or a continuous silk suture.[32] A disadvantage of these methods is that they prevent the veterinarian from clipping the animal's hair to the very edge of the wound. Another wound protection technique is to fill the wound with a sterile, water-soluble, lubricating substance* (Fig. 4–1). After preparing the surrounding area, the substance is wiped or washed from the wound along with any foreign material (e.g., hair or soap) that has adhered to it.

An ample area around the wound is clipped with electric clippers, preferably in the presence of a vacuum suction system. Hair at the wound edges may be trimmed with scissors that have been dipped in mineral oil. This causes the hair to stick to the scissor blades instead of dropping into the wound.[85] It is wise to have a separate pair of clippers to use exclusively for preparing infected wounds. This will help prevent possible contamination of elective surgical sites.

After clipping the area, the gauze sponges that had been used to pack the wound should be discarded and replaced with fresh sponges.[95] Various surgical scrub solutions and soaps are available for scrubbing the skin around the wound. Currently, a povidone-iodine scrub solution† is popular, and a new surgical scrub containing 2 per cent chlorhexidine diacetate in a stable base‡ has recently been reported to be useful. This scrub solution is capable of immediate and residual activity against gram-positive bacteria *(Staphylococcus aureus)* and gram-negative organisms *(Escherichia coli).* Following a two-minute scrub, the chlorhexidine solution was found to be comparable in

---

*K-Y Jelly is manufactured by Johnson & Johnson, New Brunswick, NJ 08903.

†Betadine Surgical Scrub is available from the Purdue Frederick Co., Norwalk, CT 06856.

‡Nolvasan Surgical Scrub is manufactured by Fort Dodge Laboratories, Inc., Fort Dodge, IA 50501.

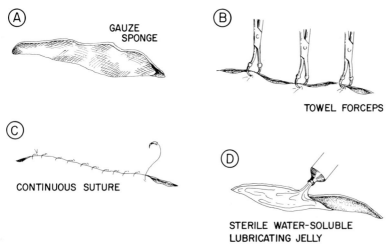

Figure 4–1: Techniques to protect a wound while the surrounding area is prepared for surgery. *A*, Packing the area with a moist, sterile gauze sponge. *B*, Closing the wound with towel forceps. *C*, Closing the area with a simple continuous suture. *D*, Filling the wound with a sterile water-soluble lubricating substance, which will be washed away following skin preparation.

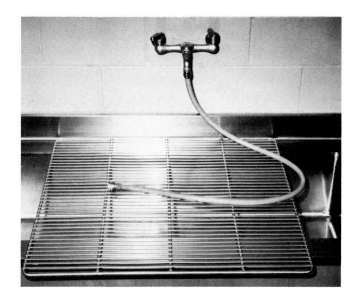

Figure 4–2: A tub with a grill work top and an adjacent water hose that is used to bathe grossly soiled animals prior to wound débridement.

activity to that of povidone-iodine against the aforementioned organisms. In tests of residual activity, the chlorhexidine solution was found to be superior to povidone-iodine against *Escherichia coli* and *Staphylococcus aureus*. This scrub has also been reported to retain a high degree of antibacterial activity in the presence of organic matter.[116]

The scrub solution should be utilized in the usual manner for preparing skin for aseptic surgery.[22] Scrubbing for five to ten minutes has been advocated.[33, 66]

Certain special preparations are necessary in some cases. If the animal is grossly soiled, a bath is indicated. A tub with a grill work top is useful (Fig. 4–2). Bathing is essential because a heavy, dirty hair coat that is soaked with exudate can complicate postoperative care.[8] Before preparing the area around wounds on the head, an eye ointment should be instilled to protect the cornea and conjunctiva.

When used, skin antiseptics should be carefully applied so that they do not enter the wound. The area is then surgically draped, leaving adequate room to extend the incision as necessary.[33, 66]

WOUND DÉBRIDEMENT

HISTORY

Cautery by fire was an early method of wound treatment. Hippocrates and later Galen perpetuated this ancient method, which was destined to persist until the 15th century. Galen fostered the notion that suppuration was essential to the healing process. This favorable regard for suppuration was not successfully challenged for nearly 14 centuries.[66]

Pierre Desault was responsible for recognizing the role of excision as a fundamental principle in treating accidental wounds. The earliest description of débridement is attributed to him.[154]

Although it had been described before the American Civil War, débridement has been stated to be the main advance in local wound therapy since that time. The technique was largely perfected during World War I and its worth was proved again during World War II.[101]

A very simple and usually very effective form of débridement occurs when a person immediately and instinctively inserts a minor cut on a finger into the mouth.[17] A similar instinctive attempt at débridement is seen in animals when they lick their wounds. The mechanics of licking undoubtedly help to remove foreign bodies and devitalized tissue from the wound; however, one must also consider the potential antibacterial effect of the basic enzyme lysozyme that is present in saliva.

DÉBRIDEMENT VS. EXCISION

The term excision has been used to describe the conversion of a wound that is not yet infected to a wound that is suitable for immediate or delayed closure. This is done by removing dead and devitalized tissue and by lavage. The term débridement has been used to describe the process that is applied to an infected wound, which includes adequate surgical drainage to remove the products of infection.[8, 22, 33] Over the years, the two terms seem to have become synonymous, and as one author has stated, " . . . it is too late to return to the more exact nomenclature."[66] With that understanding in mind, the term débridement will be used in this text.

ANESTHESIA

Patients with traumatic tissue injuries usually experience marked pain, usually at the site of injury. Cleansing the wound without anesthesia will cause further pain. The patient's natural response is withdrawal, making cleansing impossible.[37] Regional, local, or general anesthesia is indicated.

A local anesthetic agent is injected into the intact skin of the periphery of the wound with a small (27-gauge) needle. One per cent lidocaine is routinely used, since it does not impair tissue defenses or favor infection. Careful consideration should be given to the use of vasoconstrictors such as epinephrine as adjuncts to local anesthetics, especially when they are to be used in areas where the segmental blood supply is critical.[37, 117] Vasoconstrictors exert deleterious effects on tissue defenses and potentiate infection. The inhibition of tissue defenses by epinephrine can be neutralized by phentolamine, an agent that blocks the vasoactive effect of epinephrine.[37] Other disadvantages of local anesthesia include the possible dissemination of organisms through previously uncontaminated tissue planes and the possibility that the anesthesia will be limited and thus prevent wide exploration of the area. These disadvantages would be indications for using regional blocks or general anesthesia if the patient's condition will tolerate it.[33]

The author has found it beneficial to initially lavage a wound with a 2 per cent lidocaine solution. The patient appears to be more comfortable with this technique while the wound is being irrigated and manipulated to remove foreign bodies (e.g., grass, sand, and dirt). This type of topical anesthesia is insufficient for surgical débridement.

No one method is superior in all situations. The surgeon should consider the type of wound and the patient's condition in determining the most suitable type of anesthesia.

GENERAL PRINCIPLES AND OBJECTIVES

Standardization of the débridement technique is difficult, since the procedure must vary according to the type of wound, the traumatic agent, and the environment. Each wound has an individuality that will tax the surgeon's ingenuity.[66] For example, débridement of a wound that is produced by an animal's jumping through a plate glass door will be altogether different from débridement of a wound that is produced by the crushing and degloving forces of an automobile tire.

When dealing with a wound involving extensive tissue damage, certain factors should be considered. Thorough exploration may be needed to reveal the extent of the wound.[33] Thus, the skin incisions should be long enough to bare the full extent of deep tissue lacerations.[22, 66] On the limbs, skin incisions should be parallel to the long axis of the limb if possible. "Z"-shaped incisions are advisable across flexion surfaces.[66] Likewise, all fascial envelopes must be opened widely enough to expose the wound depths from end to end,[22] which helps to relieve tissue tension that is due to swelling.[8]

Two basic techniques have been described for wound débridement: (1) layered débridement,[8, 66] and (2) en bloc débridement.[66, 117] Layered débridement is advocated and involves removing devitalized tissues beginning at the surface of the wound and progressing to the wound depths (Fig. 4–3). The amount of material removed is not as extensive as that removed with en bloc débridement. This technique should be used on lesions of the limbs and feet, since moderate excision is indicated in areas where there is not much large muscle mass.[66]

En bloc or complete excision may be used in areas where there is excess tissue and has been described as the simplest and most certain way to assure elimination of damaged and contaminated tissues. One technique for ac-

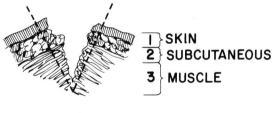

SKIN 1
SUBCUTANEOUS 2
MUSCLE 3

Figure 4–3: Layered wound débridement beginning at the surface of the wound, *1*, and progressing to the wound depths, *2* and *3*. (After Archibald, J., and Blakely, C. L.: Basic procedures and preoperative considerations, in Canine Surgery, ed. 2. Santa Barbara, Calif., American Veterinary Publications, Inc., 1974, p. 30.)

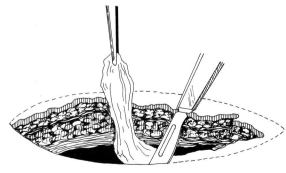

complishing this procedure is to pack the wound cavity with gauze and to place several sutures in the overlying skin to hold the gauze in the wound. The entire wound is then treated as a tumor (imagining the gauze to be the tumor mass). The mass is excised with a margin of normal tissue so that the gauze is never exposed (Fig. 4–4).[117]

It is generally accepted that wound débridement involves the removal of devitalized, contaminated, and dead tissue. If the necrotic material is not removed, it prolongs the healing process and provides a favorable environment for bacterial proliferation.[78] By removing this avascular substrate, bacterial proliferation is interrupted and the bacteria that do remain are incapable of multiplication when subjected to the defenses of viable tissue.[66]

During wound débridement all incisions should be made with a sharp scalpel.[33, 37, 76, 78, 85, 99] A study has shown that wounds made with a sharp blade are significantly more resistant to bacterial infection than wounds made with either electrical current or continuous-wave laser. Incisions made with the last two methods are bloodless, but devitalized tissue surrounds the entire area of incision.[37, 99] Another study has shown that the strengths of wounds made by a sharp blade are greater than those made by electroincision by six days after incision, and the strengths were approximately doubled from the tenth to the 12th day.[84]

Factors requiring attention during wound débridement are (1) the removal of foreign bodies from the wound; (2) adequate hemostasis; (3) the restoration of normal structure; (4) adequate lavage of the area during débridement; and (5) drainage of dead space, including counterincisions to drain deep pockets.[8, 22, 33, 66, 163]

The following should be avoided during wound débridement: (1) prolonged pressure and tearing by retractors; (2) massive ligatures, with large necrotic protions of tissue distal to the ligature; (3) plugs of necrotic tissue from electrocoagulation; and (4) extensive exploration that breaks down

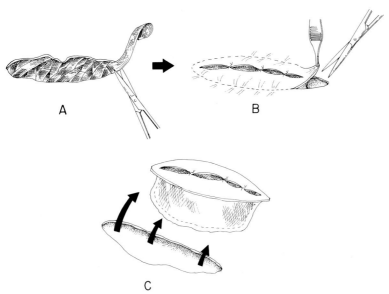

Figure 4–4: En bloc wound débridement. *A*, The wound is packed with gauze. *B*, The skin edges are temporarily sutured, and the wound is excised in the fashion of a tumor excision with a margin of normal tissue, *C*, so that the gauze is never exposed.

natural barriers to the spread of infection[8, 78] (e.g., caudal probing of a wound at the base of the neck, which could lead to intrathoracic infection via the thoracic inlet).

ASEPSIS AND DÉBRIDEMENT

Asepsis is important in wound management, and all wounds other than minor wounds should be treated in an operating room with all of the precautions that are taken with major surgery.[8, 66] Wounds are contaminated at the time of presentation to a hospital; however, it is important to remember that organisms introduced from within the hospital may be much more virulent than the original organisms.[66] Discussions that take place over wounds carry the danger of saliva droplet contamination of the wound. The bacteria from the ungloved hands of the examiner can easily contribute to infection. Regarding human surgery, it has been said, "The eleven most common causes of emergency room wound infections are the nasopharynx and ten fingers of the examiner."[37] The same holds true for veterinarians and veterinary hospitals.

To help prevent in-hospital wound contamination, the ideal course would include the use of surgical scrub, gowns, gloves, sterile drapes, and sterile instruments.[32, 37, 66, 82] The author tries to emphasize at least the use of gloves and masks to students handling accidental wounds. During the wound débridement procedure, the use of more than one set of sterile surgical instruments has been advocated.[32] Thus, as the procedure progresses, the wound is not continually contaminated by the instruments that were used in the earlier stages of the procedure. In lieu of using several sets of surgical instruments, the surgeon may use only one set, but the contaminated instruments that were used early in the procedure should be laid aside, thereby insuring that they will not be reinserted into the wound in the later stages of débridement.

SPECIFIC STRUCTURE DÉBRIDEMENT

Bones and Joints

When soft tissue injury of an extremity is associated with bone damage, splintage of the limb is valuable in preventing further tissue damage and in reducing hemorrhage and pain.[33] Certain basic principles are involved in the definitive care of denuded and fractured bone. Generally, bone encased in periosteum will survive.[33] When débriding a wound, it may be necessary to use a stiff, bristled brush or a bone curette to remove dirt from the ends of fractured bones or even to cut the bone end back a short distance.[22, 81] The following controversial statements have been made concerning the removal of bone fragments from a wound:

1. Remove detached fragments.[33]
2. Even if they are very dirty and detached, scrub and replace them.[17]
3. Remove only the bone that is completely separated from muscle and periosteum.[8]
4. If there are only a few small fragments without soft tissue attachments, remove them. If the fragments are large, replace them even if there is no soft tissue attachment.[22]

Since bone is an essential structure, it is better to err in removing too little than too much.[22] In the author's opinion, one must use clinical judgment in leaving or removing bone fragments, bearing in mind the condition of the surrounding tissues, the amount of contamination and infection, the number and size of the fragments, and the essential need for supportive bone in the area.

The fixation of compound fractures has been described for humans,[22] and the principles apply to animals. If a wound is in satisfactory condition, the use of metal implants to help immobilize bone fragments is permissible. However, such implants are contraindicated if extensive wound dissection is necessary to place them. Such dissection increases the chance of infection spreading from the original wound site. For example, placing an intramedullary pin in a compound-fractured femur would be contraindicated in the presence of infection.

One method for débridement joints entails a meticulous technique that includes wide arthrotomy, removal of debris and cartilage fragments, replacement of large articular fragments only, and closure of the capsule and ligaments without drainage.[66] The joint capsule should be closed with fine absorbable sutures; however, if the synovial membrane is extensively damaged, closure can be performed using full-thickness or split-thickness skin grafts for temporary coverage. The joints should be immobilized, systemic antibiotics should be given, and crystalline penicillin G potassium should be instilled into the joint.[82]

Tendons

In spite of contamination, tendons should not be sacrificed if they are not severed.[66] Totally exposed tendon that is denuded of paratenon is subject to slough and requires some means of temporary or permanent cover. In many degloving injuries on the limbs of animals, tendons are severed and frayed. In such instances they should be trimmed, and unless circumstances are especially favorable, repair should be deferred.[33] If the avascular ends of tendons are allowed to heal and regain their original vascularity, suturing will be more successful. Moreover, it is not always possible to determine how much of a tendon should be débrided initially.[77] It is not uncommon for tendons to be so severely severed and frayed that repair is impossible.

In small animals the superficial digital tendons are not as vital to the animal as the deep tendons, and some surgeons prefer not to repair them. If a flexor tendon is injured, it is best to immobilize the affected joint in full flexion; if an extensor tendon is involved, the converse is true.[137]

It has been stated that devitalized tendons, ligaments, and fasciae are less likely to result in infection, and they often act as a matrix for new fibroblastic activity. Owing to this property, they are often left in a wound rather than removed at the time of débridement.[46]

Muscle

Muscle tissue is considered nonviable if it appears "mushy" or friable, does not bleed when cut, does not contract when mechanically stimulated, has dirt ground into it, or is darker or paler in color than surrounding tissues.

Excision should be carried out until the exposed muscle reacts as healthy muscle tissue should.[8, 17, 33, 66, 85, 95] Muscle that bleeds but does not twitch when pinched is viable and should be trimmed of lacerated ends and separated fibers.[22]

In general, the excision of nonviable muscle should be radical, following the premise, "When in doubt, cut it out." Large masses of muscle are expendable in most areas, and it is better to sacrifice the muscle initially than to chance liquefaction necrosis and possibly the multiplication of clostridial organisms in the wound later.[17, 33] Healthy muscle tissue heals rapidly.

Dye tests for muscle viability have been described.[102, 153] An intravenous injection of sulphan blue or Kiton-fast green stains viable tissues and leaves avascular tissue unchanged. Maximum tissue staining is attained in three to five minutes, and the dye is excreted in about 48 hours by the kidneys.[153]

Five per cent methylene blue has been sprayed on the open wounds of rabbits from a distance of 15 cm. for five seconds. Color changes in the wound began between 30 and 60 minutes and reached a period of accuracy at 90 minutes postspraying. At this time, nonviable muscle was a deep blue, while viable muscle was a homogeneous light blue.[102]

Nerves

Nerves that are not severed should be cleansed gently and covered.[66] Definitive nerve repair should not be performed during wound débridement when nerves have been severed in association with contamination and trauma of the surrounding tissues.[33, 66, 77, 151] As with tendons, there may be damage on either side of the severance that cannot be visualized at the time of initial examination.[77] Temporary anastomosis of the nerve ends with a colored suture material may be performed to prevent their retraction. After the wound has healed (approximately 21 days later), the nerve may be reexposed and examined. At this time the area of interstitial damage and degeneration on either side of the point of severance can be removed, leaving viable nerve tissue for anastomosis.[151]

In some instances, definitive nerve repair may be performed at the time of initial examination. This would be in cases in which there is little surrounding soft tissue trauma and contamination (i.e., a clean laceration). As one author stated, "Those which are cut may be carefully repaired if the wound is clean, treatment is immediate, anastomosis is possible without tension, and sufficient coverage is available."[66]

Blood Vessels

In the dog, injured blood vessels seldom require more than ligation. Large vessels may be sutured; however, this is generally not necessary unless the collateral circulation has been compromised.[137] A study on dogs has shown that the collateral vessels are adequate to supply the forelimb following sudden and complete occlusion of the primary artery and vein of the thoracic limb. Hence, it appears that the clinician need not hesitate to ligate and sever the brachial vessels distal to the deep brachial branches and proximal to the bicipital branches if the need arises provided collateral vessels are intact.[27]

Similar results were reported for the pelvic limb of the dog. It was concluded that when primary collateral vessels are intact and healthy and when the dog is not in shock and has not suffered excessive blood loss, anemia, or severe cardiac insufficiency, the femoral vessels may be ligated if the need arises.[28]

Fascia

If the venous return is impaired in a structure, swelling will result. This, in turn, further occludes the vessels and results in more swelling, setting up a cycle. In such cases, it may be necessary to make full-length fascial as well as skin incisions in the area to help relieve the swelling of the limb. The aftereffects of fasciotomy are minimal.[33]

When débriding fascia, loose, ragged fragments are excised along with 5 mm. of healthy fascia.[33] Fascia is relatively avascular in its normal state and is particularly susceptible to bacterial colonization.[17]

Fat

Fat is easily devascularized and acts as a good bacterial growth medium. Contaminated fat should be liberally excised back to a healthy plane that is free of blood stains.[3, 110]

Hematomas and Seromas

As excision proceeds, tissues will begin to bleed. If there is no hemorrhage, excision has probably been inadequate. Much of the hemorrhage can be temporarily controlled by pressure packing and will have ceased by the end of the procedure; however, spurting vessels and larger veins require ligation.[33] Small-gauge stainless steel and 3–0 catgut have been advocated for ligatures.[85] The author prefers 2–0 or 3–0 beige polyglycolic acid (P.G.A.) sutures for ligation. Grasping bleeders with hemostats and touching the tip of the hemostat with an electrocautery is another means of achieving hemostasis.[85]

Insufficient hemostasis may result in a hematoma that acts as a mass of devitalized tissue.[33] It prevents proper apposition of tissues. If the hematoma is large, it can interfere with the blood supply to adjacent tissues. If it is slow to be absorbed, rigid-walled cavities containing encapsulated fluid can result.[78]

Seromas may result from (1) improperly closed dead space, (2) transection of tissue that is rich in lymphatics, (3) considerable movement of the wound, and (4) the presence of a large amount of surgical gut or other foreign material in the wound. Seromas can be prevented by (1) atraumatic techniques, (2) ligation of vessels (including lymphatics), (3) obliteration of dead space, (4) drains, and (5) compression bandages.[78]

Skin

Flaps. Clinical experience has shown that venous return, not arterial supply, is the critical factor in skin flap survival. When damaged skin is lost because of vascular insufficiency, it usually becomes turgid and dark in color. This is due to trapped blood, and restoration of venous drainage is the key to flap survival. When testing a skin flap for viability, a sharp line of color demarcation that indicates normal circulation on one end and abnormal circulation on the other is the single most important clinical observation. A flap that is a little dusky on one end but in which there is no such single point or clear line of color demarcation probably has adequate venous return. However, a sharp line of demarcation with normal color on one end and cyanosis on the other end is an undesirable sign.[117] Likewise, a skin flap that is unduly pale or bruised should be excised, since its vessels have probably been thrombosed by injury.[33] The removal of all fat from the back of a flap, followed by the excision and placement of the flap over the defect as a skin graft has been described.[13, 33] This may be performed with large, thick, devitalized flaps or partially avulsed but not contused flaps.

The tourniquet test for tissue viability has been described.[117] This test works on the principle that ischemia that is produced in an extremity by applying a proximal arterial tourniquet results in the release of various tissue amines almost immediately after the tourniquet is removed and arterial flow is reestablished. The amines can cause the closure of precapillary shunts or the opening of capillary networks or both. The result is "blushing" of the tissue for three to five minutes, after which it becomes cyanotic. This would indicate adequate circulation in the flap. However, the short period of venous congestion after the "blush" may promote thrombus formation that could be detrimental to tissue survival.[117]

Skin Edges.   Badly damaged skin edges without capillary oozing should be removed, keeping in mind that skin is precious and essential to wound closure.[17, 22] Usually, only a narrow skin margin (3 mm.) needs to be excised. However, extensively contused or undermined edges and evidence of fire or chemical damage are exceptions. Although closure will be easier if more skin is saved, skin whose viability is questionable is of no use for closure and may be the starting point for infection. If there is doubt, the wound should be inspected after 48 hours, by which time the death of the tissues will be evident and secondary excision can be undertaken.[33]

In wounds of some duration, the basal cells of the epidermis may have grown downward over the cut edge of the dermis. Suturing such edges together apposes epidermis to epidermis and healing cannot take place. Cutting a narrow strip from the skin edge is necessary before suturing.[32]

A recent report has stated that freshening the skin edges is an archaic technique and should be avoided. It was stated that skin edges that are not bleeding and are of normal color should not be excised, even in a wound several days old. The rationale for this is that healing has already started and excising the skin edge removes active cells, retarding the healing rate by several days. The exception should be the jagged wound edges that could be straightened by excision, thus facilitating closure.[95] In spite of this theory, when dealing with a wound of some duration, the author prefers to trim the skin edges in the interest of cosmesis. It is easier and produces more cosmetic results to suture squarely trimmed skin edges than to suture rounded, untrimmed skin edges.

FOREIGN BODIES

If foreign material in a wound enhances infection or causes irritation, the wound rarely heals until the material is removed or extruded. This is an example of so-called tissue intelligence, which prevents the formation of deep and spreading infection in the body. As long as the sinus from the foreign body to the surface remains open, the foreign body does no harm; however, when it seals over, a deep-seated abscess results.[78] A study has indicated that the amount of inflammation and abscess formation is directly related to the amount of foreign material present in the wound.[57]

The physical properties of the foreign material have an effect on the intensity of the body's reaction to them. Insoluble foreign bodies such as glass, gravel, and carbon particles can be inert, and if not contaminated with bacteria, they may remain in the tissues with little or no reaction. Porous materials are less well tolerated than solid and impervious ones. This is demonstrated by the body's ability to tolerate a monofilament suture better than a twisted or braided suture.[78]

The chemical composition of a foreign body also has an effect on the degree of tissue reaction. Strong acids and alkalis can cause burns, and many salts are locally or systemically poisonous. Organic materials, such as grass, straw, clothing of natural fibers, and wood, are not tolerated even if they are sterile. Talcum powder used on sterile rubber gloves is relatively insoluble and can lead to granuloma formation. To obviate the dangers of talc granulomas, a treated powder derived from corn starch has been introduced.[78]

Metallic foreign bodies may or may not cause a tissue reaction. Some metals are initially tolerated by the body, but a delayed reaction to their presence may occur. Iron may corrode, or sharp objects, such as steel needles, can migrate through tissues as a result of muscle movement and may penetrate vital organs. In other instances, objects resting against bone, blood vessels, or skin can cause erosion by pressure.[78] Bullets and shell fragments generally cause little tissue reaction. They are removed when encountered during surgery but are not diligently searched for unless they are obviously adjacent to a vital structure (near a blood vessel or a nerve or in a joint). Consequently, some restraint should be used in the search for elusive metallic foreign bodies.[17, 66]

WOUND LAVAGE

HISTORY AND BASIC FACTS

It appears to be a basic instinct of man to pour solutions into open wounds. This procedure goes back to antiquity, when various antiseptic solutions, including wine, alcohol, vinegar, and turpentine were used.[34]

There is a difference between just pouring an antiseptic solution into a wound and actually lavaging the wound. Irrigation floats away debris and separated particles of tissue, in addition to either removing, diluting, or reducing the number of bacteria within a wound.[22, 95] The volume of irrigating solution is important. A study has shown that increasing the volume of the irrigating solution decreases the incidence of infection.[146] The addition of antibiotics to the irrigating solution is beneficial, since all of the surface bacteria are more likely to be exposed to the solution than to be washed away.[142] A stated disadvantage of wound lavage is that it may obscure the extent of contamination and spread infection.[8]

In addition to the mechanical and antibacterial factors associated with wound lavage, time plays a role. A study has shown that a four-hour delay between contamination and lavage significantly increases the incidence of infection when compared with that of wounds that were lavaged one hour after contamination. This greater incidence of wound infection was effectively reduced by freshening the wounds before irrigation with normal saline solution.[146]

MODERATE-PRESSURE LAVAGE

Moderate-pressure wound lavage in the form of a thin stream of fluid has been stated to be more effective in cleaning wounds than simply flooding the wound with large quantities of fluid. This should be done by the systematic exploration of interstices, hidden planes, and pockets. A mild-pressure lavage may be accomplished by fluid whose flow is governed by gravity from an overhead enema can through rubber tubing, on the end of which is fitted a medicine dropper tip.[17] Other means of moderate-pressure wound lavage are a bulb-type syringe that exerts gentle pressure[85] or a 35-ml. syringe and a 19-gauge needle.[37] The latter apparatus delivers about 7 p.s.i. of pressure to the wound. Some recommend the ejection of surface contaminants by a turbulent swirl of liquid rather than by high-pressure lavage.[117]

HIGH-PRESSURE LAVAGE

Without Antibiotics

The use of continuous and pulsating high-pressure jets of irrigating fluids has been described for wound lavage.[17, 57, 76, 132, 157] Continuous high-pressure lavage at 10 to 15 p.s.i. has been found to remove about 84.8 per cent of the IPFs of soil from wounds. Pulsatile lavage and continuous high-pressure lavage at the same pressures have been found to be equally effective in the removal of bacteria.[132]

A Water Pik* is the device that is used for pulsating high-pressure lavage of wounds.[17, 57, 76] It has been used at 70 p.s.i. for 30 seconds, with the jet held approximately 5 cm. from the wound. This yielded approximately 4.0 gm. of force per square millimeter of tissue. The result of such lavage was a much more effective reduction in the bacterial population and a more complete removal of necrotic tissue and foreign particles than was obtained by irrigating similar wounds with a bulb syringe.[57]

The pressure at which irrigation fluid is delivered to the wound seems to be the most important determinant of successful decontamination.[132] Only by increasing the pressure can a sufficient number of bacteria be removed from a heavily contaminated wound to prevent infection.[37]

Concern has been expressed that high-pressure pulsating lavage may damage cells and tissues as well as drive bacteria into the tissues.[117] A study has shown that fluids are disseminated into adjacent tissues of the wound, predominantly in a lateral direction within the loose areolar tissue. Bacteria did not accompany the fluid and were apparently filtered out by the surface

---

*Water Pik is manufactured by Teledyne Aquatic Corp., Fort Collins, CO. 80521

tissues. Some tissue injury does occur that impairs defenses, making the wound more susceptible to infection. However, the outstanding cleansing capacity of high-pressure lavage appears to outweigh this side effect, since heavily contaminated wounds that were subjected to this treatment healed primarily without infection.[157] As stated in Jenning's work, the Water Pik has been shown to be three times more effective than a bulb syringe in removing tissue fragments and seven times more effective in removing bacteria from a wound.[76]

With Antibiotics

The addition of vancomycin and streptomycin to pulsed high-pressure irrigating fluids appears to be extremely efficient in treating contaminated wounds. This method resulted in a reduction in the incidence of wound infection when compared with the incidence of infection of control wounds that were lavaged only with saline solution.[30] As stated in Jenning's work, the addition of a combination of penicillin and streptomycin is five times more effective than water alone.[76]

WOUND LAVAGE SOLUTIONS

Water

Placing a wound under an open water tap (followed by irrigation with sterile saline solution or water) is effective in removing bacteria and tissue debris that are lying free on the surface.[117] The author has used a small shower nozzle on a hose to wash gross debris from massive wounds. When distilled water, sterile water, and tap water were compared as tissue lavage agents, microscopic evaluation revealed that distilled water and sterile water caused more tissue injury than did tap water.[16]

Saline Solution

Sterile isotonic saline solution has been recognized as effective in wound lavage.[8, 66, 119, 145] It does not cause any noteworthy tissue damage during as long as one hour of exposure, except for a tendency to slight edema.[16] The solution not only washes out visible debris but also reduces bacterial contamination by dilution.[66] Gentle irrigation with an isotonic saline solution has been found to be an effective prophylaxis in the treatment of canine incisions contaminated with approximately 110 million *Staphylococcus aureus* organisms. An increase in the volume of the lavage solution from 250 ml. to 1000 ml. further decreased the incidence of wound infection.[119] When feces-contaminated wounds were irrigated one hour after contamination, it was found that the effectiveness of irrigation with saline solution was proportional to the volume of fluid utilized. A four-hour delay between contamination and lavage lessened the success of the treatment.[145]

Others have found lavage with saline solution to be ineffective in the treatment of contaminated wounds.[34] However, in these studies only 100 to 500 ml. of saline solution were used.

Soaps and Detergents

It is generally accepted that soaps and detergents are damaging to wounded tissues. Soaps applied to uncontaminated fresh wounds irritated the tissues but did not significantly alter the wound healing process when compared with that of wounds receiving no soap. However, when soap was placed in wounds that were contaminated with *Staphylococcus aureus,* the wounds had a definite increase in the signs of infection when compared with similar wounds in which no soap had been used.[119] In order to avoid the tissue irritation caused by soap, many practitioners use only physiological saline solution for wound cleansing.[137] Others have advocated washing wounds with soaps; however, this is followed by several rinsings with sterile saline solution.[82] Detergent substances or pHisoHex* should not be used in wounds in which muscles, tendons, or blood vessels are visible because they cause chemical irritation to such structures, with resultant impaired or delayed wound healing.[79] A study has shown that detergents are also harmful to cartilage, synovia, and other soft tissues, and their use could lead to an increased susceptibility to infection, poor wound healing, and a loss of joint function.[40]

Surgical scrub solutions are a mixture of antiseptic agents and surface-active detergents. The antiseptic agent destroys viable bacteria, and the surface-active detergent reduces the surface tension between the wound and its contaminants to facilitate their removal. In addition, the detergents minimize frictional forces between the sponges and the wound surface and solubilize relatively insoluble particles, thus encouraging their removal. Unfortunately, the detergent components of surgical scrubs are toxic to tissues and impair their defenses, thereby potentiating bacterial infection rather than protecting the tissues. This is the case with pHisoHex or Betadine Surgical Scrub.[29, 135, 137]

There have been some interesting findings concerning hexachlorophene and hexachlorophene-containing detergents. One group of investigators has reported that 3 per cent hexachlorophene in saline solution causes almost no injury to wound tissues.[16] However, 3 per cent hexachlorophene has been found to cause a significant loss of cartilage ground substance, and pHisoHex causes severe tissue damage within joints, as does Betadine Surgical Scrub.[40] It is interesting to note that a study conducted in 1960 found that a pHisoHex scrub of feces-contaminated wounds was more beneficial than just instilling the solution into similar wounds and more effective than irrigating such wounds with antibiotics.[146]

One theory maintains that even though soaps are damaging to cells, their action on contaminants outweighs their adverse effects on tissues.[95] The only wound on which the author will use soap or detergent is the granulation tissue bed that is to be removed prior to primary closure.

A new detergent, Pluronic F-68, which is a poloxalene polyol with a high ethylene oxide content (80 per cent), has been described. It has no antibacterial activity; however, it allows wound scrubbing with sponges to remove bacteria, while the detergent protects the tissues from the abrasive action of the sponges.[134, 135] It also has the advantage of solubilizing relatively insoluble elemental iodine to form an iodophor. This complex has the antibacterial

---

*pHisoHex (3 per cent hexachlorophene) is manufactured by Winthrop Laboratories, New York, NY 10016.

activity of iodine and the cleansing properties of poloxalene. An intravenous injection of this solution causes no side effects, indicating that it can be used safely as a wound cleanser.[135]

Antiseptics

It has been stated in various terms[13, 16, 17, 54, 66, 109, 117, 119] and should be remembered by all who treat open wounds that any antiseptic that is strong enough to kill bacteria is also strong enough to kill tissue cells. All too often the urge to "kill germs" overlooks this truth and some toxic substances are poured into wounds. As stated by Peacock and Van Winkle, "...*a biologically oriented surgeon would never select a solution to irrigate a wound which he would not be willing, for instance, to instill into his own conjunctival sac.*"[117]

To demonstrate the detrimental effect that disinfectants have on wound tissues, three zones of injury have been described for untreated healing wounds. Zone I is the tissue defect from which the microvessels are absent. Zone II underlies zone I and is composed of severly damaged tissue with blocked capillaries. Zone III is beneath the second zone and contains vessels in which the blood flow is sluggish. Upon healing, microcirculatory function is restored in zones II and III and capillaries sprout into the tissue defect (zone I), which is being filled with invading cells and matrix material. When a disinfectant is applied to the wound, the injury extends deeper into the tissues. This adds a fourth zone of injury. There are blocked capillaries within zones II and III, and there is sluggish flow in zone IV. A delay in cell division and vascularization of the defect results, and wound healing may be delayed for twice the normal length of time (Fig. 4–5).[16]

Hydrogen Peroxide.   Three per cent hydrogen peroxide is a good cleans-

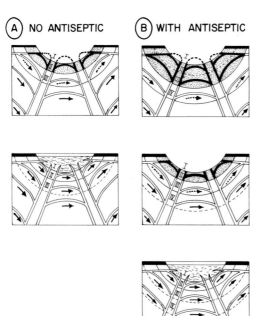

Figure 4–5: Zones of tissue damage and repair. *A,* When no antiseptic is placed on the wound, zone I includes the tissue defect with missing microvessels, zone II is composed of severely damaged tissue with blocked capillaries, and zone III contains vessels in which blood flow is sluggish. During healing, microcirculatory function is restored in zones III and II, and capillaries sprout into the tissue defect. *B,* When disinfectant is applied to the wounds, the injury extends deeper. Zone I *includes* the tissue defect from which the microvessels are absent, zones II and III are composed of blocked capillaries, and zone IV contains vessels in which blood flow is sluggish. During healing, there is a subsequent delay in cell invasion and vascularization of the area, with a resultant delay in wound healing itself. (After Branemark, P. I., Ekholm, R., Albrektsson, J, et al.: Tissue injury caused by wound disinfectants. J. Bone Joint Surg. *49A*:61, 1967.)

ing agent from the standpoint of its mechanical foaming action, which lifts debris and recently clotted blood from the wound. Its oxidizing properties have been reported to have no effect on anaerobic organisms in the wound because of its brief contact with such organisms.[76, 117] Microscopic vascular studies have shown that 3 per cent hydrogen peroxide in distilled water results in almost complete blockage of the microvascular system of the wound. If, however, saline solution is used with hydrogen peroxide, injury is much less pronounced.[16]

Povidone-Iodine. Dilute solutions of povidone-iodine* (not surgical scrub) have been described for cleansing wounds[95] and for promoting the growth of granulation tissue.[63] Various concentrations have been recommended. A 25 per cent solution has been advocated for irrigating surgical wounds; however, this was based on in vitro studies.[141] Ten milliliters in 1 liter of physiological saline solution has been used as a wound dressing on dogs.[63] A 1:100 dilution of povidone-iodine in distilled water has been found to induce only a very slight microscopic reaction in wounded tissue.[16] Povidone-iodine solutions without detergents have been mixed in a 1:1 ratio with sterile saline solution and injected into the joints of rabbits. This produced only minimal histological and no biochemical damage to the joint structure. As a result, povidone-iodine solution was recommended for irrigating and packing open wounds of the joints.[40] The use of undiluted solution has been described in one study.[34] For use in irrigating a wound, the author recommends one of the dilute solutions.

There seem to be conflicting reports on the effect of povidone-iodine in wound healing and in the prevention of sepsis. When used in a powder form, povidone-iodine did not interfere with wound healing in rats, as determined macroscopically, microscopically, and mechanically. Likewise, a clinical study found that povidone-iodine powder did not affect wound healing in any way, and it provided an antibacterial effect.[49] In contrast to this report, another study found that a 10 per cent solution of povidone-iodine was ineffective in reducing the incidence of sepsis in abdominal wounds following surgery. There was a slight increase in wound sepsis in the patients treated with povidone-iodine as compared with that in the control group. It was suggested that povidone-iodine solution may damage the tissue and predispose it to increased susceptibility to infection.[103]

This solution has the following advantages:[31]

1. It controls wound sepsis and may augment wound healing.
2. It has a broad antimicrobial spectrum and is effective in the presence of blood, pus, serum, and necrotic debris.
3. It has no untoward effects when used on mucous membranes or conjunctiva.
4. Its brown color acts as an indicator. When dressings become pale yellow or white, the solution is no longer effective.

Another advantage of povidone-iodine is the absence of bacterial resistance to the drug. A study was done with *Pseudomonas aeruginosa, Escherichia coli, Klebsiella aerogenes,* and *Serratia marcescens.* Following 20 passages under standardized conditions, no significant change was noted in the minimal inhibitory concentration, the minimal bactericidal concentration, or the killing times between parent strains and the 20th subcultures.[67]

---

*Betadine solution is available from The Purdue Frederick Co., Norwalk, CT. 06856.

Chlorhexidine. The chlorhexidine* solution that is most familiar to veterinarians is in the form of an antimicrobial concentrate that is diluted for use. In an in vitro study, the antimicrobial properties of chlorhexidine were compared with those of a quaternary ammonium disinfectant, a phenolic compound, and an iodophor. In general, the chlorhexidine had greater antibacterial activity in relatively high dilutions than the other classes of disinfectants when tested in the presence of nutrient media. It was also found effective against several strains of dermatophytes.[91]

As reported by Buckle and Seabridge, Davies found that chlorhexidine was bactericidal and capable of destroying (99.9 per cent kill) *Staphylococcus aureus*, *Streptococcus pyogenes*, *Escherichia coli*, *Pseudomonas aeruginosa* (*pyocyanea*) and *Salmonella typhi* in concentrations of 1:400,000 (0.00025 per cent); 1:20,000 (0.005 per cent); 1:50,000 (0.002 per cent); 1:17,500 (0.006 per cent); and 1:125,000 (0.008 per cent), respectively.[18] As stated in Grant and Findlay's report, Culman and Murray found that a 0.05 per cent solution (1:40 solution of a 2 per cent concentrate) is effective in killing *Pseudomonas aeruginosa* (*pyocyanea*) after a 2.5-minute exposure in fresh blood (25 per cent blood broth). *Staphylococcus aureus* (*pyogenes*), β-hemolytic streptococcus, and *Escherichia coli* were killed by even weaker concentrations.[54]

From reports it appears that chlorhexidine is nonirritating to wound tissues. In a series of 108 burn patients, topical dressing of the wounds with 0.5 per cent chlorhexidine did not destroy the regenerating epithelium or appreciably delay healing, and wound infection was rare. Likewise, animal wounds have been reported to heal readily when dressed with a 1 per cent chlorhexidine solution. However, repeated applications of a 1 per cent solution to fair skin may cause erythema, and a 0.05 per cent solution is recommended when used as a prophylaxis against infection in wounds. A 1 per cent solution is also reportedly irritating to the nasal mucosa and conjunctiva. As a result, a 0.1 per cent solution is recommended for use on delicate membranes.[54]

In light of the previously stated findings, it would appear that chlorhexidine in concentrations of 0.05 to 1 per cent could be used as an initial wound lavage agent without causing tissue damage. Mucous membranes may be more safely irrigated with a weak solution. The author has had favorable clinical results with the use of chlorhexidine as an initial wound irrigating solution and in cleansing infected wounds. A 0.05 per cent solution (1:40 dilution of the 2 per cent concentrate) is preferred.

In addition to its effectiveness at low concentrations and its relative tissue-saving quality, chlorhexidine has the advantage of being effective against a relatively broad range of gram-negative and gram-positive bacteria in the presence of body fluids. It is also advantageous in that bacteria do not develop a resistance to the solution.[54]

Acetic Acid. Attempts have been made to encourage natural enzyme activity or discourage bacterial growth by changing the pH of a wound surface. An acid pH produced by weak (0.5 per cent) acetic acid has been particularly helpful when urea-splitting organisms are prevalent, especially *Pseudomonas*.[117, 139] However, acetic acid does not affect other organisms, and when applied to wounds with *Staphylococcus aureus* and *Proteus* species, these organisms actually increased in number in many wounds.

---

*Nolvasan is manufactured by Fort Dodge Laboratories, Inc., Fort Dodge, IA 50501.

When a wound infected by *Pseudomonas* was treated with acetic acid, the following organisms either replaced the *Pseudomonas* or were present throughout the treatment: *Staphylococcus aureus*, *Proteus* species, *Streptococcus faecalis*, *Escherichia coli*, and *Streptococcus pyogenes*. When the *Pseudomonas* disappeared, the wound showed clinical improvement in most instances in spite of the presence of other organisms.[120]

Other Wound Lavage Antiseptics.   A study of the effectiveness of various wound-irrigation antiseptics has shown that a single irrigation of a contaminated wound with either 70 per cent ethyl alcohol, benzalkonium chloride, 0.25 per cent chloramine-T, aqueous iodine, povidone-iodine, or gentian violet provides significant protection against the development of infection. The effectiveness of the irrigation did not differ significantly among these solutions. There were minimal inflammatory changes in the contaminated wounds after irrigation, indicating that the bacteria were overwhelmed and minimal tissue damage was produced.[34]

Irrigating solutions of ethyl alcohol (10 and 56 per cent), chloramine-T (0.1 per cent), and carbolic acid (0.5 per cent) were ineffective in the treatment of contaminated wounds. An increased concentration (1 to 10 per cent) of carbolic acid was associated with absorption and death in guinea pigs.[34] Carbolic acid is definitely contraindicated for wound lavage in cats.

Even though silver nitrate is one of the drugs of choice in burn therapy, the results of the study on wound irrigating solutions revealed that a 0.5 per cent solution of silver nitrate potentiated wound infection. It appeared to interfere with tissue defenses and made the wounds more receptive to infection.[34]

WOUND SCRUBBING

There are varying opinions on the effectiveness of scrubbing or swabbing a wound. One theory states that swabbing a wound with saline solution–soaked surgical sponges is beneficial in that it enhances the therapeutic value of both systemic and topical antibiotics by removing bacteria or disrupting the fibrous coagulate covering of the wound.[35] The other theory maintains that mechanical cleansing with a saline solution–soaked sponge impairs the wound's ability to resist infection, with the harmful effect being directly proportional to the coarseness of the sponge used.[19, 34] With the new Pluronic F–68, a poloxalene polyol detergent, the abrasive action of the sponge is minimized and yet bacteria can be removed from the wound. A study comparing wound scrubbing utilizing this new detergent and a sponge and scrubbing utilizing saline solution and a sponge revealed a dramatic reduction in the infection rate of wounds in which Pluronic F–68 was used.[134, 135]

CHEMICAL DÉBRIDEMENT

Nonviable tissue may be removed through digestion by chemical agents. Such agents include dichloramine T and sodium hypochlorite. Damage may occur to viable cells in the area, leading to suppuration and delayed wound closure.[8]

Through the years, drugs containing sulfas and urea have been used for topical wound therapy. These drugs combine the débriding properties of urea with the antibacterial properties of the sulfas and some of the other additives. The author has used such sulfaurea compounds* to débride wounds. In addition to the débriding and antibacterial actions, the powdered form of the compound tends to remove fluid from the tissues. This latter action should be recognized when deciding whether to use this type of therapy. On a small wound that is quite edematous, sulfaurea treatment may be beneficial. However, the surgeon should consider other types of débridement when dealing with a large open wound through which the patient is already losing large quantities of fluids, electrolytes, and protein. A sulfaurea drug may complicate the situation by causing further tissue dehydration.

ENZYMATIC DÉBRIDEMENT

INDICATIONS

There are two general indications for enzymatic wound débridement: (1) Enzymatic agents may be used to débride wounds on patients that are not favorable anesthetic risks for surgical débridement.[65, 144] (2) Enzymatic agents may be used to débride wounds in which surgical débridement could result in injury to healthy tissue.[139] Both of these instances occur in veterinary surgery, and the author is not at all hesitant to utilize enzymatic débridement, especially on infected wounds or in areas of tissue sparsity. Enzymatic débridement is especially suitable for wounds on the limbs, where all available viable tissue will be needed for reconstruction. In such cases the enzyme "decides" what tissue will be removed and what tissue will remain, and the surgeon does not take the chance of removing some questionable tissue that may, with time, revitalize and be useful in reconstruction.

Other specific indications for enzymatic débridement include burns, decubital or vascular ulcers, and pyogenic or traumatic wounds.[65]

ADVANTAGES AND DISADVANTAGES

The advantages of enzymatic débridement are related to the indications. The first advantage is that it allows surgery to be postponed until hospital care improves the patient's status, and thus the patient will be a better surgical risk. The second advantage of this type of this type of débridement is the assurance that healthy tissue and granulations will not be disturbed.[144]

The disadvantages of enzymatic débridement include (1) the expense, (2) the time required to remove dead tissue, and (3) insufficient débriding action.[76, 117]

ENZYMES AND THEIR PROPERTIES

Several types of enzymes are commercially available for wound débridement, with each enzyme or enzyme combination working in its own specific

---

*Sulfaurea powder and creme are manufactured by Norden Laboratories, Lincoln, NE 68501.

TABLE 4–1 EXAMPLES OF SOME PROTEOLYTIC ENZYME DRUGS

Drug	Manufacturer	Active Ingredients
Kymar° ointment, improved	Burns-Biotec Laboratories Div. of Chromalloy Pharmaceutical, Inc. Oakland, CA 94651	Trypsin, chymotrypsin, neomycin palmitate, hydrocortisone acetate
Chymoral,° tablets—50,000 or 100,000 units	Armour Pharmaceutical Co. Scottsdale, AZ 85251	Trypsin, chymotrypsin
Elase,° lyophilized powder, ointment, and chloramphenicol ointment°	Parke-Davis Morris Plains, NJ 07950	Fibrinolysin, desoxyribonuclease (also chloramphenicol in Elase- Chloromycetin ointment)
Dornavac, solution	Merck & Co., Inc. Rahway, NJ 07065	Desoxyribonuclease
Santyl ointment	Knoll Pharmaceutical Co. Whippany, NJ 07981	Collagenase
Varidase, local or topical,	Lederle Laboratories Div. of American Cyanamid Co. Pearl River, NY 10965	Streptokinase-streptodornase
Travase ointment	Flint Laboratories Div. of Travenol Laboratories, Inc. Deerfield, IL 60015	Sutilains
Granulex° aerosol, liquid	Dow B. Hickam, Inc. Houston, TX 77085	Trypsin, balsam of Peru, castor oil
Debrisan, granules	Pharmacia Laboratories Div. of Pharmacia, Inc. Piscataway, NJ 08854	Dextranomer

°These products are currently in use at Auburn University Small Animal Clinic

way (Table 4–1). These enzymes are marketed under various brand names, and the clinician should consult an adequate drug reference source for complete information. Sather and colleagues,[139] in a review work, have summarized the properties of most of the enzymatic débriding agents.

Trypsin-Chymotrypsin

These enzymes are derived from mammalian pancreas glands and have the ability to digest necrotic tissue and pyogenic membranes and crusts.[9, 139] Early studies on trypsin have shown that it lyses fibrinous strands and coagulum on the surface of the lesion. It digests the purulent exudate's slimy and viscid coating of desoxyribonucleoprotein and then attacks the dead tissue of the lesion. With an outpouring of serum, the digested debris is floated away and the exudate becomes thin and serous. With this, viable leukocytes appear. Bacteria rapidly decrease in number and may disappear. The exudate either decreases in amount or disappears as treatment progresses, and a clean granulating surface is left.[125]

Other properties of trypsin include the following:
1. Its activity is optimal within a pH range of 6.8 to 7.5.
2. It is inactive below body temperature.

3.   It can be used with antibiotics and should be used with systemic antibiotics.
4.   It has been reported to cause a mild burning sensation topically.
5.   It loses activity with time.[125]

Although the pancreatic enzymes do not possess bactericidal properties per se, the bacterial flora of wounds has been found to decrease with their use. This is attributed to the action of the enzymes, which remove the debris that supports bacterial proliferation.[125, 144]

An ointment that combines trypsin, chymotrypsin, and neomycin is available; however, this is not the ointment of choice if rapid, active débridement is needed. An antibiotic may not be necessary, and there may be an overgrowth of nonsusceptible microorganisms.[9, 139] A product for veterinary use containing the enzymes neomycin and hydrocortisone acetate is also available. The trypsin and chymotrypsin serve to prepare the area or wound for the maximum anti-infective and anti-inflammatory actions of neomycin and hydrocortisone. As with the neomycin-containing ointment, clinically resistant strains may emerge.[21]

Trypsin and chymotrypsin are also available in enteric-coated tablet form for use in trauma cases; however, specific information on indications for this form is limited. It is contraindicated in cases of septicemia. Even though there have been no reports of it causing the spread of focal infection, an appropriate systemic antibiotic should be given in conjunction with this form of the drug.[9] The author prefers to use it in cases of severe soft tissue trauma with marked edema and inflammation.

An injectable form of chymotrypsin is also available for deep intramuscular injection. This form of the drug serves to (1) reduce inflammation; (2) reduce tissue edema, except for that of renal or cardiac origin or both; (3) prevent edema formation; (4) hasten the absorption of extravasated blood and lymph; and (5) relieve pain and aid in normal healing. The experience of the practitioner should determine whether this drug should be used in conjunction with other therapeutic agents. Though allergic and anaphylactic reactions are uncommon, the practitioner should be aware that they can occur, as with any foreign protein. The frequency of administration may be decreased as the condition improves.[21]

Fibrinolysin-Desoxyribonuclease

The fibrinolysin component of fibrinolysin-desoxyribonuclease ointment is derived from bovine plasma, and the desoxyribonuclease portion is isolated in a pure form from bovine pancreas. This combination of enzymes is said to digest exudates consisting largely of fibrinous material and nucleoprotein. Desoxyribonuclease attacks DNA, and fibrinolysin attacks the fibrin in blood clots and fibrinous exudates. This fibrinolytic activity is directed mainly against denatured protein, such as that found in devitalized tissues, while protein elements in living cells remain relatively unaffected.[9, 139] As with trypsin-chymotrypsin ointments, it has been stated that this agent is relatively ineffective in rapid and active débridement.[139]

Prior to applying the ointment, the wound should be cleansed with water, hydrogen peroxide, or normal saline solution. Dense, dry eschars should be surgically removed. After applying a thin layer of ointment, a nonadherent bandage should be applied and changed at least once, and preferably two or three times, daily. In addition to the plain ointment form, this type of drug is also available as an ointment containing chloramphenicol as a bacteriostatic agent.[9]

Fibrinolysin-desoxyribonuclease is available in a powdered form that may be reconstituted with 10 to 50 ml. of saline solution; this substance may be sprayed on a wound with an atomizer or applied with gauze strips that are saturated with the solution.[9] There is also an enzyme product that is composed of only desoxyribonuclease extracted from beef pancreas. It is available in lyophilized form. After reconstitution with sterile water or saline solution, it may be used as a wound irrigating agent or a wet dressing. It may also be injected into the infected area. The compound degrades desoxyribonucleoprotein, which may constitute 30 to 70 per cent of the total solids of purulent exudate. The degradation of the desoxyribonucleoprotein is a depolymerization reaction and not a complete breakdown. The end products are relatively large and thus less likely to be absorbed. This, along with the increased viscosity of the exudate that is produced by the enzyme, is beneficial in wound therapy.[21]

Collagenase

A collagenase enzymatic débriding agent is derived from the fermentation of *Clostridium histolyticum*. It has the unique ability to digest native as well as denatured collagen.[9, 139] This can be advantageous because the undenatured collagen fibers are involved in the retention of necrotic wound debris and thereby retard wound healing.[139]

Collagenase is primarily indicated for débriding dermal ulcers and burned areas. It is only effective in a pH range of from 6 to 8 and is inhibited by detergents, hexachlorophene, and heavy metal—containing antiseptics but not by antibiotics or hydrogen peroxide. Its ability to work with a physiological pH and temperature range make it particularly effective in the removal of eschar. It contributes to the formation of granulation tissue and the epithelialization of ulcers and burned areas. In addition, it provides a clean base for reconstructive procedures. Prior to the application of collagenase ointment, the area should be cleaned with normal saline solution, a buffer (pH 7.0 to 7.5) substance, or hydrogen peroxide. A neomycin—bacitracin—polymyxin B combination is compatible with the ointment. It can be used in powder or solution form prior to the application of the débriding ointment.[9, 139]

If collagenase comes in contact with normal skin, it has been reported to cause irritation and inflammation, especially around the margins of ulcers. Confinement to the ulcer will reverse this erythema.[9, 139] In the review by Sather and associates, it was stated that a comparative study of enzymatic débriding agents on burns revealed collagenase and papain to be more than 90 per cent effective in the digestion of wound debris and necrotic material.[139]

Sutilains

Sutilains are broad-spectrum natural proteinases derived from *Bacillus subtilis*. They function in a pH range of from 6.0 to 6.8 by degrading and liquefying the complex denatured protein of a necrotic wound to amino acids and acid-soluble peptides. They have minimal collagenolytic activity, which has been stated to be a safety factor for viable tissue.[9, 118, 139] Sutilains have been used advantageously in combination with collagenases. Eschar pretreatment with sutilains reportedly exposes the underlying collagen, which is subsequently broken down by the action of collagenase for the removal of the eschar.[139]

Water with no other additives should be used to clean a wound. This should be followed by a second cleaning with sterile saline solution prior to applying the sutilains agent. Other antiseptics and detergents (i.e., hexachlorophene, silver nitrate, benzalkonium chloride, and nitrofurazone) may inactivate the agent.[9, 65] Neomycin, mafenide (Sulfamylon) acetate, streptomycin, and penicillin do not affect the activity of sutilains.[9] For effective therapy it is advocated that wound dressings to which sutilains have been applied be changed twice a day.[65, 118] and kept moist.[9, 118] Treatment with sutilains should be discontinued if changing the dressing results in hemorrhage from the wound surface (granulation bed).[65]

Sutilains are indicated in second- and third-degree burns, decubital ulcers, incisional, traumatic, and pyogenic wounds, and ulcers secondary to peripheral vascular disease. Sutilains are contraindicated in wounds that communicate with major body cavities, neoplastic ulcers, exposed nerves and nervous tissue, and in the eyes.[9, 65]

The advantages of sutilains include rapid activity, safety, and economy.[65]

Trypsin, Balsam of Peru, and Castor Oil

This drug combination is available as an aerosol and as a liquid. The function of the trypsin is to débride the eschar and other necrotic debris. Balsam of Peru is an effective capillary bed stimulant that increases circulation to an area and provides a mild bactericidal action. The castor oil improves epithelialization by reducing premature epithelial desiccation and cornification. It also acts as a protective covering and an analgesic. The drug should be applied at least twice daily.[9]

This drug combination has been found to be extremely helpful in the healing of decubital ulcers.[160] The author has had favorable results with this compound in treating both early (e.g., infected wounds) and late (e.g., granulating) open wounds. In addition to its other properties, the protective covering that it provides is beneficial in keeping large wound surfaces soft and supple, thereby preventing the discomfort of a hard, dry eschar.

Streptokinase-Streptodornase

Another proteolytic enzyme combination that *may* be applicable in veterinary surgery is the streptokinase-streptodornase combination. It is obtained by cultivating a strain of *Streptococcus*. Streptokinase is known to activate a fibrinolytic enzyme (plasmin) of plasminogen in human serum. Activation of this fibrinolytic system results in the dissolution of blood clots and fibrinous exudates. As stated by Davis in Chapter 5, domestic animals lack adequate quantities of plasminogen (a precursor of plasmin); therefore, it is necessary to add human plasminogen to these enzymes to obtain the desired débriding activity. Streptodornase liquefies the viscous nucleoprotein of dead cells or pus and has no effect on living cells. Thus, the enzymes cause liquefaction of the viscous substances that are associated with the inflammatory or infectious processes, thereby facilitating their drainage. This drug combination is indicated in instances in which clotted blood or fibrinous or purulent exudate occurs following trauma or infectious processes that have led to ulceration or abscess formations.[9, 139]

The débriding agent is prepared by adding 10 to 20 ml. of sterile injectable water or the same quantity of physiological saline solution to a 125,000-unit vial of streptokinase-streptodornase. This provides a solution with about 5000 to 10,000 units of streptokinase and 1000 to 2000 units of streptodornase per milliliter. To be effective, this solution must be kept in contact with the wound by whatever means are feasible (e.g., gauze or other dressing). As an alternative, the contents of one vial may be dissolved with 5 ml. of saline solution and added to a carboxymethylcellulose jelly for topical application. Tetracycline, penicillin, streptomycin, and dihydrostreptomycin are compatible with the streptokinase-streptodornase solution and jelly preparation.[9]

Dextran Polymer

A new dextran polymer in the form of spherical porous beads measuring 0.1 to 0.3 mm. in diameter is available for wound débridement. The beads are formed by a three-dimensional network of dextran polymers that are highly hydrophilic. When placed in a wound, there is a flow of secretions in the interspaces between the beads that carries bacteria and granular substances from the wound into the bead layer. There is little change in pH or ionic strength.[74]

The dextran polymer beads are placed in the wound and covered with an occlusive dressing. When the beads become saturated, they are removed. The wound is cleaned with saline solution and a second dressing is applied, as described earlier. Although absorption starts at the bottom of the bead layer, wound exudate will be removed as long as dry beads are available. After the first few hours of exposure to bacteria, the number of bacteria in the bead layer is decreased, with fewer bacteria at the bottom than at the top.[74]

The advantages of this débriding agent include rapid pain relief after treatment and no allergic reactions.[74]

ANTIBIOTICS IN WOUND THERAPY

HISTORY

The low incidence of wound infection in those who were injured during the attack on Pearl Harbor has been attributed to the light sprinkling of sulfa powder into the wounds shortly after infliction. The confidence in this treatment resulted in inadequate débridement, which frequently occurred during the North African campaign. In addition, the sulfa powder was often dumped into wounds as a bolus, which then served as a foreign body. This type of local chemotherapy was a deterrent to wound healing, and thus the detrimental results that were brought about by the incorrect usage of local chemotherapy discouraged its use altogether. Penicillin became available, and although it had been used locally with apparent good results, it came to be used only systemically.[101]

In 1955 Metzger and Prigot proposed a theory for the use of antibiotics in wound treatment that holds basically true today. This theory stated that topical therapy must be considered an adjunct to the routine management of wound infections and not a replacement mechanism. For maximum benefit, topical therapy should be used in conjunction with mechanical or chemical débridement or both.[106] The present-day use of topical antibiotics in wounds as a defense against infection has encouraged the widespread misconception that wound surgery is currently less important and exacting in the prevention of local infection than it has been in previous years. It is essential that practitioners are aware of what topical antibiotics can and cannot accomplish. They have no effect on progressive tissue necrosis caused by proteolytic enzymes or on the dissolution of hematomas and dead tissue. Antibiotics cannot sterilize the dead tissue in a wound. These detrimental products must be removed by surgery. Antibiotics should be used only to limit invasive infection and to protect against septicemia.[22]

TOPICAL ANTIBIOTICS

Cytotoxicity and Treatment Intensity

The potential cytotoxicity of topical antibiotics and the intensity with which they are administered should be considered when these agents are applied to wounds. Antibiotics can be cytotoxic to host cells and can add to the damage already present in the wound. Therefore, agents should be chosen that have little or no effect on host cells but that still have an antibacterial effect.[46] Other antibiotics have been described for topical use in wounds. Some of these will be covered later in this section. Metzger and Prigot have stated that local antibiotic therapy should be intensive for short periods of time. The prolonged administration of drugs for prophylaxis should be avoided, since resistant flora become quickly established in wounds.[106]

Solutions, Ointments, and Powders

Aqueous solutions are the preferred form for applying antibiotics to wounds. A solvent that is sprayed on a wound may be absorbed or it may evaporate, leaving the antibiotic on the surface of necrosed muscle.[100, 101]

Hydrophilic antibiotic ointments are disadvantageous because they liberate the antibiotic slowly, which reduces its effective concentration. The ointment itself may cause an increase in the growth of anaerobic organisms.[100, 101] Many of the antibiotics available for veterinary use are in ointment form, and the author has not found the previously stated disadvantages to be a serious problem in wound therapy. However, when well-meaning persons place ointments in wounds that still contain foreign material, wound lavage and débridement become difficult.

Antibiotic powders usually contain filler substances and are hygroscopic. They should not be used in wound management.[46] Chlortetracycline and benzocaine, sterile talcum, and sulfa spray powder with urea were found to reduce significantly the tensile strength of experimental wounds in mice after four days of healing. The tensile strength of wounds in mice treated with nitrofurazone powder, however, did not differ from that of wounds of untreated control animals.[126] In general, antibiotic powders should not be used in wounds. In large quantities they can act as a foreign body in the wound. They tend to cake on the surface of a wound and thus shelter underlying bacteria. Powders placed in a wound containing foreign material and necrotic tissue complicate wound lavage and débridement more so than ointments.

Bacitracin, Polymyxin B, and Neomycin

Bacitracin, polymyxin B sulfate, and neomycin sulfate are all bactericidal, and, when used in combination, they can be expected to be effective against virtually the entire spectrum of pathogenic bacteria, especially since high concentrations of the drugs can be achieved locally. These agents, unlike many of the effective systemic antibiotics (especially the penicillins and cephalosporins), pose minimal hazards, either at the time of administration or subsequently.[50]

Bacitracin and polymyxin B could be toxic if given systemically; however, they are absorbed in negligible amounts during wound irrigation. Thus, it may be assumed that these two agents would be of little use in an already infected wound in which organisms had invaded the tissues. In a study on the irrigation of surgical wounds with antibiotic solutions, it was found that a solution composed of bacitracin (50 units/ml.) and polymyxin B (0.95 mg./ml.) was effective in reducing the number of microorganisms after one minute of exposure. The bacitracin solution was prepared by rehydrating the powdered contents of a 50,000-unit vial with 1 liter of saline solution. The polymyxin B solution was prepared by rehydrating the contents of a 50-mg. vial of the drug with 1 liter of saline solution. The two drugs were then mixed to produce the effective wound lavage solution.[142] From these results, it would appear that such a solution would be valuable for lavage in contaminated wounds.

A 1 per cent solution of neomycin has been found to be quite effective as a wound irrigating agent[146] and is preferred by some, since its spectrum of activity is similar to that of the mixture of bacitracin and polymyxin B and since it costs approximately one quarter of the price.[37] Neomycin also has the advantage of being effective against some of the enterobacteria (including the *Proteus* genus) that are not sensitive to polymyxin B. One reported disadvantage of neomycin is its neurotoxicity in some patients.[142]

A study of wounds inflicted during the Viet Nam conflict revealed that two different commercial preparations containing neomycin, bacitracin, and polymyxin B caused a decrease in *Staphylococcus aureus*, coliforms, and enterococci; however, they did not prevent the proliferation of *Pseudomonas* species.[111] The author has encountered similar findings in animals whose wounds were treated with preparations containing the same three drugs. *Pseudomonas* seems to be the problem organism. The author has found 0.1 per cent gentamicin sulfate ointment* to be effective in treating such infections.

---

*Garamycin ointment is manufactured by Schering Corp., Kenilworth, NJ 07033.

DMSO and Gentamicin

A recent report has indicated that dimethyl sulfoxide (DMSO) may potentiate the effectiveness of a topical antibiotic. In this study, wounds in rabbits were contaminated with *Pseudomonas aeruginosa* (10^9/ml.). Three hours after the initial infection, 90 per cent DMSO and gentamicin (5 mg./ml.) were administered topically to one group of rabbits. The control animals received gentamicin (5 mg./ml.) and normal saline solution. It was found that fewer animals that had been treated with DMSO and gentamicin developed bacteremias during the 12 hours of study. In addition, the bacterial counts of these animals decreased by 2 to 3 logs when compared with those of animals treated with the antibiotic alone.[75] This would indicate that DMSO could be a valuable adjunct in the topical antibiotic therapy of wounds.

Kanamycin and Feces-Contaminated Wounds

Research has shown that irrigation of feces-contaminated wounds with a 1 per cent kanamycin solution is as effective in preventing infection as a 1 per cent neomycin lavage.[146] These findings should be of interest to the veterinarian, since many animals seem to have a propensity for getting feces in wounds or on bandages regardless of the wound location.

Time Factor and Topical Antibiotics

The time at which topical antibiotics are applied to a wound can be important in preventing infection. As already mentioned with bacitracin and polymyxin B, these drugs have little effect once the bacteria have invaded the tissues and the wound is classified as infected.[142] In a study in which oxytetracycline was sprayed on contaminated wounds of rabbits, those animals whose wounds were sprayed within five minutes after infliction had the lowest mortality. When wounds were sprayed within one hour of wounding, the animals still had a lower mortality than that of the control animals. However, animals whose wounds were sprayed four hours after infliction had a mortality that was not significantly different from that of the control animals. This suggests the importance of the time factor in the initial use of oxytetracycline spray on the wound: it should be applied immediately after injury, prior to an increase in the bacterial count.[100]

The reason for the lack of antibiotic effect after a time lapse may be explained by the sequence of events occurring within the wound. When a clean wound is left open, an intense inflammatory response is initiated that can limit the beneficial effects of systemic and topical antibiotics. The vessels of such a wound undergo a marked increase in permeability. This allows extravasation of plasma proteins into the wound. The proteinaceous material accumulates and surrounds the bacteria, thus protecting them from contact with the antibiotic.[37] Another theory for the lack of antibiotic effect after a time lapse has been stated by Howes. It was found that contaminated crush wounds in rabbits developed infection if topical treatment with mafenide and streptomycin was delayed beyond three hours, unless the wounds were freshened by débridement. He theorized that many bacteria had entered leukocytes where the antibacterial solution could not reach them unless the leukocytes were destroyed and the bacteria were again freed. Bacteria that were freed but not destroyed were capable of reinitiating infection.[70]

Scrubbing Wounds with Antibiotics

Scrubbing wounds with antibiotics has been found to be beneficial in preventing infection. In one study, wounds on guinea pigs were contaminated with an inoculum of penicillin-resistant staphylococci and a mixture of six species of intestinal bacteria that collectively were resistant to ten commonly used antibiotics. Infections were prevented in these wounds by irrigating and scrubbing them for approximately 90 seconds one hour after contamination. The wounds were scrubbed with a mixture of bacitracin and neomycin or bacitracin, neomycin, and polymyxin B. Even in the presence of silk sutures and strangulated fat, the regimen was effective.[50]

Scrubbing contaminated wounds with a saline solution–moistened gauze sponge at the time of antibiotic treatment has been found to prolong the limited period of antibiotic effectiveness in contaminated wounds that are undergoing delayed closure. The wound scrubbing also enhanced the effectiveness of systemic antibiotics in the treatment of contaminated wounds that were closed primarily. The hypothesis to explain the therapeutic value of scrubbing as an adjunct to antibiotic therapy maintains that scrubbing mechanically cleans the wound by removing the bacteria or disrupting the coagulum covering the contaminated wound or both, thus allowing the drug more intimate contact with the organisms.[35]

Advantages and Disadvantages of Topical Antibiotics

Although topically applied antibiotics are advantageous, they are not a substitute for the proper surgical care and débridement of wounds.[8, 22, 100, 101] The advantages of topical antibiotics include the following:

1. Types and concentrations of antibiotics may be used that would be too toxic for systemic use. These drugs can be placed at the very site where they are needed.[50, 100, 101]
2. Topical antibiotics cause a reduction in the number and growth of bacteria in a wound, prolonging the golden period until débridement can be undertaken.[46, 100, 101]
3. Should débridement be incomplete, antibiotics provide early protection during the wound repair process by destroying bacteria in the necrotic tissue. After this tissue sloughs, bacteria remaining in the wound could multiply and invade the tissues. However, a better blood supply is available at this time, and the dead tissue, which is capable of stimulating a foreign-body reaction, is no longer present.[100, 101]

The primary disadvantage of topical antibiotics is that surgeons tend to rely more on a substance that kills bacteria than on the skill of their surgical technique.[154] This, unfortunately, is often true in veterinary surgery; the practitioner becomes heavily dependent upon both topical and systemic antibiotics as the result of hurried, inadequate, or too conservative débridement. Related to this is the overzealous therapeutic practice of applying antibiotics for prolonged periods, which may possibly cause the development of resistant organisms and thereby delay healing.[106] Another fault of some veterinarians is the extended and indiscriminate use of topical antibiotics without follow-up wound cultures and sensitivity examinations.

Bacteria may persist in a wound even after topical antibiotic therapy. In a study using chlortetracycline, Metzger and Prigot proposed five theories to explain why bacteria could be isolated from antibiotic-treated wounds.[106]

1. A certain number of bacteria were not reached by the drug owing to the protective action of necrotic material or because they resided in crypts.
2. The drug inhibited bacterial growth in vivo but did not kill the bacteria.
3. Organisms were successfully eliminated from the wounds following treatment; however, wounds were recontaminated by the patient or by hospital personnel.
4. The amount of the drug that was released from the chlortetracycline preparations was insufficient to cope with the bacterial flora.
5. If sufficient amounts of the drug were available, the chlortetracycline may have been antibacterial up to a certain concentration, beyond which additional amounts of the drug contributed nothing to its effectiveness.

SYSTEMIC ANTIBIOTICS

General Guidelines for Systemic Antibiotic Use

Several guidelines have been established for the use of antibiotics in the treatment of traumatic wounds in humans.[22] Many of these also apply to veterinary surgery and include the following:

1. A history of sensitivity or idiosyncratic reaction to the drug should be determined. If there is a clear history of sensitivity reaction to one or more antibiotics, it is wise to consider an effective drug that has not been used previously or to which the patient is known to have no sensitivity.
2. Almost all patients with extensive wounds should be given antibiotics. Intravenously administered aqueous penicillin G is preferable as part of preoperative resuscitation.
3. Minor wounds in patients with diabetes, extensive vascular disease, or debilitating conditions require antibiotic therapy.
4. Visceral injuries of the abdomen or chest require high-dose antibiotic therapy.
5. Massive wounds that provide ideal sites for anaerobic growth (e.g., those resulting from tetanus, clostridial myositis, or clostridial cellulitis) should receive high doses of aqueous penicillin G intravenously as soon after injury as possible. Intravenously administered tetracycline has also been recommended.
6. Animal bites, even if the wounds are small, require antibiotic therapy.

7. Extensive or excessive exposure to radiation is an indication for antibiotic therapy.
8. Antibiotic therapy should be maintained for at least five days after all clinical evidence of infection has disappeared. When there is no evidence of infection following the administration of prophylactic antibiotics, they should continue to be administered until wound healing is advanced.
9. Cultures should be taken from all contaminated areas at the time of surgery so that if infection develops, an intelligent approach to specific antibiotic therapy will be possible.
10. Prophylactic antibiotic therapy should preferably be started prior to initiating operative procedures on traumatized patients so that an effective blood level of the antibiotic will be present in the tissues and body cavities before and throughout the surgical procedures.

The last guideline has been quite helpful in preventing the "beehive" effect in dealing with infected wounds. The veterinarian is often presented with a badly infected wound. In such cases surgical débridement without an adequate blood level of the antibiotic could be like stirring up a beehive in that manipulation of the infected tissues could result in a severe septicemic condition.

The use of antibiotics should be based on the results of culture and sensitivity tests and the drug that is most specific for the pathogen should be used. It should be remembered that penicillin is still the drug of choice for most aerobic and anaerobic gram-positive wound organisms. Ampicillin has both gram-positive and gram-negative activity, including that against *Escherichia coli* and the *Proteus* spp. Gentamicin is especially useful against gram-negative infections.[76] The reader is referred to the section on wound culture for antibiotic regimens that are recommended during the time the surgeon is awaiting the culture and sensitivity results.

Systemic antibiotics should be given for at least four or five days after all clinical signs of infection have subsided. During the time the animal is receiving antibiotics, frequent temperature readings should be taken, any developing abscesses should be drained, and necrotic tissue should be removed. Should septicemia develop, a blood culture is indicated. If the organism that is recovered on culture is not sensitive to the antibiotic being given, an effective antibiotic (often penicillin) should be substituted.[82]

Abscesses and Systemic Antibiotics

For abscesses, antibiotic selection may be aided by the results of the rapid-slide technique. If the Gram stain of the homogenate reveals gram-positive organisms, a cephalosporin may be selected as the antibiotic. If gram-negative organisms are present, an aminoglycoside should be chosen.[37]

Systemic Antibiotics and Feces-Contaminated Wounds

Feces-contaminated wounds contain large numbers of strict anaerobes as well as facultative species. It has been recommended that both clindamycin and kanamycin be given systemically to treat such wounds. Clindamycin is effective against anaerobes, and kanamycin eliminates the facultative gram-negative species.[37] A factor to be considered with these drugs is their expense.

Advantages and Disadvantages of Systemic Antibiotics

The primary advantage of systemic antibiotic therapy in the treatment of traumatic wounds is the prevention of septicemia, which is associated with wound infection. This would include the prevention of the beehive effect, which has been mentioned, and the prevention of clostridial infections.

The main disadvantage of systemic antibiotics is their inability to reach the site of contamination or infection in adequate concentrations. This is due to the presence of devitalized tissue that has a poor blood supply.[46, 100, 101] Studies were conducted in which contaminated crush wounds in rabbits were treated either systemically or topically with oxytetracycline within 15 minutes after wound infliction. A 1 per cent mortality resulted and no tissue invasion by microorganisms had occurred by 72 hours after injury in the rabbits that had been treated with a 50-mg. topical spray of oxytetracycline; however, a 51 per cent mortality rate resulted and a marked tissue invasion by microorganisms had occurred by 48 hours after injury in the rabbits that had been treated with a 100-mg. intramuscular injection of oxytetracycline. This latter mortality was not significantly different from that of the control rabbits (67 per cent) in which the wounds were sprayed only with physiological saline solution.[100, 101]

The fibrin base of the granulation tissue in a healing wound can prevent systemic antibiotics from adequately penetrating the wound and from reaching its surface.[46, 128]

Other disadvantages of systemic antibiotics include (1) allergic complications, (2) toxic side effects, and (3) the disturbance of the flora of the respiratory, gastrointestinal, and urogenital tracts.[50]

COMBINATION TOPICAL AND SYSTEMIC ANTIBIOTICS

The use of both topical and systemic antibiotics can be justified from the standpoint of "attacking infection from both sides." Topical antibiotics are effective against bacteria in the devitalized tissues at the wound surface, and systemic antibiotics are effective against bacteria that have invaded the local tissues or blood stream or both. Many wounds that are seen by veterinarians have passed the contaminated state and have entered the infected state, and in many cases the infection is advanced. An example of these is the dog or cat that has disappeared from home for a few days, only to return with a well-advanced wound infection.

Studies have shown lesser numbers of bacteria in the nonviable tissues of a wound than in the viable tissues when topical oxytetracycline treatment was used. Conversely, higher counts of bacteria were noted in the nonviable tissues than in the viable tissues when oxytetracycline was injected intramuscularly.[100, 101] This suggests a lack of penetration of topical antibiotics into tissues under necrotic areas and a lack of penetration of systemic antibiotics into necrotic tissues overlying the wound surface. From this it would seem that a combination of topical and systemic antibiotics would be indicated in wound therapy to "attack infection from both sides."

DRAINS

INDICATIONS

The placement of drains in wounds is indicated in the following instances:
1. Débridement has necessarily been incomplete and foreign material is present in structures that must be left in the wound (e.g., tendons, bones, fasciae).
2. The removal of foreign material is necessary.
3. Massive contamination is inevitable (e.g., in wounds around the anus).
4. It is necessary to obliterate dead space and to prevent air pockets or the accumulation of blood, pus, and serum.
5. There is tissue of questionable viability in a wound.[8, 82, 122, 137]

PROPERTIES AND TYPES OF DRAINS

Generally, drains should be soft and pliable so that they will not encroach on important structures. They should not be irritating to the tissues and should not weaken or decompose when exposed to the drained fluid.[122]

The simplest method of wound drainage is the open technique in which the skin is left unsutured. The slight external pressure of a bandage or a cast forces edema toward the surface and prevents the accumulation of contaminated fluids.[154]

Other types of drains include
1. Penrose drains, which are made of thin latex rubber tubing from 0.5 to 1 in. in diameter and which may or may not be fenestrated. These produce the least foreign-body reaction and yet are highly effective.[8, 76, 122] Drains of 0.25 in. in diameter are also available.
2. Cigarette drains, which consist of gauze placed inside a Penrose drain for more capillary action and bulk.[76, 122]
3. Rubber or plastic tube drains, which are firm, perforated tubes or catheters of various sizes and designs.[8, 76, 122] Those made of plastic may cause less tissue reaction than those of rubber.[8]
4. Sump drains, which are double-lumen drains with the ingress portion being larger than the egress. They are used when adjacent tissues tend to seal off the openings in a single-bore drain. The sump drain allows air to enter the drained area in order to displace fluid into the drain.[76, 122]
5. Sump-Penrose drains, which are triple-lumen drains made by placing a sump drain in a Penrose drain. They are designed so that suction can be applied to one lumen, an irrigating solution introduced through a second, and air allowed to enter through the third opening.[76, 122]
6. Closed suction drains, which consist of two perforated plastic tubes sutured together at the site of infection and brought to the surface, one at each end of the wound. Antibiotic fluid is flushed into the proximal tube and necrotic debris and fluid are aspirated from the distal tube.[76]

The simpler types of drains are usually sufficient for draining wounds of the skin and its underlying structures (Fig. 4–6). A more involved drainage apparatus is used for draining the abdominal and thoracic cavities.

The packing of a wound with lengths (sometimes several feet) of gauze that have been soaked in antiseptic or antibiotic has been used as a wound drainage technique. However, this is contraindicated.[8] If the gauze breaks in a wound it may heal except for a fistulous tract leading to the embedded gauze. Another disadvantage of this type of drain is that it is possible for the animal to gain access to one end of the gauze and then to remove and eat it. The practitioner is then faced with the surgical removal of several feet of foreign body from the gastrointestinal tract of the animal. A modification of this type of drain is the seton, in which the ends of the gauze emerging from the wound are tied together outside the wound. The author does not favor this type of drain.

Penrose drains or rubber or plastic tube drains are adequate for draining the types of wounds discussed in this text. The question arises as to whether these drains should be fenestrated. Drainage occurs both through and around tubing; therefore, an unfenestrated drain probably works just as well as a fenestrated one. Fenestration may be of some benefit when flushing with an antibacterial agent. The more involved types of drains are usually used in wounds involving the body cavities.

PLACEMENT OF DRAINS

Drains should be placed such that one end is at the site to be drained. This end may be fixed in position, if necessary, by a very fine plain catgut suture. The other end of the drain passes downward via the shortest route to the exterior. At this point the drain is passed through a separate stab wound, not through the distal end of the suture line. This stab wound should be large enough to allow for adequate drainage; however, for drains in the abdominal cavity, it should not be so large that the wound contents will herniate along the side of the drain. The emergence of a drain through a separate wound allows primary closure of the entire skin wound. It also helps to prevent wound sepsis and dehiscence,

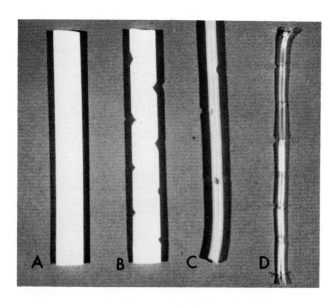

Figure 4–6: Materials that can be used as simple drains in wounds. *A,* Penrose drain; *B,* fenestrated Penrose drain; *C,* fenestrated rubber tubing drain; and *D,* fenestrated plastic tubing drain.

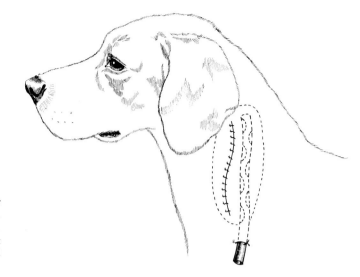

Figure 4–7: Placement of a fenestrated drain *in* a wound. One end of the tube is placed in the depths of the wound, and the other end emerges through a separate stab incision at the dependent part of the wound and is anchored with a suture.

since a drain that is left protruding between sutures may be surrounded by sepsis that could cause the entire suture line to break down. The drain should be anchored to the skin where it emerges through the separate stab wound to prevent it from slipping back into the wound (Fig. 4–7).[8, 46, 122, 137] Drains that emerge from the skin at two points are beneficial. They are placed with each end emerging from a stab incision at opposite ends of the wound (Fig. 4–8).

Antibacterial solutions may be flushed into a wound from the protruding end of the tube. When a double-ended drain is used, the solution is flushed through (if fenestrated) or around the drain tube from the highest to the lowest end.

In general, drains should be removed as soon as possible; however, they should be left in place until they have served their purpose, and this time period may vary considerably.[8, 122] It has been stated that drains should be removed when the area is cool to the touch and is healed.[137] The author prefers to follow the guideline that a drain should be removed when there is little or no

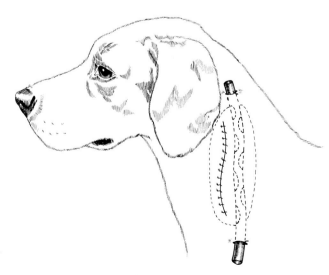

Figure 4–8: Placement of a fenestrated drain *through* a wound. The drain tubing extends through the wound, with its ends emerging from stab incisions at opposite extremities of the wound. Sutures anchor the drain in place at the stab incisions.

drainage.[46, 122] In most cases this is three to four days following surgery; however, this may vary.

A bandage should be applied over the drain if possible. This allows the surgeon to quantitate the amount of drainage with each bandage change, thus allowing good judgment as to when the drain should be removed. Bandaging also keeps the animal from licking and chewing at the drain end, which may result in an ascending infection along the drain and its premature removal.

After surgical removal of the drain, the tract should be flushed for one or two days and the wound should be bandaged during this time. An additional one or two days of bandaging is advisable after flushing has been stopped to allow the stab incisions to heal.

DISADVANTAGES OF DRAINS

The disadvantages of drains are as follows:

1. Infection may ascend around a drain and may lodge and proliferate in the drained area.[8, 122]
2. Drains may become blocked and act as foreign bodies.[8]
3. Firm drains may encroach on adjacent structures.[122]
4. Drains may tempt the surgeon to close an area that is better left open.[17]
5. A drain may slip into the wound and become lost.[122]

Regarding the last disadvantage, it is wise to measure the drain before placement and after removal to assure that the entire drain has been removed. An uneasy feeling develops when the surgeon notices that the drain is no longer protruding from the wound. The surgeon's discomfort is eased if the drain is found in its entirety in the animal's cage. If it is not, the drain has either been retracted into the wound or the animal has extracted and ingested it.

QUANTITATIVE BACTERIAL ANALYSIS OF WOUNDS

HISTORY

The concept that there exists a quantitative relationship between contamination and clinical infection is well established. French surgeons first utilized the concept in wound surgery during World War I.[129] In the late 1960s and early 1970s, Robson and co-workers reported on a quantitative bacterial analysis technique for deciding whether wounds were suitable for closure.[60, 61, 127, 129] Their reports were based on the treatment of wounds in humans. Similar studies in animals would be interesting and of possible value to the veterinarian in wound management.

WHEN TO ANALYZE AND CLOSE WOUNDS

When wounds are to be analyzed quantitatively for bacterial levels, it has been suggested that the analysis be performed on wounds more than three hours old. If the rapid-slide bacterial screening method is to be used to determine the course of therapy, it should be done following preliminary wound preparation (i.e., the use of antibacterial agents in the wound).[127]

A microbial level of 10^5 bacteria per gram of tissue or less has been associated with a significantly higher incidence of successful delayed wound closures and skin grafts. The exception to this is β-hemolytic streptococcal infections.[61, 129] Heggers and colleagues have found that 96 per cent of delayed closures and skin grafts were successful when wounds contained 10^5 organisms per gram of tissue or less at the time of closure. However, a bacterial level that is higher than 10^5 organisms per gram of tissue resulted in the average skin graft survival rate of only 20 per cent, and none of the delayed skin closures were successful.[61]

TECHNIQUE FOR RAPID-SLIDE BACTERIAL ANALYSIS

A tissue biopsy specimen is obtained aseptically by means of a dermal punch. After its weight has been determined in grams, the tissue is diluted ten-fold with thioglycolate. The tissue and the diluent are then homogenized. Using a 20-lambda Sahli pipette, exactly 0.02 ml. of the homogenized suspension is delivered to a glass slide. The inoculum is confined to an area of 15 mm. in diameter on the slide. The slide is placed in a clean, dry Petri dish and oven dried at 75°C for 15 minutes, or the slide may be fixed by gentle heat. After drying, the slide is stained with either a Gram stain or the Brown and Brenn modification of the Gram-staining technique. The smear is read under a microscope using a 1.8-mm. (magnification 97 ×) objective. All fields of the slide are examined for the presence of bacteria. If a single organism is seen on the slide, the bacterial count of the tissue is greater than the apparently critical level of 10^5 organisms per gram of tissue.[60, 61, 127, 129] The average time from excision of the biopsy specimen to the quantitative estimate report has been stated to be one hour.[61]

When the standard tube dilution pour-plate technique was compared with the rapid-slide technique on 720 cases, 170 samples contained greater than 10^5 organisms by the former technique; 164 of the 170 positive samples were also shown to be positive by the rapid-slide technique, giving an accuracy rate of 96.5 per cent. By the pour-plate evaluation, 550 of the samples contained less than 10^5 organisms; 542 of these showed the same results by the rapid-slide technique, giving an accuracy rate of 98.5 per cent.

QUANTITATIVE BACTERIAL ANALYSIS AND β-HEMOLYTIC STREPTOCOCCI

It has been found that wounds containing β-hemolytic streptococci do not progress to successful delayed closure even when the bacterial count is 10^5 or fewer organisms per gram of tissue. The reason for this has been covered at the beginning of this chapter ("Factors Related to Wound Infection"). It is better to let wounds containing β-hemolytic streptococci heal by second intention than to attempt delayed closure.[129] Likewise, skin grafting of such wounds should not be attempted.

WOUND CLOSURE

OBJECTIVE AND TIME OF CLOSURE

The objective of both surgical treatment and natural healing is the restoration of physical strength. This is accomplished by the insertion and utilization of fibers such as sutures and the synthesis of natural fibers within the wound. In the healing process, many elements contribute to the strength of the finished product, but fibers, primarily those of collagen, are the most important.[117]

Wound closure should be performed when all tissues of the wound are ready to accept closure. Closure prior to this is premature and an invitation to wound breakdown, persistent infection, and the consequences related thereto.[17]

TYPES OF WOUND CLOSURE

Primary Closure

Primary closure is accomplished either by sutures or by skin graft soon after injury.[33] Since the danger of wound infection is greater in a closed wound than in an open one, this type of closure should be performed under ideal conditions, and the surgeon should be convinced that healing will progress without interruption (Fig. 4–9A).[17, 22]

The decision regarding whether to undertake primary closure is dependent upon the time lapse since injury, the degree of contamination, the patient's condition, the amount of tissue damage, the thoroughness of excision, the status of the blood supply, the completeness of hemostasis, the possibility of closure without tension or dead space, and the certainty that observations will be made over a seven- to ten-day period following closure. If any of these conditions is in question, it may be wise to leave the wound open for a delayed primary closure.[17, 22, 66] Primary closure may be performed on wounds no later than six hours after infliction. These wounds should be débrided before closure. Wounds older than this show a marked rise in the incidence of infection.[76]

Most wounds that are caused by sharp objects (e.g., glass or knives) usually contain low levels of bacteria. After proper irrigation and meticulous débridement, these wounds will usually heal without complication following primary closure. Crush wounds containing dirt or other embedded foreign material have a greater propensity for infection. The number of bacteria and foreign bodies can be substantially reduced by high-pressure lavage, débridement, and antimicrobial prophylaxis in preparation for primary closure.[37] The placement of a drain in such wounds is strongly suggested.

In primary wound closure, layer suturing should be employed to eliminate cavities between the tissues. Every effort should be made to preserve skin. This may involve undercutting or making flaps.[8] Trimming jagged skin edges to a smooth contour has been advocated.[82] Although it is easier and faster to suture skin edges that have been smoothly débrided, it may provide a more aesthetic appearance to suture them in their irregular state, especially if the wound crosses skin tension lines.[13] Nevertheless, basic surgical principles should be adhered to, and if the irregular skin edge is obviously devitalized, it should be excised. Suturing irregular wound edges can be beneficial in preventing widened, hairless scars in short-haired dogs in which such

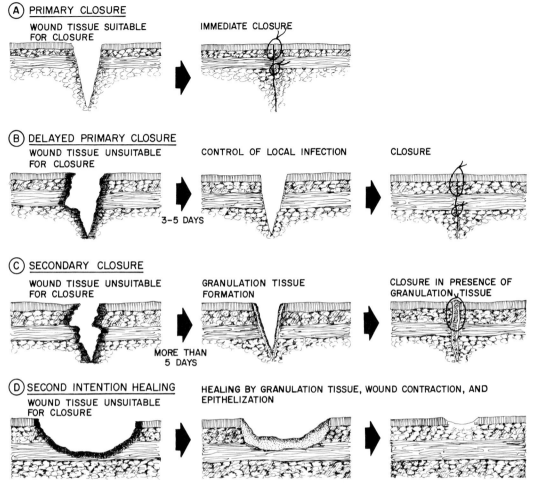

Figure 4-9: Types of wound closure and healing. See text for explanation of parts A through D.

scars would be objectionable. The reader is referred to Chapter 9 for information on the principles of W-plasty.

Skin should be sutured without tension. Tension indicates that there is a skin defect or underlying swelling, and the surgeon should consider closure by other means or delayed closure.[33] Relaxing incisions may also be considered a means of relieving tension.

Delayed Primary Closure

Animals that are presented for wound treatment several days following the injury are not favorable candidates for surgery because of their poor physical condition. Likewise, their grossly infected wounds are not suitable for immediate closure.[32] Wounds that show evidence of heavy contamination, purulent exudate, residual necrotic or questionable tissue, edema, erythema at the margins, lymphangitis, and skin tension are those in which delayed primary closure should be performed.[17, 33, 37]

Delayed primary wound closure is performed after local infection has been adequately controlled, which is usually three to five days after injury (Fig. 4–9B).[33, 38, 46, 66]

Earlier time periods have been suggested for delayed wound closure, including between 24 and 72 hours[12, 38] and between 48 and 72 hours after wounding.[8] However, a study with contaminated guinea pig wounds revealed gross infection in 73 per cent of the wounds that were closed after 24 hours, in 33 per cent of the wounds that were closed between 48 and 72 hours, and in only 3 per cent of the wounds that were closed at 96 hours (four days) after infliction.[38] From this study it would appear that four days is the optimal time for the delayed closure of *known* contaminated wounds. A study on *potentially* contaminated skin and subcutaneous tissue wounds (i.e., wounds created during operations on the gastrointestinal and biliary tracts) showed that closure between 24 and 72 hours reduced wound infection.[12]

Later time periods for delayed primary closure have been reported, including five to seven days[96] and six to seven days after wounding.[17] It should be remembered that after the fourth or fifth day, there is a progression of the proliferative or fibrotic phase of healing, which causes the wound to lose pliability, permits the formation of granulation tissue, allows epithelial fixation, and permits the establishment of fixed bacterial flora. It also becomes difficult to obliterate dead space and to close the skin. Wound contraction is starting at this time and infection has been said to be more common.[66]

Delayed primary closure is beneficial because it provides the opportunity to examine the progression of healing and allows the redébridement of any devitalized tissue that may have been missed at the first débridement.[17] During the time the wound is open, additional drainage can be provided as indicated, and when the tissue is healthy, closure can be performed.[22]

Secondary Closure

Secondary closure is that which is performed later than five days after injury. This type of closure usually implies the formation of granulation tissue.[33] Once granulation tissue starts to form, the skin edges of the wound will become adherent to the underlying tissue and approximation will be possible only by dissecting them free.[17] Suturing skin edges together in the presence of granulation tissue permits healing by secondary closure (Fig. 4–9C).[33, 79] This should not be confused with healing by second intention, which is healing of an open wound by granulation tissue and contraction (Fig. 4–9D).[79] Owing to the immobility of wound tissues in healing by second intention, the author prefers to excise the granulation tissue and a thin rim of skin at the wound margin. Then, utilizing the tissue mobility of adjacent skin, a primary type of closure is performed.

SUTURES FOR CLOSING CONTAMINATED WOUNDS

Absorbable Sutures

Catgut. Catgut is rapidly absorbed in infected wounds owing to the presence of a large number of inflammatory cells and their associated proteolytic enzymes, which destroy the catgut.[117] When more gut than is necessary (i.e., gut of large diameter or with long suture ends) is placed in a wound, excessive exudation results.[78] Chromicized catgut has been found to withstand infection better than plain catgut; therefore, plain catgut should be avoided in contaminated wounds,[1] though chromicized catgut can be used sparingly.

Polyglycolic Acid Sutures. These synthetic absorbable sutures are not affected by inflammation, since they are not attacked by enzymes.[117] Polyglycolic acid sutures have been found to have intrinsic bacteriostatic properties,[46] which are valuable in contaminated and infected wounds. When compared with catgut, these sutures evoked the least inflammatory response, and the infection rate for contaminated tissues containing P.G.A. was significantly lower than for that of tissues containing catgut.[37] Beige P.G.A. is the author's suture of choice in contaminated and infected wounds and for surgery in the oral cavity.

Nonabsorbable Sutures

Monofilament Sutures. In general, monofilament sutures withstand contamination better than multifilament sutures of the same material.[1] Monofilament stainless steel is inert in tissues and therefore a good suture for use in contaminated and infected wounds. Monofilament nylon has been found to have intrinsic bacteriostatic properties.[46] Even so, it has been reported to enhance some degree of infection in tissues contaminated with *Escherichia coli* and *Staphylococcus aureus*.[36] Others have reported a lower incidence of infection in contaminated wounds containing polypropylene or nylon sutures than in those containing other nonabsorbable sutures.[37] The author does not hesitate to place monofilament polypropylene or nylon in contaminated wounds.

Multifilament Sutures. The physical structure of multifilament suture materials is such that bacteria and tissue fluids can penetrate the interstices of the suture, but inflammatory cells cannot. The result is bacteria in a nutrient environment that is separated from the body's first line of defense, the polymorphonuclear cells and macrophages. The bacteria multiply and the wound progresses from contaminated to infected.[117] As stated by one group of investigators, the infection–potentiating effect of nonabsorbable sutures in a wound is most pronounced with silk and cotton.[37] Another study has shown no significant difference in the degree of infection that was produced by any of the nonabsorbable multifilament sutures that were tested, these being braided siliconized silk, braided waxed silk, braided untreated silk, braided nylon, twisted steel wire, and machine-twisted surgical cotton.[1] It can be concluded that multifilament nonabsorbable sutures should not be used in contaminated wounds.

For further information on suture materials, the reader is referred to Chapter 6.

Effects of Sutures on Wound Infection

The following conclusions have been drawn regarding the effects of sutures on wound infection:[37, 39]

1. Sutures that are tied tightly around deep tissue or across the edges of the wound increase the amount of infection. This enhanced infection most likely reflects strangulation and divitalization.

2. The larger the diameter of the suture, the larger will be the area of induration around the contaminated wound's edge.
3. The greater the amount of suture material that remains in the wound, the greater will be the inflammatory response in the contaminated wound.[117]

Based on the results of an investigation of sutures and infection, Edlich and associates stated that even the least reactive suture material impairs a wound's ability to resist infection. They deduced that all sutures should be avoided in dirty, contaminated wounds.[36] Though this may be ideal, it may not be practical in many instances in veterinary surgery. The author's choices for suture materials in contaminated wounds are beige P.G.A., monofilament polypropylene, nylon, or, in some cases, limited amounts of chromic catgut of small diameter.

Suture Placement

The writings of Hippocrates stated that the best dressing for one side of a wound is the healthy tissue from the other side of the wound. This is a good observation that surgeons should keep in mind today.[3]

In addition to choosing the proper suture material, selecting the tissue layer into which the sutures will be placed is important. The objectives of sutures are to obliterate dead space, to stop hemorrhage, and to give strength to the wound. Sutures that are capable of obliterating dead space, discouraging capillary hemorrhage, and making fine adjustments in tissue surfaces can be placed in any layer. It should be remembered that sutures that are placed through cells (which are approximately 90 per cent water) cannot be expected to add much in the way of physical strength to a wound, regardless of how strong the suture material is. Sutures that are expected to supply temporary strength to a wound must be placed in fibrous tissue structures.[117]

When muscle tissue is sutured, the sutures are placed predominantly through cells. However, some strength may be added to such closure by using mattress sutures, which are placed through the fascial coverings of the muscles.[85]

The effects of dead space and layered closure on the development of wound infection have been studied in dogs. Paired contaminated wounds were made on each dog. One wound was closed in four layers with 5–0 nylon. No attempt was made to close the dead space between the layers of muscles, and the subcutaneous tissue was not sutured. The second wound was closed in seven layers, including the subcutaneous tissue, and the dead space between muscle layers was closed. Eleven of the 12 wounds that were closed in four layers developed infection; however, only three of the 12 wounds that were closed in seven layers developed infection. The investigators stated that the assurance of maximum blood supply was essential to all healing. Compliance with this principle necessitates the elimination of actual or potential dead space by accurately matching tissue layers. All cells will thereby be nourished from both sides of the wound. This study indicated that the amount of suture material and the degree of trauma were of less consequence than the presence of dead space in the establishment of wound infections. It was concluded that the painstaking obliteration of potential dead space by sutures appreciably reduced the occurrence of wound infections in the presence of virulent contamination.[23]

Subcuticular and Intradermal Sutures

In the true sense of the word, subcuticular sutures are placed in the tissues under the cutis (dermis). Such sutures are placed in the subcutaneous fat to control capillary hemorrhage and to obliterate the dead space that results if the skin edges are pulled together over a subcutaneous defect. Such dead space acts as a reservoir for blood, liquefied fat, serum, and other wound contents. Even if infection does not occur, these substances can cause wound dehiscence or excessive deep scar formation.[117]

Intradermal sutures are often referred to as subcuticular sutures; however, the intradermal suture is placed in the dermis itself. One author has described the proper placement of these sutures as being superficial enough to hold the skin's edges in close approximation but deep enough to have a healthy layer of epithelium covering them. The purpose of an intradermal suture is to maintain coaptation of the cutaneous edges and to reduce the amount of new scar tissue and scar widening. When skin sutures are removed at six days, a skin wound does not have enough collagen in the scar nor is the collagen present sufficiently woven to provide the same strength that was afforded by the sutures. These wounds rarely break open. However, the scar tends to widen over the next three weeks owing to deforming forces. Intradermal sutures are an effective means of overcoming this problem, since they hold the wound edges together after the superficial skin sutures have been removed.[117] When animals lick and chew wounds, the intradermal suture has a significant advantage.

The suture materials preferred by the author for subcuticular or intradermal placement in contaminated or infected wounds are beige P.G.A. and monofilament polypropylene or nylon. The smaller sizes (2–0 to 4–0) are recommended. The reader is referred to Chapter 6 for more information on subcuticular and intradermal sutures.

Skin Sutures

Most wounds are closed by means of percutaneous skin sutures of some type. The reader is referred to Chapter 6 for more specific information on sutures and suture patterns for skin closure. A study has shown that the passage of a needle through the skin and the placement of suture material in the needle tract does inflict some trauma on the skin and increases the inflammatory response and the chance of infection in contaminated wounds.[39] It is significant to mention that the study was done using silk as a suture material. Silk is contraindicated in contaminated and infected wounds. In the author's opinion, even though needle passage and suture placement do cause some slight trauma to the skin, the advantages of skin sutures far outweigh this disadvantage. It is important to use the least traumatic needle and the suture material of smallest diameter to minimize skin trauma in suture placement.

Edema and Swelling

In many cases early closure of a properly débrided wound may be hampered by edema and swelling. In such instances skin closure results in excessive tension on the suture line. When used on limbs, relaxing incisions may be detrimental and may result in divitalization of the skin between the original and the new defect. In the presence of edema and swelling in the early stages of wound management, it is better to delay closure until the swelling recedes.[33]

In the later stages of wound healing, when swelling has subsided and the tissues have recovered from the initial trauma, relaxing incisions may be considered for wound closure, if necessary. The various types of relaxing incisions are discussed in other chapters (Chapter 9, Z-plasty and V-Y plasty; Chapter 8, simple relaxing incision or bipedicle advancement flaps).

NONHEALING WOUNDS

"PSEUDOHEALING"

Inadequate wound débridement with or without ancillary antibiotic therapy may lead to sepsis. The surgeon may have a false sense of security and close an inadequately débrided wound. The result may be a quietly progressing suppuration under well-healed skin. Antibiotic therapy will limit the spread of infection and depress the systemic signs of suppuration and may save the patient's life; however, when the accumulation of pus becomes apparent, the limb may be in jeopardy (Fig. 4–10).[22] This "pseudohealing" occurs frequently in cats in which skin puncture wounds from a bite or a scratch heal, concealing an underlying infection. Later the infection results in the loss of large amounts of tissue, including skin.

WOUND DEHISCENCE

Failure of a wound to heal is usually a sign of a local disorder. The most common factors that interfere with healing are undue tension on the skin edges, the use of improper suture material, the improper tying of knots, a poor suturing technique, necrosis and ischemia of the tissue, hematomas, infections, and the

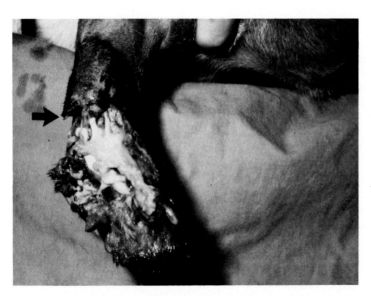

Figure 4–10: Pseudohealing. A laceration on the plantar metatarsal area (at the level of the arrow) was sutured approximately one week earlier. The laceration appeared healed until the skin, underlying soft tissues, and metatarsal foot pad sloughed. See Color Plate II–C, p. 571.

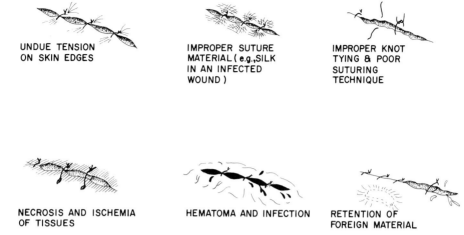

UNDUE TENSION ON SKIN EDGES

IMPROPER SUTURE MATERIAL (e.g.,SILK IN AN INFECTED WOUND)

IMPROPER KNOT TYING & POOR SUTURING TECHNIQUE

NECROSIS AND ISCHEMIA OF TISSUES

HEMATOMA AND INFECTION

RETENTION OF FOREIGN MATERIAL

Figure 4–11: Some factors that interfere with wound healing.

retention of foreign material (Fig. 4–11).[8, 117] Factors that predispose a wound to dehiscence include the failure to adhere completely to an aseptic technique, dietary deficiencies, senility, obesity, anemia, wasting diseases, excessive trauma during the surgical procedure, and improper wound closure.[8] Endocrine imbalances should alert the surgeon to the possibility of poor wound healing.

The surgeon can suspect an impending wound dehiscence when there is necrosis of the skin's edges or when palpation reveals deep collections of blood or serum. In such cases, suture removal will be followed by dehiscence.[117] A serosanguineous discharge from the suture line should also warn the surgeon of an impending wound disruption.[8]

HEALING OF DISRUPTED WOUNDS

A disrupted wound usually heals rapidly following resuturing. This is due to the fact that the lag period of healing has passed, there is an increased blood supply to the area, and phagocytosis is occurring.[78] In a study using rats, it was shown that a disrupted and resutured wound will acquire more strength by the third day than a three-day-old wound that was closed primarily. Wide excision of the wound edges after disruption greatly altered this phenomenon but did not eliminate it. The onset of fibroplasia in such wounds was earlier than in primary wounds that had to pass through the usual latent period.[140] For more information on this subject, the reader is referred to Chapter 3.

OPEN WOUND MANAGEMENT AND HEALING

INDICATIONS, ADVANTAGES, AND DISADVANTAGES

There is a "compulsion to suture" among surgeons that may be detrimental to wound healing. Leaving a wound open seems to create an uneasiness or even guilt in some surgeons. A wound left open is interpreted as an unmet challenge or incomplete treatment. However, there are many wounds in which closure should be delayed or avoided so that healing can take place by second intention. A wound that is handled in this manner usually heals quite well, and although the resultant scar may not be as cosmetic as that of a wound that has healed by primary intension, it is usually quite compatible with function. If the scar is disfiguring, it can be excised and revised after healing is complete and there is no danger of infection.[17] This is especially true in veterinary surgery in numerous instances in which many wounds are badly contaminated or infected and have such extensive tissue loss that primary or delayed primary closure is impossible.

Many inexperienced surgeons are dismayed at the size of an open wound and question whether it is possible for an extremely large wound to heal even by second intention. To ascertain the final result of open wound healing, the surgeon can simply grasp the wound edges and mechanically appose them.[117] The tension should not be excessive. In many cases the surgeon will find that the wound will be able to close itself completely by contraction. However, it may be found that the skin will cover only a portion of the wound and a graft or flap may be needed for closure of the remaining area.

Wounds of the extremities that are parallel to the long axis of the limb, no matter what their length, generally require no revision.[17] Such wounds heal by second intention and leave a minimal scar; however, they must be primarily linear, with little or no loss of skin laterally.

Healing by second intention is not without its disadvantages. One major drawback is the increased time span required as compared with that of primary wound closure.

Another disadvantage of this type of healing is the poor quality of skin

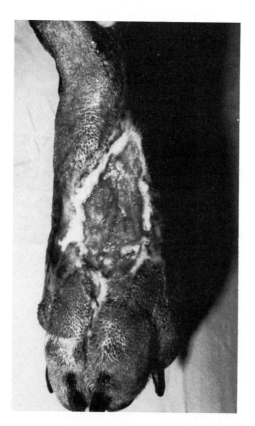

Figure 4–12: Wound on the dorsum of a dog's paw that has healed by second intention. The center of the wound has not epithelialized and remains as exposed granulation tissue.

closure. Healing by second intention requires the formation of granulation tissue, wound contraction, and epithelialization. In some instances the skin cannot contract to cover the granulation tissue of the wound. This may be due to an insufficient amount of skin in the area, such as on the lower portion of the limbs, or it may be due to chronic inflammation, causing deep scar tissue replacement that makes the skin inelastic. In such instances the only hope for an intact wound surface lies in epithelialization. The problem with this epithelial coverage, which does not overlie dermis, is that it is not induced to develop specialized structures and functions, which include the formation of keratin and the self-renewing mechanisms that are found in normal epithelium. The epithelium in these cases is poorly attached to the underlying tissue and is unable to endure environmental hazards. Almost no force is required to abrade the epithelium. The result is a wound covering that is constantly being interrupted and thus exposing underlying tissue. Secondary infection, more scar formation, and repeated epithelialization occur in these cases.[117] The reader is referred to Chapter 3 for other information concerning wound contraction and reepithelialization. This less than desirable type of healing by second intention is often encountered in dogs with large open wounds. These wounds are frequently on the lower portion of the limb where the wound either does not fully epithelialize or the epithelium is constantly being knocked or licked off (Fig. 4–12). Such wounds may require skin grafts or flaps.

MANAGEMENT OF GRANULATION TISSUE

When healing is to take place by second intention, healthy granulation tissue is necessary. A 10 per cent merbromin (Mercurochrome) solution has been described for use in decubital ulcers to stimulate the growth of granulation tissue and to débride the area. This solution has been used in large undermined, postanal pressure sores to stimulate the granulation tissue to fill in the cavities in the area. Sterile powdered gelatin foam* has been used in small decubital ulcers to promote granulation tissue formation and epithelialization and to reduce the amount of wound secretions.[139] As stated in the section on enzymatic débridement, balsam of Peru in a mixture of trypsin and castor oil stimulates capillary ingrowth into a wounded area, which is essential for granulation tissue formation. In the author's opinion, a well-nourished animal in which wound débridement has been adequate and in which there is sufficient circulation in the wound area should be capable of producing enough granulation tissue for wound healing to occur by second intention.

If a wound is to heal by contraction, the base of the wound should not be excised, particularly the area of its circumference, which, according to current information, exerts a major force in wound contraction. In instances in which the defect is large and epithelialization will be necessary in addition to contraction for wound healing, a properly applied occlusive dressing is indicated to help keep the granulation tissue below the level of the wound edge and thereby keep the surface as smooth as possible.[117] Epithelialization can then take place across this smooth, level surface.

Dogs seem to produce a greater quantity of granulation tissue than do cats. However, the problem of excessive granulation tissue formation ("proud flesh") is not as common in dogs as it is in horses. If granulation tissue pro-

---

*Gelfoam is a tradename of the Upjohn Co., Kalamazoo, MI 49001.

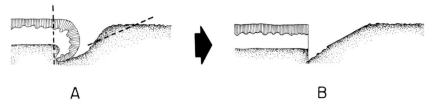

A   B

Figure 4–13: Inverted skin edge on an open, healing wound. *A*, Lines of trimming to freshen the wound edge. *B*, Trimmed wound edge.

liferates above the level of the wound edge, it may be necessary to shave or trim the tissue to reestablish a suitable condition for healing by contraction and epithelialization. After such a procedure, the previously described occlusive bandage is indicated to help maintain the granulation tissue at the proper level. Occasionally, because of the nature and location of some wounds, one edge of the skin will be inverted. Trimming this wound edge and freshening the adjacent granulation tissue are beneficial in initiating wound contraction and epithelialization along this edge (Fig. 4–13).

EXPOSED VITAL STRUCTURES IN OPEN WOUNDS

Bone that is denuded of periosteum, cartilage that is not lubricated, and tendons that are denuded of their sheaths do not tolerate exposure and tend to become desiccated. Exposed blood vessels and nerves are also vulnerable. If the extent of exposure is such that these structures will not be covered by granulation tissue within a few days, the use of a local rotation flap may be considered to cover the tissues.[17] Though grafts will not take in areas where there is no blood supply, split-thickness skin grafts have been advocated to cover exposed structures and to serve as a vapor barrier.[33] A more conservative measure, and one with which the author agrees, is simply to leave the tissues exposed and properly moistened.[17] Gauze that is saturated with petrole-

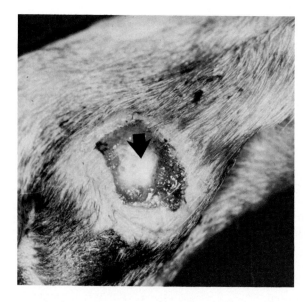

Figure 4–14: Decubital-type lesion over a flexor tendon. The lesion extends through the tendon sheath (*arrow*), resulting in continual fluid drainage from the sheath and a lack of healing.

um jelly has been recommended as an agent to cover these structures.[33] The author has found that granulation tissue nicely covers exposed structures on the limbs of animals within a few days if the wound is properly cared for and the structures are kept from drying by means of ointments and nonadherent bandages.

It has been stated that epithelial migration does not take place over exposed tendon and does so slowly over exposed fascia.[117] The author has observed a similar occurrence with decubital-type lesions over tendons. If the lesion has extended down to and through a tendon sheath, no granulation tissue will be produced over this area and consequently healing will not occur. The lack of healing is due to the constant drainage of fluid from within the tendon sheath, which acts as a fistula (Fig. 4–14).

WOUND pH AND TEMPERATURE IN WOUND HEALING

pH

Alkalinity slows wound healing by stabilizing oxyhemoglobin and preventing the dissociation of oxygen to the wound.[93] Bright pink granulation tissue in a wound may be due to locally circulating oxyhemoglobin that is not releasing oxygen to the tissues.[110]

Alkalinity may develop in an open wound as a result of respiratory alkalosis of the wound, which is produced by a loss of carbon dioxide from the wound surface into the air. The wound may have a pH of 8. Alkalinity may also be the result of ammonia-producing bacteria in a wound. In addition to raising the wound pH, ammonia causes necrosis of the tissues and can produce skin necrosis in amounts as low as 30 mg. per cent. It also causes hemolysis of red blood cells.[93, 110]

Acidification of a wound contributes to healing by increasing the release of oxygen from oxyhemoglobin. At a low P_{O_2}, even a small reduction in pH will appreciably enhance the release of oxygen from oxyhemoglobin. In fact, a shift in pH of only 0.6 releases 50 per cent more oxygen. Therefore, acidification theoretically may hasten healing by enriching the oxygen supply to the tissues.[93]

Techniques to increase wound acidity include bandaging and applying acidifying substances to the wound. Since open wounds lose carbon dioxide and become alkaline, bandaging helps to retain carbon dioxide in the tissues and thereby helps to acidify the wound (Table 4–2).[93]

TABLE 4–2 pH AND TEMPERATURE IN WOUND HEALING

	pH and Causes	Temperature	Effect	Result
Unfavorable Conditions	Alkalinity 1. CO_2 loss from wound surface 2. Ammonia-producing bacteria	Lower owing to exposed wound surface	Decreased O_2 dissociation to tissues	Inhibited wound healing
Favorable Conditions	Acidity 1. Bandaging wound to prevent CO_2 loss 2. Apply acidifying agents to wound	Higher owing to bandaging	Increased O_2 dissociation to tissues	Enhanced wound healing

The chemical acidification of wounds is the most effective means of reducing the toxicity of ammonia, which is formed by urease-producing organisms. Three substances have been evaluated for wound acidification — acetic acid, carbopol ointment, and polyacrylic acid. One per cent acetic acid maintains acidity for one hour, at which time the pH rises to neutrality or above. Consequently, it is not a good choice for wound acidification. Ideally, a wound acidifier should have a high molecular weight to prevent its absorption and a good base-binding capacity, and it must not be degraded by tissue enzymes on the wound surface. Both carbopol ointment and 20 per cent polyacrylic acid fulfill these requirements. Even after they are fully neutralized, they act as ion exchange resins and bind ammonia by exchanging Na^+ for a NH_4^+.

A study performed in 1976 suggested that infection by some organisms can result in a stronger wound. Wounds infected by *Escherichia coli* were found to be stronger than uninfected wounds. The pH in these infected wounds was lower than in uninfected wounds. It was suggested that the infection initiates an increased inflammatory response, resulting in more local tissue damage, the release of more lysozymes, and increased fibroblastic activity and vascularity, thereby producing a stronger wound. It was presumed that more oxygen was delivered because of the increased vascularity of the infected wound. Oxygen was released from oxyhemoglobin because of the greater acidosis, and this resulted in the production of more carbon dioxide, which would add to the acidosis.[124] In spite of these findings, the author would not suggest infecting a wound with *Escherichia coli*.

Temperature

Both alkalinity and low temperatures decrease oxygen dissociation.[93, 110] Therefore, it follows that bandaging a wound not only prevents the loss of carbon dioxide but retains body heat and aids in oxygen dissociation (Table 4–2).[110]

SUGAR AND INSULIN IN WOUND HEALING

Sugar

Without a clearly defined mechanism of action or rationale, sugar has been used to stimulate healing for some time. Sugar granules have an irritating effect and therefore stimulate the formation of granulation tissue. The acid pH of a sugar solution tends to increase vasodilation, which allows the increased local perfusion of blood and lymph in ulcerated areas. A hyperconcentration of sugar is also bactericidal.[10]

Sugar has been used as a débriding agent in large, necrotic, ischemic ulcers. A paste consisting of a small amount of glycerin and granulated table sugar was packed into an ulcerated area. It was postulated that the sugar, rather than the tissue, serves as a nutrient for the bacteria. It may also serve as a hydrostatic agent, reversing fluid flow in the area and thereby bringing more serum and nutrient materials into the tissue to promote healing.[26] The use of honey and comb honey has been reported in the treatment of ulcers.[71]

The author has had limited but successful experience in using granulated table sugar to treat chronic nonhealing wounds. A controlled study on the

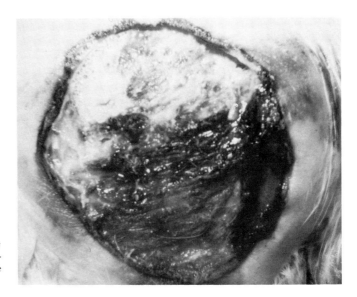

Figure 4–15: Open wound over the gluteal area of a cat exhibiting dehydrated necrotic muscle tissue. See color plate II–D, p. 569.

effects of sugar on wound healing should be undertaken to clarify the value of its use. One major problem with this form of therapy is that it increases the tendency of the animal to lick at the wound.

Insulin

Mixture. Topically applied insulin has been reported in the veterinary literature as a wound-débriding agent and a wound-healing stimulant.[11] A cream compound that is made by mixing 10 units of protamine zinc insulin suspension with 1 gm. of a base that permits the release of insulin in a sustained manner and preserves the insulin's strength did not seem to significantly reduce the amount of discharge from a *Pseudomonas*-infected wound. However, increasing the concentration of insulin to 20 units/gm. of base markedly improved the condition of the wound, as shown by a decrease in the amount of exudate and inflammation and by the appearance of new tissue at the wound periphery. Based on tests and clinical use in animals, the most effective concentration of insulin for treatment in most cases was found to be 30 units of insulin per gram of base.[11]

The author has found a mixture of 30 units of protamine zinc insulin suspension* in 28 gm. of nitrofurazone ointment base† to be effective in the topical treatment of wounds (Figs. 4–15 and 4–16). Care should be taken with the use of more than 30 units of insulin and in the treatment of large wounds, since insulin may be systemically absorbed, which can result in a systemic hypoglycemia with possible effects on the central nervous system. Although the author has not encountered signs of systemic absorption in animals in which the 30 units/28 gm. of base had been used, it should be recommended

---

*Protamine, Zinc & Iletin is available from Eli Lilly and Co., Indianapolis, IN 46206.

†Furacin is manufactured by Norwich-Eaton Pharmaceuticals, Norwich, NY 13815.

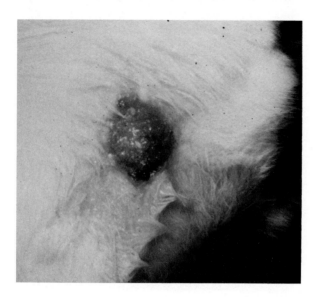

Figure 4–16: The open wound shown in Figure 4–15 approximately two weeks after topical therapy with protamine zinc insulin suspension in a nitrofurazone base. See Color plate II–E, p. 569.

to pet owners that some sugar be added to their pet's diet during this regimen. The author also recommends refrigeration of the compound to maintain its efficacy once it has been mixed.

Early Activity of Insulin. Insulin seems to be more effective in the treatment of chronic and infected wounds than it is in the treatment of fresh and noninfected wounds. In a study in which insulin was used to treat surgical wounds, fresh bite wounds, and lacerations in a series of 20 dogs and cats, there was no visible acceleration of the healing process. In a second group of animals with infected wounds (abscesses, ulcers, infected surgical wounds, and abscessed anal sacs), there was a response to topical insulin therapy. In this same study various bacteria were isolated from infected wounds. However, in no instance did the type of bacteria prevent a response to treatment with insulin. The wounds continued to contain bacteria; however, they healed faster than would have been expected with antiseptic treatment. The initial action of insulin in an infected or debilitated wound resembles that of an enzyme in that wound débridement takes place during the first 12 to 24 hours after application.[11]

Later Activity of Insulin. Insulin has the effect of increasing protein synthesis[6, 136, 158] and fat deposition.[6, 136] In one case report, these properties of insulin were used to reconstruct a depressed scar area on a woman by injecting 4 units of monocomponent porcine insulin beneath the scar three times daily. The resulting increase in fat and protein deposition under the scar raised the area to a normal level.[6] Since wound healing is dependent on collagen deposition, it follows that insulin's ability to stimulate protein synthesis may have a favorable effect on wound healing. In a study on nondiabetic rats, it was found that parenterally administered protamine zinc insulin suspension increases the tensile strength of healing incisions.[136] Topical insulin has also been found to be effective in stimulating wound healing in diabetic patients.[97]

Traumatized tissues have the capability of regenerative proliferation; however, normal metabolism is necessary. Insulin plays an important role in producing this regenerative proliferation in tissue and is believed to be a growth-promoting substance that acts in fresh wounds in which glycolysis occurs, resulting in the growth and proliferation of new tissue. Insulin conditions the cell membranes of epithelial, fat, and muscle cells so that glucose can enter the cell.[11]

It has been hypothesized that insulin does not reach the infected tissue in diabetics owing to microangiopathy. As a result, there may be an increased sugar concentration in the wound tissue, which would cause cellular dehydration and consequently decrease the resistance to infection. The local application of soluble insulin could enhance the glucose transport into the cells, thus producing a local metabolic compensation, which, together with the systemic metabolic compensation, could lead to rapid healing of ulceronecrotic lesions in diabetics.[97]

In nondiabetic individuals with chronic, nonhealing, debilitated wounds, a condition similar to that just described may occur. In debilitated wounds such as ulcers, abscesses, and infected wounds, the tissues are devitalized and impermeable and no glycolysis occurs. Therefore, there is no tissue vitality and little or no tissue proliferation. In addition, devitalized tissues have been found to contain large quantities of the enzyme insulinase, which inactivates any insulin present in the tissue. The topical application of insulin to these wounds has the initial effect of removing exudate and necrotic tissue. The insulin stimulates the tissue adjacent to the layer of necrotic tissue in the previously described manner to increase cellular metabolism, which, in turn, brings about mitosis and cell proliferation in the tissues.[11]

When comparing the effects of topical insulin therapy in the debilitated wounds of dogs and cats, the author has noted greater progress in wound healing in cats than in dogs. In addition, fresh wounds (surgical wounds or lacerations) that were treated with topical insulin have shown no increase in the rate of wound healing when compared with that of fresh wounds that have not been treated with insulin.

BANDAGING OPEN WOUNDS

Properties of a Bandage

There are four primary functions of a wound dressing: (1) protection, (2) absorption of draining material, (3) compression to prevent hematomas and the formation of dead space, and (4) stabilization.[76]

Material for Bandages

Ideally, a nonadherent material should be placed on a wound's surface to prevent disruption when the bandage is changed. Coarse-meshed gauze should not be used on epithelializing wounds, since the epithelial cells grow into the interstices of the mesh and are pulled away when the dressing is changed.[150] Removal of the gauze can also result in disruption of the surface of the granulation tissue in a wound, which causes hemorrhage. Perforated cellophane has been advocated as an excellent nonadherent covering for a wound, since it cannot be invaded by cells.[150] The author has used some of the newer, more pliable food wrapping materials as a covering for large open wounds. It is important to perforate these materials to allow drainage of the exudate. On smaller wounds, the smaller commerical nonadherent wound dressing pads* work nicely.

Pressure Bandages

In addition to preventing hematomas, dead space formation, edema, and oozing, pressure bandages may also help to prevent the accumulation of exudate in a wound, thereby decreasing the possibility of infection.[8, 82] These dressings are particularly helpful in confining the contents of a crater-like wound below its surface when the circumferential narrowing of the actively moving wound perimeter causes the underlying tissue in the wound's center to be squeezed up out of the wound.[117]

The term pressure bandage may be incorrect, unless some form of elastic material is used to maintain persistent tension. Studies in which pressure-sensitive transducers were placed in gauze or cotton dressings have shown that regardless of how the dressing is applied, pressure dissipates within 30 minutes. This is because cotton and other materials become packed, and unless an elastic material is used to exert constant tension, cotton and linen dressings do not maintain pressure on the wound's surface.[117]

Theory of Prolonged Bandaging

Dressing a wound and then applying a plaster cast that will remain over the dressing for two weeks have been advocated by Neuman. By five to seven days after application, the cast will emit an odor; however, it has been stated that the cast should not be changed until the end of two weeks. At this time the cast is removed and the wound is gently cleaned. A second cast is applied over a petrolatum-soaked gauze dressing. The cast is again left in place for two weeks, at which time it is replaced with a bandage that is to be changed every two to three weeks until healing is complete. The theory behind this mode of therapy is that it gives stability to the area, which prevents the mechanical spread of infection. It also provides an occlusive dressing that limits the loss of carbon dioxide from the wound and retains body heat. Both of these conditions favor adequate oxygenation of the healing tissues.[110] The author has not used this technique of prolonged wound dressing without change.

Wet or Dry, Hot or Cold Wound Dressings

Wet wound dressings are indicated if the debris that is to be removed from a wound is water-soluble. The use of wet compresses to rid the wound of such surface debris is biologically sound, since a wet dressing will insure the dilution and removal of thick exudate by reducing the viscosity of the secretions. Wet dressings are disadvantageous in that they cause tissue maceration, they do not increase the inflammatory response when cold, and they are uncomfortable until the body's heat raises their temperature. If a wound is

---

*Telfa pads are manufactured by The Kendall Co., Hospital Products, Boston, MA 02101.

discharging large amounts of an exudate of low viscosity that has no tendency to aggregate, a bulky, dry dressing in indicated.[117]

Wet heat is effective in increasing the inflammatory response and in producing local anesthesia. However, it is not known whether healing is enhanced by raising the temperature or whether elevated local temperatures selectively attract specialized cells or affect lymphatic function in other beneficial ways.[117] The application of hot compresses to an injured area for 15 to 20 minutes twice daily can be as beneficial as chemotherapy, and this is an underutilized aid in the topical treatment of lesions.[137]

Biological Dressings

The effectiveness of biological dressings in cleansing infected wounds will be discussed in this section. The reader is also referred to Chapter 10, where biological dressings (i.e., allografts and xenografts) are discussed further.

Biological dressings tend to sterilize infected wounds, apparently by augmenting the host's immunological defense. Skin dressings increase phagocytosis by causing a slight acidity of the wound and by raising the temperature beneath the skin coverage. Biological dressings do not significantly alter bacterial growth in the wound. They remove and prevent leukocytic accumulation on the surface of granulation tissue. It has been hypothesized that dying leukocytes or leukocytes that are active in phagocytosis may liberate a substance that reduces phagocytosis. Preventing the accumulation of this antiphagocytic substance by preventing the exudation of leukocytes may allow sterilization of the granulating bed to occur.[19]

In the study by Burleson and Eiseman, the adherence of biological dressings to granulating wound surfaces was common in the dressings that resulted in tissue sterilization. The dressings that did not adhere to the wounds did not effectively decrease the number of bacteria in the tissue. They found that bacterial counts within the wound tissue decreased significantly by the eighth day after coverage with a biological dressing. The bacterial counts decreased by 98 per cent, and the wounds were sterile in 50 to 78 per cent of the cases. Histologically, these dressings prevented the accumulation of exudate on the surface of the wound. In addition, skin dressings caused a slight (21°C) increase in wound temperature and a decrease of 0.007 units in alkalinity; however, oxygen tension was not significantly altered. It was believed that these factors in the wound environment were unlikely to have accounted for the antibacterial activity.[19]

Synthetic "Biological Dressings"

A reticulated polyurethane foam that is laminated to a microporous polypropylene film* has been developed as a substitute for homograft and heterograft skin.[2] It has the following beneficial properties:
1. It compares favorably with allograft and xenograft skin in its early adherence to the wound surface.

---

*Epigard is available from Parke-Davis, Morris Plains, NJ 07950.

2. It is thrombogenic.
3. It is impervious to bacteria and gases.
4. It is immunologically inert, sterile, and stable during extended storage.

The thrombogenic property of the material causes coagulation of the plasma exudate from the wound surface, which supplies the necessary intimate adherence of the material to the wound's surface. A structure is provided into which phagocytes can enter to entrap and kill bacteria. It was found that the synthetic material prepared a wound for grafting in the same manner as allografts and xenografts and in essentially the same amount of time. In some cases the synthetic material was found to be superior for wound débridement when compared with the biological dressings. When compared with wounds that were treated with topical antimicrobial agents, the wounds that were treated with the synthetic material were ready for grafting four to five days earlier because of more rapid and efficient débridement.[2]

It is best to change synthetic biological wound dressings daily for dirty wounds. When the granulating bed is healthy, the synthetic material can be left for two to three days between dressing changes. There is no obvious clinical advantage to using antimicrobial ointments or creams with the synthetic material. These substances prevent good contact between the synthetic material and the wound surface and in some cases have resulted in wound deterioration.[2]

The disadvantage of the synthetic material is that it lacks elasticity and does not conform to the surface of an irregular wound (Fig. 4–17).[2]

Mobilization and Immobilization

There are those who advocate early postoperative ambulation and passive physiotherapy for the patient,[46] along with the return of the injured part to as near normal function as possible.[17, 76] Physiotherapy and daily exercise minimize the occurrence of a negative nitrogen balance.[46] The early return of the

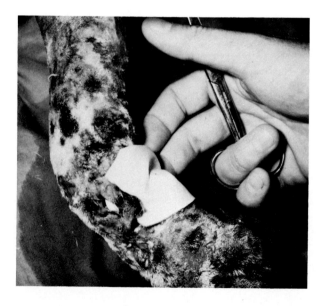

Figure 4–17: Application of a reticulated polyurethane foam laminated on microporous polypropylene film to an open wound for débridement. Note that the material does not conform well to the wound surface.

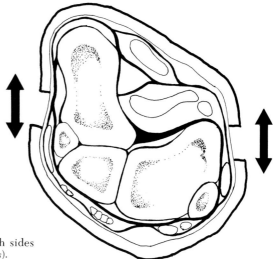

Figure 4–18: A cast that is split on both sides will allow for swelling in the limb (*arrows*).

injured part to near normal function stimulates circulation in the area, which combats infection and is essential for adequate wound healing.[17] Movement may loosen adhesions and may help to provide adequate wound drainage through a "massaging" action.[76] For these purposes, early ambulation is recommended; however, discretion should be used. If the movement of tissues disrupts the wound-healing processes and breaks down the newly forming blood vessels, which can result in hematoma formation, ambulation should be delayed.

Conversely, there are those who advocate wound immobilization for a period of time following surgery.[33, 76, 117, 137] Such immobilization may be accomplished by surface splints[117] or casts.[33] Casts should be applied with the understanding that postoperative swelling may occur. It is advisable to place padding between the digits, leaving the tips of the digits exposed so that circulation and sensation may be evaluated. If a cast is to be split, it should be split on both sides to allow for swelling (Fig. 4–18).[33, 117] The reasons for immobilization of the injured part are to (1) allow for better healing of lacerations over the olecranon, the tuber calcanei, and the antecubital, popliteal, and pretarsal areas if they are splinted for one week;[137] (2) help prevent osteomyelitis in areas of infected bone;[76] (3) provide for patient comfort;[33] (4) decrease the probability of infection;[33] (5) supply support to the tissues during collagen synthesis to prevent stress on the wound and a resultant widened scar.[117] The last factor is not as much of a problem in veterinary surgery as it is in human surgery.

Immobilization of the paws following foot pad surgery is essential. When suturing deep lacerations on foot pads, it is best to suture from the depths of the wound to the surface, using simple interrupted sutures to close dead space. This helps to immobilize the tissues internally. To appreciate the need for adequate external immobilization, one must understand the problem that can occur if the paw is not properly immobilized. If the animal is allowed to walk on the paw with no external support, the body weight tends to "splay" or flatten the pad and puts tension on the sutures. This results in wound dehiscence as the sutures tear through the tissues.

Hutton and associates have reported some interesting findings regarding the forces exerted by the foot pads of the walking dog.[72] These will help to illustrate why sutures would tend to tear through foot pads. The center of gravity is just behind the shoulder girdle of the dog. The exact position will vary with the length and width of the head and the neck and the general structure of the trunk, but in all cases it is nearer to the front than to the back. This explains the greater ratio of force to body weight for the front foot pads. The vertical force exerted by the front pads is about 1.1 times the body weight, while that of the back pads is 0.8 times the body weight. As the dog ambulates there is a "retarding force" associated with the front pads and an "accelerating force" associated with the back pads. These investigators also found that the horizontal forces that were exerted on the pads during walking were nearly ten times less than the vertical forces.[72] From these findings it can be seen that sutures in foot pads undergo considerable stress.

To prevent sutures from tearing through the tissues of the foot pad when a dog puts weight on the paw, there are two courses of action. First, the limb can be immobilized in such a way that it does not bear weight for a period of ten to 14 days. A bandage into which a metal splint* has been incorporated is then applied and left for another seven to ten days. The tendency of the foot pad to "splay" or spread out is not as great in such a splint. Second, if the limb cannot be bandaged in a position in which it will not bear weight, it should at least be bandaged adequately in a metal support.

MANAGEMENT OF SPECIFIC WOUNDS

LACERATIONS

Provided the patient is a good risk for anesthesia, uncomplicated lacerations will heal nicely if they are sutured shortly after they occur. However, it is inadvisable to risk a patient's life with anesthesia to achieve early wound closure. In some cases a small amount of opiate can be administered and a local or regional block can be performed. However, it should be remembered that local anesthetics can adversely affect the healing process. The tissue loss will probably be more than counterbalanced by the lessened risk of losing the patient.[137]

Since the general principles for suturing lacerations have been discussed elsewhere in the text, they will not be included here.

ABSCESSES

An abscess and its associated sequelae are well known to the veterinarian, and there are undoubtedly many individual preferences among practitioners in the treatment of the condition. The basics of managing infected wounds apply to this type of lesion. One author has recommended the following as a course of therapy for abscesses:

1. Lance the abscess when it comes to a head.
2. Débride and flush the lesion with an antibiotic solution or chemically cauterize it with 3 per cent iodine.

---

*Mason Meta splints are available from United Veterinary Specialties, Phoenix, AZ 85060.

3. Drain it if required.
4. Leave the area to heal by second intention or close large skin defects after inserting drains.
5. Consider systemic antibiotic therapy.[46]

DEGLOVING INJURIES

Extensive skin loss from a limb is often the result of a wringer or roller action, thus degloving the skin from the limb. Running over the limb with a vehicle tire is one of the causes of this type of injury. The injury may be anatomical, in which case the skin is actually torn off, or it may be physiological, in which case the skin is still intact, but there is complete disruption at the level of the deep fasciae, with undermining and damage to the vascular network and resultant ischemic necrosis.[104] Such wounds on the limbs of dogs and cats are usually combined with bone damage and a crushing effect.

The tissues of the wounds need to be evaluated before surgery can be undertaken. The viability of the skin is checked by pressing on it; if it blanches and then returns to a normal color, circulation is present. Dermal bleeding at the edge of the skin flaps is another indication of circulation. The occurrence of reactive hyperemia after the five-minute application of a tourniquet above a wound has also been considered evidence of the presence of circulation in the skin.[104, 105] The use of sulphan blue to evaluate tissue viability has been described[153] and is covered in an earlier section of this chapter.

Since bone damage is often associated with degloving injuries, it is advisable to use radiography to check for fractures. Manipulation of the carpus or tarsus will usually reveal an abnormal laxity, with excess angulation in the direction opposite the injury owing to loss of collateral ligaments. Torsional laxity is frequently seen in the tarsus. Occasionally a "flail" forelimb or hind limb is present that is extremely lax.[137]

Immediate treatment of degloving injuries includes ligating all points of bleeding. As soon as the patient is deemed a good anesthetic risk, the wound should be débrided. It is common to find debris that has been so forcefully ground into the tissues that it cannot be washed away. If this debris is in areolar connective tissue, the tissue can simply be removed. If it is ground into a structure that might eventually contribute to limb function, good judgment should be used in deciding whether to remove it.[137]

Tendons frequently will be frayed or torn away from their attachments. These should be cleaned as thoroughly as possible and sutured accurately in their original location.[137] Many times the tendons are so badly damaged that they are not salvageable and will have to be trimmed away. Joint capsules and ligamentous structures should be pulled over the exposed joint, but usually approximation is impossible.[137] More detailed information is available on tendon and joint débridement in their respective sections in this chapter.

The skin can frequently be sutured over the wound, even to the point of edge-to-edge approximation in some areas. The gaps that remain in the skin provide drainage and eliminate the necessity for tubes or wicks.[137] It is important to evaluate the skin as previously discussed prior to suturing it and to débride what is necessary. An avulsed skin flap that is considered to have doubtful vitality is best cleaned and properly sutured back into position, regardless of how small its pedicle is. It can be retained in this way until a line of demarcation between viable and nonviable tissue develops. More of the flap may survive than the pedicle might have suggested. The flap should not be allowed to remain until it is obviously necrotic or until a spontaneously separating slough is present. Within a day or two nonviable skin should be determinable and should be excised.[104, 105] In this type of injury, simple interrupted or continuous subcutaneous sutures of beige P.G.A. or of a monofilament synthetic (e.g., polypropylene) are indicated prior to placing skin sutures.

The limb should be immobilized in a functional, weight-bearing position. Joint stiffness may occur, but the limb may still be usable if it has been splinted properly. The splint should be changed as often as necessary (usually twice a week) to keep the draining wound clean.[137] Early in the course of events it may be necessary to sedate the animal to make bandage changing more pleasant for both the practitioner and the animal. In instances of painful superficial wounds, the author has occasionally saturated the bandage with a topical anesthetic agent (not containing epinephrine) ten minutes prior to bandage removal. This has made bandage removal from a painful wound more tolerable.

In instances in which orthopedic problems are associated with a degloving injury, the splint can usually be removed in four to six weeks. If bone and joint laxity still exists, some form of orthopedic intervention will be necessary.[137] In badly contaminated or infected wounds in which some form of internal orthopedic fixation will obviously be necessary, it is preferable to treat the wound and to provide temporary external fixation. When the infection has been controlled and healthy viable tissue is present, internal fixation can be attempted by approaching the bone through the viable tissue. Internal fixation through an infected wound can result in osteomyelitis, especially if intramedullary pins are used.

BITE WOUNDS

A dog's skin moves freely on most areas of the body, and a canine tooth will often make only a single puncture wound, resulting in a rather innocent-appearing wound on the surface. With the slashing action of a biting dog, the canine tooth can tear through muscles, separate fascial planes, sever tendons, arteries, veins, and nerves, and pull the skin away from the body to create a cavity. The skin will fall back into place, leaving only a small puncture wound on its surface that does not reflect the subcutaneous trauma.[46, 109, 137] Therefore, it is good practice to open bite puncture wounds maximally to expose the underlying damage. In most cases, a dorsoventral incision is preferable to a horizontal incision so that ventral drainage is possible.[109] A technique for opening nail puncture wounds utilizes a pair of cuticle nippers.[79] These could be used to excise a fusiform piece of skin around a dog bite wound if the skin is not too thick (Fig. 4–19). Underlying tissues can be evaluated through this opening as to the need for further débridement.

Since the tissue underlying a dog bite wound provides a good milieu for bacterial growth, it is necessary to débride thoroughly. Tissues that have lost their blood supply should be excised, especially muscle and fat. If devitalized muscle is left in the wound, the procedure may have to be repeated later under less favorable conditions. An attempt should be made to maintain an intact blood and nerve supply to the area. Fasciae, tendons, and ligaments are less likely to become infected, and they often act as a matrix for fibroblastic

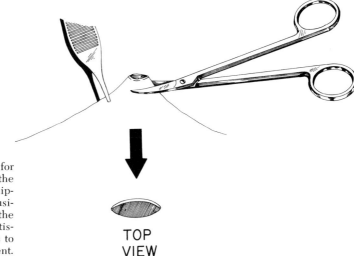

TOP VIEW

Figure 4–19: Technique for opening puncture wounds. If the skin is not too thick, cuticle nippers can be used to excise a fusiform piece of skin containing the puncture wound. Underlying tissues can then be evaluated as to the need for further débridement.

activity in the wound-healing process. Therefore, they may not need to be as extensively débrided.[109] An alternative or an adjunct to débridement is to establish drainage from the dorsalmost to the ventralmost limit of the subcutaneous separation.[46]

The lavage of bite wounds with copious amounts of saline solution or irrigation with hydrogen peroxide has been suggested.[92] However, Furneaux has advised against wound lavage because it could spread organisms and extend cellulitis.[46] The author prefers to flush such wounds with a dilute solution (0.05 per cent) of commercial chlorhexidine (1:40 dilution of a 2 per cent solution).

After débridement, dead space should be closed. If the wound can be completely débrided, it can be totally closed. If there is incomplete débridement, contamination, or a compromised blood supply, provisions should be made for drainage. The dorsal aspect of the wound may be closed, while the ventral portion may be left unsutured to allow for drainage. If there is a pocket at the ventral aspect of the wound, an opening should be made at its ventralmost portion to permit drainage. Setons or preferably latex drainage tubes can be placed in the wound.[109]

Hemostasis should be accomplished using a minimal number of absorbable sutures of small diameter. Synthetic absorbable sutures are preferable to catgut, and, when needed, nonabsorbable monofilament sutures such as nylon or stainless steel are preferable to multifilament sutures (silk, cotton, and Vetafil) for burying in tissues.[109]

Skin lacerations should be trimmed back to healthy skin and should be closed either primarily[46, 109] or by delayed primary closure.[46] In cases in which devitalized skin has been removed, it may not be possible to close the entire wound. In such instances it is best to close the dorsal aspect of the wound and to leave the ventral portion open to heal by second intention. If the removal of nonviable skin means leaving a large area uncovered, it is better to leave some of the nonviable skin to cover the wound, thereby providing some protection while the deeper tissues begin to heal. When the skin begins to slough in a few days, it can be trimmed away, and the exposed area can be allowed to heal as an open wound or it can be repaired by grafting.[109] As with degloving injuries, it is possible that some questionably viable skin that is sutured may become viable and thus provide adequate wound coverage. An alternative to suturing the skin whose viability is questioned would be to excise it and to provide wound coverage with a nonadherent dressing while healing by second intention progresses.

Systemic and local antibiotic therapy should be considered in the treatment of bite wounds.[46] The systemic antibiotics that have been advocated include procaine penicillin G (65,000 to 110,000 units/kg. of body weight) at the time of wound treatment, followed by ampicillin, which is to be administered for three to five more days.[109] Cloxacillin sodium or ampicillin has been recommended by Leith.[92] The author prefers to dispense ampicillin for a five-day course of therapy following the surgical repair of the wound.

The blood supply to the injured area is a primary factor in the healing of bite wounds. Although massive cervical, facial, and leg wounds may heal well because of an ample blood supply, back, lateral thoracic, and flank wounds tend to heal less ideally in many cases. Skin and subcutaneous wounds on the cranium develop seromas more readily than wounds in other areas. Consequently, it is best to leave sutures in these areas for at least two weeks to prevent dehiscence when they are removed.[109]

SNAKEBITE WOUNDS

Grades of Venenation

A grading system has been established for evaluating the degree of venenation that is produced by a snakebite. Although the following grades apply to humans, they probably also pertain to some degree to animals.

1. Grade 0
   A. No venenation
   B. Fang or tooth marks
   C. Minimal pain
   D. Less than 1 in. of surrounding edema and erythema
   E. No systemic involvement
2. Grade I
   A. Minimal venenation
   B. Fang or tooth marks
   C. Severe pain
   D. 1 to 5 in. of surrounding edema and erythema in the first 12 hours after the bite
   E. Systemic involvement usually not present
3. Grade II
   A. Moderate venenation
   B. Fang or tooth marks
   C. Severe pain
   D. 6 to 12 in. of surrounding edema and erythema in the first 12 hours after the bite
   E. Systemic involvement possibly present
   F. Nausea, vomiting, giddiness, shock, or neurotoxic symptoms

4. Grade III
   A. Severe venenation
   B. Fang or tooth marks
   C. Severe pain
   D. More than 12 in. of surrounding edema and erythema in the first 12 hours after the bite
   E. Systemic involvement usually present, as in grade II.[79]

Tourniquets

A snake injects venom into the subcutaneous tissues and it is absorbed via the lymphatics.[79] For this reason tourniquets are applied to incarcerate the venom. The proper placement and maintenance of a tourniquet entails the following:

1. A flat tourniquet should be used (e.g., a flat latex rubber drain tube).[7, 45, 86, 148]
2. It should be applied proximal to the bite wound.[45, 86, 115]
3. The tourniquet should be tight enough to occlude only the superficial lymphatics, tissue spaces, and veins.[45, 79, 86, 113, 115] It should not shut off the arterial supply. If a finger can be inserted easily under the tourniquet, it is properly applied (Fig. 4–20).[45, 79, 86, 148]
4. Some advocate leaving the tourniquet in place for two hours,[7, 86, 115] while others recommend 45 to 60 minutes.[45] Still others advise removing the tourniquet every 20 minutes.[113, 148]
5. The tourniquet should be advanced periodically to keep it ahead of the swelling.[79, 115]

The use of a modified Robert Jones' dressing has been advocated to immobilize the limb, absorb tissue fluids and venom from the incisions that

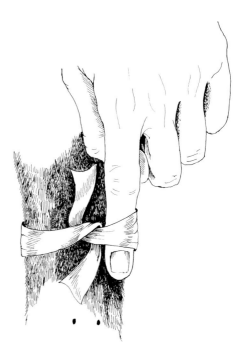

Figure 4–20: A flat latex rubber drain tube is applied proximal to a snakebite wound. The tourniquet should not be applied too tightly; it should be possible to easily insert a finger under it.

are made over the bite wounds, reduce the lymphatic flow, and minimize the pain.[45]

Incision and Suction of Snakebites

The technique of making incisions over the fang marks and applying suction is widely recognized.[7, 22, 42, 45, 73, 79, 86, 115, 148] Studies on dogs have shown that 53 per cent of the venom can be removed in 15 minutes by this technique. Wide excision of the entire area around the snakebite within ten minutes of the time of injection has been found to remove 79 per cent of the venom.[79] Another study has shown that dogs receiving as high as four minimal lethal doses of venom will recover when incision and suction are performed one hour after the injection of venom.[73]

There are varying opinions as to the type of incision to be used for venom removal. The use of cruciate incisions is generally condemned, since the tips of the flaps that are created may undergo necrosis, and such a wound is subject to anaerobic contaminants and clostridial infections.[7, 45, 86, 148] The types of incisions that have been advocated include the following:

A.   A continuous linear incision can be made through both fang marks extending to the fascia covering the muscle. Care is taken not to sever vital structures, such as tendons, motor nerves, or major blood vessels (Fig. 4–21A).[7, 86]

B.   A single linear incision that is carried to a depth of at least 5 mm. may be made to connect the fang marks (Fig. 4–21B).[45]

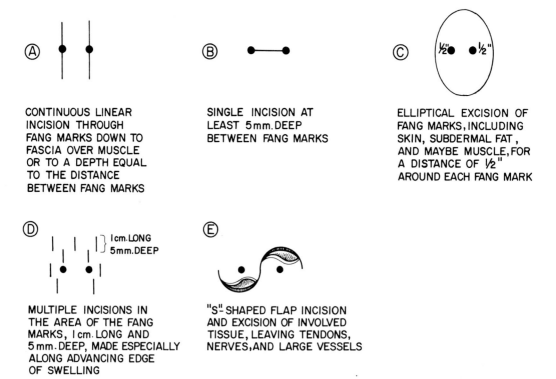

ⒶCONTINUOUS LINEAR INCISION THROUGH FANG MARKS DOWN TO FASCIA OVER MUSCLE OR TO A DEPTH EQUAL TO THE DISTANCE BETWEEN FANG MARKS

ⒷSINGLE INCISION AT LEAST 5 mm. DEEP BETWEEN FANG MARKS

ⒸELLIPTICAL EXCISION OF FANG MARKS, INCLUDING SKIN, SUBDERMAL FAT, AND MAYBE MUSCLE, FOR A DISTANCE OF ½" AROUND EACH FANG MARK

ⒹMULTIPLE INCISIONS IN THE AREA OF THE FANG MARKS, 1 cm. LONG AND 5 mm. DEEP, MADE ESPECIALLY ALONG ADVANCING EDGE OF SWELLING

Ⓔ"S"- SHAPED FLAP INCISION AND EXCISION OF INVOLVED TISSUE, LEAVING TENDONS, NERVES, AND LARGE VESSELS

Figure 4–21: Various incisions for treatment of snakebites. See text for explanation of parts *A* through *E*.

C. The depth to which the venom has been injected is generally considered to be three fourths of the distance between the fang marks. A rule of thumb is to incise the skin and subcutaneous tissue to the same depth as the distance between the fang marks (Fig. 4–21A).[79]

D. An elliptical excision of the fang marks, including the skin and subdermal fat to the depth of the muscle fascia and sometimes a section of muscle but not of nerves, blood vessels, or tendons, has been suggested.[7, 86, 148] The excision should include the circumferential area within 12 mm. (0.5 in.) of each fang mark. This method is effective for removing venom from a wound on the trunk if it is done within a few minutes after infliction of the bite (Fig. 4–21C).[7]

E. Multiple incisions in the area have been described;[42, 45, 115] however, these may increase the possibility of subsequent infection.[115] Multiple incisions should be considered when swelling progresses rapidly in spite of ancillary treatment. They are most advantageous when made longitudinally 1 cm. long and 5 mm. deep and should be made along the front of advancing swelling to allow for serum to ooze from them as cellulitis develops (Fig. 4–21D).[45]

Cutter suction cups provide an easy and effective means of removing venom. If several of these are available, they can be alternated over the incisions every 15 minutes. Suction should be continued vigorously for two hours and then maintained for 30 minutes of each hour for an additional two or three hours, depending on the bite severity.[115] Suction by mouth is not recommended since this could endanger the individual performing the suction.[7, 86]

A more radical approach has been reported. This technique entails the surgical removal of all affected tissue around the bite. After a linear or an "S"-shaped flap incision is made, all hemorrhagic tissue is excised except tendons, nerves, and large blood vessels (Fig. 4–21E). The resulting wound is closed immediately or closure is delayed until the viability of the underlying tissue and skin flaps has been determined to be adequate. Although polyvalent antivenin has been the mainstay in the medical management of snakebite, it does not prevent the tissue-destructive effects of the venom. The early surgical removal of venom-laden tissue has been shown to markedly reduce the amount of tissue necrosis. Of 22 patients who were treated with polyvalent antivenin either alone or in conjunction with cryotherapy, steroids, and incision and suction methods, 15 developed tissue necrosis around the bite area. In contrast to this, the incidence of tissue necrosis among those who were treated primarily by excisional therapy was only five of 61. An added advantage of excisional therapy is the reduction of delayed systemic intoxication by the venom.[68]

Cryotherapy

The use of ice-pack cryotherapy has been described for the treatment of snakebite.[45, 79] Plastic bags filled with ice and water help to keep the extremity dry during the period of therapy. A previously applied tourniquet should not be released until the extremity has been packed in ice for approximately five minutes, and the tourniquet should never be reapplied to the limb after the limb has been placed in the ice. The extremity must be observed at frequent intervals until it can be left out of the ice packs without an increase in the severity of the signs. In addition, hypothermia helps to relieve the intense pain associated with snakebites. Cooling is usually not necessary for more than 24 to 48 hours. It would appear that cryotherapy has its greatest effect as an early (before one hour has elapsed) emergency measure before the patient is transported to a hospital. Cooling also helps to prevent the spread of venom.[79]

Cryotherapy is not without its disadvantages and contraindications. It may increase local necrosis in the area where the venom was injected.[79] Local frostbite and the freezing of already damaged tissues can be prevented by wrapping the ice packs in towels.[45] Cryotherapy is contraindicated in peripheral vascular disease, diabetes, and cases in which the patient is advanced in age or not cooperative.[79] The last factor presents a major limitation in the use of cryotherapy in animals, since they tend to move about and might withdraw the limb from the ice packs.

Antivenin

Polyvalent antivenins that are available are specific for neutralizing the venom of viperine snakes.* These include all North American species of rattlesnakes, copperheads, and water moccasins in which the venoms are predominantly hematotoxic.[7, 79, 113] The antivenin should be stored at 35 to 45°C and used immediately after it is reconstituted.[7] Since antivenin contains horse serum, it is wise to skin test an individual prior to antivenin therapy.[79] Should anaphylaxis occur as a result of antivenin therapy, epinephrine should be administered.[7]

The dose of antivenin that is required will vary, depending upon the size of the animal, the size of the snake, and the amount of venom injected by the snake. Generally speaking, smaller individuals require higher doses of antivenin, since they receive a proportionally larger dose of venom.[7, 79, 115] If widely spaced fang puncture wounds are present, it can be assumed that the snake was large and therefore a relatively large volume of venom would have been injected. Consequently, a correspondingly large amount of antivenin may be required for neutralization.[45] The actual dose may vary from one to five vials (10 to 50 ml.) of reconstituted antivenin.[7, 113, 115]

Various routes of administration have been recommended:
1. The intravenous route is recommended by one manufacturer, since less time is required for the antivenin to reach the venom than with other routes, especially that of intramuscular injection.[7]
2. Another suggested route of administration is a combination of intramuscular and intravenous injection, without injection into the actual bite areas.[45]
3. Local infiltration of the bite area with 10 ml. of antivenin, followed by an intramuscular injection of the remainder of the drug, has been suggested.[115]
4. The subcutaneous injection of half of a vial of antivenin around or just proximal to the bite and the deep intramuscular injection of the remaining half of the vial have been advocated. Following this, a

---

*Antivenin (Crotalidae) Polyvalent is available from Fort Dodge Laboratories, Inc., Fort Dodge, IA 50501 and from Wyeth Laboratories, Philadelphia, PA 19101.

second vial of antivenin in normal saline solution is started as an intravenous drip.[79]

5. Intra-arterial injection of antivenin has been suggested. One vial of antivenin is mixed with 100 ml. of normal saline solution, and this substance is pumped into a regional artery using a sphygmomanometer bulb. A tight tourniquet that is applied proximal to the injection site keeps the antivenin in the area of the bite. About 20 minutes is required for injection of the mixture. If there is a history of allergic reaction, 100 ml. of hydrocortisone sodium succinate should be added to the intra-arterial solution.[86, 148] With any antivenin, carefully read the manufacturer's recommendations prior to using the product.

Antibiotics and Supportive Therapy

Antibiotics. Antibiotics should be given to patients with snakebite to help prevent secondary infections.[17, 45, 79, 115] Penicillin and streptomycin combinations have been reported to be effective in combating bacterial infections secondary to snakebites. Wide-spectrum antibiotics may also be used.[115]

Supportive Therapy. Steroid therapy for snakebite victims has its proponents and opponents. Steroids have been advocated in cases of severe envenomation to help reduce both local and widespread systemic effects.[45] In addition, they may be beneficial in reducing the serum reactions associated with antivenin therapy,[7, 79, 86] minimizing pain, improving the patient's sense of well-being, promoting the even distribution of edema, and minimizing the possibility of slough.[7, 86] Prednisone has been suggested in an initial dosage of 2.2 mg./kg. of body weight, followed by 1.1 mg./kg. every 12 hours.[86] Knapp and Flowers have stated that snakebitten dogs that had been treated with cortisone acetate had a lesser degree of tissue necrosis and slough and a prolonged survival time, showed less pain, were more active, ate better, and were in better physical condition than dogs that did not receive the drug.[83] Others have reported that cortisone is not lifesaving, but it does prolong life and prevent sloughing.[115] The prolonging of life may enable other medicaments to exert their beneficial effects.[7, 86]

Antihistamine therapy is reported to be contraindicated in the treatment of snakebite in animals, as this is said to potentiate the venom's toxicity.[7, 114, 115, 148] In contrast to this, Frye has reported beneficial results with antihistamines such as diphenhydramine hydrochloride, tripelennamine (Pyribenzamine) hydrochloride, and chlorpheniramine maleate.[45]

Tranquilizers have also been reported to potentiate the effect of snake venom. However, morphine and meperidine hydrochloride* may be used to control the pain associated with snakebite.[113] Since morphine tends to depress respiration, meperidine would be the drug of choice and should be continued until the pain has subsided.[45, 86] The exception to this rule is the use of meperidine to treat the pain associated with the venom of the Gila monster. There appears to be a synergism between the venom and the drug that compounds the venom's toxicity.[45] In general, sedatives and analgesics should be employed with discretion because large doses may mask important clinical signs.[7]

---

*Demerol Hydrochloride is available from Winthrop Laboratories, New York, NY 10016.

Intravenously administered fluids such as lactated Ringer's solution may be needed to bolster fluid volume and electrolyte levels and to replace the extracellular fluid that has been lost as a result of edema formation.[79, 86] Calcium gluconate has been suggested as a means of combating hemolysis and preventing muscular twitching;[86, 115] however, its use is controversial.[45] A blood transfusion may be necessary to bolster fluid volume and electrolyte levels[86] as well as to help counteract the anemia that may result from the hemolytic effect of the venom.[79]

When treating a case of snakebite the clinician should consider the size of the animal, the degree of envenomation, the location of the lesion, and the animal's condition upon presentation in deciding on the proper therapeutic agents and methods to be used in treatment. A more severe envenomation in a small dog may require some of the more aggressive methods that have been described in this section whereas a less severe envenomation in a large dog may not require as aggressive an approach to save life and limb.

GUNSHOT WOUNDS

Wounds Inflicted by High-Velocity or Unknown Velocity Missiles

High-velocity missiles will produce more severe internal damage than those of low velocity. If the veterinarian knows that the wound has been produced by a high-velocity missile or if he does not know the velocity of the wounding missile, it is best to follow the recommendation of one author who advocates opening the wound tract and inspecting the involved tissues.[163] Using this technique may require enlarging the wound or joining the entrance and exit wounds.[96] This will allow the surgeon to decide whether and how much débridement is necessary (Fig. 4–22). Any other method may be insufficient and may lead to wound complications. If, at the time of exploration, no foreign bodies or tissue devitalization is found, the wound may be primarily closed. However, if devitalization is present, the wound should be opened a

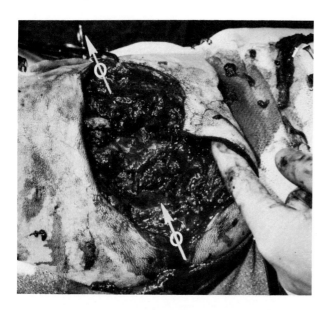

Figure 4–22: Gunshot wound across the lumbar region of a dog. The missile velocity was unknown. There were relatively small holes of entry and exit (*arrows*). The entrance and exit wounds were joined to create one large wound, which revealed massive damage to muscle tissue and one vertebral dorsal spinous process. Thorough débridement and the application of a drain were necessary.

sufficient length to permit exploration of the entire area. Wounds on the extremities should be opened longitudinally to facilitate closure, and wounds in flexion creases should be opened transversely.[163] The devitalized tissue should be thoroughly débrided, and the wound should be left unsutured and bandaged for a period of time, followed by delayed primary closure in four to ten days.[96, 163] The author has closed such wounds; however, adequate drainage was afforded, and the drains were flushed daily with an antibacterial solution. Systemic antibiotics were also administered.

A more conservative approach to early wound débridement has been suggested. Immediately after an injury, wounds do not show a clear line of demarcation between viable and devitalized tissue. Caution has been advocated in débriding such wounds; as much skin as possible should be saved and only severely discolored tissue should be removed.[95] The author emphasizes that the potential for infection and complications in a conservatively débrided contaminated wound is greater, and such a wound should be managed with this in mind (i.e., the wound should be left open or provisions for adequate drainage should be made).

Gas gangrene has been reported in gunshot wounds that have been sutured primarily. Treatment included wide excision of the involved tissue, the intramuscular injection of gentamicin, and the use of hyperbaric oxygen.[96]

The principles of wound débridement have been discussed in an earlier section of this chapter, and these principles apply to gunshot wounds. At this point, some variations and specific factors relative to débriding gunshot wounds will be mentioned. When gunshot wounds involve fractures as well as soft tissue damage, it is desirable to delay fracture repair in favor of treating soft tissues, using splints and external devices to immobilize the fracture until the soft tissues have been adequately treated.[95]

Exploration for missile fragments and other foreign materials should not invade tissues far from the wound tract; however, if foreign materials are intra-articular or adjacent to vital structures, they should be sought out and removed.[95] As mentioned earlier, there is usually little tissue reaction to bullet and shell fragments.

The entire missile tract should be explored, removing as much hair and debris as possible. Nerves, vessels, and tendons must be identified, preserved, and covered with protective tissue.[95] The particulars of muscle débridement have been covered in an earlier section of this chapter. Loose-lying small fragments of fascia must be removed. Perforated fascia should be incised the full length of the skin incision to permit exposure of the more extensively damaged underlying muscle. Since fascia is relatively resistant to the devitalizing effects of missile perforation, excision is usually limited to removing that which has been shredded or is badly contaminated.[95]

As mentioned in Chapter 2, high-velocity missiles cause more tissue damage than do low-velocity missiles. Therefore, débridement of high-velocity missile tracts will be more extensive, and it is advisable to leave the wound open.[96, 163]

Low-Velocity Missile Wounds

Since wounds that are caused by low-velocity missiles do not result in the internal tissue damage that is associated with high-velocity missiles, their treatment may be more conservative. In a series of 105 gunshot wounds in humans that were caused by low-velocity missiles, the treatment consisted of cleansing the surrounding skin, applying a dry, sterile pressure bandage, splinting and elevating the extremity, administering systemic antibiotics in all but six cases, and bed rest. The wounds were not incised, probed, or irrigated. All wounds healed without infection.[108]

The "pull-through technique" has been described for treating through-and-through gunshot wounds that are caused by low-velocity missiles. Forceps are passed through the wound tract and a swab that has been soaked in mild antiseptic is then pulled through the tract.[96]

In dogs, clipping the hair, thoroughly cleansing the superficial portion of the wound and the adjacent skin, and changing the bandages daily may be all that is required to treat wounds with minimal tissue damage. Antibiotics may be given as necessary.[95]

Although the majority of low-velocity bullet wounds require no real surgery, an aggressive surgical approach should be taken when the characteristics of the wound indicate the need for such.[58] The veterinarian may use a more conservative approach to this type of wound when it is known that a low-velocity weapon produced the injury and tissue damage does not appear to be great. However, if there is doubt as to the velocity of the wounding missile or the amount of internal tissue damage, a more radical approach should be taken.

BURNS

Chapter 5 is devoted to the management of burns. Burn cases are not often encountered in veterinary medicine; however, when they occur the clinician is presented with the challenge of treating and reconstructing the burned area as well as treating the accompanying systemic complications. Some of the aspects of topical burn therapy will be covered in this section. The reader is referred to Chapter 5 for information on the systemic aspects of burns.

Organisms and Burns

Staphylococcus aureus (pyogenes), Streptococcus pyogenes, Pseudomonas aeruginosa (pyocyanea), and *Proteus* organisms are all common burn contaminants.[54] A report in 1968 stated that the primary gram-positive organism that had been causing septicemia in burn patients since 1960 was the coagulase-positive *Staphylococcus aureus.* The gram-negative organisms that had been causing septicemia included *Pseudomonas aeruginosa, Proteus mirabilis, Paracolobactrum aerogenoides,* the *Aerobacter* group, and the *Klebsiella* group. Since 1960 a decrease in the number of gram-positive organisms and an increase in the number of gram-negative organisms causing septicemia have been reported.[5]

Pseudomonas organisms are the most troublesome in burn wounds. They can cause death without leukocytosis, fever, or positive blood cultures, as is typical with other gram-negative organisms. The bacterial counts of *Pseudomonas* from under the burn eschar more closely reflect the mortality than do bacterial counts from other organs. It was found in a study using rats that mortality is directly proportional to the bacterial concentration in the burn wound.[147] Walker, and co-workers have stated that it is possible to produce active immunization against burn wound infections with some strains of *Pseudomonas*. However, treatment with serum from immunized animals does not protect against mortality. They also found that polymyxin B therapy can fail to prevent death in infected animals, even though the infecting organism is sensitive in vitro and the doses used are maximal.[155]

Mycotic infections that were caused by *Phycomycetes* or an *Aspergillus* sp. have been reported in human burn wounds.[138] The infections occurred in burns that had been treated topically with mafenide and systemically with penicillin. The signs of infection included inflammation, rapid change in the color and character of the burn wound, eschar separation earlier than expected, and unexplained toxemia. The sudden appearance of violaceous or black spots in second-degree burn areas was also noted. Early separation of the eschar is highly suggestive of fungal infection. Infections that are caused by *Phycomycetes* and *Aspergillus* invade blood vessels, producing thrombosis, ischemia, and gangrene. In addition, these infections may invade the tissue along nerves, vessels, and fascial planes and spread extensively beneath intact skin. The radical excision of infected tissues and of the adjacent unburned tissue is recommended if the organisms have invaded subcutaneously. Amphotericin B has been suggested for patients with disseminated fungal disease.[138] Although mycotic burn infection has been reported only in humans, it is also possible in animals, in which case the aforementioned treatment would be applicable.

Problem with Systemic and Topical Burn Therapy

The main difficulty that is encountered with topical antibacterial or antimicrobial compounds is the fact that most of them do not penetrate the eschar deeply enough to cause a significant therapeutic effect at the interface between the viable and nonviable tissues. Likewise, systemic antibiotics and other antimicrobial agents that are administered parenterally are not carried into the interface in therapeutic concentrations because of the inadequate circulation in the area. Since 1965 several compounds have been utilized that have the ability to penetrate the eschar with sufficient antibacterial activity to control burn wound sepsis. These compounds include (1) a 0.5 per cent solution of silver nitrate, (2) 10 per cent mafenide acetate, (3) silver sulfadiazine, and (4) Neosporin.[98]

Compounds for Topical Burn Therapy

Silver Nitrate Solution. A thick bandage is first applied over the burn and then it is saturated with 0.5 per cent silver nitrate solution.[98, 107] The inner dressings are moistened continuously with the solution and are changed every 12 hours or at least daily. If they are allowed to dry, the silver nitrate in the dressing becomes caustic to the open wound.[98]

The advantages of 0.5 per cent silver nitrate solution, as stated by various sources,[5, 80, 87, 98, 107, 162] include the following:

1. It has bacteriostatic and fungicidal properties.
2. It is not as toxic as some drugs and is safer than many.
3. Cleaner wounds with less odor result.
4. There is no need for anesthesia when changing dressings.
5. It prevents the infection from converting second-degree wounds to third-degree wounds.
6. The wet dressings permit joint mobility.
7. Wound epithelialization is not impaired.
8. It is nonallergenic, inexpensive, readily available, and chemically stable.

The following disadvantages of 0.5 per cent silver nitrate solution have also been stated:[5, 80, 87, 98, 107]

1. It stains the area and environment deep black.
2. Electrolyte derangements occur (deficiencies of sodium, potassium, chloride, calcium, and magnesium) and may result in dilutional hyponatremia and convulsions.
3. It is ineffective in combating established infections and over a greasy coating or dead epidermis.
4. It may cause methemoglobinemia and clostridial myositis.
5. It has an adverse effect on donor sites and dermatomes.
6. The dressings are expensive, even though nitrate itself is inexpensive.
7. There is difficulty judging burn depth and evaluating the burn.
8. It causes delayed eschar separation.

Mafenide.   This drug is applied twice daily as a 10 per cent cream to a depth of 0.5 cm. on the burn with a gloved hand or tongue blade. In humans the wound may be left exposed or may be bandaged.[98] For veterinary use the wound would have to be bandaged because of the nature of the patient. Twice daily dressing changes help to débride the wound. Burns should be cleansed thoroughly each day to allow for visual inspection and reapplication of the mafenide.[98] In a 1967 report using rats, the addition of 90 per cent DMSO to serve as a vehicle for 10 per cent mafenide had no added effect in controlling *Pseudomonas* infections in burn wounds. When 10 per cent mafenide and mafenide in a DMSO vehicle were compared as to mortality and quantitative bacterial levels, only the former was found to be effective.[88]

Several sources have stated the following advantages of mafenide therapy:[5, 80, 94, 98]

1. Safety.
2. Effectiveness in suppressing bacterial colonization (bacteriostatic).
3. Ease in handling and application.
4. Ample penetration of the eschar.
5. Lack of staining.
6. Low toxicity.

Mafenide's disadvantages include the following:[5, 87, 94, 98, 147].
1. Sensitivity reactions.
2. The formation of hematomas beneath the burn eschar.
3. The emergence of a resistant strain of *Staphylococcus* and *Pseudomonas*.
4. Irritation and pain on application.
5. Delayed eschar separation owing to a suppressed microbial débriding action.
6. Increased insensible water loss.
7. Acidosis (more marked with the hydrochloride than with the acetate salt).
8. Inhibition of carbonic anhydrase, with an increased respiratory rate.
9. Retarded epithelial regeneration.

Silver Sulfadiazine.   The advantages of silver sulfadiazine outnumber its disadvantages. These advantages include:[87, 98]

1. Low to nonexistent toxicity.
2. A wide range of bacteriostatic activity.
3. A lack of staining.

4. Less painful application than with mafenide.
5. Ease in application and incorporation into the dressings.
6. Ample penetration of the eschar.

The main disadvantage of silver sulfadiazine is that it delays eschar separation.[98] A study on rats has shown that a combination of silver sulfadiazine and sutilains was ineffective in reducing bacterial counts. However, when the sutilains were applied once daily in the morning and the silver sulfadiazine was applied twice daily at eight-hour intervals, bacterial counts were reduced.[89] Since cerium compounds exert measurable antimicrobial action in vitro, cerous nitrate has been added to silver sulfadiazine cream. The cerous nitrate strikingly enhances the topical antiseptic effect of the cream on burn wounds without increasing its toxicity.[43]

Povidone-Iodine. Povidone-iodine possesses a broad antimicrobial spectrum, which is basically that of iodine; it is lethal to both gram-positive and gram-negative bacteria. It is also active against many yeasts, fungi, protozoa, and viruses.[47] A study has revealed that povidone-iodine ointment is quite effective as a prophylactic topical antibacterial agent when used early in the treatment of burn wounds, i.e., within minutes after thermal injury. At this time the burn has not yet been exposed to a great deal of bacterial contamination. When the treatment of burns is delayed, the area may already be heavily colonized by bacteria and may have burn wound sepsis. In a case in which subeschar colonization has occurred, povidone-iodine ointment is not effective.[131] When burn wounds or other wounds involving skin loss are sprayed with povidone-iodine immediately after injury, the crust that forms over the wound provides a protective cover against infection. The epithelium may then heal in an ideal environment.[159]

Two studies have shown that the frequent application of povidone-iodine is necessary to control burn wound sepsis.[43, 131] To control *Pseudomonas* infection, the application of povidone-iodine ointment four times daily was found superior to the daily or alternate-day application of the drug.[47]

In the study by Georgiade and Harris, povidone-iodine was reported to cause no toxic, allergic, or skin sensitivity reactions, nor were there signs of electrolyte or metabolic imbalance in the series of patients.[47] However, systemic absorption of povidone-iodine from burn wounds has been reported in two cases of severe burns (35 per cent burn and 75 per cent burn). Both patients had severe metabolic acidosis and serum-iodine levels far in excess of normal. Sodium bicarbonate therapy was necessary to control the acidosis, and hemodialysis was effective in reducing the serum-iodine concentration. The authors recommended that povidone-iodine should not be used topically on burns covering greater than 20 per cent of the body area.[121]

A mild burning or stinging sensation has been reported with the application of povidone-iodine to burns.[47]

Chlorhexidine. A 0.5 per cent solution of chlorhexidine was used in a series of 108 burn patients who were treated over a 14-month period. Gauze soaked in the solution was applied to the burn, followed by further bandaging. Infection was rare in the cases that were treated in this manner, and the chlorhexidine did not destroy regenerating epithelium or appreciably delay healing.[54] A 1 per cent chlorhexidine ointment* is available for veterinary use and could possibly be used for burn therapy. However, it should be kept in mind that a 1 per cent solution applied repeatedly to the fair skin of humans has

---

*Nolvasan ointment is available from Fort Dodge Laboratories, Inc., Fort Dodge, IA 50501.

been reported to cause some erythema.[54] For further information on the use of chlorhexidine in the treatment of wounds, the reader is referred to the section in this chapter dealing with wound lavage.

Gentamicin. A 0.1 per cent gentamicin sulfate ointment has been reported to be a safe broad-spectrum antibiotic to which resistance has rarely developed. In the ointment form, the absorption rate is low, and when it is used with systemic therapy, it has been found to reduce the effects of *Pseudomonas* exotoxin.[5] When treating *Pseudomonas*-infected wounds other than burn wounds, the author has noted a marked change in the wound shortly after initiating topical gentamicin therapy. A factor that should be considered in using this drug is the expense of the medication.

Proteolytic Enzymes. The use of proteolytic enzymes to treat burn wounds has its advantages and disadvantages. Sutilains have been reported to be more effective than other enzymes in the débridement of burn eschar. The sutilains ointment tended to lyse the eschar of a fresh burn more quickly and completely than the dry, leathery eschar of an old burn. It did not damage viable epithelium or inhibit reepithelialization of the wound, nor did it have any adverse effect on the success of the skin grafts.[118]

A disadvantage of enzymatic débriding solutions is that they provide a wet, warm medium with dead protein tissue in various stages of denaturation, which is ideal for bacterial growth.[24] In addition, enzymatic débriding agents may open new routes of bacterial invasion.[147]

Although sutilains have been reported to increase eschar separation as previously mentioned, they also have certain disadvantages. These include the following:

1. Sutilains have been reported to predispose the burn wound to sepsis, and the addition of mafenide or silver sulfadiazine is of questionable value in preventing burn wound sepsis.[89, 161] The addition of silver sulfadiazine cream to the sutilains ointment has been associated with a reduction in purulence, dermal necrosis, weight loss, and damage to epithelial cells. Sutilains may also harm tissue that is injured but not immediately coagulated by heat.[161]
2. A mild, transient, burning pain has been associated with the topical application of sutilains ointment.[118]
3. The application of sutilains requires that the wound be kept moist.[98]
4. Sutilains ointment should be applied only to limited areas of the body (not exceeding 10 per cent of the body surface at one time).[98]
5. The ointment is most effective early in the course of therapy and becomes less effective later on a leathery, dry eschar.[98]
6. The enzymes are inactivated by heavy metals, such as silver.[98]

Mechanical Burn Therapy

In addition to the chemotherapeutic approach to burns, the mechanical removal of burn eschar has its place in burn therapy. Burn eschar is considered to be the residue of skin elements that have been coagulated by heat.[24] It is composed almost entirely of tough collagen fibers in various states of radiant energy denaturation.[117] The eschar differs from a scab, which contains dead cells and flimsy fibrin,[117] and from the fibrinous crust that forms secondarily to partial-thickness burns.[24] One mechanical approach to eschar removal entails cutting the eschar into 1-in. squares to increase the surface area for débridement. An electrocautery is used to make the cuts through the eschar only.

Tangential eschar removal has been performed with a dermatome or a knife that is used for skin grafts by taking parallel slices through the eschar until a bleeding surface appears.[98]

Summary

In summary, burns do not occur with great frequency in animals; however, when they do, they can present the veterinarian with some formidable problems. The problems that a veterinarian encounters in burn therapy can be even greater than those encountered by a physician owing to the contrary or noncooperative nature of the patient. For example, keeping the wound as clean as possible can be more of a problem when dealing with an animal, since it has no concept of infection. Urine and fecal contamination of the wound are frequent. In addition, animals often chew off a bandage so that they can lick and chew at the wound or consume the skin graft.

DECUBITAL ULCERS

Decubital ulcers are occasionally seen in dogs and require therapy, either surgical or nonsurgical. Sather and colleagues have published an in-depth review of the various means that are used to treat decubital ulcers in humans.[139] This section will cover the techniques that the author has found to be beneficial in treating decubital ulcers.[152] The best approach to decubital ulcers in animals is to prevent them. Factors that are beneficial in their prevention include the following:

1. The patient's position should be changed frequently.[48, 56, 112, 152]
2. The animal should rest on sufficient padding. This may be in the form of foam rubber mattresses, air mattresses, water mattresses, sheepskin pads, or sawdust beds.[48, 56, 62, 117, 152] Artificial sheepskin pads* have been found to be beneficial by the author and are used routinely at the Auburn University Small Animal Clinic (Fig. 4–23).
3. The animal should be fed a high-protein, high-carbohydrate diet that is supplemented with vitamins. Androgenic steroids may help to reverse tissue breakdown.[44, 48, 53, 56, 62]
4. The skin should be kept clean, dry, and free of excreta. Whirlpool or warm water baths two or three times daily help to keep the skin clean and to promote circulation (Fig. 4–24).[48, 62, 152]

---

*Decubicrest Pads are available from Hillcrest Mills, Inc., Janesville, WI 53545.

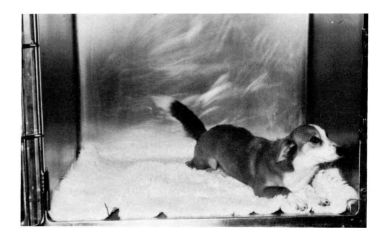

Figure 4–23: Bedding a dog on an artificial sheepskin pad to help prevent decubital ulcers.

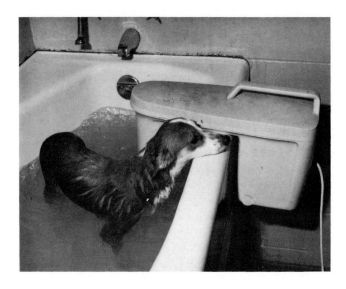

Figure 4–24: Whirlpool baths in warm water keep skin clean and promote circulation.

The nonsurgical treatment of decubital ulcers includes the use of many topical compounds, as stated in Sather and associates' review.[139] The author has had beneficial results using topical protamine zinc insulin suspension or a compound containing trypsin, balsam of Peru, and castor oil.* The mixture of insulin that is currently used contains 30 units of protamine zinc insulin suspension in 28 gm. of nitrofurazone ointment base. The following regimen has proved to be beneficial:

1. Lavage the ulcer with hydrogen peroxide.
2. Apply infrared light to the ulcer for about 15 minutes three times daily.
3. Apply the insulin mixture to the ulcer twice daily.
4. Place a "doughnut" bandage around the ulcer to prevent pressure on the ulcer (Fig. 4–25).[152]

---

*Granulex is manufactured by Dow B. Hickam, Inc., Houston, TX 77085.

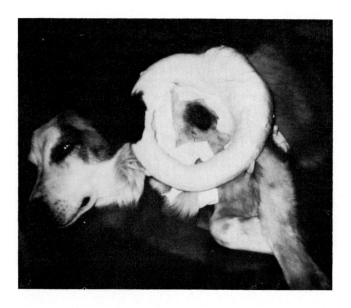

Figure 4–25: Doughnut bandage helps to keep pressure off a decubital ulcer or off the site of surgical repair. (From Swaim, S.F., and Votau, K.: Prevention and treatment of decubital ulcers in the dog. Vet. Med. Small Anim. Clin. *70*:1071, 1975.)

Using a doughnut bandage and spraying the ulcer with the trypsin, balsam of Peru, and castor oil compound are effective in treating decubital ulcers. It should be emphasized that the aforementioned regimen is to be used in conjunction with the previously suggested methods for the prevention of decubital ulcers (i.e., sufficiently padded bedding, a good diet, and adequate skin hygiene).

Decubital ulcers are often treated surgically, which can provide rapid primary healing in the area. Since most decubital ulcers are basically circular in shape, the wound can be débrided to this shape and closed by one of the methods described in Chapter 7. The technique that is preferred by the author is the conversion of the circular wound to a fusiform shape by removing two triangular pieces of skin from opposite sides of the circle, followed by routine closure. A doughnut bandage is applied to prevent pressure on the surgical site so that healing can take place. Large decubital ulcers may be treated nonsurgically until they reach a size that is small enough to allow closure as previously described, or the large defect can be corrected by using some type of skin flap, as described in Chapter 8.[152] The surgical removal of bony prominences underlying decubital ulcers has been recommended in the treatment of cases in which severe debility and loss of soft tissue mass have resulted in extreme protrusion of the prominence.[56, 112, 149, 152]

CLOSTRIDIAL INFECTIONS

Clostridial Myositis and Gangrene

"Dirty" wounds are more apt to harbor gas gangrene–producing anaerobic bacilli than are "clean" wounds. However, even clean wounds contain these organisms and hemolytic streptococci with sufficient frequency to suspect their presence in every case.[123] Clostridial infections are the result of a sizable amount of dead, unoxygenated tissue that is caused by direct injury or some deficiency in the blood supply, such as would occur with a blood vessel injury or a tight cast.[101]

The pathogenicity of a clostridial infection starts with a damaged blood supply and a traumatized muscle mass. With no blood supply or an inadequate supply the tissue mass becomes anoxic. The breakdown products of the traumatized tissue provide an excellent growth medium for the clostridia that are present. To further complicate the situation, the interrupted blood supply prevents polymorphonuclear leukocytes and other substances that are important in the body's defense mechanisms from entering the anoxic, devitalized tissue.[143] Thus, the conditions are present for clostridial infection.

The signs of clostridial myositis or gas gangrene as described in humans are usually recognized in the first 48 to 72 hours after injury. These signs include a general illness (not necessarily associated with fever) that is not commensurate with the extent of injury, severe local pain, edema, a foul seropurulent discharge, and, in the late stages, gas in the tissues as evidenced by crepitus or radiographic findings.[33] It would be wise for the veterinarian to be aware of these signs, since similar conditions may exist in animals.

The treatment of clostridial infections must be radical; the wound should be opened, the necrotic tissue should be removed, and the dead muscle bellies should be widely excised. Penicillin is the drug of choice and should be administered in high doses.[33] Amputation of a limb may be indicated in some severe cases.

Tetanus

Tetanus is not a common infection in dogs; however, it does occur in association with lacerations and puncture wounds.[41, 62] Deep wounds provide a more favorable anaerobic environment for the growth of *Clostridium tetani* than do superficial wounds. In some cases the wound may be small, and it is not always possible to find the portal of entry.[41]

Of the two toxins that are produced by the organism, tetanospasmin and tetanolysin, the former is the more important in the production of typical muscle spasms.[41] The signs of tetanus usually appear within five to eight days after the introduction of the organism,[41, 62] but they may appear as early as three days or as late as ten days after introduction.[41] The signs include muscle hyperexcitability with chronic spasms and tonic contractions of the face and auricular muscles (Fig. 4–26). These spasms produce a "smiling" appearance, wrinkling of the skin on the forehead, and pulling up of the ears. Other signs include spasticity, trismus, an inability to stand, protrusion of the nictitating membrane, opisthotonos, and hypersensitivity to external stimuli.[41, 62]

The treatment of tetanus includes wound débridement, cleansing, and the use of hydrogen peroxide to flush the wound. High doses of penicillin and intravenous antitoxin are indicated.[41, 62] Antitoxin should be given intravenously in a dose of 30,000 to 100,000 units after a subcutaneous test dose of 0.1 to 0.2 ml. has been given to check for reactions to horse serum.[41] Other means of supportive therapy include muscle relaxants, tranquilizers, and barbiturates.[41, 62]

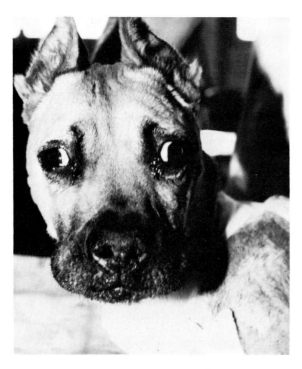

Figure 4–26: Tonic muscle spasms of the facial and auricular muscles resulting from tetanus infection.

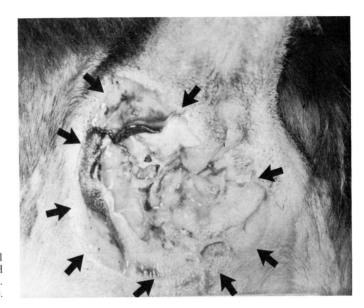

Figure 4–27: Necrosis of perianal tissue (*arrows*) that has been treated with cryosurgery. (Courtesy of P. A. Bushby.) See color plate II–F, p. 569.

CRYOSURGERY

GENERAL INFORMATION

Cryosurgery is included in this chapter, since the final stage of this procedure is the healing of an open wound. Cryosurgery has been described as a means of removing skin tumors.[14, 15, 25, 52, 55, 59, 90] This type of tumor removal is a form of trauma in itself in that the pathological tissue is subjected to cryotrauma, which causes the loss of this tissue and results in a skin defect that heals as an open wound. Cryosurgery has been described as causing a frostbite effect in which heat is extracted from the tissue until it is no longer viable. The temperature at which this occurs is generally accepted to be −20° C and below.[14, 90] The cryobiological and physiological changes and the microscopic tissue alterations that occur within the tissues have been adequately described,[20, 52, 55, 90] and the reader is referred to these sources for detailed information on these subjects. After cryosurgery, swelling and mild hyperthermia become apparent within two to three hours. The edema may last for up to four days, during which time superficial necrosis with marked discoloration becomes obvious.[90] Necrosis may appear as early as 12 to 24 hours postoperatively and is usually complete by the seventh day after treatment;[14] however, slough separation may take up to 20 days (Fig. 4–27).[90] Following the slough of pathological tissues, a clean granulation tissue bed is left, and healing occurs by epithelialization over this bed (Fig. 4–28).[14, 90]

In general, there is an orderly progression of tissue change: edema and erythema, infiltration of inflammatory cells, tissue necrosis, tissue slough, and repair by granulation and reepithelialization. Healing has been found to occur from the margins of frozen areas inward. Granulation tissue develops on all exposed surfaces and epithelialization begins from the periphery of the lesions. This epithelial tissue has been found to be strong, viable, hypopigmented, and lacking in adnexal structures.[20]

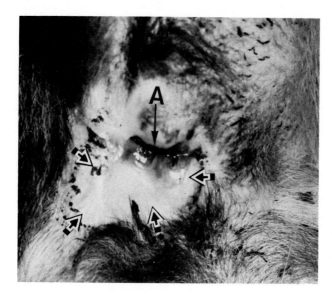

Figure 4–28: Perianal lesion shown in Figure 4–27 is healed. The epithelium over the healed lesion is indicated by the arrows. A designates the anus. (Courtesy of P. A. Bushby.) See color plate II–G, p. 569.

INDICATIONS

Owing to the nature of this type of treatment, it can only be applied in areas where there exists a suitable route by which the necrotic material can be discharged;[90] consequently, the technique has been used to treat various superficial pathological conditions. Cryosurgery has been stated to be particularly useful in treating locally invasive, nonmetastatic soft tissue lesions of the distal extremity in cases in which conventional excision may have prevented primary skin closure.[55, 59] The technique has been used to remove various benign and malignant tumors from the skin and eyelids as well as to treat perianal fistulas, lick and eosinophilic granulomas, interdigital and sebaceous cysts, proliferative lesions of the ear canal, tumors and lesions of the oral cavity, and pharyngeal and nasal tumors. It is also used in tonsillectomies and in performing biopsies for malignant neoplasms.[15, 20, 52, 55, 90] Most mammary tumors are removed using routine surgical techniques, but some selected mammary tumors are treated cryosurgically. Animals with ulcerative, infected tumors and animals that are high surgical risks are candidates for the cryosurgical removal of mammary tumors.[52]

TECHNIQUE

The purpose of this section is to acquaint the practitioner with the basic aspects of cryosurgery as it would apply to surgery of the skin. For more detailed information on the subject, the reader is referred to the various texts and publications that deal with the subject in detail.

Several media have been described for cryosurgical procedures. These include Freon, carbon dioxide, nitrous oxide, and liquid nitrogen.[14, 52, 55] Freon has been described for cataract removal. Carbon dioxide is applied as a "snow" or as a pressurized "pencil." It does not penetrate tissue deeply (only 5 mm.) and is useful in the removal of surface tumors.[52] Nitrous oxide is one of the "warmer" cryogens and does not penetrate as deeply as others. It is used as a gas under pressure that is allowed to expand through a small orifice. This agent is more predictable than others in relation to the extent of tissue freezing that it will accomplish, and the use of thermocouples to gauge the amount of freezing in surrounding tissue may not be as important with this medium as with others. This would apply to areas of tumor removal where surrounding vital tissues would not be harmed, as in the case of isolated skin tumors. An advantage of this medium is that nitrous oxide units offer a defrost mechanism that allows the operator to disengage the cryoprobe from the frozen tissue. Nitrous oxide is also readily available to veterinarians.[51, 52] Liquid nitrogen is capable of freezing rapidly and penetrating deeply. It is the medium that is most used for tumor removal. It can be used in probe, spray, or swab forms.[52]

The basic guidelines for cryosurgery are as follows:
1. The tissue must be frozen to at least −20°C.
2. The rate of freezing must be rapid and the rate of thawing must be slow and unassisted.
3. Two or three freeze-thaw cycles must be used to achieve maximum cell death in those areas where cells tend to survive the freeze-thaw cycle.[52]

Various methods may be used to apply the cryosurgical medium. These include swabbing the lesion with the medium, pouring it on the lesion, spraying it on the lesion, and using a cryoprobe to freeze the lesion.[51, 52, 55, 90] Thermocouples that are placed in the tissue surrounding the lesion and in the lesion itself monitor the extent of tissue freezing and protect the surrounding vital structures (Fig. 4–29). Placing a thermocouple in the lesion assures that the tissue in the depths of the lesion reaches −20°C. When dealing with a neoplastic condition, it is recommended that a 5-mm. margin of normal tissue be included in the frozen area. When dealing with an infiltrating tumor, a 1-cm. margin of normal tissue is recommended.[52, 55]

When spraying or pouring the cryosurgical medium onto a lesion or swabbing a lesion with it, it is essential to protect the surrounding normal tissue. This protection may be afforded by applying a thick coating of petroleum jelly around the lesion's periphery to act as an insulator. A Styrofoam or tin container with both ends removed and of a diameter that is equal to that of the tumor may be placed over the tumor and sealed to the skin with petroleum jelly (Fig. 4–30).[55] Endotracheal tube adapters and plastic syringe covers may also be used as protectors. Gauze sponges, cotton, and water-soluble surgical lubricant have also been described as insulating substances.[52]

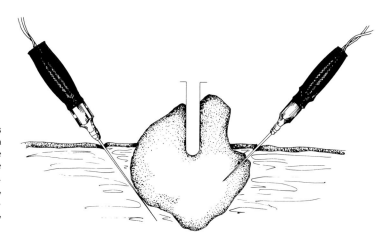

Figure 4–29: Thermocouples placed in and adjacent to a lesion monitor the extent of tissue freezing and help to protect the surrounding vital structures. (After Greiner, T.P., Liska, W.D., and Withrow, S.J.: Cryosurgery. Vet. Clin. North Am. 5:5715, 1975.)

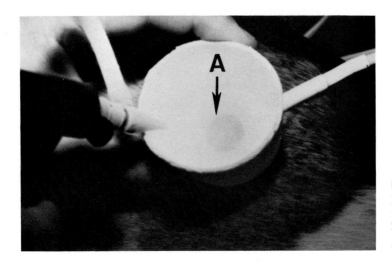

Figure 4–30: Styrofoam cup with a hole cut in the bottom, A, has been placed over a lesion, and the cryosurgical medium is being sprayed into the cup. (Courtesy of P. A. Bushby.)

A cotton swab may be soaked in liquid nitrogen and directly applied to a small mass until it is frozen. Liquid nitrogen may also be poured directly onto the mass after proper insulating procedures have been accomplished.[55] Liquid nitrogen or nitrous oxide may be sprayed on the lesion, but again, the proper insulation must be provided to protect surrounding tissues from the "scatter" of the medium.[52, 55]

The use of a cryoprobe is a little more involved than the spray, swab, or pouring techniques. First, the thermocouples should be placed in and around the lesion. The probe is applied in or on the lesion before freezing is begun; otherwise cryoadhesion makes accurate repositioning of the tip difficult.[90] As freezing progresses, an "ice ball" forms in the tissue that will increase in size until equilibrium is reached between the heat that is gained from the surrounding tissues and the local blood vessels and the heat that is lost to the probe (Fig.

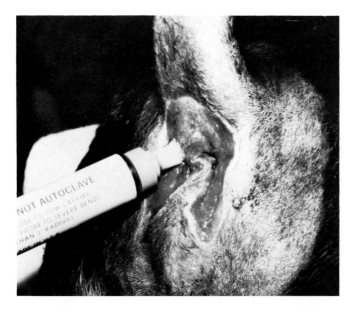

Figure 4–31: Use a cryoprobe to produce an ice ball in a lesion. (Courtesy of P. A. Bushby.)

4–31).[90] Other factors governing the size of the ice ball are (1) the surface area for heat exchange of the cryosurgical instrument, (2) the length of time that the cryoprobe is applied, (3) the temperature that is employed, and (4) the vascularity and ambient temperature of the tissue that is being treated.[14] Depending on the site and the nature of the lesion, tissue destruction usually takes from one to five minutes.[90] Once freezing is complete, the cryoprobe, which will adhere to the tissues, should be allowed to release spontaneously in an unassisted thaw.[52, 90] An "escape" zone has been described, which is a subliminal layer of cells that has the potential for survival. This is undesirable. For this reason at least one and possibly three repeated freeze-thaw cycles have been advocated and are described in the literature.[52, 55, 90] This procedure achieves maximum cell death in areas where the cells have survived the first freeze-thaw cycle.

Three methods that have been described for applying cryosurgery are (1) the overlapping-probe method, (2) the base method, and (3) the punch method. The overlapping-probe method entails producing several overlapping ice balls to form one large ice ball. This increases the total area of necrosis and kills cells that would be present in the escape zone.[51, 90] The base method requires removing the bulk of a large lesion by conventional surgery and freezing the remaining base. This procedure, like the overlapping-probe method, insures maximum cell death.[51] The punch method is performed by placing the cryoprobe into the hole that is made by a punch biopsy of the lesion. This allows the ice ball to penetrate deeper into the lesion.[51, 52]

ADVANTAGES AND DISADVANTAGES

The advocates of cryosurgery have stated the following numerous advantages of this technique.[14, 52, 55, 90]

1. It is safe and simple.
2. The time required for anesthesia is brief.
3. It produces minimal hemorrhage.
4. It allows the removal of tumors that would be difficult to remove by conventional means owing to their location or proximity to vital tissues.
5. It may be used as a palliative measure in cases with a grave prognosis.
6. It may be used as an adjunct to chemotherapy and immunotherapy.
7. Antigens that are associated with killed tumor cells are left in situ after cryosurgery. Such antigens help to stimulate an immune response against malignant cells.
8. There is a sharp delineation between frozen (destroyed) cells and viable tissue.
9. The danger of metastasis from handling tumors during surgery is decreased.
10. Cryosurgery can remove tumors in certain areas without permanently damaging these tissues as a result of freezing (e.g., tumors in or around bones, large blood vessels, and nerves).
11. Lesions may be removed from areas that do not heal well following surgical excision (e.g., areas around joints, interdigital spaces, and the distal portion of limbs).

The following disadvantages of cryosurgery have also been stated:[51, 52, 55, 59, 90]

1. The lesion is aesthetically unpleasing as a result of the foul odor and discharge from the necrosing tissue.
2. Damage may be done to normal vital tissue surrounding the lesion as the result of overfreezing the lesion, especially when liquid nitrogen is used.
3. Excessive freezing will produce excessive scarring.
4. The healing time is slower than that required for healing of a surgical incision by first intention.
5. A different color hair will grow when the lesion heals.

REFERENCES

1. Alexander, J.W., Kaplan, J.Z., and Altemeier, W.A.: Role of suture materials in the development of wound infection. Ann. Surg. 165:192, 1967.
2. Alexander, J.W., Wheeler, L.M., Rooney, R.C., et al.: Clinical evaluation of Epigard, a new synthetic substitute for homograft and heterograft skin. J. Trauma 13:374, 1973.
3. Altemeier, W.A.: Wound Healing in Surgery: Proceedings of the Panel Discussion. Somerville, N.J., Ethicon, Inc., 1970, p. 14.
4. Altemeier, W.A., and Gibbs, E.W.: Bacterial flora of fresh accidental wounds. Surg. Gynecol. Obstet. 78:164, 1944.
5. Altemeier, W.A., and MacMillan, B.G.: Comparative studies of topical silver nitrate, Sulfamylon, and gentamicin. Ann. N.Y. Acad. Sci. 150:966, 1968.
6. Amroliwalla, F.K.: Vaccination scar with soft tissue atrophy restored by local insulin treatment. Br. Med. J. 1:1389, 1977.
7. Snake venom poisoning: Its pathogenesis and clinical management. Fort Dodge Laboratories, Fort Dodge, Iowa 1976.
8. Archibald, J., and Blakely, C.L.: Basic procedures and preoperative considerations, in Archibald, J. (ed.): Santa Barbara, Calif., Canine surgery, ed. 2. American Veterinary Publications, Inc., 1974, pp. 17–106.
9. Baker, C.E.: Physician's Desk Reference, ed. 32. Oradell, N.J., Medical Economics Co., 1978.
10. Barnes, J.W.: Sugar sweetens the lot of patients with bedsores. J.A.M.A. 225:22, 1973.
11. Belfield, W.O., Golinsky, S., and Compton, M.D.: The use of insulin in open-wound healing. Vet. Med. Small Anim. Clin. 5:455, 1970.
12. Bernard, H.R., and Cole, W.R.: Wound infections following potentially contaminated operations: Effect of delayed primary closure of the skin and subcutaneous tissue. J.A.M.A. 184:118, 1963.
13. Borge, A.F.: Elective Incisions and Scar Revision. Boston, Little, Brown and Co., 1973.
14. Borthwick, R.: Cryosurgery and its role in the treatment of malignant neoplasms. J. Small Anim. Pract. 13:369, 1972.
15. Borthwick, R.: Cryosurgery in veterinary practice: A preliminary report. Vet. Rec. 86:683, 1970.
16. Branemark, P.I., Ekholm, R., Albrektsson, J., et al.: Tissue injury caused by wound disinfectants. J. Bone Joint Surg. Am. 49A:48, 1967.
17. Brown, P.W.: The prevention of infection in open wounds. Clin. Orthop. 96:42, 1973.
18. Buckle, R.C., and Seabridge, C.E.: The effect of chlorhexidine in the peritoneal cavity: An experimental study. Lancet 1:193, 1963.
19. Burleson, R., and Eiseman, B.: Mechanisms of antibacterial effect of biologic dressings. Ann. Surg. 177:181, 1973.
20. Bushby, P.A., Hoff, E.S., and Hankes, G.H.: Microscopic tissue alterations following cryosurgery of canine skin. J. Am. Vet. Med. Assoc. 173:177, 1978.
21. Charles, W.: Veterinarian's Product and Therapeutic Reference: A Guide to Pharmaceuticals and Biologicals. Caldwell, N.J., Therapeutic Communications, Inc., 1976.
22. Committee on Trauma, American College of Surgeons.: Early Care of the Injured Patient, ed. 2. Philadelphia, W. B. Saunders Co., 1976.
23. Condie, J.D., and Ferguson, D.J.: Experimental wound infections: Contamination versus surgical technique. Surgery 50:367, 1961.
24. Connell, J.F. Jr., and Rousselot, L.M.: The use of proteolytic enzymes in the debridement of the burn eschar. Surg. Forum. 4:422, 1953.
25. Conroy, J.D.: Neoplasms of the skin and subcutis, in Kirk, R.W. (ed.): Current Veterinary Therapy: V. Small Animal Medicine. Philadelphia, W. B. Saunders Co., 1974.

26. Cress, R.H., and Busza, A.: The conservative management of ischemic ulcers. J. Med. Assoc. Ala. 37:905, 1968.
27. Cummings, B.C.: Collateral circulation of the canine thoracic limb, in Some Techniques and Procedures in Small Animal Surgery. Bonner Springs, Kans., Veterinary Medical Publishing Co., Inc., 1963, pp. 144–152.
28. Cummings, B.C.: Collateral circulation of the canine pelvic limb, in Some Techniques and Procedures in Small Animal Surgery. Bonner Springs, Kans., Veterinary Medical Publishing Co., Inc., 1963, pp. 153–161.
29. Custer, J., Edlich,R.F., Prusak, M., et al.: Studies in the management of the contaminated wound: V. An assessment of the effectiveness of PhisoHex and Betadine surgical scrub solutions. Am. J. Surg. 121:572, 1971.
30. Cutright, D.E., Bhaskar, S.N., Gross, A., et al.: Effect of vancomycin, streptomycin, and tetracycline pulsating jet lavage on contaminated wounds. Milit. Med. 136:810, 1971.
31. Dedo, D.D., Alonso, W.A., and Ogura, J.H.: Povidone-iodine: An adjunct in the treatment of wound infections, dehiscences, and fistulas in head and neck surgery. Trans. Am. Acad. Ophthalmol. Otolaryngol. 84:68, 1977.
32. Dixon, A.C.: The secondary closure of wounds. Vet. Rec. 75:1133, 1963.
33. Dudley, H.A.F.: Wounds and their treatment, in McNair, T.J. (ed.): Hamilton Bailey's Emergency Surgery, ed. 9. Baltimore, Williams & Wilkins Co., 1972, pp. 47–57.
34. Edlich, R.F., Custer, J., Madden, J., et al.: Studies in management of the contaminated wound: III. Assessment of the effectiveness of irrigation with antiseptic agents. Am. J. Surg. 118:21, 1969.
35. Edlich, R.F., Madden, J.E., Prusak, M., et al.: Studies on the management of the contaminated wounds: VI. The therapeutic value of gentle scrubbing in prolonging the limited period of effectiveness of antibiotics in contaminated wounds. Am. J. Surg. 121:668, 1971.
36. Edlich, R.F., Panek, P.H., Rodeheaver, G.T., et al.: Physical and chemical configuration of sutures in the development of surgical infection. Ann. Surg. 177:679, 1973.
37. Edlich, R.F., Rodeheaver, G.T., Thacker, J.G., et al.: Management of soft tissue injury. Clin. Plast. Surg. 4:191, 1977.
38. Edlich, R.F., Rogers, W., Kasper, G., et al.: Studies in the management of the contaminated wound: I. Optimal time for closure of contaminated open wounds: II. Comparison of resistance to infection of open and closed wounds during healing. Am. J. Surg. 117:323, 1969.
39. Edlich, R.F., Tsung, M.S., Rogers, W., et al.: Studies in the management of the contaminated wound: I. Technique of closure of such wounds together with a note on a reproducible experimental model. J. Surg. Res. 8:585, 1968.
40. Faddis, D., Daniel, D., and Boyer, J.: Tissue toxicity of antiseptic solutions: A study of rabbit articular and periarticular tissues. J. Trauma 7:895, 1977.
41. Farrow, B.R.H., and Love, D.N.: Infectious diseases, in Ettinger, S.J. (ed.): Textbook of Veterinary Internal Medicine. Philadelphia, W. B. Saunders, 1975, pp. 221–222.
42. Fillmore, R.S.: The early local treatment of snakebite. Tex. State J. Med. 37:311, 1941.
43. Fox, C.L. Jr., Monafo, W.W. Jr., Vatche, H.A., et al.: Topical chemotherapy for burns using cerium salts and silver sulfadiazine. Surg. Gynecol. Obstet. 144:668, 1977.
44. Freeman, B.S.: Treatment of bedsores in paraplegic patients. Surgery 21:668, 1947.
45. Frye, F.L.: Bites and stings of venomous animals, in Kirk, R.W. (ed.): Current Veterinary Therapy: VI. Small Animal Practice. Philadelphia, W. B. Saunders Co., 1977, pp. 166–173.
46. Furneaux, R.W.: Management of contaminated wounds. Canine Pract. 2:22, 1975.
47. Georgiade, N.G., and Harris, W.A.: Open and closed treatment of burns with povidone-iodine. Plast. Reconstr. Surg. 52:640, 1973.
48. Gibbon, J.H., and Freeman, L.W.: The primary closure of decubitus ulcers. Ann. Surg. 124:1148, 1946.
49. Gilmore, O.J.A., Reid, C., and Strokon, A.: A study of the effect of povidone-iodine on wound healing. Postgrad. Med. J. 53:122, 1977.
50. Glotzer, D.J., Goodman, W.S., and Geronimus, L.H.: Topical antibiotic prophylaxis in contaminated wounds. Arch. Surg. 100:589, 1970.
51. Goldstein, R.S.: Nitrous oxide cryosurgical units: Their use in veterinary practice. Vet. Med. Small Anim. Clin. 72:1587, 1977.
52. Goldstein, R.S., and Hess, P.W.: Cryosurgery of canine and feline tumors. J. Am. Anim. Hosp. Assoc. 12:340, 1976.
53. Groce, E.S., Schullinger, R.N., and Shearer, T.P.: The operative treatment of decubitus ulcers. Ann. Surg. 123:53, 1946.
54. Grant, J.C., and Findlay, J.C.: Local treatment of burns and scalds using chlorhexidine. Lancet 272:862, 1957.
55. Greiner, T.P., Liska, W.D., and Withrow, S.J.: Cryosurgery. Vet. Clin. North Am. 5:565, 1975.
56. Griffith, B.H.: Pressure sores, in Ruge, D. (ed.): Spinal Cord Injuries. Springfield, Ill., Charles C Thomas Publishers, 1969, pp. 135–144.

57. Gross, A., Cutright, D.E., and Bhaskar, S.: Effectiveness of pulsating water jet lavage in treatment of contaminated crushed wounds. Am. J. Surg. *124*:373, 1972.
58. Hampton, O.P.: The indications for debridement of gunshot (bullet) wounds of the extremities in civilian practice. J. Trauma *1*:368, 1961.
59. Harvey, H.J.: General principles of veterinary oncologic surgery. J. Am. Anim. Hosp. Assoc. *12*:335, 1976.
60. Heggers, J.P., Robson, M.C., and Doran, E.T.: Quantitative assessment of bacterial contamination of open wounds by a slide technique. Trans. R. Soc. Trop. Med. Hyg. *63*:532, 1969.
61. Heggers, J.P., Robson, M.C., and Ristroph, J.D.: A rapid method of performing quantitative wound cultures. Milit. Med. *134*:666, 1969.
62. Hoerlein, B.F., and Bowen, J.M.: Clinical disorders of nerves and muscles, in Hoerlein, B.F. (ed.): Canine Neurology: Diagnosis and Treatment, ed. 3. Philadelphia, W. B. Saunders Co., 1978, pp. 286–287.
63. Hoffer, R.E., and Alexander, J.W.: Pinch grafting. J. Am. Anim. Hosp. Assoc. *12*:644, 1976.
64. Hohn, D.C., Granelli, S.G., Burton, R.W., et al.: Antimicrobial systems of the surgical wound: II. Detection of antimicrobial protein in cell-free wound fluid. Am. J. Surg. *133*:601, 1977.
65. Holobek, J.: Clinical experience with a proteolytic enzyme. Vet. Med. Small Anim. Clin. *68*:148, 1973.
66. Hoover, N.W., and Ivins, J.C.: Wound debridement. Arch. Surg. *79*:701, 1959.
67. Houang, E.T., Gilmore, O.J.A., Reid, C., et al.: Absence of bacterial resistance to povidone-iodine. J. Clin. Pathol. *29*:752, 1976.
68. Huang, T.T., Blackwell, S.J., and Lewis, S.R.: Hand deformities in patients with snakebites. Plast. Reconstr. Surg. *62*:32, 1978.
69. Howe, C.W.: Experimental studies on determinants of wound infection: II. Surgery *60*:1072, 1966.
70. Howes, E.L.: Topical streptomycin in wounds. Am. J. Med. *2*:449, 1947.
71. Hutton, D.J.: Treatment of pressure sores. Nurs. Times *62*:1533, 1966.
72. Hutton, W.C., Freeman, M.A.R., and Swanson, S.A.V.: The forces exerted by the pads of the walking dog. J. Small Anim. Pract. *10*:71, 1969.
73. Jackson, D., and Harrison, W.T.: Mechanical treatment of experimental rattlesnake venom poisoning. J.A.M.A. *90*:1928, 1928.
74. Jacobsson, S., Rothman, G., Arturson, K., et al.: A new principle for cleansing of infected wounds. Scand. J. Plast. Reconstr. Surg. *10*:65, 1976.
75. Jennings, P. B.: Use of dimethylsulfoxide as an adjunct to topical antimicrobial therapy. Proceedings of the 12th annual meeting of the American College of Veterinary Surgeons: Advances in Veterinary Surgery and Surgical Education. Des Moines, Iowa. February 2, 1977.
76. Jennings, P.B.: Surgical techniques utilized in the presence of infection. Arch. Offic. J. Am. Coll. Vet. Surg. *4*:43, 1975.
77. Johnston, D.E.: Wound healing and reconstructive surgery. Am. Anim. Hosp. Assoc. Sci. Proc. *2*:383, 1975.
78. Johnston, D.E.: Wound healing. Arch. Offic. J. Am. Coll. Vet. Surg. *3*:30, 1974.
79. Jones, R.C., and Shires, G.T.: Principles in the management of wounds, in Schwartz, S.I., Hume, D.M., Lillehei, R.C., et al. (eds.): Principles of Surgery. New York, McGraw-Hill Book Co., 1969, p. 162.
80. Kaplan, M.F., and Berggren, R.B.: Comparative clinical study of local burn wound therapy. Ann. N.Y. Acad. Sci. *150*:961, 1968.
81. King, M.K.: Immediate skin grafting following injuries. Surg. Gynecol. Obstet. *81*:75, 1945.
82. Kirk, R. W., and Bistner, S.I.: Handbook of Veterinary Procedures and Emergency Treatment, ed. 2. Philadelphia, W. B. Saunders Co., 1975, pp. 181–183.
83. Knapp, W.A., and Flowers, H.H.: Treatment of poisonous snakebite in the dog with cortisone acetate. Vet. Med. *51*:475, 1956.
84. Knecht, C.D., Clark, R.L., and Fletcher, O.J.: Healing of sharp incisions and electroincisions in dogs. J. Am. Vet. Med. Assoc. *159*:1447, 1971.
85. Knowles, R.P.: Injuries to skin, muscle, and tendon, in Some Techniques and Procedures in Small Animal Surgery. Bonner Springs, Kans., Veterinary Medical Publishing Co., Inc., 1963, pp. 153–161.
86. Knowles, R.P., Snyder, C.C., Glenn, J.L., et al.: Bites of venomous snakes, in Kirk, R.W. (ed.): Current Veterinary Therapy: IV. Small Animal Practice. Philadelphia, W. B. Saunders Co., 1971, pp. 111–113.
87. Krizek, T.J., and Cossman, D.V.: Experimental burn wound sepsis: Variations in response to topical agents. J. Trauma. *12*:553, 1972.
88. Krizek, T.J., and Davis, J.H.: Experimental *Pseudomonas* burn sepsis: Evaluation of topical therapy. J. Trauma *7*:433, 1967.
89. Krizek, T.J., Robson, M.C., and Groskin, M.G.: Experimental burn wound sepsis: Evaluation of enzymatic debridement. J. Surg. Res. *17*:219, 1974.

90. Lane, J.G.: Practical cryosurgery: An introduction for small animal clinicians. J. Small Anim. Pract. *15*:715, 1974.
91. Lawrence, C.A.: Antimicrobial activity, in vitro, of chlorhexidine. Ft. Dodge Biochem. Rev. *30*:3, 1961.
92. Leith, D.G.: Bite wounds. Am. Fam. Physician *11*:93, 1975.
93. Leveen, H.H., Faik, G., Borek, B., et al.: Chemical acidification of wounds: An adjuvant to healing and the unfavorable action of alkalinity and ammonia. Ann. Surg. *178*:745, 1973.
94. Lindberg, R.B., Moncrief, J.A., and Mason, A.D.: Control of experimental and clinical burn wound sepsis by topical application of Sulfamylon compounds. Ann. N.Y. Acad. Sci. *150*:950, 1968.
95. Lipowitz, A.J.: Management of gunshot wounds of the soft tissues and extremities. J. Am. Anim. Hosp. Assoc. *12*:813, 1976.
96. Livingstone, R.H., and Wilson, R.T.: Gunshot wounds of the limbs. Br. Med. J. *1*:667, 1975.
97. Lopez, J.E., and Mena, B.: Local insulin for diabetic gangrene. Lancet *1*:1199, 1968.
98. Lynch, J.B., and Blocker, T.G.: Thermal burns, in Converse, J.M. (ed.): Reconstructive Plastic Surgery: Principles and Procedures in Correction, Reconstruction, and Transplantation, ed, 2. Philadelphia, W. B. Saunders Co., 1977, Vol. 1.
99. Madden, J.E., Edlich, R.F., Custer, J.R., et al.: Studies in the management of the contaminated wound: IV. Resistance to infection of surgical wounds made by knife, electrosurgery, and laser. Am. J. Surg. *119*:222, 1970.
100. Matsumoto, T., Dobek, A.S., Kovaric, J.J., et al.: Topical antibiotic spray in contaminated crush wounds in animals. Milit. Med. *133*:869, 1968.
101. Matsumoto, T., Hardaway, R.M., Dobek, A.S., et al.: Antibiotic topical spray applied in a simulated combat wound. Arch. Surg. 95:288, 1967.
102. Matsumoto, T., Hardaway, R.M., and Heisterkamp, C.A.: Determination of the viability of muscle soon after wounding. Arch. Surg., *94*:794, 1967.
103. McCluskey, B.: A prospective trial povidone-iodine solution in the prevention of wound sepsis. Aust. N.Z. J. Surg. *46*:254, 1976.
104. McGregor, I.A.: Fundamental Techniques of Plastic Surgery, ed. 6. Edinburgh, Churchill Livingstone, 1975.
105. McGregor, I.A.: Degloving injuries: Hand. *2*:130, 1970.
106. Metzger, W.I., and Prigot, A.: The effect of local antibiotic therapy upon the survival of wound bacteria. Antibiot. Chemother. *5*:423, 1955.
107. Monafo, W.W., and Moyer, C.A.: The treatment of extensive thermal burns with 0.5% silver nitrate solution. Ann. N.Y. Acad. Sci. *150*:937, 1968.
108. Morgan, M.M., Spencer, A.D., and Hershy, F.B.: Debridement of civilian gunshot wounds of soft tissue. J. Trauma *1*:354, 1961.
109. Neal, T.M., and Key, J.C.: Principles of treatment of dog bite wounds. J. Am. Anim. Hosp. Assoc. *12*:657, 1976.
110. Neuman, N.B.: Management of contaminated wounds of the extremities. Vet. Med. Small Anim. Clin. *69*:1275, 1974.
111. Noyes, H.E., Chi, N.H., Linh, L.T., et al.: Delayed topical antimicrobials as adjuncts to systemic antibiotic therapy of war wounds: Bacteriologic studies. Milit. Med. *132*:461, 1967.
112. Olivari, N., Schrudde, J., and Wahle, H.: The surgical treatment of bedsores in paraplegics. Plast. Reconstr. Surg. *50*:477, 1972.
113. Parrish, H.M., and Scatterday, J.E.: A survey of poisonous snakebites among domestic animals in Florida. Vet. Med. *52*:135, 1957.
114. Parrish, H.M., Scatterday, J.E., and Moore, W.: The use of antihistamine (Phenergan) in experimental snake venom poisoning in dogs. J. Am. Vet. Med. Assoc. *129*:522, 1956.
115. Parrish, H.M., Scatterday, J.E., and Pollard, C.B.: The clinical management of snake venom poisoning in domestic animals. J. Am. Vet. Med. Assoc. *130*:548, 1957.
116. Paul, J.W., and Gorden, M.A.: Efficacy of chlorhexidine surgical scrub compared to that of hexachlorophene and povidone-iodine. Vet. Med. Small Anim. Clin. *73*:573, 1978.
117. Peacock, E.E. Jr., and Van Winkle, W. Jr.: Wound Repair, ed. 2. Philadelphia. W. B. Saunders Co., 1976.
118. Pennisi, V.R., Capozzi, A., and Friedman, G.: Travase, an effective enzyme for burn debridement. Plast. Reconstr. Surg. *51*:371, 1973.
119. Peterson, L.W.: Prophylaxis of wound infection: Studies with particular references to soaps with irrigation. Arch. Surg. *50*:177, 1945.
120. Phillips, I., Lobo, A.Z., Fernandes, R., et al.: Acetic acid in the treatment of superficial wounds infected by *Pseudomonas aeruginosa*. Lancet *1*:11, 1968.
121. Pietsch, J., and Meakins, J.L.: Complications of povidone-iodine absorption in topically treated burn patients. Lancet *1*:280, 1976.
122. Postlethwait, R.W.: Principles of operative surgery: Antisepsis, techniques, sutures, and drains, in Sabiston, D.C. (ed.): Davis-Christopher: Textbook of Surgery, ed. 11. Philadelphia. W. B. Saunders Co., 1973, pp. 323–339.

123. Pulaski, E.J., Meleney, F.L., and Spaeth, W.L.C.: Bacterial flora of acute traumatic wounds. Surg. Gynecol. Obstet. 72:982, 1941.
124. Raghava, R., Matei, W., and Enquist, I.F.: Quantitation of local acidosis and hypoxia produced by infection. Am. J. Surg. 132:64, 1976.
125. Reiser, H.G., Patton, R., and Roetting, L.C.: Tryptic debridement of necrotic tissue. Arch. Surg. 63:568, 1951.
126. Robertson, R.D., Ritter, C., and Hance, H.: The relative influence of three topical antibacterial drugs on tensile strength of wounds. Vet. Med. Small Anim. Clin. 69:36, 1974.
127. Robson, M.C., Duke, W.F., and Krizek, T.J.: Rapid bacterial screening in the treatment of civilian wounds. J. Surg. Res. 14:426, 1973.
128. Robson, M.C., Edstrom, L.E., Krizek, T.J., et al.: Efficacy of systemic antibiotics in treatment of granulating wounds. J. Surg. Res. 16:299, 1974.
129. Robson, M.C., and Heggers, J.P.: Delayed wound closures based on bacterial counts. J. Surg. Oncol. 2:379, 1970.
130. Robson, M.C., and Heggers, J.P.: Surgical infection: II. The β-hemolytic streptococcus. J. Surg. Res. 9:289, 1969.
131. Robson, M.C., Schaerf, R.H.M., and Krizek, T.J.: Evaluation of topical povidone-iodine ointment in experimental burn wound sepsis. Plast. Reconstr. Surg. 54:328, 1974.
132. Rodeheaver, G.T., Pettry, D., Thacker, J.G., et al.: Wound cleansing by high pressure irrigation. Surg. Gynecol. Obstet. 141:357, 1975.
133. Rodeheaver, G., Pettry, D., Turnbull, V., et al.: Identification of the wound infection-promoting factors in soil. Am. J. Surg. 128:8, 1974.
134. Rodeheaver, G.T., Smith, S.L., Thacker, J.G., et al.: Mechanical cleansing of contaminated wounds with a surfactant. Am. J. Surg. 129:241, 1975.
135. Rodeheaver, G., Turnbull, V., Edgerton, M.T., et al.: Pharmacokinetics of a new skin wound cleanser. Am. J. Surg. 132:67, 1976.
136. Rosenthal, S.P.: Insulin accelerates wound healing. Arch. Surg. 96:53, 1968.
137. Roush, J.C.: Trauma to the extremities. Canine Pract. 2:38, 1975.
138. Salisbury, R.E., Silverstein, P., and Goodwin, M.N. Jr.: Upper extremity fungus invasions secondary to large burns. Plast. Reconstr. Surg. 54:654, 1974.
139. Sather, M.R., Weber, C.E., and George, J.: Pressure sores and the spinal cord injury patient. Drug Intelligence Clin. Pharmacol. 11:154, 1977.
140. Savlov, E.D., Dunphy, J.E., and Anderson, M.A.: The healing of the disrupted and resutured wound. Surgery 36:362, 1954.
141. Scherr, D.D., and Dodd, T.A.: In vitro bacteriological evaluation of the effectiveness of antimicrobial irrigating solutions. J. Bone Joint Surg. 58A:119, 1976.
142. Scherr, D.D., Dodd, T.A., and Buckingham, W.W.: Prophylactic use of topical antibiotic irrigation in uninfected surgical wounds. J. Bone Joint Surg. 54A:634, 1972.
143. Schaeffer, J.R., Brown, R.B., and Gold, D.: Emergency War Surgery: NATO Handbook. Washington, D.C., United States Government Printing Office, 1958.
144. Shelby, R.W., Taylor, L.E., Garnes, A.L., et al.: Enzymatic debridement with activated whole pancreas. Am. J. Surg. 96:545, 1958.
145. Singleton, A.O. Jr., Davis, D., and Julian, J.: The prevention of wound infection following contamination with colon organisms. Surg. Gynecol. Obstet. 108:389, 1959.
146. Singleton, A.O., and Julian, J.: An experimental evaluation of methods used to prevent infection in wounds which have been contaminated with feces. Ann. Surg. 151:912, 1960.
147. Skornik, W.A., and Dressler, D.P.: Topical antisepsis studies in the burned rat. Arch. Surg. 103:469 1971.
148. Snyder, C.C., Knowles, R.P., Pickens, J.E., et al.: Pathogenesis and treatment of poisonous snakebites. J. Am. Vet. Med. Assoc. 151:1635, 1967.
149. Spanos, P.K., and McQuarrie, D.G.: Early total ischiectomy with primary closure of decubitus ulcer. Am. J. Surg. 126:98, 1973.
150. Stark, R.B.: Plastic Surgery. New York, Harper & Row Publishers, Inc., 1962.
151. Swaim, S.F.: Isolated peripheral nerves, in Bojrab, M.J. (ed.): Current Techniques in Small Animal Surgery. Philadelphia, Lea & Febiger, 1975, pp. 10–14.
152. Swaim, S.F., and Votau, K.: Prevention and treatment of decubital ulcers in the dog. Vet. Med. Small Anim. Clin. 70:1069, 1975.
153. Tempest, N.M.: The use of intravenous dye technique in the assessment of tissue viability. J. Bone Joint Surg. 2B:646, 1960.
154. Trueta, J.: Reflections on the past and present treatment of war wounds and fractures. Milit. Med. 141:255, 1976.
155. Walker, H.L., Mason, A.D., and Raulston, G.L.: Surface infection with Pseudomonas aeruginosa. Ann. Surg. 160:297, 1964.
156. Ward, C.G., Clarkson, J.G., Taplin, D., et al.: Wood's light fluorescence and Pseudomonas burn wound infection. J. Am. Med. Assoc. 202:127, 1967.
157. Wheeler, C.B., Rodeheaver, G.T., Thacker, J.G., et al.: Side effects of high pressure irrigation. Surg. Gynecol. Obstet. 143:775, 1976.

158. Wool, I.G., Rampersad, O.R., and Moyer, A.N.: Effect of insulin and diabetes on protein synthesis by ribosomes from heart muscle: Significance for the hormones mechanism of action. Am. J. Med. *40:*716, 1966.
159. Wynn-Williams, D., and Monballiv, G.: The effects of povidone-iodine in the treatment of burns and traumatic losses of skin. Br. J. Plast. Surg. *18:*146, 1965.
160. Yucel, V.E., and Basmajian, J.V.: Decubitus ulcers: Healing effect of an enzymatic spray. Arch. Phys. Med. Rehabil. *55:*517, 1974.
161. Zawacki, B.E.: Effect of Travase on heat injured skin. Surgery 77:132, 1975.
162. Ziffren, S.E.: Results of the treatment of burns with silver nitrate. Ann. N.Y. Acad. Sci. *150:*946, 1968.
163. Ziperman, H.H.: The management of soft tissue missile wounds in war and peace. J. Trauma *1:*361, 1961.

5

THERMAL BURNS

Lloyd E. Davis, D.V.M., Ph.D.

The subject of thermal burns will only occasionally concern the veterinarian, since burns are somewhat uncommon in the animal population. The widespread alterations in structure and function that are produced by a severe thermal burn provide a real challenge to the ingenuity and knowledge of the attending veterinarian, as few forms of injury equal the intensity of the metabolic response of thermal trauma.

The literature pertaining to burns is extensive and much of it relates to thermal trauma in humans; however, considerable research has been performed in which the domesticated species were employed as experimental subjects. A review of the experimental literature provides the basis for this chapter. This review is not exhaustive by any means, but it is believed to be thorough enough to provide a firm foundation for the clinical management of thermal burns in dogs.

CLASSIFICATION OF BURNS

Burns of human skin have classically been categorized into three degrees according to the severity and the type of lesion produced. The first degree indicates damage to the epithelium, with transient erythema and subsequent desquamation. Burns of the second degree involve the entire epidermis and variable depths of the dermis, with some damage to accessory skin structures, and are accompanied by the formation of vesicles. In third-degree burns the full thickness of the skin is completely destroyed, with variable amounts of damage to subcutaneous structures, and the sequelae are ulceration and sloughing. This system of classification is only applicable to humans and swine; however, it is not entirely adequate for use even in these species because it does not differentiate among the more severe burns and provides little information relative to treatment and prognosis.

Lehman[55] suggested a classification of burns based on observations of the wound slough. He classified them into group I, group II, and group III. Group I pertains to superficial burns and combines the old classifications of the first and second degrees. There is little difference in the treatment and no difference in the prognosis of burns in this group. Group II involves burns of the full thickness of the skin. This group requires protection from damage and contamination but no skin grafts. Group III refers to burns in which there is both destruction of the full thickness of the skin and damage to the underlying structures. These burns require grafting. This classification, with a different terminology, is frequently encountered in the more recent literature in which burns are described as superficial, partial thickness, or full thickness; this terminology will be employed throughout this discussion.

PATHOLOGY OF BURNS

SKIN

Following a superficial burn the skin is slightly erythematous and thickened owing to hyperemia and edema in the deeper layers. Various depths of the epidermis may coagulate as a result of the heat. In very superficial burns the surface layers of the epidermis will desquamate, but these will be rapidly replaced from the intact stratum germinativum. A deeper superficial burn will produce complete loss of the epidermis, and healing will rapidly occur by the proliferation of the epithelial cells that are located in the accessory skin structures of the dermis.

Partial-thickness burns produce severe damage to the epidermis and the superficial half of the dermis. The capillaries and venules become dilated and congested and allow plasma to leak from them. This results in massive edema of the subcutaneous tissues. Leukocytes adhere to one another and to the endothelium of the capillaries. Margination is first noted on the side of the vessel closest to the site of injury.[10] The platelets and erythrocytes share in this general "stickiness," suggesting the presence of a plasma factor.[3] Leukocytes migrate from the damaged vessels into the surrounding tissues. The epithelium of the deeper portions of the skin appendages remains viable and healing will commence from these cells. Several days after the injury is sustained, plasma exuding from the damaged surface will dry to form a tan crust.

In a full-thickness burn the entire skin coagulates into a somewhat homogeneous mass as a result of the action of heat on the proteins. The superficial blood vessels of the subcutis are thrombosed and the deeper vessels become excessively permeable. This results in severe edema of the subcutaneous tissues and dry gangrene of the damaged tissues. The eschar that develops is dark brown and leathery. Grossly, the burned area will be either pearly white or charred (Fig. 5–1). The tissue will be insensitive because the cutaneous nerve endings have been destroyed. Full-thickness burns heal slowly if not grafted because healing depends on epithelialization from the wound edges.

Electrical burns are categorized separately because the combined effects of heat and electrical current produce a lesion that is significantly different from that produced by heat alone.[50, 66, 68] The amount of damage produced by an electrical current will depend principally on the amperage and duration of contact with the wire. The passage of current through the tissues will follow Ohm's law, i.e., at a constant voltage the current conduction will be a function of the resistance of the conductor. The tissue fluids, by virtue of their electrolytic nature, are good conductors, and the principal impediment to current flow is provided by the skin or mucosa. Dry skin provides a high degree of resistance that is markedly decreased in wet skin.

The skin lesion is well circumscribed at the point of contact and this area is dead. Deep to the site of contact the injury extends toward the other point of

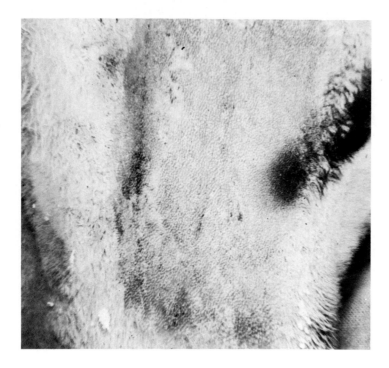

Figure 5–1:   Appearance of the skin surface immediately following a full-thickness burn. See color plate III–A, p. 570.

contact, with resultant destruction of the deeper tissues. The main blood vessels in the area are good conductors and thrombosis may occur, with resultant gangrene of the area served by them. An electrical burn is characterized by a lesion that is cold, bloodless, pale yellow, and painless; the sloughs are slow to separate and the lesion is slow to heal. If the burn is produced by arcing of the current, a copper deposit may be left on the affected surface. The extent of damage is often difficult to assess because small areas of skin damage may accompany severe damage to the underlying structures.

LIVER

The pathological changes in the liver following severe burns have been studied by Dexter and Petersen,[30] Buis and Hartman,[14] James and associates,[52] and Erb and co-workers.[34] These authors found that cloudy swelling, dilation of sinusoids, some centrolobular degeneration, and an increased amount of pigment in reticuloendothelial cells were present by the third day after burning. In fatal cases the liver showed marked congestion, extensive necrosis and fatty infiltration.

KIDNEYS

Severe thermal trauma produces reflex renal vasoconstriction that results in renal damage when accompanied by burn shock.[49] The lesions are granular, with vacuolar degeneration of the tubular epithelium and little damage to the glomeruli.[14, 49] Free hemoglobin is usually present in the tubules.

OTHER ORGANS

Other common postmortem findings are vascular congestion and edema of the central nervous system and petechiae in the myocardium, intestinal tract, and kidneys.[34] The adrenals are often swollen and hemorrhagic and are characterized microscopically by hypertrophy and lipoid depletion.[29] Ulceration of the duodenum, which is subject to perforation and hemorrhage, is a frequent concomitant of severe thermal trauma. This particular type of ulcer is named after its discoverer, Curling. The genesis of Curling's ulcer was studied in dogs by Hartman[48] and Friesen.[38] They showed that hemoconcentration was important as a predisposing factor in the genesis of experimental gastroduodenal ulcer and that proper fluid therapy prevented its occurrence. High gastric acidity tended to increase the incidence of ulceration. Some of the animals died as a result of internal hemorrhage or peritonitis following perforation.

Kabat and Levine[53] noted that a small proportion of cats died within a matter of minutes after burning. They observed that respiration was arrested but the heart continued to beat for a few minutes prior to death. Attempts at resuscitation were unsuccessful. This condition was shown to be due to widespread and numerous fibrin emboli in the pulmonary capillaries. They were able to reproduce this syndrome in healthy cats by injecting 3 to 4 ml. of feline blood that had been heated to 65° C.

A frequent and severe complication of burns around the face is respiratory tract damage.[57] This problem was investigated in dogs by Moritz and colleagues.[64] Hot, dry air has little effect on the lungs because of its low specific heat, but it does produce a severe tracheitis and may cause rapid death by means of the resultant obstructive edema of the larynx (Fig. 5–2). If

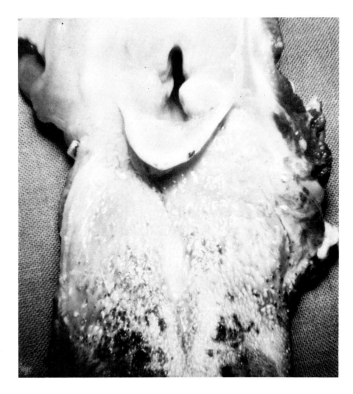

Figure 5–2: Laryngeal edema produced by inhalation of flame. See color plate III–B, p. 570.

edema of the larynx does not develop, the tracheitis may predispose the animal to bronchopneumonia. Exposure to live steam may produce severe pulmonary damage with hemorrhage and edema. Steam is most active in this respect because of its high specific heat. The centrally located alveoli are most severely affected because they have the shortest and most direct connections with the primary bronchi.

PATHOLOGICAL PHYSIOLOGY

The pathological physiology accompanying thermal trauma has been reviewed by Harkins.[46] Excellent accounts of various aspects of the pathological physiology of burns are found in the textbook by Artz and colleagues[6] and in the *Symposium on Burns,* which is published by the National Research Council of the National Academy of Sciences.[24, 77]

CARDIOVASCULAR SYSTEM

At the time of burning and immediately following thermal injury to the dog, there is a rise in arterial blood pressure as a result of constriction of arteries, arterioles, and larger veins.[1, 70] This is probably due to the release of epinephrine by the adrenal medulla and to general sympathetic nervous system activity. During this initial phase, the heart rate may be increased, the cardiac output nearly normal, and the spleen contracted.

Following this initial phase, the animal enters a transitional phase that is characterized by a fall in blood pressure, decreased cardiac output, and an enhanced response to pressor drugs.[40, 41, 70] In this phase, sludging of the blood cells passing through or near burned tissues occurs, resulting in a reduced blood flow to the tissues and a slowing of blood flow in the larger veins.[1, 11] The inadequate venous return to the heart causes a decreased cardiac output, which in turn produces a fall in systolic blood pressure. The slowing of blood flow to the tissues results in an endothelial anoxia of the stagnant type, and capillary permeability becomes greatly increased.

After a short period the untreated, severely burned animal enters a terminal phase in which Page[70] noted that the peripheral vascular bed and myocardium were completely refractory to pressor drugs. The cardiac output may decrease to half its normal value, there is a marked reduction in plasma and blood volumes and a decrease in urine flow, and blood pressure falls to shock levels.[40, 41]

FLUID AND ELECTROLYTE SHIFTS

Most animals that have severe burns of more than 50 per cent of their body surface die as a result of water and electrolyte shifts. The magnitude of these losses is directly related to the extent and severity of the burn.[6] As has been previously indicated, there is damage to the capillaries, increasing their permeability, and the destruction of nerves to the arterioles allows them to open widely. These factors combine to allow a rapid translocation of incredibly large volumes of protein-rich fluid from the vascular system into the subcutaneous tissues. In the words of Cope,[24] "The burn wound is a parasite on the surface of the body. Like a leech the wound sucks water, protein and electroytes from the plasma circulating through its depths, and it swells with edema." In an attempt to simplify the problems associated with thermal burns, Cameron and associates[18] studied the effects of acute anhydremia produced by the subcutaneous injection of hypertonic solutions. They observed that this procedure resulted in severe local edema, leading to hemoconcentration, circulatory collapse, and many metabolic changes that are normally associated with severe thermal trauma. The problem of capillary permeability was investigated by Netsky and Leiter[67] and Cope and Moore.[26] It was demonstrated that in burns the capillary membrane becomes as permeable to colloids as it formerly was to ions. Cope and colleagues[27] observed that the total protein concentration of the edematous fluid was always lower than that of the plasma, indicating that more water than protein is lost from the capillaries. They further discovered that the albumin-globulin ratio was decreased in the plasma and increased in the lymph, indicating a differential permeability of the damaged membrane. Perlmann and co-workers[73] and Prendergast and associates[75] observed this same shift in the albumin-globulin ratio and further demonstrated a marked elevation in the gamma globulin fraction of the plasma.

In addition to the water and protein shifts that occur with burns, there is a marked alteration in the electroyte distribution. Fox and Baer[37] showed that burned tissue cells lose their potassium and gain sodium and water. There is a loss of sodium and a gain of potassium by the extracellular fluid of normal tissues, which points to extracellular dehydration with intracellular swelling. This acquisition of water by uninjured cells throughout the body leads to a further reduction in extracellular fluid and blood volumes. It also explains the frequent occurrence of cerebral and pulmonary edema accompanying burns and the fact that the burned patient is particularly susceptible to water intoxication.

The most rapid rate of loss and translocation of water and electrolytes occurs in the first few hours after injury. This loss is of the order of one milliliter per kilogram of body weight per per cent of area burned at the sixth hour following injury.[77] Salzberg and Evans[82] found that a partial-thickness burn of 20 per cent of the body surface of dogs produced a loss of 28 per cent of the plasma volume at six hours. The plasma volume returned to control values by the 27th hour, and by one week postburn it had risen to 25 per cent above normal.

There is generally a positive nitrogen balance if intensive blood and plasma therapy is administered. There is an extremely positive sodium balance soon after injury owing to excessive sodium conservation by the kidneys and accumulation of the ion in the damaged tissues. After the phase of translocation of fluid and electrolytes, the nitrogen balance becomes strongly negative if renal function is normal. This will begin on the third day and may last for as long as a month. There is a correlation between the severity of the burn and the duration of negative nitrogen balance.

About the third to fifth day the large accumulation of edema in the wound begins to shift to extracellular water and diuresis occurs. If the animal has developed an acute renal insufficiency, the reabsorbed water is imposed on the circulating blood volume and such complications as congestive heart failure and pulmonary edema may intervene.

Throughout the remainder of the clinical course, there is a gradual tendency toward anabolic activity. Electrolyte, water, and protein balances are easily maintained and epithelialization of the wound takes place.

BLOOD

There are significant changes in the hemogram as a result of a severe burn. Severe anemia generally accompanies widespread burning. Raker and Rovit[79] found that a moderate 50 per cent burn would decrease the red blood cell volume by 8 per cent and a severe 50 per cent burn would destroy, on the average, 40 per cent of the red blood cell volume. Marked hemolysis occurs shortly after injury because of an increase in mechanical and osmotic fragilities of the erythrocytes. The appearance of spherocytosis coincides with the development of increased fragility.[45] Hemoglobinemia and hemoglobinuria are prominent shortly after injury. There is an increase in urobilinogen excretion and urinary coproporphyrin levels.[51, 52] The anemia becomes more severe during the clinical course as a result of a considerable depression in hemoglobin formation.[50, 51] The packed cell volume increases during the first few hours because of splenic contraction; this is followed by a decrease that is attributable to hemolysis and decreased erythropoiesis. There is a gradual return to normal at 54 days. The erythrocyte count follows this same general pattern.[12]

The total white blood count may rise to 36,000/cu. mm. in 12 hours.[12] This primary wave of neutrophilia is accompanied by lymphocytopenia and eosinopenia and its magnitude is related to the extent of surface area injured. A further neutrophilic leukocytosis develops five to ten days after burning.[85] There is a shift to the left in the Schilling index during this period. The white blood cell count returns to normal by the 43rd day (Fig. 5–3).[12]

The change in the number of eosinophils was studied by Wight and colleagues.[90] They observed a rapid decline in the number of circulating eosinophils immediately after trauma that was not correlated with the extent or severity of the burn. The count began to rise by the third day in patients who were making satisfactory clinical progress. The failure of eosinophils to reappear by the third day was considered a grave prognostic sign. In later weeks of convalescence, a marked elevation of eosinophils to 2000/cu. mm. of blood was noted in patients who were making satisfactory progress. Of course, systemic therapy with adrenal corticoids will alter this pattern entirely because of the suppression of eosinophil production that is caused by the drug.

MISCELLANEOUS CHANGES

Following injury there are greatly increased blood levels of adrenocorticotropic hormone (ACTH) and consequently an increased secretion of adrenal corticoids.[39, 89] Instances of acute adrenal medullary insufficiency following severe thermal trauma have been reported by Goodall.[42] Pseudodiabetes may result from the intense response to stress and will be aggravated by a high-caloric, high-carbohydrate intake too soon after injury.[35] Glyconeogenesis is enhanced by the increased corticoid secretion, and glucose utilization is inhibited following thermal trauma.[91] The bicarbonate content of the plasma

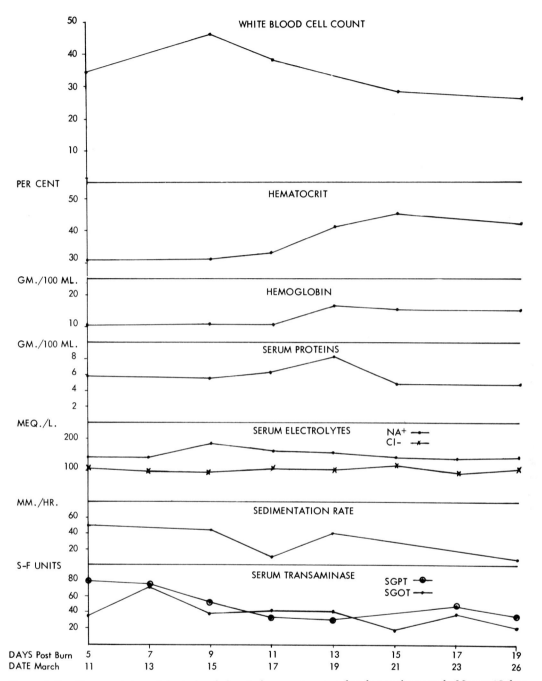

Figure 5–3: Changes in hematological and chemical parameters in a dog during the period of five to 19 days following a 20 per cent partial-thickness burn.

is decreased and there is an increase in the lactic acid level of the blood owing to the damaged liver's inability to convert the acid.[87] These changes result in metabolic acidosis. There is a marked increase in plasma fibrin and cholesterol levels.[19] Osteoporosis may be produced following burns as a result of the excessive secretion of adrenocortical hormones and prolonged immobilization.[6]

Dziemian[31] studied the effects of burns on renal function in goats. After severe burning, the effective plasma flow was greatly decreased. There was constriction of the efferent arterioles and decrease in the glomerular filtration rate and maximal tubular reabsorption.

CLINICAL MANAGEMENT OF THERMAL BURNS

ESTIMATION OF THE EXTENT AND SEVERITY OF INJURY

The magnitude of fluid and electrolyte losses and metabolic disturbances is dependent on the extent and severity of injury to the body surface, as has already been indicated. As a consequence, the proper decisions concerning

TABLE 5–1 CONVERSION OF BODY WEIGHT TO SURFACE AREA

Body Weight		Surface Area[*]	
Kilograms	Pounds	Square Meters	Square Centimeters
2	4.4	0.16	1600
4	8.8	0.25	2500
6	13.2	0.33	3800
8	17.6	0.40	4000
10	22.0	0.46	4600
12	26.5	0.52	5200
14	30.9	0.58	5800
16	35.3	0.64	6400
18	39.7	0.69	6900
20	44.1	0.74	7400
22	48.5	0.79	7900
24	52.9	0.83	8300
26	57.3	0.88	8800
28	61.7	0.92	9200
30	66.1	0.97	9700
32	70.6	1.01	10,100
34	75.0	1.05	10,500
36	79.4	1.09	10,900
38	83.8	1.13	11,300
40	88.2	1.17	11,700
42	92.6	1.21	12,100
44	97.0	1.25	12,500
46	101.4	1.28	12,800
48	105.6	1.32	13,200
50	110.0	1.35	13,500
52	114.4	1.39	13,900
54	118.8	1.43	14,300
56	123.2	1.47	14,700
58	127.6	1.50	15,000
60	132.0	1.53	15,300
62	136.4	1.57	15,700
64	140.8	1.60	16,000
66	145.2	1.63	16,300
68	149.6	1.66	16,600
70	154.0	1.70	17,000

[*] Calculated with the following equation:
Area (in meters)$^2 = 0.1 \times$ Wt.$^{2/3}$ (in kilograms).

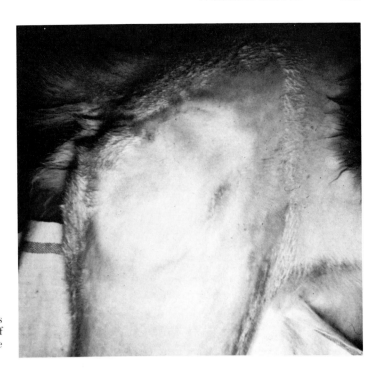

Figure 5–4: Partial-thickness burn surrounded by areas of superficial injury. See color plate III–C, p. 572.

the nature and extent of therapy will depend on the clinician's ability to ascertain the extent and depth of the injury.

The extent of surface injury may be estimated by measuring the area of burned skin with a metric ruler or tape, dividing that area by the total surface area of the animal, and multiplying by 100. Table 5–1 lists the values for the conversion of body weight (Wt) to surface area (S) based on the well-known formula, $S = 0.1 \times Wt^{2/3}$.

To illustrate the calculation of the extent of burn in a dog, consider a 30-lb. (13.6 kg.) dog that has been scalded with hot water. The area of injury is clipped and the limits of the injury are observed. The area is divided into subareas that are convenient to measure, the dimensions of the subareas are recorded, and their areas are calculated and then added together to give us the total surface area of the injury. We arrive at a figure of 1160 sq. cm. for the area of injury. We then consult Table 5–1 and find that a 30-lb. dog will have a total surface area of approximately 5800 sq. cm., and 1160/5800 × 100 gives us a value of 20 per cent for the extent of injury.

The depth of burn is difficult to determine, particularly if the dog is seen immediately after injury. In general, there is a tendency to overestimate rather than underestimate the severity of the trauma. Artz and associates[6] indicated some generalizations that are useful in this regard. Superficial burns are usually caused by exposure to a minor flash or are located at the periphery of more severe damage; these lesions are characteristically hyperesthetic (Fig. 5–4). Partial-thickness burns are usually the result of exposure to flash and scalding and are painful but show decreased sensitivity. Full-thickness burns are generally produced by flame and are anesthetic and leather-like.

Patey and Scarff[72] developed a method that should be useful to the veterinarian in determining the depth of cutaneous damage. They employed a modified van Gieson's stain consisting of 0.2 per cent acid fuchsin and 1 per cent picric acid in aqueous solution. If this stain is applied to the injured area, it will stain normal skin red, areas of minor necrosis a pale yellow, and areas of marked necrosis a bright yellow without any red. Ham[44] observed that a simple method for differentiating between a superficial burn and a deeper injury is to pull the hairs. If the hair offers normal resistance, the burn is superficial; if it is easily removed, the injury is considered to be deep.

The relation of severity of partial- and full-thickness burns was studied by Bull and Squire.[15] In a review of their case records, they found that mortality was best related to the extent of full thickness plus one fourth of the partial-thickness burn. In other words, for the same area a full-thickness burn was four times as serious as a partial-thickness burn.

INITIAL CARE OF THE BURN PATIENT

When the animal is presented, a careful history should be taken with particular attention to the circumstances surrounding the accident. Morphine sulfate can be injected intravenously in low doses. Narcotics or sedatives should be given intravenously because of poor absorption from subcutaneous areas in the presence in incipient peripheral circulatory failure. Higher doses that are given subcutaneously without effecting pain relief may suddenly be absorbed into the circulation as circulatory integrity is restored. This may lead to serious respiratory center depression.

After analgesia is effected, the hair is clipped from the injured area and the extent and severity of the wound are estimated as described earlier. If the wound area is less than 15 per cent of the total surface area and largely a superficial or partial-thickness burn, only a minimum of supportive therapy will be required. An area of greater than 15 per cent or the presence of full-thickness injury will call for rigorous initial fluid replacement.[7] Patients with severe burns of more than 50 per cent of their body surface rarely survive for more than ten days under the most ideal circumstances. The most merciful treatment for these patients is euthanasia.

Doubt regarding the severity of the condition may be partially resolved by collecting urine and blood samples and observing them for free hemoglobin. The presence of "pink plasma" or hemoglobinuria generally denotes a deep, extensive burn (Fig. 5–5). The history and an examination for the sensitivity of the lesion will also be helpful in this regard, as was previously indicated. Care must be taken not to overlook possible respiratory involvement in burns around the face. This will be manifested by redness of the oral and pharyngeal mucous membranes and the presence of an intractable cough. If these signs are present, the practitioner should be prepared to perform an emergency tracheostomy and to administer oxygen to combat anoxia. In the presence of pulmonary damage, fluid and electrolytes must be kept at the minimal effective levels to avoid the complication of pulmonary edema.[35]

After the animal has been examined and the extent of injury has been determined, there will be two courses of action, depending on the extent and severity of injury. If the lesions are superficial or involve less than 15 per cent of the body surface, local treatment of the burn may be instituted. If the burns are more severe, the jugular vein should be cannulated and fluid therapy should be started immediately. If the animal is in shock when presented and it is impossible to raise a vein, it is imperative that a vein be surgically exposed and cannulated because intravenous fluids are most urgently re-

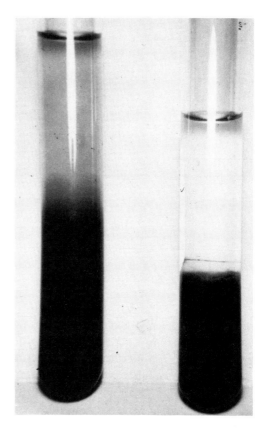

Figure 5–5: Centrifuged blood samples before (*right*) and after (*left*) extensive thermal injury. See color plate III–D, p. 570.

quired at this time. This cannula will literally serve as a "life line" to the animal. Polyethylene tubing should not be left in the vein for more than seven days because of the possibility of thrombosis and consequent pulmonary embolism.[7]

The fluids of choice for replacement of water and electrolytes are a saline bicarbonate or lactated Ringer's solution.[36] A regimen for meeting the fluid, electroyte, and colloid requirements for the first few days following injury has been outlined by several investigators.[6, 7, 35] The requirements are calculated as follows: body weight (in kilograms) × per cent burn × 4 ml. = the amount of lactated Ringer's solution or saline bicarbonate solution that is required in the first 24 hours. A 5 per cent dextrose solution should be administered at the rate of 45 ml./kg. of body weight in addition to the electrolyte solution to replace insensible cutaneous loss, obligatory water for renal function, and pulmonary losses. One half of this total calculated volume should be given within the first eight hours after injury, one fourth in the next eight hours, and one fourth in the last eight hours. Thereafter, the electrolyte dosage should be decreased to half while maintaining the dosage of dextrose solution; these quantities of fluids should be administered until diuresis becomes evident. At this point, parenterally administered fluids should be sharply curtailed and electrolyte solutions should be administered orally if the animal exhibits thirst. There is a real danger in allowing the animal to consume large amounts of water alone, as the burned patient is particularly liable to suffer water intoxication.

To illustrate how to calculate this regimen for fluid therapy, reconsider the example cited previously in which the dog weighed 30 lbs. and had a 20 per cent burn. By converting the weight to kilograms, we obtain $30 \div 2.2$ or 13.6 kg.; 13.6 kg. $\times$ 20 per cent $\times$ 4 ml. = 1088 ml. of lactated Ringer's solution or saline bicarbonate solution, and 13.6 $\times$ 45 ml. = 612/ml. of 5 per cent dextrose solution. This gives us the total amount for each fluid that is required in the first 24 hours. One half of this quantity of electrolyte solution and the same volume of dextrose solution would be administered in each consecutive 24-hour period until diuresis is established.

Recent work by several investigators[36, 54] has shown that the greatest need during the immediate postburn period is for large quantities of sodium and water. Colloids administered during this time did not significantly increase survival time and were actually deleterious because they decreased renal function and reduced capillary filtration in peripheral tissues, thereby aggravating tissue hypoxia. The need for plasma or whole blood should be assessed after the patient's condition has stabilized. If the animal is severely hypoproteinemic or anemic at this time, adequate quantities of blood or plasma should be administered.[63]

At the time treatment is instituted, it may be advantageous to heparinize the animal (1 mg./kg., given intravenously). It has been shown that heparin will markedly enhance the effectiveness of the repair mechanisms, delay the onset of dry gangrene, and diminish the amount of tissue loss.[59, 71]

If anuria supervenes, the intravenous administration of an isotonic sodium sulfate solution is recommended, as it has been shown to be the most effective agent with which to reestablish renal function.[69] After diuresis has commenced the level of potassium excretion may be high and this ion should be included in the parenterally or orally administered solution as potassium chloride.

The most important aspect in the treatment of shock from burns is the careful and frequent observation of the patient's progress.[43] The unburned skin should be warm and of near-normal turgor. The veins should fill and empty easily and the mucous membranes should be moist and pink. The urinary output should be in the range of 15 to 25 ml./hr. for a large dog. Unusual thirst and restlessness indicate the need for more intensive fluid therapy and not the administration of sedatives. An increase in pulse rate and a decrease in blood pressure occur late in cardiovascular collapse, and the failure of veins to fill suggests a contracted plasma volume and advancing shock. Oliguria indicates that therapy has failed to keep pace with losses or that acute renal insufficiency is occurring.

Corticosteroids may be administered during this period to shield the adrenal cortex from the effects of excessive ACTH by inhibiting the pituitary gland and to provide adequate quantities of adrenocorticosteroids during stress.[2] It has been demonstrated by Crassweller and associates[29] that adrenal exhaustion may occur after severe burns and that mortality may be decreased by the administration of corticosteroids. It was further shown by Whitelaw[89] that the circulating endogenous ACTH is present in quantities that are insufficient to meet the acute stress of severe burns. Cortisol and ACTH decrease capillary permeability in inflammation but are ineffective in limiting the leakage of proteins from the capillaries of burned tissues.[8, 25] The administration of corticotropin is advisable in order to restimulate the adrenal cortex after the most stressful period. Tetanus toxoid should be administered prophylactically.

It has been demonstrated that placing the burned part of an animal in ice water will reduce the rate and amount of edema formation and the degree of hemoconcentration.[28] This method of treatment is to be criticized, however, when it is applied to an extensive injury because the undesirable effects of a fall in body temperature would outweigh the possible advantages.

The effect of environmental temperature on the 24-hour mortality following a severe cutaneous burn was studied by Elman and coworkers.[33] It was observed that the lowest mortality occurred at an ambient temperature of 75° F and mortality increased to 100 per cent with either an increase or a decrease of 20° F. This factor should be considered, particularly in the summertime, and the animal should be placed in an air-conditioned room, if available.

LOCAL TREATMENT OF THE WOUND

When the initial emergency procedures have been completed, the clinician's attention should be directed to the treatment of the wound. The burned surface and the surrounding normal skin should be gently washed with a bland white soap or a hexachlorophene detergent. This will remove much of the foreign matter and many of the transient organisms that are present in the area. It has been shown that hexachlorophene in bar or liquid soap has no untoward effects on the lesion, whereas tincture of green soap produces a tissue reaction as a result of its alcoholic content.[9]

Many of the older drugs employed in the local treatment of burns have been discarded. Oils and greasy salves macerate tissue and delay healing. Picric acid, butyl aminobenzoate, gentian violet, acriflavine, and tannic acid destroy viable cells and delay healing.[13, 58] Tannic acid should not be applied to extensive burns for the added reason that it is absorbed and produces extensive liver damage.[7] Petrolatum in small quantities was shown to have no effect on healing.[13] Rovatti and Brennan[81] studied an ointment that contained aloe. They found that it prevented the separation of the eschar in deep dermal burns and shortened the healing time. Hydrophilic ointments containing mafenide (Sulfamylon) acetate or silver sulfadiazine (Silvadene) may be applied to the lesion to prevent infection. Care should be employed in the use of ointments containing sulfonamides or topical anesthetics because of the possibility of absorption and the resultant systemic toxicity.

The cutaneous lesion may be treated by either of the following methods: the closed method in which the wound is cleansed and a dressing is applied and left in place until healing commences, and the exposure method in which the lesion is left uncovered and exposed to the air.

Several different approaches to the closed method could be employed in the dog. Wet dressings of sterile isotonic saline solution or Dakin's solution may be applied.[5] These tend to limit the fluid loss through the surface, keep the eschar soft, and in the case of Dakin's solution, inhibit the multiplication of microorganisms. An alternative method is the application of a single layer of sterile gauze that is lightly impregnated with petrolatum. This is then covered with sterile compresses and a retaining bandage. The advantage of this dressing is that it permits viewing the progress of wound healing without disturbing the injured surface. It is important to avoid large quantities of petrolatum, since they macerate the tissues and delay healing. The advantages of the closed method are that it keeps the wound clean and prevents the animal from licking or biting the injured area.

The exposure method as described by Pulaski and Artz[76] is generally inapplicable for use in animals, since the eschar must remain intact until healing commences. Movement by the animal tends to cause the division of the eschar and the formation of fissures through which bacterial contaminants may gain entrance. Modifications of the exposure method may be employed and, indeed, may be necessary in certain locations of the body. Choy and Wendt[21] described the use of polyvinyl plastic, which is dispensed as an aerosol, as a dressing for burns. This procedure should be useful in the treatment of burns in animals. Figure 5–6 shows a case managed by the exposure method.

Although enzymes have been investigated for the débridement of the burn eschar, the principal difficulty has been the requirement of a broad spectrum of enzymatic activity. Most enzymes possess a high degree of substrate specificity, and the eschar is composed of a great variety of substrates,

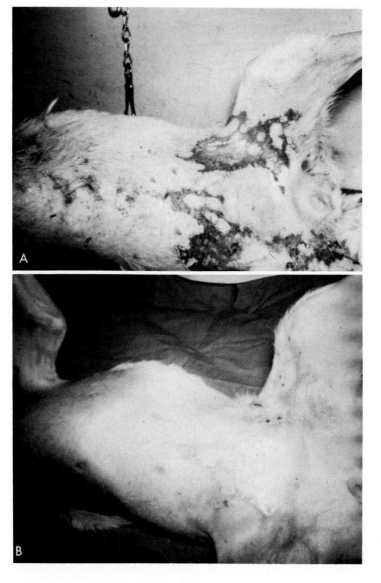

Figure 5–6: A, Healing partial-thickness burn 14 days after injury. B, Same case 21 days after injury. See color plate III–E, p. 570.

e.g., fibrin, collagen, coagulated proteins, and purulent exudate. Streptoki-nase-streptodornase,[22, 23] trypsin,[80] and an enzyme produced by *Clostridium histolyticum*[4] are several of the enzymes that have been studied. Streptoki-nase-streptodornase is effective in breaking down fibrin and pus in humans. For use in animals, human plasminogen must be added to the enzymes, since the domestic animals lack adequate quantities of this precursor. Trypsin is active against necrotic tissue in general but has no effect on viable cells, since they possess intracellular antitryptic substances.[80] The enzymes produced by *Clostridium histolyticum* are active against collagen and aid in the separation of the eschar. Schales[83] studied the inhibitory effects of a series of compounds on the activity of pepsin, trypsin, and chymotrypsin. The local enzymatic treatment of the lesion requires that the eschar be surgically crosshatched in order that the enzymes may reach their specific substrates.[23]

The principal aims in local treatment are the prevention of infection, the promotion of rapid healing, the minimization of scar formation, and the prevention of mutilation of the wound by the patient.

CONVALESCENT CARE OF THE PATIENT

The problem of nutrition in the burned patient has been extensively investigated. Harper[47] indicated that the extremely negative nitrogen balance in burned patients was attributable to the endocrine response to trauma and stress, losses of protein-rich exudate, and excessive catabolism of the tissues. The increased caloric requirement is a consequence of the increased rate of metabolism resulting from infection and fever. An increase in caloric intake is also desirable because of its protein-sparing effect. The effect of environmental temperature on the state of nutrition of burned rats was studied by Caldwell.[16] He found that rats that were maintained at 20° C with their diet fixed at preburn levels lost weight, had a sustained negative nitrogen balance, did not deposit body fat, and had a high mortality. These changes were not evident in rats that were kept at a temperature of 30° C. If the two groups were allowed free access to food, this marked difference was not observed. Again, the problem of ambient temperature becomes important. The requirement for and the utilization of B vitamins are increased following an extensive burn.

At the earlist possible time, high-calorie substances and nitrogen should be given in quantity. If the animal refuses to eat and drink, these may be administered parenterally as protein hydrolysate and dextrose solution. Taylor and colleagues[86] have shown that 80 to 100 per cent of the amino acids from intravenously administered protein hydrolysate or amino acids are utilized. Protein hydrolysate is preferable to amino acids because parenterally administered amino acids tend to aggravate the acidosis. In addition to calories and nitrogen, the animal should be supplied with therapeutic amounts of B vitamins, ascorbic acid, and vitamin A to provide adequate quantities for metabolism and optimum wound healing.

If the animal will eat, these nutrients should be fed in quantity. The animal should not be force-fed, however, because this procedure is poorly tolerated by the burned dog even though it does improve the nitrogen balance.[62] Some practical considerations have been pointed out by Elman:[32] skimmed milk can be fed in larger amounts than whole milk and still provide equivalent quantities of protein; lean meat and egg white are excellent sources of protein; and large amounts of fat tend to satiate the hunger drive and thereby prevent the ingestion of adequate amounts of protein. Any commercial high-protein, high-calorie, low-fat diet that is supplemented with vitamins should provide adequate nutritional care for the animal during convalescence. The requirements during this period are 2 to 3 gm. of protein and 50 to 80 calories/kg. of body weight per day.[47, 86]

Testosterone propionate has been shown to reduce the nitrogen loss following a burn.[62] Anabolic steroids are a useful adjunct to the nutritional care of the burned patient, as they reduce the time necessary to regain positive nitrogen balance and would decrease the incidence of osteoporosis.

Some other problems that may prove troublesome during the period of convalescence are persistent anemia and wound infection.. The anemia should be treated with whole blood transfusions as indicated. Infection seems to be almost inevitable as a concomitant of burns. The nature of the eschar and the abundance of plasma, together with a poor blood supply in the region of the burn, provide a rich medium for bacterial growth. Most studies of the microbiology of burns have been performed on human patients and hence are not applicable to this discussion. It could be reasonably assumed, however, that streptococci and staphylococci would be common invaders, since they are part of the normal flora of the skin and the mucous membranes of the dog. *Pseudomonas aeruginosa* infections are a common and serious complication of burns in human patients and could conceivably be a problem in animal patients.

Extensive full-thickness burns will require surgical treatment following separation of the burn slough. This is especially true of lesions located over flexion surfaces, since widespread cicatrix formation in these areas will produce extreme functional disability. Muir[66] and Hyslop and Miller[50] recommend the excision of electrical burns back to healthy tissues within the first 12 hours. The site of excision should then be closed by primary closure or with a split-skin graft. They believe that this treatment decreases the period of disability, lessens suffering, and provides a better functional and cosmetic result. Nunn,[68] on the other hand, believes that débridement should not be attempted until sloughing is complete, because one cannot determine exactly the limits of injury.

Pinch grafts would seem to be the most practical method of skin grafting in most practices because the technique requires only those instruments that every practitioner has at hand.

SUMMARY

There are few forms of trauma that equal the magnitude and intensity of response of thermal injury. In order to rationally treat a severe, extensive burn, it is necessary for the veterinarian to understand the multitude of changes in structure and function that are produced by this physical agent. The greatest problems that are encountered in the clinical management are the prevention of shock and infection.

REFERENCES

1. Abell, R. G., and Page, I. H.: A study of the smaller blood vessels in burned dogs and cats. Surg. Gynecol. Obstet., 77:348, 1943.
2. Alexander, W. G.: The use of cortisone in the treatment of a severe burn in a dog. S.W. Vet., 4:10, 1951.
3. Allison, F., Jr., Smith, M. R., and Wood, W. B., Jr.: Studies on the pathogenesis of acute inflammation. J. Exp. Med., 102:655, 1955.
4. Altemeier, W. A., Coith, R., Culbertson, W., et al.: Enzymatic debridement of burns. Ann. Surg., 134:581, 1951.
5. Armistead, W. W.: Thermal burns. North Am. Vet. 36:453, 1955.
6. Artz, C. P., Moncrief, J. A., and Pruitt, B. A.: Burns: A Team Approach. Philadelphia, W. B. Saunders Co., 1979.
7. Artz, C. P., and Soreff, H. S.: Modern concepts in the treatment of burns. J.A.M.A., 159:411, 1955.
8. Baker, J. W., Wight, A., Michel, A. J. D., et al.: A clinical and experimental evaluation of the influence of ACTH on the need for fluid therapy of the burned patient. Ann. Surg., 134:614, 1951.
9. Best, R. R., Coe, J. D., and McMurtrey, G. B.: The effect of soaps containing hexachlorophene on wounds and burned surfaces. Arch. Surg., 62:895, 1951.
10. Brånemark, P.-I., Breine, U., Joshi, M., et al.: Microvascular pathophysiology of burned tissue. Ann. N. Y. Acad. Sci., 150:474, 1968.
11. Brooks, F. H., Dragstedt, L. R., Warner, L., et al.: The sequence of circulatory changes following severe thermal burns. Anat. Rec., 100:644, 1948.
12. Brooks, J. W., Robinett, P., Largen, T. L., et al.: A standard contact burn: Method of production and observations on the blood picture following its production in dogs. Surg. Gynecol. Obstet., 93:543, 1951.
13. Brush, B. E., Lam, C. R., and Ponka, J. L.: Wound healing studies on several substances recommended for the treatment of burns. Surgery, 21:662, 1947.
14. Buis, L. J., and Hartman, F. W.: Histopathology of the liver following superficial burns. Am. J. Clin. Pathol., 11:275, 1941.
15. Bull, J. P., and Squire, J. R.: A study of mortality in a burns unit: Standards for the evaluation of alternative methods of treatment. Ann. Surg., 130:160, 1949.
16. Caldwell, F. T.: Metabolic response to thermal trauma: II. Nutritional studies with rats at two environmental temperatures. Ann. Surg., 155:119, 1962.
17. Cameron, G. R.: Experimental pathology of burns. Br. Med. Bull., 3:88, 1945.
18. Cameron, G. R., Burgess, F., and Trenwith, V.: An experimental study of some effects of acute anhydraemia. J. Pathol. Bacteriol., 58:213, 1946.
19. Chanutin, A., and Ludewig, S.: The effect of B-chloroethyl vesicants, thermal injury, and turpentine on plasma fibrin, cholesterol, and sugar of dogs and rats. J. Biol. Chem., 167:313, 1947.
20. Chardack, W. M., Brueske, D. A., Santomauro, A. P., et al.: Experimental studies on the synthetic substitutes for skin and their use in the treatment of burns. Ann. Surg., 155:127, 1962.
21. Choy, S. J., and Wendt, W. E.: A new local treatment of burns. Abstracted from U.S. Armed Forces Med. J., 1952, in J. Am. Vet. Med. Assoc., 125:203, 1954.
22. Connell, J. F., Jr., and Rousselot, L. M.: The use of proteolytic enzymes in the debridement of the burn eschar. Surg. Forum, 4:422, 1953.
23. Connell, J. F. Jr., and Rousselot, L. M.: The use of enzymatic agents in the debridement of burn and wound sloughs. Surgery, 30:43, 1951.
24. Cope, O.: in Symposium on Burns. National Research Council, National Academy of Sciences, 1951, p. 33.
25. Cope, O., Graham, J. B., Mixter, G., Jr., et al.: Threshold of thermal trauma and influence of adrenal cortical and posterior pituitary extracts on the capillary and chemical changes: An experimental study. Arch. Surg., 59:1015, 1949.
26. Cope, O., and Moore, F. D.: A study of capillary permeability in experimental burns and burn shock using radioactive dyes in blood and lymph. J. Clin. Invest., 23:241, 1944.
27. Cope, O., Graham, J. B., Moore, F. D., et al.: The nature of the shift of plasma protein to the extravascular space following thermal trauma. Ann. Surg., 128:1041, 1948.
28. Courtice, F. C.: The effect of local temperature on fluid loss in thermal burns. J. Physiol., 104:321, 1946.
29. Crassweller, P. O., Farmer, A. W., and Franks, W. R.: Experimental burn studies including treatment with cortisone-active material extracted from urine. Br. Med. J., 2:242, 1950.
30. Dexter, F. E., and Petersen, R. E.: Changes in the liver and pancreas following superficial burns. Bios., 12:187, 1941.
31. Dziemian, A. J.: The effects of burns on kidney function. Fed. Proc., 7:29, 1948.
32. Elman, R.: Physiologic problems of burns. J. Mo. Med. Assoc., 41:1, 1944.

33. Elman, R., Cox, W. M., Jr., Lischer, C., et al.: Mortality in severe experimental burns as affected by environmental temperature. Proc. Soc. Exp. Biol. Med., 51:350, 1942.
34. Erb, I. H., Morgan, E. M., and Farmer, A. W.: The pathology of burns. Ann. Surg., 117:234, 1943.
35. Evans, E. I.: The early management of the severely burned patient. Surg. Gynecol. Obstet., 94:273, 1952.
36. Fox, C. L., Jr.: The role of alkaline sodium salt solutions in the treatment of severe burns. Ann. N. Y.. Acad. Sci., 150:823, 1968.
37. Fox, C. L., Jr., and Baer, H.: Redistribution of potassium, sodium, and water in burns and trauma, and its relation to the phenomena of shock. Am. J. Physiol, 151:155, 1947.
38. Friesen, S. R.: The genesis of gastroduodenal ulcer following burns: An experimental study. Surgery, 28:123, 1950.
39. Gann, D. S., Kingsbury, B., Drucker, W. R., et al.: Diminished adrenal corticoid response to burn and ACTH in the nephrectomized dog. Proc. Soc. Exp. Biol. Med., 108:99, 1961.
40. Gilmore, J. P.: Cardiovascular changes in the burned dog following the infusion of IV fluids. Am. J. Physiol., 190:513, 1957.
41. Gilmore, J. P., and Handford, S. W.: Hemodynamic response of the dog to thermal radiation. J. Appl. Physiol., 8:393, 1956.
42. Goodall, M.: Adrenal medullary insufficiency in severe thermal burn. J. Clin. Invest., 39: 1927, 1960.
43. Griffith, C. A.: Burns: II. Burn shock. N.W. Med., 55:167, 1956.
44. Ham, A. W.: Experimental study of the histopathology of burns with particular reference to sites of fluid loss in burns of different depths. Ann. Surg., 120:689, 1944.
45. Ham, T. H., Shen, S. C., Fleming, E. M., et al.: Studies on the destruction of red blood cells: IV. Thermal injury. Blood, 3:373, 1948.
46. Harkins, H. N.: The present status of the problem of thermal burns. Physiol. Rev., 25:531, 1945.
47. Harper, H. A.: Nutritional aspects of the care of the burned patient. Plast. Reconstr. Surg., 21:389, 1958.
48. Hartman, F. W.: Curling's ulcer in experimental burns. Ann. Surg., 121:54, 1945.
49. Hueston, J. T., Hossack, D. W., and Taft, L. I.: Renal changes in fetal burns: A clinico-pathologic study of four cases. Aust. N. Z. J. Surg., 26:289, 1957.
50. Hyslop, V. B., and Miller, E. W.: Treatment of electric burns. J. Int. Coll. Surg., 23:481, 1955.
51. James, G. W., III, Abbott, L. D., Brooks, J. W., et al.: The anemia of thermal injury. J. Clin. Invest., 33:150, 1954.
52. James, G. W., III, Purnell, O. J., and Evans, E.,I.: The anemia of thermal injury: II. Studies of liver function. J. Clin. Invest., 30:191, 1951.
53. Kabat, H., and Levine, M.: Capillary emboli as a lethal factor in burns. Science, 96:476, 1942.
54. Kessler, E., Hughes, R. C., Orlando, C., et al.: Comparative effects of saline and isooncotic albumin in saline on sodium excretion. Proc. Soc. Exp. Biol. Med., 125:543, 1967.
55. Lehman, E. P.: The delayed classification of burns. Surgery, 12:651, 1942.
56. Lovell, J. E., and Al-Bagdadi, F.: The integument. In Evans, H. E., and Christensen, G. C.: Miller's Anatomy of the Dog. ed. 2. Philadelphia, W. B. Saunders Co., 1979.
57. Mallory, T. B., and Brickley, W. J.: Pathology with special reference to the pulmonary lesions. Ann. Surg., 117:865, 1943.
58. Maun, M. E., Schneider, R. C., Pilling, M. A., et al.: Tissue reactions to medicaments used in the local treatment of burns. Surgery, 14:229, 1943.
59. McCleery, R. S., Schaffarzick, W. R., and Light, R. A.: An experimental study of the effect of heparin on the local pathology of burns. Surgery, 26:548, 1949.
60. McClure, R. D.: Liver injury in burns, in Josiah Macy, Jr., Foundation's Second Conference on Liver Injury. New York, 1944, pp. 87–89.
61. Meloy, W. C.: Histopathology, chemistry and supportive treatment of burns. Med. Ann. D. C., 16:426, 1947.
62. Meyer, F. L., Hirshfeld, J. W., and Abbott, W. E.: Metabolic alterations following thermal burns: VII. Effect of force feeding, methionine and testosterone propionate on nitrogen balance in experimental burns. J. Clin. Invest., 26:796, 1947.
63. Moncrief, J. A.: Burns. N. Engl. J. Med., 288:444, 1973.
64. Moritz, A. R., Henriques, F. C., Jr., and McLean, R.: The effects of inhaled heat on the air passages and lungs. Am. J. Pathol., 21:311, 1945.
65. Moyer, C. A., Coller, F. A., Iob, V., et al.: A study of the interrelationship of salt solutions, serum and defibrinated blood in the treatment of severely scalded, anesthetized dogs. Ann. Surg., 120:367, 1944.
66. Muir, I. F.: The management of electrical burns. Postgrad. Med. J., 33:219, 1957.
67. Netsky, M. G., and Leiter, S. S.: Capillary permeability to horse proteins in burn shock. Am. J. Physiol., 130:1, 1943/1944.
68. Nunn, L. L.: Severe electrical burns. N.W. Med., 56:691, 1957.

69. Olson, W. H., and Nechles, H.: Studies of anuria: Effect of infusion fluids and diuretics on the anuria resulting from severe burns. Surg. Gynecol. Obstet., 84:283, 1947.

70. Page, I. H.: Cardiovascular changes resulting from severe scalds. Am. J. Physiol., 142:366, 1944.

71. Parsons, R., Jr., Alrich, E. M., and Lehman, E. P.: Studies on burns: V. Experimental study of the effect of heparinization and gravity on tissue loss resulting from third degree burns. Surg. Gynecol. Obstet., 90:722, 1950.

72. Patey, D. H., and Scarff, R. W.: The diagnosis of the depth of skin destruction in burns and its bearing on treatment. Br. J. Surg., 32:32, 1944-1945.

73. Perlmann, G. E., Glenn, W. W. L., and Kaufman, D.: Changes in the electrophoretic pattern in lymph and serum in experimental burns. J. Clin. Invest., 22:627, 1943.

74. Peters, R. A.: The biochemical lesion in thermal burns. Br. Med. Bull., 3:81, 1945.

75. Prendergast, J. J., Fenichel, R. L., and Daly, B. M.: Albumin and globulin changes in burns as demonstrated by electrophoresis. Arch. Surg., 64:733, 1952.

76. Pulaski, E. J., and Artz, C. P.: Exposure (open) treatment of burns. U.S. Armed Forces Med. J., 2:769, 1951.

77. Purnell, O. J., and Evans, E. I.: in Symposium on Burns. National Research Council, National Academy of Sciences, 1951, p. 40.

78. Quinby, W. C., Jr., and Cope, O.: Blood viscosity and the whole blood therapy of burns. Surgery, 32:316, 1952.

79. Raker, J. W., and Rovit, R. L.: The acute red blood cell destruction following severe thermal trauma in dogs. Surg. Gynecol. Obstet., 98:169, 1954.

80. Reiser, H. G., Patton, R., and Roettig, L. C.: Tryptic debridement of necrotic tissue. Arch. Surg., 63:568, 1951.

81. Rovatti, B., and Brennan, R. J.: Experimental thermal burn. Indust. Med. Surg., 28:364, 1959.

82. Salzberg, A. M., and Evans, E. I.: Blood volumes in normal and burned dogs: A comparative study with radioactive phosphorus-tagged red cells and T-1824 dye. Ann. Surg., 132:746, 1950.

83. Schales, O.: New inhibitors of enzymatic proteolysis. Proc. Soc. Exp. Biol. Med., 79:75, 1951.

84. Schwartz, L. G.: Use of lyophilized canine plasma for treatment of shock in dogs. J. Am. Vet. Med. Assoc., 140:145, 1962.

85. Sevitt, S.: Eosinophile and other leucocyte changes in burned patients. Br. Med. J., 1:976, 1951.

86. Taylor, F. H. L., Davidson, C. S., and Levenson, S. M.: The problems of nutrition in the presence of excessive nitrogen requirement in seriously ill patients with particular reference to thermal burns. Conn. State Med. J., 8:141, 1944.

87. Walker, J., Jr.: The pathologic physiology of the extensive superficial burn. Surg. Clin. North Am., 26:1488, 1946.

88. Wallace, A. B.: A present (1957) outlook on burns. Plast. Reconstr. Surg., 21:243, 1958.

89. Whitelaw, J. J.: Physiological reaction to pituitary adrenocorticotropic hormone in severe burns. J.A.M.A., 145:85, 1951.

90. Wight, A., Raker, J. W., Merrington, W. R., et al.: The ebb and flow of the eosinophiles in the burned patient and their use in the clinical management. Ann. Surg., 137:175, 1953.

91. Young, M. K., Jr., Seraile, L. G., and Brown, W. L.: Inhibition of glucose utilization following thermal injury. Am. J. Physiol., 191:119, 1957.

SECTION III

RECONSTRUCTION OF TRAUMATIZED SKIN

6

GENERAL PRINCIPLES OF DELAYED WOUND EXCISION AND CLOSURE

DELAYED WOUND EXCISION

Prior to undertaking reconstruction of the skin, it is necessary to prepare the area. In some instances, reconstruction of the wound may be indicated at the time of initial excision or as soon as possible after the inciting trauma (i.e., primary or delayed primary closure). However, in many cases of massive soft tissue trauma with contamination or infection, it is necessary to allow the wound to heal sufficiently by means of granulation tissue, epithelialization, and wound contraction (i.e., healing by second intention) before undertaking reconstruction. When the wound is adequately healed, the surgeon may assess its shape and then decide upon the proper reconstructive technique (Figs. 6–1 and 6–2). An area in which cutaneous neoplasms or cysts have been excised will also need reconstruction. Regardless of the

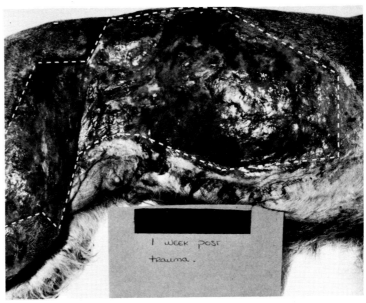

Figure 6–1: A large, open wound soon after infliction.

237

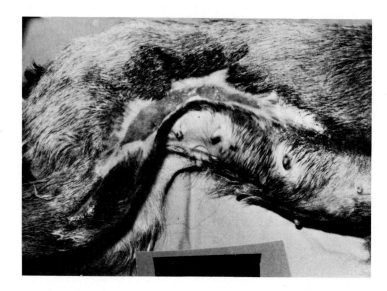

Figure 6–2: The wound in Figure 6–1 after healing by contraction and epithelialization.

nature of the lesion, the goal of the surgeon should be to remove the offending lesion while providing the best possible cosmetic result.[18]

The technique for débridement of a fresh wound has been described previously in Chapter 4. When excising a large wound that has healed by contraction and epithelialization, the author prefers to incise around the wound at the junction of normal, haired skin and the unhaired epithelium using a sharp scalpel blade (No. 10 or No. 15). A light outlining incision is

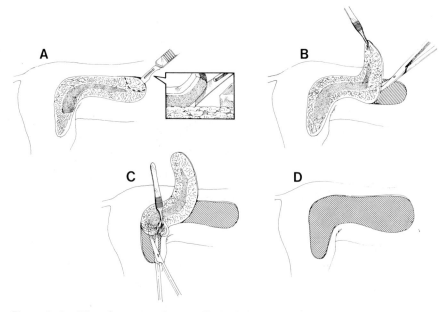

Figure 6–3: Wound excision of a partially healed wound. *A*, The epithelialized granulation tissue along one side of the lesion is undermined. *B*, Tissue forceps and scissors are used to excise half of the wound. *C*, Second half of the wound is excised. *D*, The excision is completed.

made through the epidermis first. The incision through the remainder of the dermis is completed following the outlining. A small area along one side of the lesion, which has been undermined to a depth of 2 to 3 mm., is picked up with forceps. Excision of the remainder of the lesion (the unhaired epithelium and granulation tissue) is carried out toward the center of the lesion with a scalpel or curved, blunt-pointed scissors at an initial starting depth of 2 to 3 mm. At this point, the procedure is repeated from the opposite side of the lesion (Figs. 6–3 and 6–4).[18] Another technique for excising such a lesion is to remove the unhaired epithelium only, followed by scraping or shaving the superficial surface of the central granulation tissue with a scalpel blade (Fig. 6–5). Following the excision of a lesion, the surgeon may evaluate the shape of the lesion. If the surrounding skin is to be moved into the lesion for reconstruction, the surgeon must decide (1) whether the wound is sufficiently geometrical so that further excision will be unnecessary; (2) whether further tissue needs to be re-

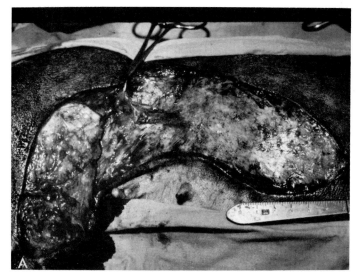

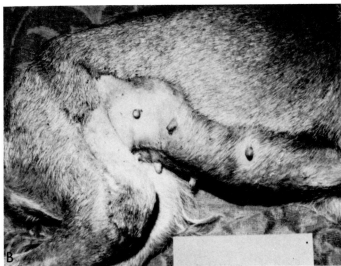

Figure 6–4: *A,* Excised wound shown in Figure 6–2. *B,* Final result after reconstructive surgery.

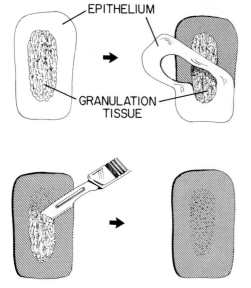

Figure 6–5: Wound excision by removing epithelial tissue and shaving the top off the remaining granulation tissue.

moved to convert the wound to a geometrical shape that will facilitate closure; or (3) whether the wound may be closed easily enough without having to rely on a geometrical shape for closure.

Skin lesions can be removed by elliptical, wedge, or circular excision.[26] In the dog these would apply more to smaller traumatic and tumorous lesions. However, larger lesions could also be removed in these ways.

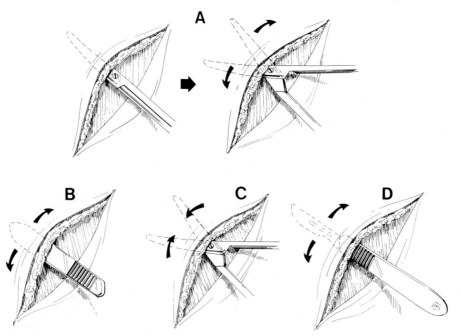

Figure 6–6: Tissue undermining techniques. *A* and *B*, Blunt techniques. *C* and *D*, Sharp techniques.

UNDERMINING

After wound excision, it is often necessary to undermine the skin in the surrounding area to facilitate its movement for wound closure. Small defects can frequently be closed by simple sutures; however, undermining and sliding the skin are necessary for larger defects.[5]

Undermining is performed by blunt or sharp dissection with scissors in order to find the natural cleavage line in the loose subcutaneous connective tissue.[35] With blunt dissection the points of the scissors are closed when they are inserted and then spread after they have reached the depth of the wound. This helps prevent damage to blood vessels in the area. Blunt dissection can also be performed with the blunt end of a scalpel handle.[18] Sharp dissection entails snipping the tissue with the scissor blades as they are advanced through the tissue. This technique increases the risk of hemorrhage. Undermining may also be done with a sharp scalpel held parallel to the skin surface.[18, 26, 50] Here, again, the chances of hemorrhage may be greater (Fig. 6–6).

If the surgeon prefers to gauge the depth of undermining by a sense other than sight, he can elevate the skin edge with a skin hook held between the thumb and middle finger of one hand. As the other hand operates the scissors, he can feel the depth of undermining with the forefinger of the hand that is holding the skin hook (Fig. 6–7).[78]

Undermining is particularly useful on the trunk of an animal because of the mobility of the skin.[35] However, the technique is also quite useful in other areas. Undermining about the face should be very superficial, just under the dermis, since deeper undercutting could result in damage to branches of the facial nerve, especially in the labial area (Fig. 6–8).[50, 78] On the limbs and trunk, undermining should be deeper to utilize the cleavage between subcuticular tissue and deep fascia (Fig. 6–9).[50]

The extent to which undermining can be carried without damaging the skin's blood supply is a matter that needs controlled study in the dog and cat. Undermining may be quite extensive and yet may result in little or no harm.[13, 66] The primary disadvantage of undermining is the possibility of hematoma formation in the space that is created.[50] As previously mentioned, the chances of this occurring are greater if a sharp dissection technique is used.

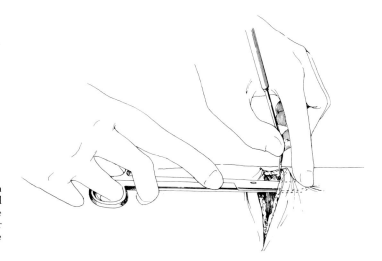

Figure 6–7: Gauging the depth of undermining. Skin is elevated with a skin hook held between the thumb and the middle finger while the forefinger gauges the depth of undermining.

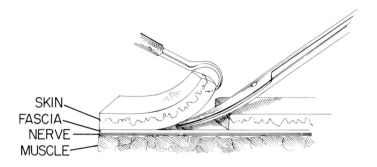

SKIN
FASCIA
NERVE
MUSCLE

Figure 6–8: Undermining skin on the face just under the dermis avoids facial nerve damage. (After McGregor, I. A.: Fundamental Techniques of Plastic Surgery, ed. 5. Edinburgh, Churchill Livingstone, 1972, p. 13.)

HEMOSTASIS

At the time a wound is excised, either initially or after a delay, hemorrhage will be encountered that needs to be controlled. Various means are available to accomplish hemostasis.

PRESSURE AND TIME

When hemorrhage is the result of capillary oozing, it can be effectively controlled by sustained pressure. Such pressure probably acts to occlude the capillaries until coagulation occurs. It is best to apply pressure for five minutes while watching the clock, since there is generally a tendency to underestimate the time elapsed.[6, 26]

CLAMPING AND TWISTING SMALL VESSELS

Clamping and twisting small vessels prevent the introduction of foreign material into a wound. However, these methods are not truly reliable for hemostasis.[6, 9, 18, 26]

LIGATION

After bleeding vessels are clamped accurately with fine-pointed hemostats, they are tied with fine suture materials. Chromic catgut (4–0) is strong, causes little tissue reaction, and has been advocated for use as a ligature. Owing to the lack of tensile strength and the increased inflammation asso-

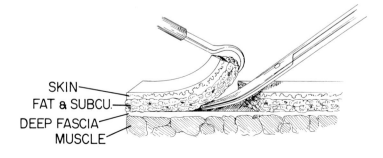

SKIN
FAT & SUBCU.
DEEP FASCIA
MUSCLE

Figure 6–9: Undermining on the limbs and trunk between the subcuticular tissue and deep fascia. (After McGregor, I. A.: Fundamental Techniques of Plastic Surgery, ed. 5. Edinburgh, Churchill Livingstone, 1972, p. 13.)

ciated with it, plain catgut should not be used.[6] The ligature may be simply tied about the vessel, or it may be transfixed in surrounding tissue for more security.[18, 26]

ELECTROSURGERY

Electrosurgical techniques probably provide the most rapid and effective means of achieving hemostasis of blood vessels of small to medium diameters. An electrical current of high frequency (2 to 18 million cycles/sec.), relatively high amperage, and low voltage will coagulate the walls of blood vessels to produce hemostasis. A fine-tipped electrode may be applied to the end of a severed vessel to coagulate the walls. This may cause some thermal damage to surrounding tissues. To minimize such trauma, coagulation may be accomplished by bringing the active electrode of the electrosurgical apparatus into contact with a small hemostat or forceps that is accurately gripping the vessel.[9, 18, 26]

TOPICAL VASOCONSTRICTORS

Surgical sponges that are moistened with epinephrine (1:10,000),[26] epinephrine hydrochloride (1:1000),[6, 18] or phenylephrine hydrochloride (Neo-Synephrine, 1:20,000)[26] can be applied to a wound to diminish bleeding from capillaries and small vessels. These topical agents produce an initial vasoconstriction; however, once the action of the drug is completed, a reflex hyperemia follows that may be great enough to cause further bleeding.[26]

FIBRIN AND GELATIN FOAM

Fibrin[26] and gelatin foam[18, 26] can be used to pack small cavities from which there is constant oozing. Small pieces of these materials are readily absorbed into the tissues with minimal reaction. However, neither substance should be left on a bed where a skin graft is to be placed, since it will delay vascularization of the graft.[26]

CHEMICALS

Certain cauterizing chemicals, such as trichloroacetic acid, phenol, and silver nitrate, will control hemorrhage by sealing small blood vessels.[18] However, such chemicals are caustic to surrounding tissues and should be used with discretion. Other forms of hemostasis should usually be considered before using cauterizing chemicals.

WOUND CLOSURE AND PRESSURE BANDAGES

Closing a wound with sutures will control most minor hemorrhage. This, in conjunction with a pressure bandage, may be quite helpful in attaining hemostasis.[18] The art of applying a pressure bandage that results in hemostasis and yet does not cause ischemia of the area is something that comes with experience. It is better to apply a bandage too loosely and have the pet owner return to have the bandage replaced than to apply a bandage too tightly and have the pet owner return with an animal suffering from ischemic necrosis.

WOUND CLOSURE

SURGICAL INSTRUMENTS

An elaborate array of surgical instruments is not needed to perform skin closure in the dog and cat. In fact, every practicing veterinarian has the basic instruments (needle holder, scissors, and thumb forceps) needed for skin closure. Certain instruments have been suggested to make skin closure a more refined technique (Fig. 6–10). A needle holder–scissors combination has been advocated for use in skin closure.[50] This is particularly helpful to the surgeon who does not have an assistant to cut sutures. The author has found small ophthalmic needle holders to be useful in skin closure. To avoid breaking the needle,[3] needle holders should not be clamped near the eye of the needle. Grasping the needle in an area one-quarter to one-half the distance between the end and the point of the needle has

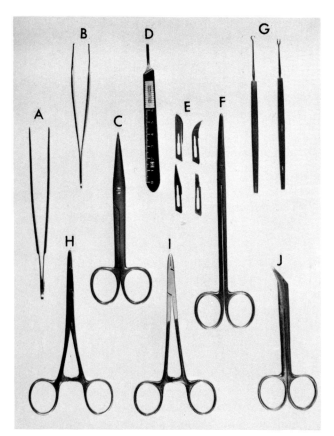

Figure 6–10: Examples of instruments that could be used for skin surgery. *A*, Dressing forceps. *B*, Brown-Adson forceps, one vs. two delicate teeth. *C*, Straight, sharp-sharp scissors. *D*, Bard-Parker No. 3 metric scalpel handle. *E*, No. 10, 11, 12, and 15 scalpel blades. *F*, Metzenbaum scissors (curved). *G*, Skin hooks. *H*, Olsen-Hegar combined needle holder and scissors. *I*, Hegar-Baumgartner needle holders (bulldog jaws). *J*, Suture wire–cutting scissors.

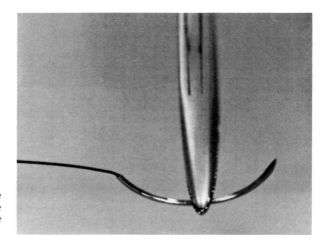

Figure 6–11: The proper grasp of a needle in needle holders is halfway between the base and tip of the needle, near the tip of the needle holders.

been recommended.[19] Curved needles should be held near the tip of the needle holders, since clamping the broad portion of the jaws on a curved needle will tend to bend (straighten) the needle (Fig. 6–11).[3, 19]

Two types of scissors have been advocated for use in skin closure — straight, sharp-pointed scissors for cutting wound margins and sutures, and curved, blunt-pointed scissors for undermining edges.[50] However, scissors used on the skin tend to have a crushing action; skin incisions made by a scalpel are preferable.[2] The surgeon should also have a pair of scissors for cutting wire sutures.

Manipulation of the skin when placing sutures should be done as atraumatically as possible. The least traumatic means of manipulating the skin edges is by using the fingers only. With some practice, the thumb and index finger of one hand can be utilized to tense the skin while the needle is inserted with the other hand using needle holders (Fig. 6–12).[3] The skin hook causes a minimal amount of trauma to the skin; however, coordination

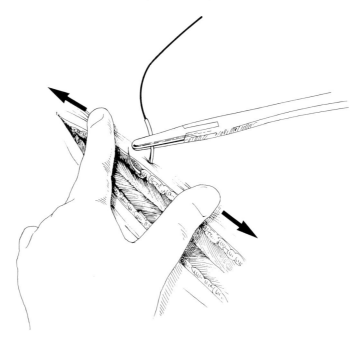

Figure 6–12: The least traumatic way to steady skin edges for suture placement is to tense the skin with the thumb and the finger.

and speed may be difficult to attain with this instrument.[2, 6, 50] The author has found that a suture needle held in needle holders may be used as a type of skin hook. Because of the difficulty that may be encountered in using skin hooks, dissecting thumb forceps are more routinely used. The decision to use toothed or nontoothed forceps should be made with regard to the amount of trauma that each may cause. Toothed Adson tissue forceps will hold without slipping or undue pressure and with minimal trauma.[3, 6] Tissue forceps without teeth require more pressure to hold the tissue, thereby causing more trauma.[6]

Regardless of the instruments used to suture tissues, the surgeon should bear in mind the use of an atraumatic technique. The simple crushing effect of a forceps or hemostat causes appreciable trauma to both cells and vessels. This results in a loss of protoplasm, blood, and lymph into the interstitial spaces. Destroyed or damaged cells thus provide a media upon which bacteria can multiply, create sepsis, and destroy more tissue. An atraumatic technique helps keep this damage to a minimum. It can thus be seen that the use of sharp instruments as well as sutures of the proper size and a swaged needle are important in accomplishing an atraumatic technique.[26]

MANAGEMENT OF DAMAGED DEEP STRUCTURES AND CLOSURE OF DEAD SPACE

The initial management of severed and damaged tendons and nerves has been discussed in Chapter 4. When such damage is present, a wound that has been allowed to heal as an open wound or that has been closed after initial excision or débridement will require reopening and exposure of the tendons and nerves following the initial surgery, at which time definitive repair may be undertaken. In the case of damage to peripheral nerves, approximately 21 days should elapse before reexposure and definitive repair of the nerve are undertaken.[72] This time lapse allows the avascular ends of nerves and tendons to heal and regain their vascularity so that suturing may be more successful.[35] In addition, the area of damaged nerve and tendon will be more readily visible and can be removed before anastomosing the remaining viable tissue.[35, 72] Since nonabsorbable suture materials will be needed to anastomose the nerves and tendons and since many of these wounds are contaminated, it is advisable to delay the definitive repair until such contamination or infection has been eliminated. Stainless steel wire sutures may be used to overcome the problem of nonabsorbable sutures in a contaminated wound;[35] however, stainless steel is not a recommended suture material for peripheral nerve repair. Because it is not the purpose of this text to describe the techniques for definitive nerve and tendon repair, the reader is referred to texts and periodicals that deal with these subjects.

After excision or débridement or after reexposure and repair of deeper structures, it is necessary to close dead space in a wound before final closure of the skin is undertaken. Methods for eliminating dead space include buried sutures, bandages, and drains.[34] When lacerations are deep and involve the division of muscles, it is advisable to approximate the muscle tissue prior to skin closure to prevent pocketing and seroma formation.[62] When placing sutures to close dead space, the surgeon should be careful

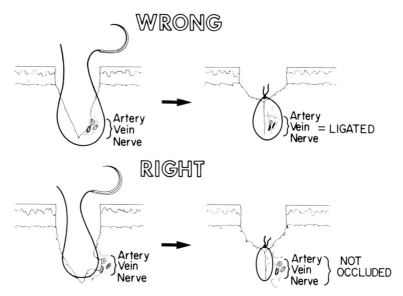

Figure 6–13: Sutures closing dead space should not ligate arteries, veins, or nerves.

not to include major vessels or nerves in the suture because they would essentially be ligated as the suture is tied. Such ligation could lead to impaired innervation or circulation or both to surrounding tissues, which could further impede healing (Fig. 6–13). Another factor that should be kept in mind is that closure of dead space by sutures has been found to increase the incidence of infection. The number of buried sutures should be kept to a minimum in accidental wounds, and only fine material, such as 3–0 chromic surgical gut, should be used.[35] The author prefers polyglycolic acid (P.G.A.) sutures in such instances. Sutures should be placed to close dead space without creating pockets in which infection could begin. If there is any doubt, a drain should be placed in the wound at the time of closure.

SUTURES

History

Knecht and colleagues included a brief review of the history of suture materials in a recent veterinary text.[36] In this review it was stated that according to Celsus in the first century A.D., sutures were well known and had been in use for many years. In the second century A.D., Galen recommended the use of silk for sutures. After having been in a state of disuse during the Middle Ages, the use of sutures was revived by Paré in the 1500s. In the 1800s kid and buckskin were used as absorbable sutures, and suture sterilization became a part of the aseptic technique. Further advances brought stainless steel sutures in 1934 and synthetic suture materials in the 1940s.[36]

A recent review of the history of sutures by Snyder stated that suture materials have been taken from every source imaginable, including ores, plants, fowl, animals, plastics, and humans. Some of the more interesting materials include ant pincers, animal sinews (tendons from the falcon, kangaroo, deer, whale, buffalo, moose, caribou, steer, and jack rabbit), human and animal fascia, silkworm gut, and horsehair. Horsehair was widely used by plastic surgeons in the United States until about 1940 and is still used in Russia to close cleft lips. Metallic sutures have included gold wires, silver wires, metal hooks, and, more recently, steel and tantalum wires.[67] Numerous suture materials, either natural or synthetic and absorbable or nonabsorbable, are currently available to the surgeon. Some of the more commonly used materials will be discussed in this chapter.

The Ideal Material

As yet, the perfect suture material has not been found. Each of the presently available suture materials has advantages and disadvantages. The ideal suture material should have the following properties: (1) It should be suitable for use in any operation, with the only variable being the size as determined by the tensile strength. (2) The surgeon should be able to handle it naturally and comfortably. (3) There should be minimal reaction to the suture material, and it should not create a situation favorable to bacterial growth. (4) It should have high tensile strength in a small caliber. (5) A knot in the material should hold securely without fraying or cutting. (6) The material should be easy to thread and sterilize, and it should not shrink in the tissue. (7) It should be nonelectrolytic, noncapillary, nonallergenic, and noncarcinogenic. (8) The material should be absorbed with minimal tissue reaction after it has served its purpose.[3, 61] Other desirable qualities of suture materials include a monofilament composition and low cost.[36] Until the perfect suture material is developed, the surgeon should be familiar with advantages and disadvantages of the available suture materials.

The surgeon must bear in mind that if biological processes reduce the sutures' tensile strength, this loss of strength must be proportional to the gain in wound strength. It should also be realized that sutures may alter the healing process. These factors, the presence or absence of infection or drainage, and personal preferences based on handling and clinical results will govern the choice of suture materials.[36]

Choosing Sutures

The Proper Type.   In general, surgeons are not well informed about suture materials,[61] and the choice of suture material in most cases is based on what and how the surgeon was taught and personal preference rather than scientific fact. Until the ideal suture material is available, sutures should be selected with regard to their chemical and physical characteristics and the known biological reaction to each suture material. Analysis of a wound and the various materials that are available to close it will usually lead the surgeon to the suture material best suited to the particular situation.[37, 58] The surgeon should not hesitate to use several different types of suture materials in one operation. The tissue, the pathology, the patient, and the wound should be the determinants in the wise choice of suture material.[65] The surgeon's technique, however, is of more importance than the choice of suture material in closing a wound.[3, 14, 22, 61] In essence, a good surgeon can usually achieve satisfactory results with any type of suture material.[58]

The Proper Size. The surgeon must also select the proper diameter of suture material. In doing so, it should be remembered that the holding power of the tissue in which sutures are placed rather than the strength of the suture material itself determines the strength of the union.[31] Of the soft tissues, skin and fascia have the greatest suture-holding power and fat has the least. In fact, it has been stated that sutures pull out of fat at 0.125 lb. of tension, out of muscle at 0.25 lb. of tension, out of fascia at 8 lb. of tension, and out of skin at 10 lb. of tension.[3] Taylor has stated that it takes 0.44 lb. of tension to pull sutures out of fat, 2.8 lb. of tension to pull sutures through muscle, and 8.3 lb. of tension to pull sutures through fascia.[73] Although the figures differ, the principle is the same—fat is weaker than fascia.

In the interest of cosmesis and the atraumatic technique, it is advisable to use a noncapillary suture material of as small a diameter as possible.[2] It has been stated that the tensile strength of a suture need not be appreciably greater than that of the tissues it is intended to support.[13, 26, 36, 62] Oversize suture material does not add to the strength of the repaired wound, and, in fact, it may weaken it by causing excessive tissue reaction. Conversely, sutures of a smaller diameter are less traumatic to tissues; the knots are smaller, and the surgeon is compelled to handle the suture material more gently. Consequently, he is less likely to strangulate tissue.[36] If a suture breaks while being tied, it is probably because it is being pulled too tightly. It *is not* the function of a suture to drag the skin into place when it will not advance easily over a wound. It *is* the function of the suture to hold the wound edges lightly together.[13, 66] Using a material of small diameter for skin sutures will prevent the surgeon from dragging skin edges together and thereby producing tension; this is because material of small diameter is generally weaker and tends to break under extreme tension, whereas material of larger diameter does not have this tendency. Increasing the number of sutures and using sutures of small diameter could alleviate tension in a wound, since it has been found that the tension or strain that must be overcome to hold the wound edges together is divided into smaller portions as the number of sutures is increased. The stress on each one of the sutures decreases with the addition of each new one.[22, 31, 69] It is better to increase the number of sutures than to increase the size of the suture material (Fig. 6–14).[6]

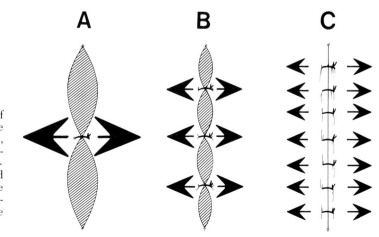

Figure 6–14: As the number of sutures in a wound increases, the tension per suture decreases. A, There is a great degree of tension on one suture. B, The tension on the suture is reduced with the addition of two more sutures and even further reduced with the addition of more sutures, C.

TABLE 6–1   RECOMMENDED SIZES FOR LIGATIONS AND SUTURES[32, 62]

Use	Size
Ligatures	
Larger vessels and pedicles	1–0 to 2–0
Smaller vessels	3–0 to 4–0
Sutures	
Blood vessels	3–0 to 6–0
Nerve sheaths	5–0 to 6–0
Fasciae and dense connective tissue	1–0 to 3–0
Subcutaneous fasciae	3–0 to 4–0
Thick skin (dorsal cervical area)	2–0 to 3–0
Thin skin (ventral abdomen and medial thigh)	3–0 to 5–0
Skin grafts	3–0 to 4–0
Facial and eyelid skin	5–0 to 6–0

Also of interest is the fact that the mere passage of a needle and a suture through the skin produces trauma. On microscopic examination it has been found that even minimal trauma, such as that caused by the prick of a needle, produced a distinct local reaction and a typical aseptic inflammation with slight exudation that lasted for about five days after infliction. This was followed by proliferation and cicatrization that was complete after ten to 15 days. The scar could still be seen after 20 days. The compression trauma caused by tying a knot in the suture material produced a considerably increased zone of tissue reaction, and the exudation was somewhat prolonged. Fibroplasia was predominant on the tenth postoperative day, and the scar occupied a distinctly wider area (about twice as wide) than the scar that was produced by the needle prick.[46] It can be seen that additional trauma caused by a traumatic needle, traumatic tissue handling, a suture material of large diameter, and knot tying under tension add to these pathological changes. This lends support to the use of an atraumatic technique and atraumatic materials, including suture material of relatively small diameter in closing wounds.

Guidelines have been stated for the size of ligature and suture to use for various purposes and in various areas.[36, 62] Those that are applicable in reconstructing traumatized skin and underlying soft tissues are shown in Table 6–1.

Commonly Used Suture Materials

Numerous suture materials are available to the surgeon today in the form of both natural and synthetic products that are either absorbable or nonabsorbable. The properties of some of the more common suture materials that are used in skin closure will be dealt with in the following section.

Absorbable Sutures

Natural

Catgut.   The word catgut, which is a misnomer, comes from "kit-gut" (meaning fiddle string), the kit being a small fiddle or violin.[18] The absorbable suture is, in most cases, obtained from the submucosa of the small intestine of sheep;[18, 26, 36] surgical gut is also obtained from the serosal layer of the small intestine of cattle.[26] The gut can be treated with chromium salts which will slow the absorption process of the gut in situ.[18, 26, 36] This process also reduces the soft tissue reaction to catgut. Surgical gut is classified in the following manner according to the extent that it has been chromicized: Type A, plain or untreated; Type B, mild treatment; Type C, medium treatment (usually referred to as chromic gut); and, Type D, prolonged treatment.[36]

The absorption rate of surgical gut is quite variable and depends upon many factors; however, certain basic conclusions have been drawn. Medium chromic gut will usually remain intact in muscle tissue for ten to 20 days. In some unusual circumstances, it may be absorbed in six to ten days.[3] It should be remembered that allergic reactions to catgut as well as the normal tissue reaction to it may affect its rate of absorption;[33] chromic gut may be rapidly absorbed in patients that are sensitive to it or to chromic acid.[3] Sutures placed in certain tissues will be absorbed more rapidly than those placed in other tissues. For example, sutures in serous and mucous membranes will be absorbed considerably faster than those in muscle.[26] In general, catgut placed in an area of abundant blood supply will be absorbed more rapidly, whereas sutures placed in avascular tissues will remain intact for as long as three months or more.[3]

A study in 1942 reported variations in the absorption rate within individual lots of the same type of catgut. It was also found that catgut that was supposed to be slowly or intermediately absorbed was rapidly absorbed instead. Knots were the last part to be absorbed in this type of catgut.[33] A separate study also found that knotted catgut was absorbed more slowly than unknotted catgut. This was believed to be because the fibers of the catgut are brought into more intimate contact when knotted, and therefore cellular invasion is more difficult.[46] In slowly absorbed catgut, the knots were found to be absorbed at about the same rate as the rest of the suture.[33] To add another variable to the matter of surgical gut absorption, some investigators have stated that gut of smaller diameter is absorbed more rapidly than that of larger diameter,[26] while others have found that catgut of large diameter is absorbed as fast as, or faster than, catgut of small diameter.[46] In addition to those factors already stated, variations in pH, tissue enzymes, physical stress, and properties that are not so well understood are undoubtedly responsible for what appears now to be an unpredictable absorption time.[58]

The tensile strength and knot-holding abilities of catgut are subject to change. The dry tensile strength of chromic catgut exceeds that of cotton or silk sutures of the same size; however, it loses strength more rapidly than either of these when implanted in tissue.[3] When wet, chromic catgut loses 19 per cent of its strength, and plain catgut loses 39 per cent of its strength.[30] Even though catgut loses its tensile strength early, it may take a while for it to be absorbed. The tensile strength may be lost by 25 to 28 days, but the material is not absorbed for 90 days or longer.[22] Studies have shown a tendency for catgut that loses its tensile strength early to be absorbed earlier than catgut that maintains tensile strength for a longer time.[33] It has been found that placing chromic catgut in a protein-depleted animal can hasten the loss of tensile strength, even to the point that it is totally unreliable.[37]

As with tensile strength, the knot-holding ability of gut decreases when it becomes wet.[3, 27, 28, 30, 33, 36] The coefficient of friction has been found to be a reliable expression of a suture's knot-holding ability. Stainless steel has the best coefficient of friction (0.288), followed by catgut (0.260) in the dry state;[3, 61] however, catgut decreases in knot-holding ability when it is wet. Consequently, it is advisable to place three throws when tying a knot with gut, and the ends should be cut long to assure knot stability.[36]

Gut has some elasticity, which makes it unlikely to strangulate tissues. It has also been stated to have good handling qualities.[3, 36]

When buried in tissue, surgical gut stimulates an inflammatory reaction that results in its absorption. The beneficial effects of this material come from the fibroblastic reaction that it causes rather than from the transitory phagocytic effect that it creates.[3] The fibroblastic reaction is appreciable during the period of absorption, and it is doubtful that wound healing is adversely affected by the phagocytic action.[3, 61] When the sutures are removed, the phagocytic cells leave the area; however, if the sutures remain, these cells remain and contribute to the fibrosis.[3]

It has been adequately documented that the tissue reaction to plain (unchromicized) catgut is greater than the reaction to chromic catgut.[26, 27, 33, 45, 46, 58] In fact, a study that was done on rabbits in which various suture materials and other foreign bodies were buried subcutaneously showed that the inflammatory reaction around plain gut was similar to that around pieces of sterile wood.[46] The progression of this reaction is from an early, intense, inflammatory reaction to fibroplasia and scar formation in eight to ten days.[73] However, it has been said that the tissue reaction to catgut sutures is much less intense than what has been previously stated in the literature.[17] One author has likened the reaction to surgical gut to that seen with heterografts.[58] Factors other than the reaction to the gut itself may add to tissue reaction. Irritating chemicals used in the chromicizing process or unfixed or unstable chromic compounds that have not been removed from the catgut could possibly add to tissue irritation. In addition, the alcoholic tubing fluid may contain a liquid that is not water-soluble, which may be a source of irritation.[33]

Surgical gut may be buried even in the presence of infection.[3] Since the braided and twisted nonabsorbable sutures have interstices that provide refuge for devitalized tissue, blood, and bacteria, they are not good sutures to use in infected wounds. Absorbable sutures are preferred in wounds in which surgical débridement cannot be carried out without endangering important structures.[58] Even though surgical gut can be used in infected wounds, it should be remembered that gut is capillary, which makes it capable of absorbing and spreading tissue fluids and exudate. The serous exudate that it causes may provide a growth medium for bacteria.[3, 36]

In spite of the variations in absorption, tensile strength, and knot-holding ability, surgical gut has two characteristics of the ideal suture.[3] It is relatively well tolerated by the tissues, and it is eventually absorbed.[3] When used in repairing wounds of the skin and underlying structures, catgut is advantageous in that it can approximate the subcutaneous tissue and superficial fascia; since it is buried beneath the skin, it does not require removal.[18]

The disadvantages of catgut are its expense and the fact that it can not be resterilized.[3] Plain catgut elicits an intense inflammatory reaction and remains structurally stable for a relatively short period; therefore, it is considered unacceptable for subcuticular suturing.[58]

Extruded Collagen. This relatively new absorbable suture material is made from the reconstituted collagen of the flexor tendons of cattle.[26, 36, 58] Although there is no great biological difference between this material and the collagen obtained from sheep intestines,[58] it is more uniform, pliable, and stronger.[26] Since these sutures contain less mucopolysaccharides and glycoproteins than gut sutures, they produce slightly less of a reaction than plain gut sutures of comparable size.[58] However, they do not retain strength for a long period in vivo and, in some instances, are prematurely absorbed.[36] The dry, straight breaking strength of an extruded collagen suture exceeds that of a surgical gut suture of the same size; however, the wet knot strength exceeds that of gut only slightly. The material handles well and is smooth, strong, and pliable; its resilience permits easy knot tying. The first half hitch sinks together easily and tightly so that the entwined pieces of suture hold well. Because of this, it is not necessary to use tension to keep the half hitch from slipping while the remainder of the knot is tied. Fraying and breaking occur much less often with this type of suture than with catgut sutures of comparable size.[53]

Synthetic

Polyglycolic Acid. Polyglycolic acid (P.G.A.) is a noncollagenous, nonantigenic, nonpyrogenic synthetic absorbable suture.[1] Sutures of this material have tensile strength similar to that of polyester sutures (Dacron).[1, 28] Thus, the initial breaking strength is high; however, strength is rapidly lost after one week following implantation. Initially, 2–0 P.G.A. must be 25 per cent stronger than 2–0 chromic catgut to equal the gut in strength after six days in vivo.[36] A study has shown that the loss of strength with P.G.A. was more rapid than with catgut.[60] It loses one third of its strength in one week and 80 per cent of its strength in two weeks, whereas catgut loses 80 per cent of its strength in two months.[3, 60, 61]

Polyglycolic acid does not have the tendency to swell when it is wet that plain and chromic catgut have.[30, 73] In vivo testing has shown a 66 per cent incidence of knot slippage with plain catgut, a 50 per cent incidence of slippage with chromic catgut, and only an 11 per cent incidence of slippage with P.G.A.[73] Howes has stated that the wet knot strength of P.G.A. should be about 1.4 times as great as that of chromic catgut and two times as great as that of plain catgut.[30] However, this material does have a low coefficient of friction, and it is necessary to use a surgeon's knot or multiple throws to prevent slippage of the knots.[3, 36]

The multifilament, braided structure of P.G.A. gives it handling qualities similar to those of silk.[4, 7, 36, 58] or linen.[29] The tissue drag associated with the material helps to prevent its slippage in wound edges.[29] This drag seems to be caused by an angular rather than a straight passage through tissues,[7] a factor that could be important in placing intradermal sutures. The light-colored P.G.A. becomes difficult to see when it is coated with blood;[7] this problem is eliminated when green P.G.A. sutures are used. Polyglycolic acid causes a minimal bland tissue reaction.[1, 3, 11, 58, 60, 61]

There are varying opinions as to how P.G.A. is absorbed. One theory is that absorption is due to an enzymatic mechanism rather than to the inflammatory response elicited by catgut.[28] Another theory is that P.G.A. is absorbed by a process of hydrolysis in which tissue esterases release the glycolic acid.[15, 36, 44] The end products of this hydrolysis are natural body metabolites,[58] which are completely and uniformly absorbed over 40 to 60 days.[36]

Polyglycolic acid is well tolerated in clean as well as grossly infected wounds.[11] In vitro studies have indicated that the degradation products of P.G.A. sutures are potent antibacterial agents. Likewise, in vivo studies have shown infection rates in tissues containing P.G.A. sutures to be significantly lower than those in tissues containing gut sutures.[15] Microscopic examination of P.G.A. in the oral cavity revealed an absence of bacteria within the interstices of the P.G.A. sutures, thus suggesting that the suture inhibits bacterial penetration.[43] Findings such as these would certainly indicate that P.G.A. sutures could be recommended for closing a contaminated or infected wound.

The use of P.G.A. sutures in oral tissues is promising.[43, 77] They cause less tissue reaction than other multifilament, nonabsorbable materials or catgut.[43, 77] In addition, the knots remain small, and the suture does not tend to swell, fragment, or collect necrotic debris and exudate ("wicking action") as silk does. These sutures are absorbed between 16 and 20 days after placement.[77]

Some investigators have advocated the use of P.G.A. for intradermal sutures,[29] while others have reported a tendency toward widened, raised, hypertrophic scars when it is used for this purpose.[64] When used as a skin suture, P.G.A. was found to cause less reaction than nylon but more reaction than silk.[4] When left in place as skin sutures in dogs, P.G.A. sutures produced only a slight reddening around the sutures and were shed between 20 and 60 days.[7]

Polyglactin 910. This absorbable suture material is produced by a co-polymerization of highly purified lactide and glycolide. It is braided to facilitate handling and is available in violet to enhance its visibility in the surgical field.[48]

Compared with P.G.A. and nonabsorbable polyester sutures, polyglactin 910 has been shown to exhibit the highest tensile and knot strengths.[48] Animal studies have shown that when its surgical function is complete and all tensile strength is lost, this material absorbs more rapidly than any other synthetic absorbable suture, and thus a prolonged foreign-body reaction is minimized.[12, 48]

Polyglactin 910 handles and ties easily.[12] However, because it is braided, its passage through tissue is rough and it tends to cut soft organs. Knot tying requires some accuracy; the first knot must be placed in the precise position in order to complete the knot.[48]

This suture material's nonreactivity is similar to that of nylon,[12] and its absorption is by controlled hydrolysis of its two polymers. Relatively few leukocytes localize around the suture during its absorption.[48]

Polyglactin 910 has been used for subcutaneous and intradermal sutures, with a resultant comfortable thin-line scar of superior strength.[12, 48] Because of this, the surgeon may choose to use this material in the closure of skin wounds.

Nonabsorbable Sutures

Natural

Silk. Silk is one of the oldest and most widely used suture materials. It is generally classified as a nonabsorbable natural suture material; however, it may be absorbed over a period of time.[59] It is prepared from threads spun by silkworm larvae and is either braided or twisted to form the suture.[36]

Other suture materials have a greater tensile strength than silk, and it is generally accepted that silk loses its tensile strength when placed in vivo.[51, 52, 58, 59, 73] When wet, silk becomes 10 to 15 per cent weaker,[58] and one researcher has shown that by one month after placement, silk has lost 59 per cent of the tensile strength that it had at one week. The loss of strength continues until none remains at 24 months.[51, 52] Accompanying this loss of tensile strength is the slower absorption of silk, which occurs at a variable rate.[59] At times silk may be absorbed within a year, but it more often persists for many years.[60]

One of the most favorable characteristics of silk is its good knot-holding ability,[18, 26, 36, 50] which is attributed to its relatively rough surface.[50] Another property of silk that makes it desirable is the ease with which it handles.[36, 50, 58, 61] It has been said to have the best "feel" of any available suture material.[58]

As with all suture materials, silk has its disadvantages, and one of these is the tissue reaction that it incites.[3, 36, 58, 61, 73] The reaction to silk is not severe, but it is greater than that caused by plastics or stainless steel. Buried silk sutures generally become encapsulated and cause no problem; however, they can cause cysts that rupture or produce fistulas that do not heal until the offending piece of silk is removed. Such reactions may be caused by the irritating substances used in preparing the suture.[3]

Silk is capillary, with many interstices between the fibers that permit serum and blood to penetrate the suture and form a refuge for bacteria.[3, 36, 58] In addition, silk has been found to potentiate infection; this has been related to the tissue reaction incited by silk. Thus, silk should be avoided in wounds having known gross bacterial contamination.[15, 36] In fact, the introduction of staphylococci on a silk suture can enhance the development of infection by as much as 10,000-fold.[15]

Silk has been advocated for various purposes in wound closure. It may be buried in noninfected wounds.[3, 18] Size 3–0 silk is frequently used for skin closure.[18] In lieu of silk, some have recommended a dermal suture made from fibers that are finished by a special process.[36] Owing to its good knot-holding ability and lack of stiff suture ends, it has been recommended for use in mucous membranes of the genital area[18] and on the tongue.[26] However, it should be remembered that silk sutures in the oral cavity may swell and fragment as well as collect necrotic debris and exudate.[77] Silk has also been recommended for suturing wounds adjacent to the eyes, since its pliability allows the suture ends to lie flat after the knots are tied. For tie-over dressings it is the easiest suture material to handle.[26]

Cotton. Cotton is in the same classification and has many of the same properties as silk. The tensile strength of cotton is similar to that of silk except that it does not decrease when wet.[28, 73] One investigator found that cotton kept its tensile strength for up to one month in vivo, but it decreased to 59 per cent of its original strength by two years.[51, 52] Although it may show a decrease in strength over a two-year period, it is not absorbed.[59] Others have stated that it actually gains tensile strength when wet.[36] The knot security of cotton is better than that of silk[28, 73] and actually increases when it is wet.[28] Other advantages of cotton include its low cost,[3, 18] pliability, smoothness, stability during sterilization, and, unlike silk, decreased tendency to untwist.[3]

One disadvantage of cotton is its inferior handling quality;[3, 28, 73] this is related to its electrostatic properties, which cause it to cling to gloves and surgical linen.[3, 36] Cotton also incites a tissue reaction.[3, 36, 61] In addition, cotton is capillary, like silk, and subject to the same problems. It is not recommended for skin closure[3] and, like silk, has been found to potentiate infection. Thus, it should not be used in wounds having known gross bacterial contamination.[15] As with silk, contaminated cotton may cause pustules and fistulae that must be removed before healing will occur.[3]

Stainless steel. Stainless steel is a metallic suture material that is available in monofilament and multifilament forms. It has been said to have the greatest tensile strength and knot security of all the suture materials,[73] and these strengths do not decrease when the suture is placed in vivo.[3, 28] Steel, however, has a poor handling quality.[3, 18, 36, 61, 73] This is especially true for monofilament wire, which kinks easily, lacks elasticity, and produces bulky knots.[36]

Metallic sutures have been advocated for use intradermally[18] but may be too stiff to conform to the topography of the suture pathway; this results in considerable mechanical irritation to the tissue as the patient moves.[15] The inflexibility of wire may lead to the breaking of buried continuous wire sutures. The multifilament wire is more resistant to fragmentation than the monofilament, but it is not recommended for continuous buried sutures or for use in infected wounds. If a continuous wire suture is buried, it should be placed in a loose spiral pattern and brought out through the skin to facilitate removal. To circumvent the problems of a buried continuous wire suture interrupted sutures may be used. This is not without disadvantage either in that the cut ends of buried steel can cause irritation by pricking the skin or by forming a prominence that is subject to irritation.[3, 36] In addition, the migration of buried metal sutures through tissues may occur.[3] Interrupted steel sutures should not be used close to large vessels because of the potential hazard of their sharp ends cutting the vessel.

An advantage of steel sutures is that they incite virtually no inflammatory reaction.[3, 36, 61] These sutures can remain in the body indefinitely and not be absorbed; however, this factor can cause difficulty if the wound must be entered again.[3]

Owing to its noncapillary structure, steel can be effectively used in contaminated and infected wounds, since it does not support infection.[3, 36] This can be a distinct advantage when dealing with many of the open wounds encountered in veterinary surgery. Steel is also good for suturing tissues that heal slowly and are subject to physical stress.[3]

Steel has a tendency to cut not only tissues[3, 36, 61] but also surgeon's gloves.[3] This may lead the surgeon to include so much tissue in the suture that strangulation may occur. Cutting of the tissues seems to be more prevalent with the finer gauge wires. Despite its tendency to cut through tissue, the steel suture has been described for use in tension sutures.[3]

Synthetic

Several synthetic nonabsorbable suture materials have been developed over the years. These materials include polyesters (Dacron), polyolefins (polyethylene, polypropylene),[15, 73] and polyamides (nylon,[15, 73] polymerized caprolactam[24]).

Polyesters (Dacron). The polyester fiber suture materials are available in a braided form and have a good tensile strength,[18, 36] second only to metallic sutures.[28, 73] Such sutures have the added advantage of prolonged strength when placed in vivo,[28] maintaining their original tensile strength for two years.[73]

The knot-holding ability and the handling quality of polyesters are closely related. Dacron polyester has a high coefficient of friction; this excessive friction between the surfaces of the suture causes problems in tying. The multifilament Dacron grabs, sticks, and does not slip into place easily.[15, 73] In this untreated state, polyester sutures have good knot security,[28] second only to that of stainless steel sutures.[73] To increase the ease with which polyester sutures slip into a knot, they can be coated with textile finishes.[15] However, coating polyester with Teflon and silicone reduces knot security markedly.[28, 36, 47, 61] Teflon-coated Dacron sutures will still slip after placing six well-tied knots.[73]

There is relatively little tissue reaction to polyesters.[28] Although they may cause less tissue reaction than nylon,[18] cotton, or silk,[36] they cause more reaction than other synthetic sutures.[36] The coated polyester seems to cause slightly more reaction than does the uncoated because of the dislodgement of fragments of Teflon from the suture.[51, 59] However, the difference in tissue reactions between the two types of polyester has been stated to be minimal.[15, 59]

Studies showed that the incidence of infection when uncoated polyester (Dacron) sutures were used in contaminated wounds was not significantly different from the incidence of inflammatory response of tissues in which sutures coated with either Teflon, silicone, or wax were used.[15]

Polyolefins (Polyethylene, Polypropylene).   Although they possess an excellent tensile strength that remains even after numerous autoclavings,[39, 75] the monofilament polyethylene sutures have very poor knot retention.[75] This is generally attributed to the "memory" or "plastic memory" (tendency of certain plastics to assume their original shapes following twisting or torsion) of the suture material. Others report that monofilament polyethylene handles and ties with relative ease.[36] Braiding the polyethylene imparts sufficient roughness to it to provide good knot retention. In addition, the braided material handles well, with a somewhat rigid feel and the resilience of catgut. A nominal foreign-body reaction to polyethylene is another of its advantages.[75] Studies in which polyethylene sutures were placed in infected abdominal wounds of dogs demonstrated that such sutures were well tolerated in the presence of infection.[39, 75]

Polypropylene is a polyolefin that has been melted and extruded to form monofilament strands.[73] It has a high tensile strength[76] that is reportedly equal to that of nylon and greater than that of polyethylene, cotton, and silk.[73] This tensile strength is maintained in vivo for long periods.[52, 61] Like polyester, it maintains its original strength for two years.[52, 73]

Knot security is greater with polypropylene than with other monofilament synthetic materials;[52] in one study it was found to be equal to uncoated polyester, lightly coated polyester, and silk.[47] The first throw with polypropylene tends to slip unless tension is maintained on both ends of the suture. However, this throw may be tightened with the second throw.[52]

Related to the handling qualities of polypropylene is its flexibility;[76] it will stretch three times the length of other synthetics.[47] Even though polypropylene does not have the tensile strength of polyesters, its ability to absorb more energy than these fibers is important in that polypropylene can give with tissue as swelling occurs postoperatively. This reduces the likelihood of sutures cutting through the tissues when the wound is under stress.[27]

Experiments have shown that polypropylene provokes a moderate to minimal foreign-body reaction that is only slightly greater than that of polyethylene.[52, 59, 76] The response consists of an early, acute, inflammatory reaction that is limited to neutrophils. This response is similar to that elicited by other nonabsorbable suture materials but considerably less in degree and more transient. A connective tissue capsule forms around the sutures and is believed to add some support to the wound.[51, 52] After two years in vivo, polypropylene becomes slightly stiff and may fragment between 18 and 24 months.[59, 61]

Polypropylene sutures can be buried in infected wounds[16, 51, 52, 76] and elicit less infection in contaminated tissue than do metallic sutures. This is also true of monofilament nylon.[15]

Polypropylene may be used for continuous subcuticular (intradermal) sutures. Because of its smoothness, the suture passes through the tissues easily and can be placed rapidly. Size 2–0 has been recommended for this type of suture pattern, since it is strong enough to withstand the pull necessary for removal. Such sutures may remain in place for ten to 14 days or longer.[52]

Polyamides (Nylon, Polymerized Caprolactam). Nylon sutures are made from a polyamide that is heated and forced through a spinneret to form fine monofilament strands.[73] The tensile strength of this material is high,[18, 36, 61] and it is maintained in vivo.[61] One of the disadvantages of nylon is its poor knotting ability. Owing to its hardness, knots tend to slip and untie;[18, 36, 50, 61] however, this problem can be overcome by using multiple knots.[18] This poor knotting ability may be advantageous in regard to suture tension in that knots would tend to slip to the proper tension when they have been tied too tightly.[18]

Monofilament nylon tends to be pliable[50] but may kink or fray.[18, 36] Generally, its handling qualities have been classified as relatively poor.[36, 73]

Nylon sutures are relatively inert. When compared with Dacron polyester and polypropylene, they cause the least tissue reaction.[51] What reaction occurs is in the form of a thin capsule of connective tissue that develops around the suture.[52]

Monofilament nylon can be used in infected wounds and has been advocated for use in the mouth.[18] As with polypropylene, nylon has been found to elicit less infection in contaminated tissue than do metallic sutures.[15] Although it is a nonabsorbable suture material, the results from in vitro studies have suggested that the degradation products of nylon sutures are potent antibacterial agents;[15] this property is also attributed to the absorbable P.G.A. sutures.

In comparing continuous sutures of 3–0 silk with those of 3–0 nylon, it was found that wounds closed with nylon were stronger than those sutured with silk when the sutures were left in place throughout the healing process.[37]

A polymerized caprolactam suture has become popular in veterinary surgery and is widely used as a skin suture, it can also be buried in tissues after heat sterilization.[36] This suture is a multifilament polyamide suture material of the nylon family.[28] The filaments are neither braided nor twisted but are in a bundle enclosed in a smooth, seamless cover.[24, 32] The material has a superior tensile strength.[24, 28, 32, 36] When compared with catgut and black braided silk of the same diameter, it was the strongest.[24] However, its wet strength is 15 to 20 per cent less than its dry strength.[32] In vivo studies of this material have demonstrated only a slight reduction in strength after it has been in situ.[24] Repeated boiling in water, sterilization by autoclaving, and storage in water or alcohol have no perceptible effect on the physical properties of caprolactam.[24, 32] Its knot security is reportedly good, but it requires three knots for a secure tie,[24] undoubtedly because of its smoothness. It is also pliable.[24, 32] When compared with silk and catgut sutures, polymerized caprolactam sutures caused the least cellular reaction.[24]

Summary of the Properties of Suture Materials

Catgut.   The main advantage of this suture material is its ultimate absorption by the tissues. It does not have the favorable handling qualities of other suture materials, and it does elicit a definite inflammatory reaction. Because of most surgeons' experience and familiarity with this material it will undoubtedly remain popular despite the advent of new synthetic absorbable suture materials.[27, 37]

Absorbable Synthetics.   The P.G.A. suture and the lactide-glycolide copolymer suture materials appear to be significant breakthroughs in suture technology. They are strong, inert, flexible sutures that provide excellent knot security. Their rate of tensile strength loss in tissues is similar to that of chromic catgut. They appear to be suitable for ligatures and for joining soft tissues in which a prolonged tensile strength is not essential. The handling quality of these sutures is fair, especially with regard to the ease of tying knots.[27, 37]

Silk and Cotton.   Although they are inferior to modern synthetics in many ways, silk and cotton often have better handling qualities and allow accurate knot placement without the constriction of tissues.[27, 37] However, these sutures have a propensity to increase tissue infection when placed in contaminated wounds. The intensity of infection has been shown to be greater with these suture materials than with other multifilament materials (stainless steel, polyester, and nylon). This would indicate that the chemical nature of the suture is a more significant factor in this respect than the physical form.[15]

Metallic Sutures.   The main advantages of stainless steel sutures are strength, knot security, and nonreactivity in tissues. The disadvantages include extreme stiffness, poor handling characteristics, and fragmentation under cyclic stress. These sutures are mainly used in areas that require strength, security, lack of elasticity, and minimal tissue reaction.[27, 37]

Polyesters.   The primary advantages of these suture materials are strength, nonreactivity, and good handling characteristics. However, when they are coated with Teflon or silicone for smoothness, knot security decreases. Prolonged retention of strength has made this the suture material of choice in most cardiac surgery.[27, 37]

Synthetic Monofilament Sutures.   The advantages of these nonabsorbable sutures include strength, elasticity, noncapillarity, monofilament structure, and smoothness.[3] They are also resistant to infection.[27] Polypropylene is the best of the synthetic monofilaments with regard to strength, knot security, lack of deterioration in tissue, and low tissue reactivity.[27, 37] In addition, polypropylene has the ability to give with tissue, and it does not elicit any appreciable sinus tract formation.[27] Knot security may be a problem with synthetic monofilament sutures, since they have a "memory." This is the property of these fibers to straighten out or unkink after loops have been formed by tying knots.[58] As a result, knots tend to slip.[3] It has been stated that many surgeons put in one knot for every day they would like the suture to remain in place.[58] This could make a rather cumbersome knot if the sutures are to remain in place for any length of time. Another disadvantage of nylon is the sensitivity that some individudals have to it, which results in a tissue reaction.[3]

Some general rules should be kept in mind when using synthetic nonabsorbable sutures. Before they are buried in tissues, they should be autoclaved, and an aseptic surgical technique should be used. When they are buried, a continuous suture pattern should not be used unless the suture is of a monofilament type. Many of the synthetic nonabsorbable sutures have a low coefficient of friction and thus poor knot-holding ability. Therefore, four single throws or a surgeon's knot followed by a square knot is recommended to prevent knot slippage.[36]

OTHER MATERIALS USED FOR WOUND CLOSURE

Metal Clips

Michel wound clips are short bands of malleable metal with a point at each end. They are applied to the wound with a special forceps that bends each band, causing the points to pierce the skin on either side of the incision. Thus, the clips hold the wound edges together.[3] The clips are easy to sterilize and apply, and they can be used in infected wounds.[36] They are applied quickly, do not enter the wound, and cause no discernible scar.[3] While one end of the forceps is designed to apply the clips, the other end is designed to remove them (Fig. 6–15).

The disadvantages of the clips are that they tend to pucker the edges of the incision, they lack the strength to support the apposed tissues, and animals can remove them with ease.[3] If a bandage is placed over them clips may catch on the gauze of the bandage and cause pain.[18] In addition to these disadvantages, they tend to increase scarring if they are not removed early enough.[36] Recently, other types of metal wound clips and applicators have been designed and used for skin closure. (The Proximate* wound staple applicator has been used at the Auburn University Small Animal Clinic.)

Surgical Adhesive Tape

Surgical adhesive strips have several advantages; however, their use is limited in veterinary surgery. Positive features of wound closure by tape include no tissue irritation or maceration by the tapes, good adherence to the

---

*The Proximate disposable skin stapler is manufactured by Ethicon, Inc., Somerville, N.J. 08876.

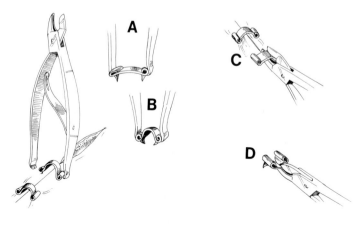

Figure 6–15: A and B, Application of Michel wound clips for wound closure. C and D, Wound clip removal. (After Archibald, J., and Blakely, C. L.: Sutures, in Archibald, J. [ed.]: Canine Surgery, ed. 2. Santa Barbara, Calif, American Veterinary Publications, Inc., 1974, p. 38.)

skin even in the presence of fluid, a lack of creeping and shifting in position, nonreactivity to x-rays, and painless removal. Strips may be sterilized by all standard measures and are easily handled with surgical gloves.[25, 66] From the standpoint of wound healing, taping eliminates many of the problems that accompany suture closure, including tissue strangulation and necrosis, subcutaneous inoculation by surface organisms when placing sutures,[25, 66] wound infection, needle tracks, and suture canal scarring.[8] Wounds closed by tape have been found to be stronger than those closed by sutures according to testing performed between ten and 150 days. Wounds closed by tape achieved 90 per cent of the strength of unwounded skin at 150 days, whereas wounds closed by sutures reached only 75 per cent of the strength of unwounded skin at this time.[37]

Tapes are not used in veterinary surgery for two main reasons: animals can easily remove them before adequate wound healing has occurred,[66] and tape closure is contraindicated on haired areas of the body.[8] It has been found that tapes are forced off the skin by growing hair over a period of five to seven days.[26]

Wound Adhesives

Methyl 2-cyanocrylate is a tissue adhesive that has been investigated for closing skin. This material is a self-sterilizing liquid monomer that is converted to a solid state by polymerization.[26] It solidifies under a pressure of 10 lb./sq. in.[16] When it is pressed into a thin film between the surfaces to be joined, the polymerization, which occurs at room temperatures, is catalyzed by small amounts of water from the air or the surface of the wound;[9, 26] weak bases also catalyze the polymerization.[9] The adhesive will set in two to 60 seconds, depending upon the thickness of the film and the moisture present.[9] Others have found setting times to vary from 30 to 60 seconds,[16] and from one-half to three minutes.[26] Absolute hemostasis is important, since excessive blood or other fluid prevents adhesion.[26]

Buried sutures should be placed to close deeper tissues before applying the adhesive.[25] The adhesive is usually applied with a camel's-hair brush, and instruments are used to appose and press together the surfaces that are to be joined.[16] It should be remembered that application of the adhesive below the surface of the skin may create a barrier to healing.[26]

When adhesive is used to hold a skin graft in place, it should be applied to the surrounding skin margin that will be overlapped by the graft. If the adhesive is applied to either the graft bed or the raw surface of the graft, the graft will not take, since the adhesive will prevent nutrients and capillary buds from entering the graft to nourish it.[26]

Special care must be taken when handling the adhesive, since its adhesive power is so great and there is no solvent to reverse the polymerization. If care is not used, instruments or gloves may become permanently attached to the skin or to each other.[26] To help protect instruments, they may be siliconized prior to use.[16]

SUTURE NEEDLES

The surgeon must choose not only the proper suture material but also the proper suture needle. Needles may be either circumferential or linear; the circumferential suture needles are available in $1/4$, $3/8$, $1/2$, and $5/8$ circle and $1/2$

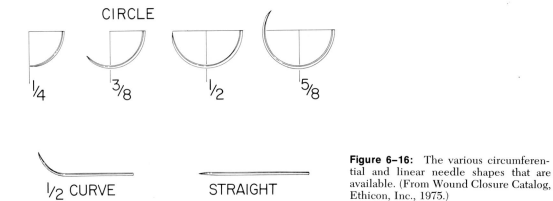

Figure 6-16: The various circumferential and linear needle shapes that are available. (From Wound Closure Catalog, Ethicon, Inc., 1975.)

curve (Fig. 6–16).[19, 20] In addition, different manufacturers have described various designs for needle points and shafts. The three manufacturers that most commonly supply the Auburn University Small Animal Clinic have needle designs as illustrated in Figure 6–17.

The attachment of the suture to the needle may be by passage of the suture through an eye in the needle or by fixation of the suture directly into the end of

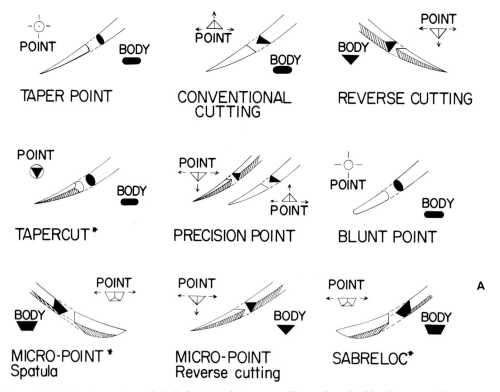

Figure 6-17: Various point and shaft designs of suture needles as described by three manufacturers. (A, From the Selection, Handling and Use of Needles and Needle Holders, Ethicon, Inc., 1975. Tapercut, Micro-Points, and Sabreloc are manufactured by Ethicon, Inc.

NEEDLE POINT DESIGNS- DAVIS & GECK

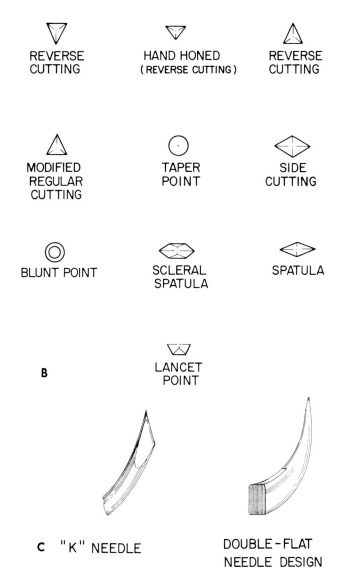

Figure 6–17 Continued: *B*, After Davis and Geck Needle Catalog, Davis and Geck, American Cyanamid Co., Pearl River, NY 10965. *C*, After Deknatel Sutures Hospital Specialties, Deknatel, Inc., 1973. K and Double-flat needles are manufactured by Deknatel, Inc.)

the needle (swaged needle). The latter type of suture-needle combination has several advantages. These needles need no threading, they do not become unthreaded during suturing, and they are sterilely prepackaged.[6] However, the principal advantage of this type of suture and needle is the lack of trauma associated with its passage through the tissues when compared with that caused by a threaded eyed needle pulling a double thickness or a knot of suture through the tissue (Fig. 6–18).[6, 18, 42, 49, 67] Such trauma may predispose to small abscesses and result in a painful surgical site.[49]

Eyed needles should be of a size and type consistent with the size of suture being used and the density of tissue being sutured. When suturing dense structures such as the skin, a cutting-edge needle should be used. The needle should be large enough to accommodate the suture material but the smallest that

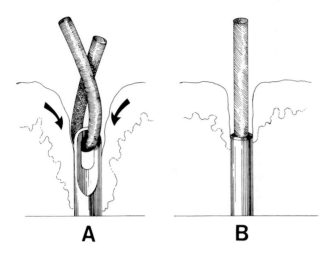

Figure 6–18: Tissue trauma caused by a threaded eyed needle, *A*, is greater than that caused by a swaged needle, *B*.

will penetrate the tissue.[3] In some patients, the tissues may be tougher or more fibrosed than normal and may require the use of a heavier gauge needle.[19]

Generally speaking, needles of $1/4$, $3/8$, or $1/2$ circle with either a cutting or a noncutting point should be used to close subcuticular tissues. The same type of needles but with a cutting point should be used to close the skin.[3] Swaged needles are preferable and, in the interest of the atraumatic technique, should be the smallest that will penetrate the tissue.

SURGEON'S POSTURE

The surgeon should be in a comfortable, relaxed position, with his elbows braced against his body or otherwise supported so that movement is primarily from the wrists and fingers.[26, 50] Bracing the hands against the patient has also been suggested;[26] however, the veterinary surgeon should consider the size of the patient and use discretion in this matter. The "heavy" hand of a surgeon or an assisting surgeon resting on the thorax or abdomen of a small dog or cat for any length of time could result in respiratory embarrassment for the patient. A seated position has also been advocated[6] and is preferred by the author when performing surgical techniques of some delicacy.

PLACEMENT OF SUTURES

The procedure of suturing wound edges together is one that is performed almost daily by veterinary surgeons and is therefore considered simple and is often taken for granted. However, there have been many statements, rules, and guidelines presented on the procedure. The following section will deal with some of the general principles of suturing wounds.

Handling Wound Edges

Manipulation of the skin edges while placing sutures was discussed in the section on surgical instruments. Let it suffice at this point to say that regardless of the technique used to manipulate the skin edges, it should be as atraumatic as possible. Allis' tissue forceps should not be used as skin retractors.[6] The use of dissecting thumb forceps is probably the most common way of handling skin, but skin hooks and fingers are even less traumatic. One technique for placing sutures without the use of forceps entails passing the needle through the first skin border, utilizing the underlying structures for support. The second skin border is held by skin tension and the aid of a gauze sponge. The needle is then passed from beneath up through the skin.[6]

The aim in closing skin wounds is to have the skin edges square and to bring them together accurately with no overlapping of the edges. Slight eversion of the suture line helps to insure good dermal apposition and avoids inversion of the skin edges.[50] If wound edges are at an angle through the skin, it is best to excise the edges in such a manner as to make them perpendicular to the skin's surface (Fig. 6–19).[62] Wound edges should also be accurately apposed in a horizontal plane. Anatomical landmarks and points of reference created by a wound's irregularities can be used to bring tissues together in the same relationship that they had prior to laceration.[6] For example, the wound edges of a laceration through a large pigmented spot on a dog may be aligned accurately by aligning the edges of the spot. In linear wounds, traction at the commissures of the wound will help align the edges accurately.[6] Accurate alignment of the wound edges helps prevent an excess of skin on one side of the wound when suturing reaches the commissure. Such excess skin forms a "dog ear," the correction of which is discussed in Chapter 7.

Placement and Tying of Sutures

Passage of the Needle.   When a curved needle is used, it should be passed through the tissue in a curved fashion, since it moves most readily in this manner.[19, 50] Large bites of tissue should not be taken with an inadequately small needle, nor should needles be forced or twisted in an effort to bring the point through the tissue.[19] Such maneuvers may result in the bending or breaking of the needle. When pulling a needle through the tissue with needle holders, the needle holders should not damage the point or cutting edge of the needle. The grasp should be as far back on the needle as possible.[19]

The purpose of a skin suture is to hold the edges of the wound together while the wound heals. The sutures should be placed squarely across the wound.[66] In general, sutures should take equal bites into both sides of the

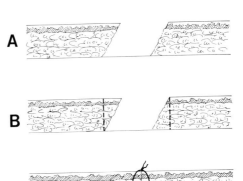

Figure 6–19:   Uneven skin edges, *A*, are trimmed, *B*, so that they appose squarely when sutured, *C*. (After Curtin, J. W.: Basic plastic surgical techniques in repair of facial laceration. Surg. Clin. North Am. 53:40, 1973.)

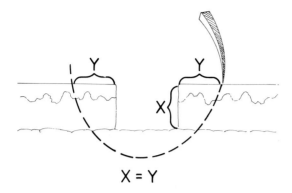

Figure 6–20: The distance of needle insertion away from the skin edge (*Y*) is equal to the skin thickness (*X*). (After Borges, A. F.: Elective Incisions and Scar Revision. Boston, Little, Brown and Co., 1973, p. 66.)

wound edge and should be carried well into the tissue to give an even closure throughout the wound.[38] It has been stated that the distance between the needle puncture site and the wound edge should be equal to the thickness of the skin (Fig. 6–20).[6, 13] Others have reported that sutures should be placed from 1 to 5 mm. from the wound edge.[22, 26, 36, 62, 78] It should be remembered that when large bites of tissue are taken, large suture marks can result because a large segment of tissue will be subjected to the constricting effect of the suture and its possible consequences.[10, 26]

Passing the needle through the skin perpendicular to the skin's surface on both sides of the wound has been advocated.[13] However, others describe passing the needle at a slight angle so that a slightly greater bite of the deeper part of the dermis or fat is taken. When the needle is passed through the second side of the wound, it is again passed at a slight angle so that it includes more tissue in the deeper aspects of the wound.[6, 9, 18, 26, 50] Placing the suture in this manner tends to create a moderate eversion of the skin edges or at least prevents inversion (Fig. 6–21). Inverted scars do not present the problem in veterinary surgery that they do in human surgery owing to the hair coat that covers the scar. However, such scars could be objectionable in very short haired breeds or on areas of the body where the hair is short. Moderate eversion

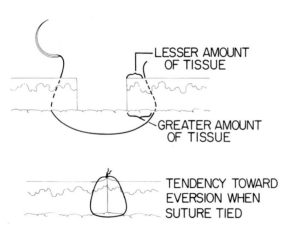

LESSER AMOUNT OF TISSUE

GREATER AMOUNT OF TISSUE

TENDENCY TOWARD EVERSION WHEN SUTURE TIED

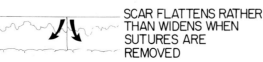

SCAR FLATTENS RATHER THAN WIDENS WHEN SUTURES ARE REMOVED

Figure 6–21: Advantage of passing a needle at a slight angle through the skin. (After McGregor, I. A.: Fundamental Techniques of Plastic Surgery, ed. 5. Edinburgh, Churchill Livingstone, 1972, p. 21.)

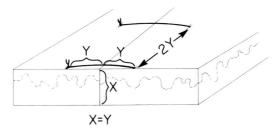

X=Y

Figure 6–22: A guideline for the proper distance between skin sutures.

DISTANCE BETWEEN SUTURES= 2 TIMES SKIN THICKNESS

of an incision tends to flatten in time because of the skin tension that is present after the sutures are removed,[26] whereas flat scars or inverted scars tend to invert further.

Tissue drag may be reduced by coating the suture with a sterile antibiotic ointment. This is done by drawing the suture material through a folded gauze sponge onto which the ointment has been placed.[37] This could also help prevent infections that might accompany twisted or braided sutures owing to their capillary properties.

Distance Between Sutures.   In determining the best distance between sutures, one guideline states that there should be the same distance between sutures as the sutures are wide. In other words, the distance between sutures should be twice the skin's thickness (Fig. 6–22).[13] Sutures may range from 1 to 5 mm. apart.[3, 18, 23, 26, 36, 62, 68, 69, 78] In general, the spacing between sutures may be increased in thick-skinned areas.[6, 62] Tension on individual sutures may be relieved by increasing the number of sutures to close a wound; however, too many sutures placed near the wound margins may delay healing by causing excess tissue reaction and producing necrosis as a result of impaired blood supply. On the other hand, too few sutures may interfere with healing because the wound edges are not in complete apposition.[3] A good rule of thumb to use when spacing sutures would be to place as many sutures as close together as necessary for satisfactory coaptation of the wound edges. It should be remembered that wounds following skin tension lines will need fewer sutures than those cutting across these lines.[6]

Order of Placement.   The order of placing sutures may be helpful in distributing wound tension evenly among the sutures. Two orders of suture placement have been described (Fig. 6–23). When the first suture is placed in the center of the wound, it should not be tied too tightly. This may result in incomplete approximation of the wound edges at this point until the other sutures have been placed.[6]

Suturing Unequal Wound Edges.   It is occasionally necessary to suture wound edges of unequal thickness or wound edges that do not lie on exactly the same level. When the two skin edges are of unequal thickness, both edges should be undermined at the same depth in the superficial subcutaneous tissue. A subcutaneous tissue flap of the desired thickness can then be advanced from the thicker side across and under the thinner side, where it will be sutured (Fig. 6–24).[26] When one skin edge lies slightly below the other, an attempt may be made to place them on the same level by passing the suture needle down through the side that is higher and up through the side that is lower. Catching a small amount of subcutaneous fascia with the needle and pulling it up under the lower skin edge helps to bolster it (Fig. 6–25).[13] When

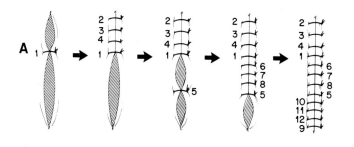

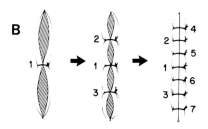

Figure 6–23: *A* and *B*, Two orders of suture placement for even distribution of wound tension. Numbers indicate the order of suture placement. (*A*, After Borges, A. F.: Elective Incisions and Scar Revision. Boston, Little, Brown and Co., 1973, p. 67.)

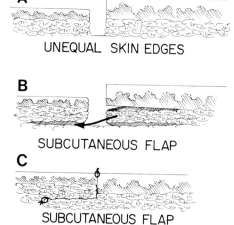

Figure 6–24: A technique for suturing skin edges of unequal thickness, *A*, utilizing a flap of subcutaneous tissue, *B*, to raise the thinner side, *C*.

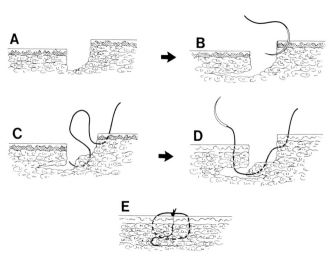

Figure 6–25: *A*, A technique for suturing skin edges that are on *slightly* different levels. *B*, The needle passes *down* through the higher side. *C*, It gets a bite of subcutaneous tissue, and *D*, is passed *up* through the lower side. *E*, Tying the suture levels the skin edges.

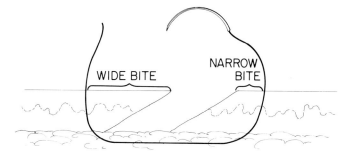

Figure 6–26: Suture placement when suturing uneven skin edges resulting from an angular cut through the skin. (After Knowles, R. P.: Injuries to skin, muscle and tendon, in Some Techniques and Procedures in Small Animal Surgery. Bonner Springs, Kans., Veterinary Medicine Publishing Co., Inc., 1963, p. 141.)

the wound edges are uneven because of an angular cut through the skin and cannot be trimmed to lie at right angles to the surface, they may be sutured by unequal placement of the needle. In such a wound, the needle passes through the obtuse side near the skin edge and through the acute side at some distance from the skin edge. This minimizes sloughing but usually necessitates a snug bandage or stent suture to prevent distortion of the wound edges (Fig. 6–26).[38]

Handling Suture Material.   Sutures made of resilient material should be carefully handled to avoid kinking, which weakens the suture material. Twisting that may lead to fraying should also be avoided. Forceps should not be clamped on any part of a suture that will remain in the tissue.[3, 36] When forceps are used to tie knots, only the ends of the suture strands should be grasped. Knots should be tied with care so that there is minimal friction between the strands, because friction weakens the strand by breaking some fibers and stretching others.[3]

Knots

Security.   Tying a secure knot is most important. The coefficient of friction of a suture material has been found to correlate closely with knot security, and each suture material has its own coefficient of friction. Monofilament steel has the highest coefficient of friction, followed, in descending order by gut, Dacron, cotton, nylon, and Teflon-coated materials. When a knot is tied under tension, the first throw may loosen before the second throw can be placed owing to the smoothness of some suture materials.[3] As a general rule, the smallest suture material of adequate strength should be used for wound closure, since knots tied with smaller-sized materials are more secure.[28, 36]

The length of the cut ends of a suture will vary with the suture material used and the location of the suture. If a knot has been tied squarely and securely, the ends do not have to be long. When sutures are buried the ends should be cut close to the knot, since long ends are irritating, cause additional separation of tissue, and act like foreign material.[3, 36] It is particularly advisable to cut the end of steel sutures close to the knot when they are buried. Owing to its knot security, there is little danger of a steel knot untying if the ends are cut short. Because of the change in tensile strength and knot security of surgical gut when it is buried, the author and others[36] prefer to leave the suture ends a little longer. In general, the greater the knot security, the shorter the suture ends may be.

The knots of skin sutures should be placed on one side of the incision to prevent irritation and to keep them from being pushed between the wound edges.[3] In addition, this maneuver serves as a "fine adjustment" of the wound edges. It is not uncommon for one edge of the wound to be slightly higher than the other. The lower side can be raised by manipulating the knot to that side of the wound.[50] Placement of the knot on one side of the incision also facilitates removal of the sutures without contamination of the tissues beneath the surface.[3]

Suture Tension.   Sutures tied too tightly can lead to problems: cut or torn tissues, excessive exudation, strangulation of tissues with subsequent necrosis, delayed healing, infection, pain, wound disruption, and unsightly scars.[3] From a pathophysiological standpoint, sutures that are too tight interfere with the circulation and thus the oxygen supply to the tissues. The trauma is increased, and the collagen synthesis needed for wound healing is depressed.[22]

When tying a knot, instruments should be used to allow better regulation of tension and to achieve greater finesse in knot placement.[50] Knots should be tied by pulling opposing suture ends perpendicular to the wound in the same plane and with the same amount of tension. The needle holders should remain parallel to the wound and move back and forth perpendicular to it. Such measures will help prevent loosening of the first throw of a suture, which occurs when the first loop is lifted or when there is uneven tension applied to either suture end. This results in inadequate tissue apposition.[36]

Many factors contribute to the formation of suture marks around a closed wound; however, tension is the major factor in producing such marks. There are two kinds of suture tension: intrinsic and extrinsic. Intrinsic tension is the constricting tension within the suture loop and is dependent on the tightness of the suture in relation to the encompassed tissue mass. If a suture is too tight, it causes local pressure, ischemia, and then necrosis, with subsequent scar formation and visible suture marks that may be punctate or linear. Edema of the encompassed tissue indirectly increases the tightness of the suture. The size of the suture material has a bearing on intrinsic tension in that the heavier the suture material, the easier it is to apply greater tension. The mass of tissue included in a skin suture also affects intrinsic tension. The larger the tissue bulk (or the farther from the skin edge the suture is placed), the greater is the force needed to appose the edges. Increased tissue mass within the suture allows that much more tissue to become edematous after the suture is in place (Fig. 6–27).[10]

Extrinsic tension is the pulling tension from outside the suture loop. It pertains to the tensions applied to the cut surfaces themselves. Since the sutures sustain the approximated wound edges, any force applied against the cut surfaces is thus transmitted through the sutures to the tissue encompassed by the tied sutures. The tension in the area is influenced by the direction of the incision in relation to skin tension lines and by tension on the edges that are being apposed. The latter is partly related to the size of the gap being sutured

INTRINSIC

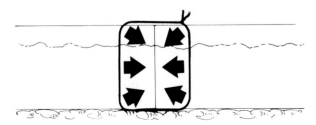

Figure 6–27: Intrinsic suture tension is the constricting tension within the suture loop. Tight sutures may result in suture marks. (After Crikelair, G. F.: Skin suture marks. Am. J. Surg. 96:633, 1958.)

EXTRINSIC

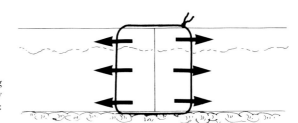

Figure 6-28: Extrinsic tension is the pulling tension from outside the suture loop. This may contribute to suture marks. (After Crikelair, G. F.: Skin suture marks. Am. J. Surg. 96:634, 1958.)

and the looseness of the cut edges. Movement of a sutured incision that runs at right angles to skin tension lines exerts force away from the center, with possible resultant necrosis (Fig. 6–28).[10] Some of the postoperative edema can be reduced by pressure dressings; however, allowance should be made for edema when tying the sutures. A good guideline is to tie sutures so that they *just* approximate the skin edges.[26]

Selection of the appropriate suture material and prevention of lateral pull on a wound will be helpful in eliminating suture tension. As mentioned previously, fine sutures will encourage closures with less tension than those in which heavier sutures are used. In fact, the suture material should be *slightly* stronger than what is necessary to maintain closure of the wound.[13, 26, 36, 62] Lateral pull on a wound closure results from closing wound edges from which a large segment of skin has been removed either traumatically or surgically. Much of this lateral pull can be eliminated by using subcutaneous sutures to take the tension off the skin sutures.[26] The reader is referred to Chapter 7 for the techniques used to advance tissues into place. Making the long axis of excisions parallel to skin tension lines is also helpful in eliminating tension in wound closure.[26]

Types of Knots

Square Knots. There are several knots that the surgeon can use in wound closure, the most common of which is the square knot (Fig. 6–29). When using this knot, certain fundamental rules must be considered. First, it should be used as a binder knot, i.e., one that lies in close contact with an object. This would be the case in wound closure. Secondly, the strain on the two ends of the knot should be continuous and not intermittent. Care should be taken so that the knot assumes the correct shape when tied. It has been noted that over half of

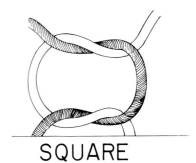

Figure 6-29: Square knot.   SQUARE

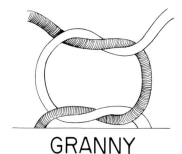

GRANNY

Figure 6–30: Granny knot.

the supposed square knots that are tied during surgery are in fact not square knots. The motions for making the knot are correctly performed, but the result is not quite right, the reason being that the square knot collapses very easily when the strain on the two ends is unequal.[21, 26] If the pull on both ends of the suture is not equal when the first half of the knot is tied, a half hitch results, which will not lie flat and will have no holding power.[26, 36] When tying the second half of the knot, the free ends must lie in opposite directions to prevent the knot from untying when the suture is cut. To avoid untying, it is wise to place an added half knot on top of the square knot. Even if this last throw were to come untied, the underlying square knot should remain secure.[26] When using suture materials with a high coefficient of friction and minimal tension, these three throws are generally sufficient to secure knots. However, when synthetic or monofilament suture materials or other suture materials with a low coefficient of friction are used, four or more throws or combinations of a surgeon's knot with additional throws may be needed to prevent knot slippage.[28, 36] The incidence of knot slippage has been found to increase with the size of the suture material.[28]

Granny Knot. The granny knot, which is formed in two halves like the square knot, is an unsafe knot that is prone to slip, especially if the strain on the two ends of the suture is unequal (Fig. 6–30).[21, 36] This knot should be avoided. A modified granny knot has been described in which two identical half knots are first tied to form the granny knot, which permits a slight adjustment after the knot has been drawn up, this is followed by a third throw placed on the knot. The third throw is in the opposite direction from the last throw of the granny knot, thus forming a square knot.[21] However, a report on knot security stated

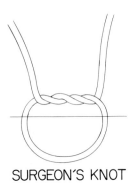

SURGEON'S KNOT

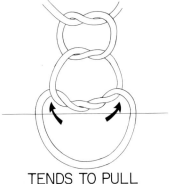

TENDS TO PULL
UP AT ENDS

Figure 6–31: A surgeon's knot may become unsightly as additional throws are placed on top of it.

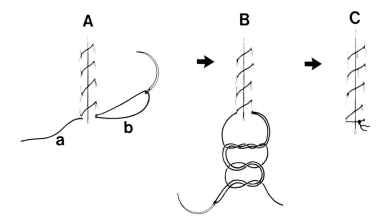

Figure 6–32: The technique for ending a continuous suture when an eyed needle–suture combination is used. A, The suture end, a, is tied to the loop, b. B, The knot is created and, C, completed.

that knots with all throws squared were more secure than granny knots with square throws added.[47]

Surgeon's Knot. The surgeon's knot is especially good when security is needed, as with materials with a low coefficient of friction.[21] In such instances, it may be necessary to overlay a surgeon's knot with a square knot or to use two surgeon's knots.[36] However, the surgeon's knot takes longer to tie and places more suture material in the wound than does a square knot. This knot does not make a good ligature knot, since it does not place the proper tension upon small blood vessels owing to the bulk of the suture material used in the first throw.[36] It may also produce a rather unsightly knot when other throws are placed on the top of it (Fig. 6–31).[21]

Techniques for Tying Square Knots. There are two techniques for tying a square knot at the end of a continuous suture. When using an eyed needle–suture combination , the suture strand near the needle is doubled. As the end of the wound is approached, this double strand is taken directly through the final stitch and tied to the free end of the double strand that has not been pulled through (Fig. 6–32).[21, 36] This technique cannot be used with a swaged needle–

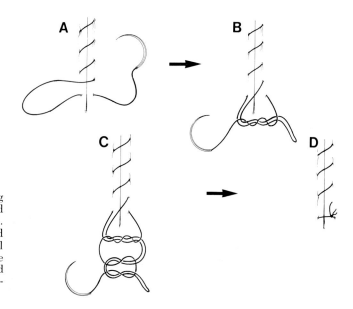

Figure 6–33: The technique for ending a continuous suture when a swaged needle–suture combination is used. This may also be used with an eyed needle–suture combination. A, The final loop is created in the suture. B, The loop and single suture strand are tied together. C and D, The knot is completed.

suture combination. The second technique can be utilized with a swaged needle–suture combination. With this technique, wound closure is completed and the suture strand near the needle is tied to the last loop in the suture line (Fig. 6–33).[21, 36] Both techniques require tying a single strand to a double strand.[21] In either technique, three to four throws should be placed to secure the end of the suture line.[36]

SUTURE PATTERNS

Of the many suture patterns available to the surgeon, those that are used most often when closing skin wounds are the intradermal suture patterns and the simple interrupted suture.

Intradermal Sutures

The terms subcuticular suture and intradermal suture have been used somewhat loosely in the literature. What has often been referred to as a subcuticular suture is actually an intradermal suture, since it is placed in the lower portion of the dermis or in the area where the dermis blends into the subcutaneous tissues.[3] A subcuticular suture is one that is placed in subcutaneous tissues. The main objective of such sutures is to control capillary hemorrhage and to obliterate dead space that is caused by pulling skin edges together over the top of a subcutaneous defect. Blood, liquefied fat, serum, and other wound contents provide a good medium for bacteria, and a subcutaneous space acts as a reservoir for such material. Even if infection does not develop, this material may lead to complications in healing. Subcutaneous sutures will help eliminate these spaces and their potential problems.[58]

If the skin is sutured after closing the subcutaneous tissues, the scar may have a tendency to widen after the skin sutures are removed.[58, 78] Since wounds sutured under tension tend to disrupt, widen, and produce stretch marks, it would be advisable to place an intradermal suture in these wounds.[6] The need for such a suture is greatest during the period following the removal of skin sutures and during the remodeling of newly synthesized collagen. If the intradermal sutures are absorbed or weakened during this time, widening of the scar will occur.[58]

It is important to place intradermal sutures superficially enough to hold the skin edges together, yet deep enough to have a healthy layer of epithelium covering them. If an intradermal suture passes into the deeper layers of the epidermis, problems could arise. Any foreign fiber that passes through the epithelium and causes interruption of intercellular bridges and cell surfaces provides both the initiating stimulus and the physical pattern for mitosis and migration. Epithelial cells then grow along the suture line, following it through the dermis and up to the opposite epithelial surface, where contact inhibition stops the cell growth. The wound is then traversed by a suture and an epithelium-lined tract. Such tracts may not cause problems, but they may develop closed epithelial sinuses, cysts, or internal tracts. Ideally, then, an intradermal suture should remain confined to the dermis. After insertion of a row of intradermal sutures, the epithelial edges should be apposed closely enough so that additional skin sutures seem unnecessary. However, some fine sutures are generally needed for final adjustment of the skin edges.[58]

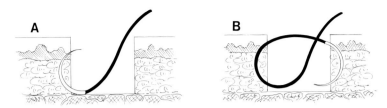

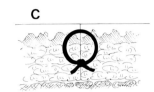

Figure 6–34: Placement and tying of an interrupted intradermal suture. A, The needle is first passed from the deep to the superficial layers. B, The needle is then passed from the superficial to the deep layers on the opposite side of the wound. C, The suture is completed.

It seems that each surgeon has a preferred material for intradermal sutures. In general, it should be small in diameter, strong, and light in color and should produce little tissue reaction.[58] In addition, it should be noncapillary[42] and have a low coefficient of friction that allows easy removal.[26, 42] Some feel that the suture material should have soft, natural fibers rather than stiff fibers,[58] while others believe that the suture should lend some stiffness to the wound.[26, 42] The suture materials that have been advocated for intradermal use have ranged in size from 3–0 to 6–0 and have included such substances as monofilament nylon,[6, 18, 26, 42, 50, 70] monofilament steel,[6, 26, 42, 78] white silk,[58] silkworm gut,[50] polyethylene,[42] chromic catgut,[50, 68, 78] plain catgut,[26] and polyesters.[26]

Two basic types of intradermal suture patterns are most used. In one type, the needle is inserted into the deeper edge of the wound first, incorporating a small amount of subcutaneous tissue and the deeper portion of the dermis. On the other side of the wound the direction of needle passage is reversed so that the needle passes through the dermis first and then the subcutaneous tissue. When this suture is tied, the knot is buried deep in the subcutaneous tissue rather than close to the skin's surface (Fig. 6–34).[9, 42, 50, 62, 78] If the knot is large and is not buried, it may cause pressure and local necrosis of the skin.[36]

The second type of intradermal suture pattern is continuous.[3, 5, 6, 9, 18, 26, 36, 42, 50, 62, 78] It can be placed rapidly and utilizes little suture material: however, it does not have the strength of a normal skin suture pattern.[36] The needle is passed horizontally through the dermis, taking small bites alternately from each side. As suturing is continued, care should be taken to place sutures at the same level. The entrance site of each bite should be backed up slightly from the previous point of exit to prevent the two sites from being directly opposite each other.[18, 26, 42] If this suture is to be removed at a later date, removal may be facilitated by passing the suture through the skin to the outside at intervals along its length. These outside loops may be from 1 to 3 in. apart, depending upon the ease with which the suture material slides through the dermis when pulled after the loops have been cut (Fig. 6–35).[6, 9, 26, 42, 70] When steel is used, it has been suggested that the suture be interrupted at 1.5- to 2-inch intervals and the steel be knotted loosely instead of leaving loops.[78] To further facilitate suture removal, each needle entrance point should be opposite the last exit site instead of backed up slightly, as previously described.[36]

These continuous intradermal sutures may be started and ended in several fashions. Fixation of the suture ends may not be necessary at all.[6, 18, 26, 42, 78] One

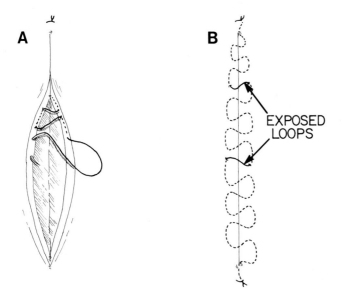

Figure 6–35: Placement of a continuous intradermal suture, leaving a few loops exposed to facilitate suture removal. *A*, Placement of suture. *B*, Completed suture with two loops of exposed suture material.

technique involves anchoring the starting end of the suture with a simple suture taken just beyond one commissure of the wound and passing the suture from this point through the commissure of the wound. To end this suture, the needle passes out through the other commissure of the wound. The suture is cut, a simple interrupted suture is placed in line with the wound, and the cut end of the running stitch is tied to it (Fig. 6–36).[62] A similar pattern can be placed without cutting the suture to tie it at its end; instead, a bite is taken through the skin from the outside and the suture is tied back on itself (Fig. 6–36,

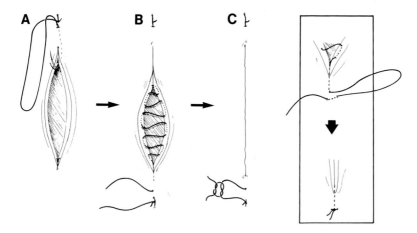

Figure 6–36: A technique for beginning and ending a continuous intradermal suture. *A*, A simple interrupted suture is placed beyond the commissure of the wound, and the needle is passed through the commissure. *B*, The suture is passed through the other commissure of the wound and completed. *C*, The final suture end is tied to a simple interrupted suture that is placed in line with the wound. *Insert*, An alternative technique for ending a continuous intradermal suture is shown. (*A*, *B*, and *C*, After Pullen, C. M.: Reconstruction of the skin, in Bojrab, M. J. (ed.): Current Techniques in Small Animal Surgery. Philadelphia, Lea & Febiger, 1975, p. 281.)

Figure 6–37: Burying the first knot of an intradermal suture. *A,* The suture is placed from the deep to the superficial layer, and then from the superficial to the deep layers. *B,* The beginning suture is completed (After Archibald, J., and Blakely, C. L.: Sutures, in Archibald, J. (ed.): Canine Surgery. ed. 2. Santa Barbara, Calif., American Veterinary Publications, Inc., 1974, p. 48.)

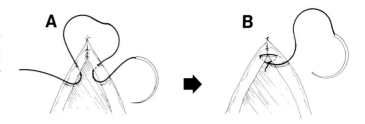

insert).[36] This technique may also be used to begin the suture. A modification of this method entails anchoring the suture slightly beyond the wound ends by means of a knot tied on the surface of the skin.[5, 9, 18] The ends of this type of intradermal suture may also be anchored over small drain tubes or pieces of gauze.[5, 42]

When an absorbable suture material is used intradermally, the beginning and ending knots may be buried at either end of the wound.[3] To bury the beginning knot, the first bite is taken from the deep through the superficial layers of the dermis. The second bite is taken just across from the first from the superficial through the deep layers. Tying places the knot deep to the dermis (Fig. 6–37). The method used to complete suturing depends on the type of needle used. When using a swaged needle, Knecht and associates have described a technique in which the needle is inserted from the superficial through the deep layers; following this a loop of suture is lifted from the wound. The needle is then introduced from the deep through the superficial layers on one side, crosses the wound, and is inserted into the tissue from the superficial through the deep layers toward the previously created loop. Tying the suture end to the loop results in a buried knot (Fig. 6–38).[36] When an eyed needle is used, Archibald and Blakely have described a technique in which the needle is inserted under the opposite skin edge from the deep through the superficial layers, and a double strand of suture is drawn through the skin. The needle is then inserted in the opposite edge of the wound from the superficial through the deep layers, and the double suture strand is brought from beneath the skin.

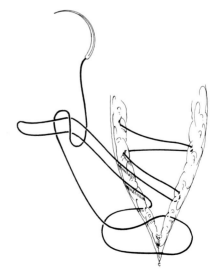

Figure 6–38: A technique for ending a continuous intradermal suture when using a swaged needle–suture combination. (After Knecht, C. D., Welser, J. R., Allen, A. R., et al.: Fundamental Techniques in Veterinary Surgery. Philadelphia, W. B. Saunders Co., 1975, p. 43.)

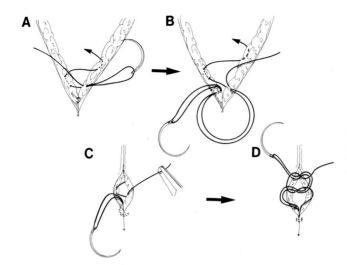

Figure 6–39: A technique for ending a continuous intradermal suture when using an eyed needle–suture combination. A, The needle is passed from the deep to the superficial layers on one side of the wound. B, The needle is then passed from the superficial to the deep layers on the opposite side of the wound. C, The wound is closed and ready for tying the free suture end to the needled loop. D, The knot is completed.

The single strand of suture protruding from the wound is held while the double strand is drawn tight. The single strand and the double strand are then tied together. The suture ends are cut near the knot, resulting in a buried knot (Fig. 6–39).[3]

There are two other types of intradermal sutures, one of which is a combination of the continuous and the interrupted patterns.[70] Such a suture has additional strength and requires a minimum of external skin fixation. However, it is dependent upon having skin of sufficient thickness to allow the placement of two rows of sutures in the dermis. The other type of intradermal suture pattern is composed of horizontal mattress sutures of fine chromic catgut placed deep in the dermis.[68]

Even though skin edges appear to be well apposed following intradermal suturing, it is still advisable to place some skin sutures to provide a finer approximation of the skin edges.[6, 18, 26, 70] Additional sutures would also be indicated to prevent wound dehiscence, since many dogs will remove sutures by licking. Should subcuticular sutures alone be used to close the skin, the animal should be hospitalized to insure restricted activity and prevent self-mutilation.[36]

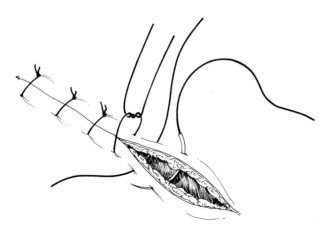

Figure 6–40: Simple interrupted sutures.

Simple Interrupted Sutures

The other commonly used suture pattern in closing skin wounds is the simple interrupted suture.[62, 69] This pattern is composed of a single loop of suture material passed perpendicular to the plane of the tissues, with the ends of the suture emerging on opposite sides of the wound (Fig. 6–40). Many of the characteristics and principles for the proper placement of simple interrupted sutures have been covered in the section on the placement and tying of sutures, to which the reader is referred. This type of suture can be used in both deep and superficial tissues. It can also be used as a type of tension suture.[3, 18] One advantage of an interrupted suture over a continuous suture in skin closure is that the surgeon can more precisely adjust the tension of each suture at each segment of the wound according to the spreading forces that are present.[6] Interrupted sutures also have their disadvantages, including the use of a greater amount of suture material, the increased time that is required for tying and cutting each suture, and the increased amount of suture material that remains in the wound (e.g., knots) when sutures are buried. The simple interrupted suture is an apposing suture; however, too much tension can result in inversion of the wound edges when eversion would be more desirable.[36]

Simple Continuous Sutures

A simple continuous suture pattern consists of a progressive series of sutures inserted without interruption perpendicular to the plane of the tissues, with only the beginning and the end of the suture being tied. These sutures can be placed so that the suture advances above or beneath the skin. When the suture advances above the skin, the portions of the suture beneath the skin are perpendicular to the wound edge, and the portions of the suture material above the skin are angular to the skin edge.[3, 36] The reverse is true when the suture is advanced below the skin.[3] A modification of this suture pattern is called the "running suture" in which both the deep and the superficial portions of the suture are advanced (Fig. 6–41). Although running sutures can be placed more quickly, regularity of stitching is difficult to achieve.[36]

Simple continuous sutures are occasionally used for skin closure and can be applied more rapidly than interrupted sutures.[6, 18, 50] This suture pattern is also useful for the closure of subcutaneous tissues and fasciae in nontension

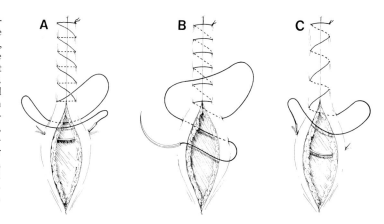

Figure 6–41: Simple continuous suture patterns. *A,* Suture advancement above the skin. *B,* Suture advancement below the skin. *C,* Suture advancement above and below the skin. (*A* and *B,* After Archibald, J., and Blakely, C.L.: Sutures, in Archibald, J. [ed.]: Canine Surgery, ed. 2. Santa Barbara, Calif., American Veterinary Publications, Inc., 1974, p. 44. *C,* After Knecht, C.D., Welser, J.R., Allen, A. R., et al.: Fundamental Techniques in Veterinary Surgery. Philadelphia, W. B. Saunders Co., 1975, p. 42.)

planes.[36] This pattern is more advantageous than the continuous lock suture pattern in that it better allows tension adjustment after placement than does the continuous lock suture pattern.[6] These sutures are weaker than simple interrupted sutures,[23, 69] and tend to pucker the skin,[18, 50] and strangulate the skin edges;[18] if there is a break anywhere along the suture, the entire wound may break down.[18, 31] The tendency to strangulate wound edges is due to pulling the suture too tightly rather than any inherent defect of the method.[50] In summary, this is a rapid technique for closing the skin, although the results never surpass those of the simple interrupted suture method.[6]

Vertical Mattress Sutures

A vertical mattress suture is an interrupted loop of suture material inserted perpendicular to the plane of the tissues, with both suture ends emerging on one side of the wound (Fig. 6–42A). The needle is introduced approximately 8 mm. from the incision. It passes across the wound and exits at a corresponding point on the opposite side. From this point the needle is advanced 4 mm. toward the skin edge, is reinserted through the skin, and is passed back across the incision to a point that is about 4 mm. from the skin edge on the original side. These sutures are usually placed 5 mm. apart.[36] This pattern is useful as a tension suture[6] and as an everting skin suture.[6, 26, 50] When placed into the fascia underlying the skin, it serves as a hemostatic suture by eliminating dead space under the undermined skin.[9] When the skin edges have been undermined for some distance and the surgeon does not wish to place any deeper sutures to approximate the deep layers of tissue, the vertical mattress suture may be used as a tension suture.[6] In these instances and in other instances in which there is minor skin tension, the vertical mattress sutures are used along with simple interrupted sutures to close the wound.[3, 6, 26] Caution should be taken so that these sutures are tight enough to bring the skin borders closer to each other but not so tight as to completely coapt them. Final approximation of the skin edges should be accomplished with the simple interrupted sutures.[6] In general, the ratio of vertical mattress sutures to interrupted sutures should not exceed 1:5 (Fig. 6–42B).[68] However,

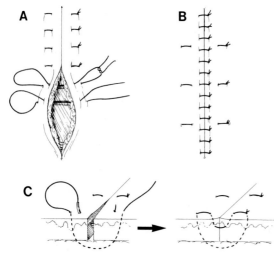

Figure 6–42: Vertical mattress sutures. A, Placement of vertical mattress sutures. B, Combination of vertical mattress and simple interrupted sutures. C, A modified vertical mattress suture with the second bite taken 1 mm. deep in the dermis and 2 mm. back from the skin edge. (C, After Pullen, C.M.: Reconstruction of the skin, in Bojrab, M.J. (ed.): Current Techniques in Small Animal Surgery. Philadelphia, Lea & Febiger, 1975, p. 280.)

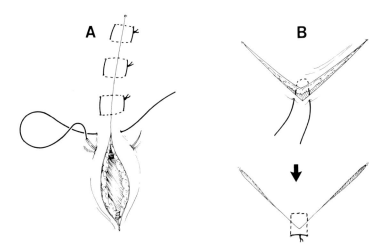

Figure 6–43: *A,* Interrupted horizontal mattress sutures. *B,* A half-buried horizontal mattress (three-point) suture at the tip of a "V"-shaped wound. (*B,* After McGregor, I. A.: Fundamental Techniques of Plastic Surgery, ed. 5. Edinburgh, Churchill Livingstone, 1972, p. 25.)

the alternate use of vertical mattress and simple interrupted sutures has also been described.[69] In most cases, the vertical mattress sutures are removed before the simple interrupted sutures, generally on the third postoperative day, since their purpose is accomplished before that of the simple interrupted sutures and also because they tend to produce suture marks if left in too long.[6, 68]

When skin is thin, poorly supported, or mobile on its deep surface and has a tendency to invert, vertical mattress sutures may be used to help evert the skin edges.[3, 50] On small animals, such skin is located on the abdomen and medial surfaces of the upper parts of the limbs.[3]

A modified vertical mattress suture has been described that provides edge-to-edge apposition with a slight tendency toward eversion. Instead of placing the second portion of the suture deep in the tissue, it is placed 1 mm. deep in the dermis and about 2 mm. back from the skin edge (Fig. 6–42C).[62, 69]

The vertical mattress suture is stronger than the horizontal mattress suture in tissues that are under tension. However, it has the disadvantages of requiring an increased amount of suture material and of being time-consuming to apply.[36]

Interrupted Horizontal Mattress Sutures

The interrupted horizontal mattress suture is a loop of suture material placed interruptedly in the same plane as the tissues, with both ends of the suture emerging on the same side of the wound. As described by Knecht and colleagues, this suture is placed by inserting the needle 2 to 3 mm. from the edge on one side of the wound. The needle is passed angularly through the tissue below the edge of the tissue plane to prevent excessive eversion of the tissues. It crosses the incision and exits in an angular pattern on the opposite side. The suture is advanced 8 mm. along this side of the wound, reintroduced into the skin, passed back across the wound as previously described, and tied (Fig. 6–43A). These sutures are usually placed 4 mm. apart, but the distance depends on the subject and the tissue being sutured.[36]

These sutures are valuable for closing dead space,[18] everting skin edges,[6, 18, 26, 69] and relieving tension.[18, 36] They are not needed for good approximation of the skin and may tend to cut through the skin and become embedded.[6] Because of their geometric design, these sutures have a tendency to reduce the blood supply to the wound edges, especially when they are tied under tension.[69]

A half-buried horizontal mattress suture has been found to be effective in closing the point of a "V"-shaped wound. The portion of the suture that passes through the point of the "V" is buried in the dermis and runs in the same plane as the skin (Fig. 6–43B). This often helps prevent necrosis of the tip of the "V," which could occur following the use of a simple interrupted suture. The suture may also be advantageous for suturing a skin flap into position. The buried portion of the suture lies within the flap so that it effectively holds the flap in place, and yet the danger of damaging the skin by inserting sutures through it is avoided.[26] This type of suture has also been called a three-point suture.[50]

Continuous Horizontal Mattress Sutures

A continuous horizontal mattress suture pattern consists of a progressive series of sutures placed uninterruptedly in the same plane as the tissue, with only the beginning and the end of the suture being tied (Fig. 6–44). It is started with a simple interrupted suture and is advanced from 7 to 8 mm. above the skin and parallel to the incision line between each passage of the suture under the skin and perpendicular to the incision line.[36] Such a pattern can be used as a subcutaneous suture pattern to close deep tissues. This is also the pattern of the continuous intradermal suture. When used to close the skin, the suture penetrates the full thickness of the skin with each bite and permits accurate approximation of the wound edges with reduced tension.[5]

Continuous Lock Sutures

A continuous lock suture pattern, also called a "blanket stitch," is a progressive series of sutures inserted uninterruptedly in the same plane as the tissue. The needle passes above the unused suture material following each suture. Only the beginning and end of the suture are tied. When an eyed

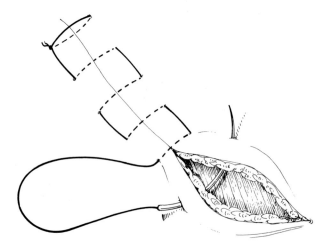

Figure 6–44: Continuous horizontal mattress suture.

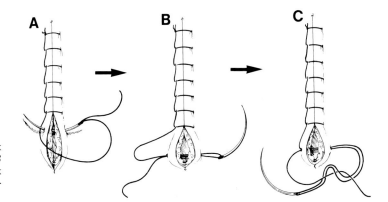

Figure 6–45: Continuous lock suture. *A,* Placing the suture. *B* and *C,* Ending a continuous lock suture when an eyed needle–suture combination is used.

needle is used to place this suture pattern, the suture should be ended by inserting the needle in the direction opposite that previously used. The remaining free end of the suture is held on the side of insertion. The loop of suture formed on the side opposite that of insertion is tied to a single end (Fig. 6–45).[36] An advantage of this suture pattern is its greater stability in the event of a partial failure. It has the disadvantage of requiring an increased amount of suture material.[36] The other advantages and disadvantages of this pattern are the same as those of the simple continuous suture pattern.[50]

Cross Sutures

The cross-stich or "baseball" stitch is a double simple continuous suture pattern; one suture line is placed, followed by the placement of a second suture line from the opposite direction (Fig. 6–46). This pattern is indicated when the skin is thick and when some haste is required. The first row of sutures is placed deep, wide, and loose to approximate the full thickness of the skin edges. The second row is used for fine approximation of the superficial edges of the wound. If the wound appears almost completely closed after

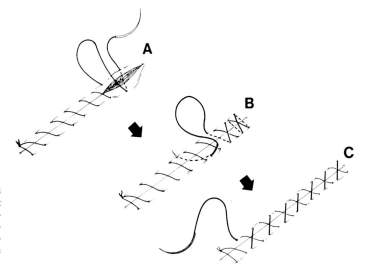

Figure 6–46: Placement of cross sutures. *A,* Placement of the first row of continuous sutures. *B,* Placement of the second row of continuous sutures in the opposite direction. *C,* Final appearance of cross sutures.

the first row of sutures has been placed, the returning second row of sutures may skip over a number of loops until the starting knot is reached. It is better to have the loops too loose than too tight. If the loops are loose, a few simple interrupted sutures may be added to complete the skin approximation where needed. If the cross-stitch is too tight, there is not much that can be done.[6] This pattern is not commonly used in veterinary surgery.

X Mattress Suture

Related to the cross-stitch is the X mattress suture. The needle is inserted 3 to 4 mm. from the wound edge on one side and passed to the opposite side of the wound in the manner of placing a simple interrupted suture. The needle is then advanced about 5 mm. and crosses the wound without penetrating the tissue. The needle is passed a second time through the tissues parallel to the first passage. The suture ends, which are on opposite sides of the wound, are tied together, thus forming an "X" on the skin surface. This type of suture is a tension suture that provides strength and prevents eversion of the wound edges. It is particularly useful in suturing the skin of stumps (Fig. 6–47).[36]

Tension Sutures

Indications. Occasionally wounds cannot be closed without excessive tension being placed on the sutures because of tissue loss. The tension may cause the sutures to cut through the tissues, with resultant strangulation and eventual wound disruption. Specific indications for tension sutures would include wounds in aged and debilitated animals when delayed wound healing is anticipated, abdominal wounds, and wounds over joints where joint movement might break the suture line. When the suturing of contaminated wounds is delayed, tension sutures that do not pass through the wound cavity can be used to help in closure without risking contamination of the suture.[3] It has been found in dogs that as long as there is a good blood supply to the skin, the wound may be closed under marked tension without fear of necrosis.[55]

Basic Techniques. Generally speaking, tension sutures should be placed well away from the skin edges to reduce the chances of strangulation and marginal necrosis. After drawing the wound edges closer together with either towel forceps or with the tension sutures themselves, interrupted sutures can be used to complete the closure without the risk of excessive strain on these sutures.[3, 69]

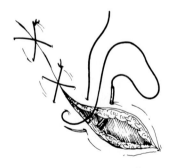

Figure 6–47: Placement of an X mattress sutures. (After Knecht, C. D., Welser, J. R., Allen, A. R., et al.: Fundamental Techniques in Veterinary Surgery. Philadelphia, W. B. Saunders Co., 1975, p. 40.)

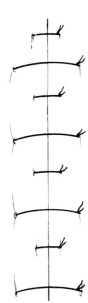

Figure 6–48: Alternating wide and narrow bites with simple interrupted sutures for a tension suture. (After Archibald, J., and Blakely, C. L.: Sutures, in Archibald, J. (ed.): Canine Surgery, ed. 2. Santa Barbara, Calif., American Veterinary Publications, Inc., 1974, p. 47.)

The addition of supports such as rubber tubing, buttons, or gauze placed under the sutures before they are tied will reduce the tendency of sutures to cut through the tissues. Sutures with such supports are frequently called quilled sutures.[36, 69] Under a pressure bandage, areas of necrosis corresponding to the surface areas of these supports may occur. Therefore it would be preferable to place two or three rows of some type of tension suture without supports under pressure bandages.[69]

Types

Simple Interrupted Tension Sutures. In addition to being the most commonly used suture for the closure of skin wounds, the simple interrupted suture may also be used as a tension suture. By alternating the size of the bite of tissue taken when placing the sutures (wide bite — narrow bite — wide bite), the danger of marginal necrosis owing to tissue strangulation is minimized (Fig. 6–48).[3]

Horizontal Mattress Tension Sutures. Interrupted horizontal mattress sutures by themselves may serve as tension sutures.[18] When used as such, they are placed well away from the skin edges, and simple interrupted sutures are used to approximate the skin edges.[3] A potential disadvantage of such sutures as compared with vertical mattress sutures is their tendency to interfere with the circulation of the skin edge (Fig. 6–49A).[69] The horizontal mattress tension suture may be modified in an effort to overcome its tendency to cut into tissue and to interfere with the circulation by placing stents under the suture. These stents may be segments of rubber tubing[57] or buttons (Fig. 6–49B).[3, 5] This technique has been described as an effective way to close the lesion that remains after the surgical excision of an elbow hygroma.[57]

An adjustable tension suture that utilizes the interrupted horizontal mattress suture and rubber stents has been described for eyelid closure in ophthalmologic work and as a tension suture in other types of wounds. To make an adjustable horizontal mattress tension suture, 2–0 monofilament nylon has been found to be the best suture material. Bungs (stents) made of latex rubber

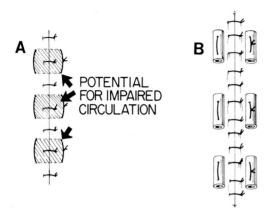

Figure 6–49: *A*, Horizontal mattress tension sutures may impair circulation at the wound's edge. *B*, Rubber tubing stents placed under the sutures help to prevent circulatory impairment.

tubing with an outside diameter of ⅜ in. and an inside diameter of ³/₁₆ in. are also necessary. These are quartered longitudinally and cut into lengths of 10 to 12 mm. The horizontal mattress tension suture is placed through the bungs in the usual fashion. The manner in which the knot is tied is responsible for the facility in adjusting the suture. A surgeon's knot is placed next to the bung. Approximately 1 cm. above this a second knot is tied using three squared throws (Fig. 6–50*A*). The suture may be tightened by placing the jaws of a hemostat between the two knots and opening the jaws, thus pulling the surgeon's knot tighter (Fig. 6–50*B*). To loosen the suture, the jaws of the hemostat are inserted *under* the surgeon's knot and opened, thus loosening the suture (Fig. 6–50*C*). The advantages of this suture include the ability to alter suture pressure, the avoidance of pressure sloughing, and, when it is used in ophthalmic surgery, the opportunity to review occasionally the condition of the eyeball. The primary disadvantage is the danger of the animal's "adjusting" the suture by licking, chewing, or scratching.[63]

Vertical Mattress Tension Sutures. The use of vertical mattress sutures as tension sutures in wounds with minimal tension has been discussed in the section on vertical mattress sutures. These sutures may also be used as tension sutures in wounds in which tension is greater. When closing such wounds, strong, nonirritating material such as monofilament nylon (2–0 to 1) is used along with stents placed under the loops of the suture.[34, 35] The

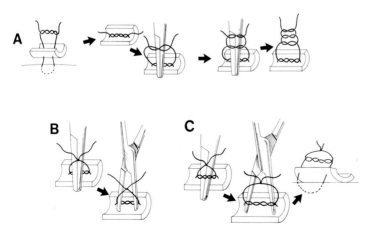

Figure 6–50: *A*, Placement of an adjustable horizontal mattress suture. *B*, Tightening the suture. The forceps spread apart *above* the surgeon's knot. *C*, Loosening the suture. The forceps spread apart *below* the surgeon's knot. (After Rickards, D. A.: An adjustable suture: A technique for altering the tension of stitches postoperatively, especially in third lid flaps. Vet. Med. Small Anim. Clin. 68:88, 1973.)

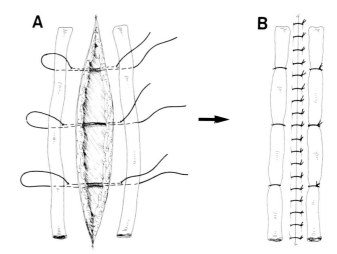

Figure 6–51: *A*, Vertical mattress tension sutures placed over soft rubber tubing. *B*, Simple interrupted skin apposition sutures used with tension sutures.

stent material may be firm[3] or soft rubber tubing (Penrose drains).[34] Soft aluminum welding–rod stents have been used in large animals.[74] This type of tension suture is used in conjunction with simple interrupted sutures to approximate the skin edges (Fig. 6–51). The tension sutures are removed three days postoperatively, by which time the tissues have been stabilized by strands of fibrin.[34, 35, 68] This type of suture has also been found to be effective in closing wound defects left by the surgical correction of elbow hygroma in dogs.[34]

Far-Near-Near-Far (Pulley) Sutures. This suture has been described as a combination of tension and approximating sutures.[3, 41, 62, 69, 78] It is indicated in wounds in which the skin edges are widely separated. This pattern provides the necessary tension for approximating the wound edges without applying tension at the incision line. The "far" component of the suture supplies the tension, while the "near" component apposes the skin edges.[36, 62] The far component of the suture is the first to be placed so that the knot does not lie on the suture line. The near component is placed only 1 to 2 mm. from the far component.[62] The first needle insertion is made at some distance from the incision. The needle passes through the skin and subcutaneous tissue, crosses the wound, and exits through the skin on the opposite side of the incision near the wound edge. The needle is then returned externally across the wound to the side of entrance. It enters the skin near the wound edge and passes through the skin and subcutaneous tissues. The needle advances across the wound and exits at a distance equal to that of the original far component.[36] Excessive tightening of the suture should be avoided to prevent inversion of the suture line (Fig. 6–52A).[62] The mean tensile strength of this pattern has been reported to be greater than that of simple interrupted and mattress suture patterns.[41, 69] However, as stated by Knecht and co-workers, the disadvantage of this pattern is that an excessive amount of suture material is placed in the area, with double sutures in the incision and an overlapping suture pattern on the skin.[36]

Far-Far-Near-Near Sutures. This suture is placed in the order of its name and is similar to the far-near-near-far suture in its advantages and disadvantages. As explained by Knecht and associates, the needle is inserted at a point distant from the skin edge and passed to a corresponding point on

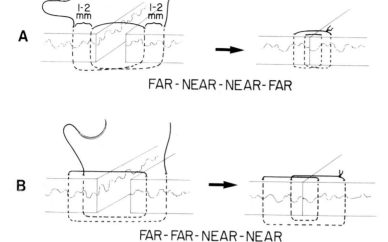

Figure 6–52: *A*, Far-near-near-far suture. *B*, Far-far-near-near suture. (*A*, After Pullen, C. M.: Reconstruction of the skin, in Bojrab, M. J. [ed.]: Current Techniques in Small Animal Surgery. Philadelphia, Lea & Febiger, 1975, p. 279. *B*, After Knecht, C. D., Welser, J. R., Allen, A. R., et al.: Fundamental Techniques in Veterinary Surgery. Philadelphia, W. B. Saunders Co., 1975, p. 49.)

the opposite side of the incision. After returning the needle across the incision externally, it is passed from a point closer to the incision on the original side to a similar close point on the opposite side (Fig. 6–52*B*).[36]

Stent Sutures. Stent sutures are effective tension sutures. They provide a means of obliterating dead space when there has been massive tissue excision.[66] They are also effective in reducing postoperative edema and hemorrhage.[66, 78] A large curved needle and monofilament stainless steel are used to place the sutures from 0.50 to 0.75 in. apart along the wound, with the needle entering the skin 0.25 to 0.50 in. from the wound edge. The needle is passed deep into the underlying tissues and emerges 0.25 to 0.50 in. from the opposite wound edge. These sutures are left untied, and the wound edges are closed, usually with simple interrupted sutures; however, a simple continuous or lock suture pattern can be used. A gauze roll of 0.50 in. width is then placed over the closed incision, and the stent wires are closed firmly over the roll (Fig. 6–53).[38, 66] This type of bandage exerts even pressure between

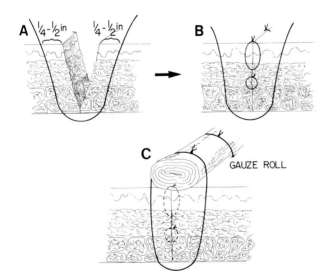

Figure 6–53: *A*, Placement of stent sutures. *B*, Closure of subcutaneous tissue and skin. *C*, Placement of gauze roll and tying of stent sutures.

wound edges and underlying tissues, eliminates dead space, and acts as a self-retaining bandage. It also prevents the animal from molesting the wound.[38] Removal of the stent bandage seven days postoperatively, followed three days later by removal of the remaining skin sutures, is recommended for animals.[66]

Intradermal Tension Sutures.   Intradermal sutures are actually a form of tension suture in that they help appose the skin edges and prevent the widening of scars after the skin sutures are removed. In humans a wound closed with only subcutaneous sutures and skin sutures will tend to have a widened scar, whereas the scar of a wound closed with subcutaneous sutures, intradermal sutures, and skin sutures does not tend to widen after the skin sutures are removed. The intradermal suture helps to overcome the tension and prevents the widening.[58]

"Walking" Sutures.   A buried tension suture has been described that evenly distributes tension to tissues around the wound. In addition, it moves skin over a large defect and obliterates dead space. These sutures are placed with absorbable suture material. The first bite is taken in the deep portion of the dermis; the second bite is taken in the deeper tissues toward the center or toward one side of the wound.[71] For further details and illustrations of the "walking" suture, the reader is referred to Chapter 7.

MINIMIZING WOUND SCARRING

Scarring of the skin is not the problem in veterinary surgery that it is in human surgery owing to the overlying hair coat of animals. However, in short-haired breeds and on regions of the body where hair is typically short in other breeds, scarring may be evident. Scarring may be the result of tension, which can lead to separation of the wound edges or an abnormal amount of scar tissue.[18, 26] In animals this would usually be in the form of a widened scar. Tension also causes sutures to cut their way through the skin and subcutaneous tissue by pressure necrosis (Fig. 6–54).[6, 10, 18, 68] The longer the time the

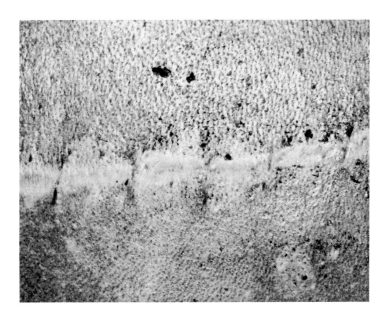

Figure 6–54: A widened scar with suture marks resulting from tension on the wound.

sutures are left in, the greater are the chances of a more severe scar.[3, 5, 6, 10, 18, 26, 58, 68] The relationship of the sutures to the wound edge and the region of the body in which the wound is located will affect the amount of scar tissue.[26]

A study has shown that the size of the suture and of the suture needle are not offenders per se in the production of suture marks. However, heavy suture material may be indirectly responsible for excessive suture tension that can lead to suture marks. If sutures are placed properly without tension and if all other causes of suture marks are eliminated, sutures that are left in longer than seven days are more likely to cause suture marks.[10]

Infection is also a major contributing factor in scar formation.[18, 26] Epithelium-lined pits and sinus tracts frequently become infected, causing stitch abscesses.[6, 58] Infection around a suture can lead to a suture mark.[26, 68] When this develops, it is best to remove the suture and treat the wound with moist dressings. This eliminates the constricting effect, removes the foreign body, increases the circulation to the area, and improves drainage.[26]

The following practices are important in minimizing scar formation: (1) relieving tension on the wound; (2) placing skin sutures near the edge of the wound; (3) removing sutures at the appropriate time; and (4) preventing infection, both during (by using an aseptic technique) and after surgery. Proper bandaging is a major factor in keeping an animal from licking and chewing a wound. It also helps prevent urinary and fecal contamination.

SUTURE REMOVAL

Many theories have been presented as to when sutures should be removed. The overall principle is to remove sutures at the earliest time that it is judged to be safe. This decision, of course, is dependent upon the surgeon's experience and judgment and factors related to the wound itself, such as the site of the wound, the line of the wound, and the tension on the wound.[50] Thus, it can be seen that no specific time can be set for suture removal.[6, 50] In general sutures should be left in longer when healing has been delayed, in weight-bearing incisions such as midline abdominal incisions, in older patients, and in wounds in which disruption is more likely (areas of tension).[3, 6] On the other hand, sutures may be removed sooner (about six or seven days postoperatively) in wounds that have healed by first intention, are supported by underlying sutures, or are in an area of slight movement or flaccid skin.[3, 6, 18]

There have been varying reports as to the effect that early suture removal has on wounds. It has been stated that by six days postoperatively a wound has not accumulated enough collagen to produce a scar with the same strength as that of the sutures holding the wound. Removal of the sutures at this time subjects the skin edges to a deforming force that is resisted only by fibrin and cells. The wound rarely breaks open at this stage; however, the width of the scar gradually increases over the next three weeks, since there is little to resist deformation other than a gelatinous intradermal matrix. Such wounds are relatively fragile and often undergo considerable changes in size and appearance during the two-to-three-week period after suture removal.[58] In contrast to this, another study revealed that wounds from which sutures were removed four days postoperatively were stronger at seven days than wounds in which the sutures had been left in place the entire seven days. The study also indicated that the increase in tensile strength was due to increased tension on the wound interface after suture removal rather than to removal of the suture itself. A histological examination demonstrated more fibroblastic proliferation when the sutures had been removed four days postoperatively.[54] The differences may be due to species variation. A controlled study in dogs and cats is necessary before any statement can be made concerning the effects of early suture removal in these species.

In order to allow earlier suture removal and yet maintain support for the wound, a compromising technique has been used: every other suture is removed from a wound early in the postoperative period, followed by removal of the remaining sutures at the prescribed time.[6, 18, 26] Varying times (three days postoperatively,[26] or five to six days postoperatively[6]) have been stated for removal of the first sutures.

In summary, sutures should be removed when the wound is sufficiently healed. Earlier removal invites dehiscence and widening of the scar. Leaving sutures in longer than necessary increases the chances of epithelium-lined tracts, infection, and scars. If there is some question about whether a wound is healed sufficiently for suture removal, a few sutures may be removed and the skin edges should be carefully tested. Thus it can be ascertained whether healing is only the result of epithelialization or whether significant fibrous protein synthesis has occurred between the dermal edges.[58]

One of two instruments may be used for removing sutures — scissors or a scalpel. In both, manipulation of the suture is basically the same. Contamination of the wound must be prevented. Ideally, the scar and the exposed portions of the suture should be painted with an antiseptic solution. The suture end is grasped and drawn straight upward from the skin. This exposes a portion of the suture buried in the skin beneath the knot. When the suture is cut at this point, only clean material is drawn through the tissue as it is removed.[3, 6] The ideal pull on the suture is *toward* the incision (Fig. 6–55).[6, 50]

When scissors are used to cut the suture, they should be sharp and should cut to the point.[50] If stainless steel wire has been used for closure, special

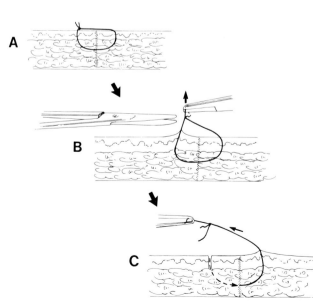

Figure 6–55: Proper technique for removing skin sutures. *A,* A skin suture in place in a healed wound. *B,* The suture end is drawn straight upward from the skin and cut below the knot. *C,* The suture is pulled *toward* the incision site for removal. (After Archibald, J., and Blakely, C. L.: Sutures, in Archibald, J. [ed.]: Canine Surgery, ed 2. Santa Barbara, Calif., American Veterinary Publications, Inc., 1974, p. 40.)

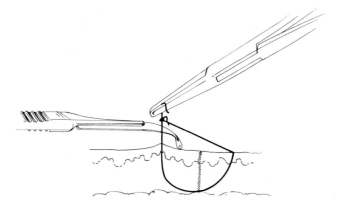

Figure 6–56: A No. 12 scalpel blade with a drop of epoxy resin on its tip being used for suture removal.

wire-cutting scissors should be used. A No. 11[40, 50] or a No. 12[40] scalpel blade may be used for suture removal. The tips of these blades may be dipped in commercial epoxy resin to make suture removal safer and more comfortable for the patient (Fig. 6–56).[40] If the surgeon questions the strength of a wound after the sutures have been removed, it is wise to bandage or protect the wound for an additional week.[50]

With regard to wound strength, it has been found that incisions that are made through a previous scar heal faster and with greater strength than do similar incisions made in unscarred skin. The amount of collagen in the final scar is less, and the appearance of the scar is better than in primary wounds of the same age.[58]

WOUND DRESSING

In veterinary surgery, a bandage plays an important role in providing a suitable atmosphere for wound healing. The purposes of a bandage are (1) to protect the wound from contamination,[70] (2) to prevent tension on the wound margins,[70] (3) to obliterate dead space,[35] (4) to supply sufficient pressure to minimize postoperative hemorrhage and edema;[6, 35, 70] (5) to restrict motion;[6, 35, 70] and (6) to prevent trauma to the wound.[6]

Bandages are relatively easy to apply to the extremities of animals but difficult to apply to the head and trunk.[35] One technique for bandaging includes the application of a nonirritant material, such as sterile gauze soaked in petroleum jelly, followed by a thick, resilient dressing that is bound loosely to preclude discomfort and constriction, and finally adhesive bandages to prevent slippage.[35] The author prefers to apply a sterile, nonadherent, perforated material,* followed by circumferential wrapping of some type of soft, rolled bandage material, and a final application of adhesive tape to cover the bandage and anchor it to the hair on either end of the bandage. When placing a dressing other than a pressure bandage on an extremity, the authors prefers to almost "hang" the bandage on the limb. To accomplish this, the topical pads and circumferential wrappings are applied with no pressure at all. Likewise, the adhesive tape is applied with no pressure. To help assure this, the strips of tape are torn prior to placing them on the bandage rather than

---

*Telfa surgical dressing, which is supplied by Kendall Hospital Products Division, Chicago.

rolling the tape directly from the roll onto the bandage. The holding power of the bandage comes from two or three strips of tape at the proximal aspect of the bandage that are well adhered to the bandage and the surrounding hair.

It is desirable to keep both the bandage and wound dry, and attempts may be made to waterproof bandages by applying rubber or plastic sheeting over the bandage. In doing so, it should be remembered that unless these materials are made watertight, they will hold any moisture that does get in. A bandage placed in a plastic bag should be checked periodically, since normal body moisture accumulates inside the bag and moistens the bandage. When well-meaning pet owners waterproof a pet's bandage by covering it with a plastic bag, they should be cautioned not to use rubber bands to secure the bag. It is possible for a rubber band to slip off the bag and to move up under the hair of the limb, remaining unnoticed until its constricting effects become visible.

Waterproofing may be accomplished by applying collodion to the wound; however, this substance should not be placed on a wound immediately after closure, since it can cause chemical irritation to the subcutaneous tissue and interpose an impregnable wall between the healing skin edges.[70]

Pressure bandages are often indicated, especially for the prevention of hematomas and postoperative edema.[50, 70] In addition to controlling these conditions, pressure bandages provide immobility and splinting, which are favorable for rapid, uneventful healing.[50] The application of these bandages requires a fine touch so that the dressing is secured tightly enough to accomplish its purpose and yet not so tightly that it impedes circulation, which can lead to severe soft tissue damage and even slough. An animal that continually licks and chews at a bandage may just be that type of animal, or such behavior may indicate a problem that is not obvious to the veterinarian.

Occasionally, plaster casts or splints of plaster, wood, aluminum, plastic, or other synthetic materials are needed to immobilize an area in order to attain good wound healing. The patient's habits and activity as well as the type and location of the wound need to be evaluated when this type of dressing is considered.[70]

The statement, "The younger and more irresponsible the patient, the larger and more secure the bandage must be,"[70] would certainly apply to animals. The veterinarian has the problem of preventing an animal from chewing at bandages and wounds. Many measures have been devised to prevent wound and bandage molestation. Such measures include muzzles, Elizabethan collars placed around an animal's neck, a plastic bucket with a hole in the bottom placed around an animal's head, and "side boards" to prevent a dog from turning and molesting the hindquarters. The application of offensive substances, such as hot pepper sauce or distasteful chemicals, to the bandage or around the wound has been used to prevent animals from molesting wounds and bandages.

Frequent evaluation of bandages is necessary, and they should be changed as needed. This is especially true when the bandage has a tendency to become wet, as this provides a favorable medium for bacterial growth. Dogs' urinating on and in bandages is a source of irritation for both the wound and the veterinarian. In the author's opinion, a bandage with dirt on the outer layer of adhesive tape but clean and dry from that point inward does not provide as great a potential for infection as does the wet bandage.

When a bandage is removed, it is not uncommon to have some adhesion between the dressing and the wound. Moistening the dressing with sterile normal saline solution and softening crusts with hydrogen peroxide facilitate bandage removal. A moist applicator stick has also been found useful in teasing a dressing away from the wound.[68]

The application of topical antibiotics to a wound is left to the discretion of the surgeon. The effects of topical antibiotics on wound healing have been covered in Chapter 4.

REFERENCES

1. Allman, F. L.: Polyglycolic acid suture in routine sports injury surgical practice. Surg. Gynecol. Obstet. *136*:607, 1973.
2. Archibald, J.: Procedures in plastic surgery. J. Am. Vet. Med. Assoc. *147*:1461, 1965.
3. Archibald, J., and Blakely, C. L.: Sutures, in Archibald, J. (ed.): Canine Surgery, ed. 2. Santa Barbara, Calif., American Veterinary Publications, Inc., 1974, pp. 35–52.
4. Auerbach, R., and Pearlstein, M. M.: A comparison of polyglycolic acid (Dexon), nylon and silk sutures in skin surgery. J. Dermatol. Surg. *1*:38, 1975.
5. Berson, M. I.: Atlas of Plastic Surgery, ed. 2. New York, Grune & Stratton, Inc., 1963.
6. Borges, A. F.: Elective Incisions and Scar Revision. Boston, Little, Brown and Co., 1973.
7. Brothwick, R.: Use of polyglycolic acid suture material. Vet. Rec. *92*:386, 1973.
8. Conolly, W. B., Hunt, T. K., Zederfeldt, B., et al.: Clinical comparison of surgical wounds closed by suture and adhesive tape. Am. J. Surg. *117*:318, 1969.
9. Converse, J. M.: Introduction to plastic surgery, in Converse, J. M. (ed.): Reconstructive Plastic Surgery: Principles and Procedures in Correction, Reconstruction, and Transplantation, ed. 2. W. B. Saunders Co., 1977, Vol. 1.
10. Crikelair, G. F.: Skin suture marks. Am. J. Surg. *96*:631, 1958.
11. Dardik, H., Dardik, I., and Laufman, H.: Clinical use of polyglycolic acid polymer as a new absorbable synthetic suture. Am. J. Surg. *121*:656, 1971.
12. Deutsch, H. L.: Observations on a new absorbable suture material. J. Dermatol. Surg. *1*:49, 1975.
13. Dixon, A. C.: The secondary closure of wounds. Vet. Rec. 75:1133, 1963.
14. Dunphy, J. E.: Wound Healing in Surgery: Proceedings of the Panel Discussion. Somerville, N.J., Ethicon, Inc., 1970, p. 27.
15. Edlich, R. F., Panek, P. H., Rodeheaver, G. T., et al.: Physical and chemical configuration of sutures in the development of surgical infection. Ann. Surg. *177*:679, 1973.
16. Ellett, E. W.: Nonsuture closure of wounds with an acrylic cohesive. Mod. Vet. Pract. *45*:46, 1964.
17. Enquist, I. F.: Wound Healing in Surgery: Proceedings of the Panel Discussion. Somerville, N.J., Ethicon, Inc., 1970, p. 10.
18. Epstein, E.: Skin Surgery. Philadelphia, Lea & Febiger, 1962.
19. The Selection, Handling and Use of Needles and Needleholders. Somerville, N.J., Ethicon, Inc., 1975.
20. Wound Closure Catalog. Somerville, N.J., Ethicon, Inc., 1975.
21. Flinn, R. M.: Knotting in medicine and surgery. Practitioner *183*:322, 1959.
22. Forrester, J. C.: Quantity and quality in wound repair, in International Symposium: Sutures in Wound Repair. Somerville, N. J., Ethicon, Inc., 1972, pp. 9–10.
23. Forrester, J. C.: Suture materials and their uses. Nurs. Mirror *140*:48, 1975.
24. Fox, M., and Young, W.: Experimental evaluation of a new synthetic polymer suture material, supramid extra. Surgery *52*:913, 1962.
25. Golden, T., Levy, A. H., and O'Connor, W. T.: Threadless suture for skin wounds and incisions. Am. J. Surg. *104*:603, 1962.
26. Grabb, W. C., and Smith, J. W.: Basic techniques of plastic surgery, in Grabb, W. C., and Smith, J. W. (eds.): Plastic Surgery: A Concise Guide to Clinical Practice. Boston, Little, Brown and Co., 1968.
27. Herrmann, J. B.: Modern surgical sutures: Their characteristics and applications, in International Symposium: Sutures in Wound Repair. Somerville, N.J., Ethicon, Inc., 1972, pp. 30–31.
28. Herrmann, J. B.: Tensile strength and knot security of surgical suture material. Am. Surg. *37*:209, 1971.
29. Herron, J.: Skin closure with subcuticular polyglycolic acid sutures. Med. J. Aust. *2*:535, 1974.
30. Howes, E. L.: Strength studies of polyglycolic acid versus catgut sutures of the same size. Surg. Gynecol. Obstet. *137*:15, 1973.
31. Howes, E. L.: The immediate strength of the sutured wound. Surgery 7:24, 1940.
32. Jackson, S.: Supramid Extra. Washington, D.C., S. Jackson, Inc.
33. Jenkins, H. P., Hrdina, L. S., Owens, F. M., et al.: Absorption of surgical gut (catgut): III. Duration in the tissue after loss of tensile strength. Arch. Surg. *45*:74, 1942.

34. Johnston, D. E.: Hygroma of the elbow in dogs. J. Am. Vet. Med. Assoc. *167*:213, 1975.
35. Johnston, D. E.: Wound healing and reconstructive surgery. Am. Anim. Hosp. Assoc. Sci. Proc. *2*:383, 1975.
36. Knecht, C. D., Welser, J. R., Allen, A. R., et al.: Fundamental Techniques in Veterinary Surgery. Philadelphia, W. B. Saunders Co., 1975.
37. Knowles, R. P.: Critique of suture materials in small animal surgery. J. Am. Anim. Hosp. Assoc. *12*:670, 1976.
38. Knowles, R. P.: Injuries to skin, muscle, and tendon, in Some Techniques and Procedures in Small Animal Surgery. Bonner Springs, Kans., Veterinary Medicine Publishing Co., Inc., 1963.
39. Koontz, A. R., and Kimberly, R. C.: Marlex — an ideal suture material. Arch. Surg. *86*:162, 1963.
40. Larsen, J. S.: Epoxy-tipped scalpel blades for removing sutures. Vet. Med. Small Anim. Clin. *66*:468, 1971.
41. Larsen, J. S., and Ulin, A. W.: Tensile strength advantage of the far-and-near suture technique. Surg. Gynecol. Obstet. *131*:123, 1970.
42, Lewis, J. R.: The Surgery of Scars. New York, McGraw-Hill Book Co. 1973.
43. Lilly, G. E., Cutcher, J. L., Jones, J. C., et al.: Reaction of oral tissue to suture materials: IV. Oral Surg. *33*:152, 1972.
44. Longo, T.: A comparative study of catgut and P.G.A. suture material, in International Symposium: Sutures in Wound Repair. Somerville, N. J., Ethicon, Inc., 1972, p. 34.
45. Madden, J. L.: Wound Healing in Surgery: Proceedings of the Panel Discussion. Somerville, N.J., Ethicon, Inc., 1970, p. 7.
46. Madsen, E. T.: An experimental and clinical evaluation of surgical suture materials. Surg. Gynecol. Obstet. *97*:73, 1956.
47. Magilligan, D. J., and DeWeese, J. A.: Knot security and synthetic suture material. Am. J. Surg. *127*:355, 1974.
48. Martyn, J. W.: Clinical experience with a synthetic absorbable surgical suture. Surg. Gynecol. Obstet. *140*:747, 1975.
49. McCashin, F.: Atraloc needles: An advancement in atraumatic, aseptic surgery. Pract. Vet. *145*:8, 1973.
50. McGregor, I. A.: Fundamental Techniques of Plastic Surgery, ed. 5. Edinburgh, Churchill Livingstone, 1972.
51. Miller, J. M.: A new era of non-absorbable sutures. Exp. Med. Surg. *28*:274, 1970.
52. Miller, J. M.: Evaluation of a new surgical suture (Prolene). Am. Surg. *39*:31, 1973.
53. Miller, J. M., Zoll, D. R., Brown, E. O., et al.: Clinical observation on the use of an extruded collagen suture. Arch. Surg. *88*:167, 1964.
54. Myers, M. B., Cherry, G., and Heinburger, S.: Augmentation of wound tensile strength by early removal of sutures. Am. J. Surg. *117*:338, 1969.
55. Myers, M. B., Combs, B., and Cohen, G.: Wound tension and wound sloughs: A negative correlation. Am. J. Surg. *109*:711, 1965.
56. Nelson, J.: Wound repair in patients following irradiation, in International Symposium: Sutures in Wound Repair. Somerville, N. J., Ethicon, Inc., 1972, p. 21.
57. Newton, C. D., Wilson, G. P., Allen, H. L., et al.: Surgical closure of elbow hygroma in the dog. J. Am. Vet. Med. Assoc. *164*:147, 1974.
58. Peacock, E. E., Jr., and Van Winkle, W.: Surgery and Biology of Wound Repair. Philadelphia, W. B. Saunders Co., 1970.
59. Postlethwait, R. W.: Long-term comparative study of non-absorbable sutures. Ann. Surg. *171*:892, 1970.
60. Postlethwait, R. W.: Polyglycolic acid surgical suture. Arch. Surg. *101*:489, 1970.
61. Postlethwait, R. W.: Wound Healing in Surgery: Proceedings of the Panel Discussion. Somerville, N.J., Ethicon, Inc., 1970, p. 8.
62. Pullen, C. M.: Reconstruction of the skin, in Bojrab, M. J. (ed.): Current Techniques in Small Animal Surgery. Philadelphia, Lea & Febiger, 1975.
63. Rickards, D. A.: An adjustable suture: A technique for altering the tension of stitches postoperatively, especially in third-lid flaps. Vet. Med. Small Anim. Clin. *68*:880, 1973.
64. Rose, T. F.: Skin closure with subcuticular polyglycolic acid sutures. Med. J. Aust. *627*:146, 1975.
65. Schilling, J. A.: Wound Healing in Surgery: Proceedings of the Panel Discussion. Somerville, N. J., Ethicon, Inc., 1970, p. 10.
66. Smithcors, J. F.: New methods of skin closure. Mod. Vet. Pract. *47*:118, 1966.
67. Snyder, C. C.: On the history of the suture. Plast. Reconstr. Surg. *58*:401, 1976.
68. Stark, R. B.: Plastic surgery. New York, Harper & Row Publishers, Inc., 1962.
69. Stashak, T. S.: Reconstructive surgery in the horse. J. Am. Vet. Med. Assoc. *170*:143, 1977.
70. Straith, R. E., Lawson, J. M., and Hipps, J. C.: The subcuticular suture. Postgrad. Med. *29*:164, 1961.
71. Swaim, S. F.: A "walking" suture technique for closure of large skin defects in the dog and cat. J. Am. Anim. Hosp. Assoc. *12*:597, 1976.

72. Swaim, S. F.: Isolated peripheral nerves, in Bojrab, M. J. (Ed.): Current Techniques in Small Animal Surgery. Philadelphia, Lea & Febiger, 1975.
73. Taylor, T. L.: Suture material: A comprehensive review of the literature. J. Am. Podiatry Assoc. 65:649, 1975.
74. Treat, L. A.: Wire suturing technique for the repair of large wounds in horses. Vet. Med. Small Anim. Clin. 64:76, 1969.
75. Usher, F. C.: Braided Marlex suture. Arch. Surg. 83:203, 1961.
76. Usher, F. C., Allen, J. E., Crosthwait, R. W., et al.: Polyprolene monofilament: A new biologically inert suture for closing contaminated wounds. J.A.M.A. 179:780, 1962.
77. Wallace, W. R., Maxwell, G. R., and Cavalaris, C. J.: Comparison of polyglycolic acid suture to black silk, chromic, and plain catgut in human oral tissues. J. Oral Surg. 28:739, 1970.
78. Zovickian, A.: Closure of soft tissue surface wounds, surgical and traumatic, in Cooper, P. (ed.): The Craft of Surgery, ed. 2. Boston, Little, Brown and Co., 1971, vol. 1.

7

MOVING LOCAL TISSUES TO CLOSE SURFACE DEFECTS

INTRODUCTION

The veterinarian has an advantage over the physician in correcting skin defects, since the skin of small animals is elastic and abundant, with ample hair.[17] These qualities enable the veterinarian to perform the simplest form of transplant, viz., the sliding of skin over a defect by direct traction.[22] In this way many defects can be repaired merely by undermining and directly approximating the wound's edges.[17, 26] Small skin defects can frequently be closed following simple excision of the denuded or scarred area and suturing of the skin's edges. Undermining and sliding the skin or relaxing incisions are needed for closure of larger lesions. Still larger defects or defects that are in certain areas (e.g., around the eyes, ears, anogenital area, or distal limbs) may require skin grafts or pedicle flaps for adequate closure.[3] The skin on the head, neck, trunk, and proximal aspects of the limbs of small animals is relatively mobile and lends itself readily to the primary closure of most lesions (Fig. 7–1). Because this type of reconstruction is accomplished with such ease, it is preferred to the more complicated techniques.[22] It has been stated that lesions of the thoracic skin that are smaller than 3×3 in. will close completely in three to five weeks with very little

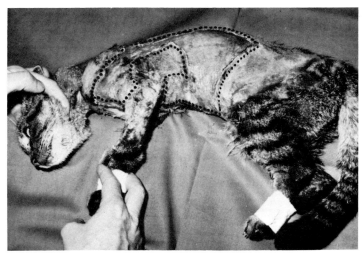

Figure 7–1: A large, open, infected wound (inside dotted line) resulting from an automobile accident.

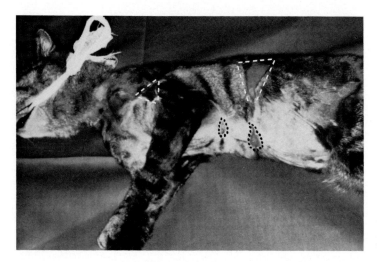

Figure 7–2. The result of the wound (inside dotted lines) in Figure 7–1 healing by contraction and epithelialization.

scarring as a result of the looseness of the skin in this area.[14] In the author's experience, lesions that are larger than this on the trunk of a dog or cat heal remarkably well. However, in some large wounds healing progresses to a certain extent and ceases. The main reason for performing primary closure on large wounds is to avoid the long waiting period and the inconvenience of treating an open wound. In some cases, owing to a lack of available skin, it is necessary to let large lesions on the trunk heal and contract as much as possible before undertaking surgical closure (Figs. 7–1 and 7–2).

TENSION LINES

As stated by Kraissl, a report was published in 1861 on the presence and patterns of tension lines within the skin of human cadavers.[18] This report was the result of a study in which multiple cutaneous stab wounds had been made over the body. Further work was performed on this topic in the 20th century, and in 1941 a report stated that connective tissue in the skin is oriented in parallel sheets or strands, with lesser amounts of connective tissue arranged at right angles to these. These sheets or strands run in the lines of increased tension, thus forming lines of cleavage.[9]

When a blade cuts the skin, it is the tension of the skin that causes the skin edges to separate. Skin tension is also the force that pulls on a linear scar, causing it to widen. At times this tension may stimulate the scar and cause it to hypertrophy. In most areas of the body there is skin tension in all directions; however, the degree of tension is greatest in one direction.[5]

In 1951 a study was conducted to determine the difference between tension lines and wrinkle lines in the skin. The former were believed to be the result of static forces being exerted on the skin of a cadaver, whereas wrinkle lines were stated to be the result of dynamic forces acting on living skin.[18] Wrinkle lines were found to run uniformly at right angles to the action of the muscles upon which they were dependent for their formation.[12, 18] Gravity was also found to have an influence on these lines.[18]

Tension lines have been studied in dogs (cadavers and anesthetized animals) by making multiple cutaneous stab wounds over various parts of the body and noting the predominant direction in which the long axis of the stab wounds becomes oriented within an area. These lines were mapped on the cadavers and on outline drawings. There was general agreement with regard to the main features of tension lines in the dog (Figs. 7–3A through C).[13] It has been stated that the stripes of the zebra and the tiger follow a pattern similar to the resting skin tension lines on most parts of their body.[5] It must be kept in mind that differences in breed, sex, age,[13] and body conformation[9] will affect tension lines.

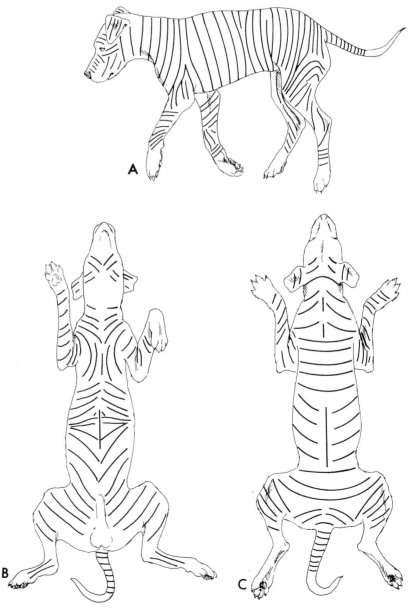

Figure 7–3: A, Lateral, B, ventral, and C, dorsal views of a dog showing the direction of the skin tension lines. (From Irwin, D. H. G.: Tension lines in the skin of the dog. J. Small Anim. Pract., 7:595 and 596, 1966.)

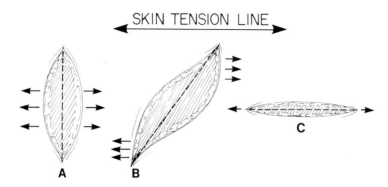

SKIN TENSION LINE

A   B   C

Figure 7–4: Degree and shape of divergence of skin edges with incisions made at different angles to the skin tension lines. Broken line in the center of each wound shows the direction of the original incision. *A*, An incision made perpendicular to skin tension lines tends to gape widely. *B*, An incision made at an angle to skin tension lines tends to take a curvilinear shape. *C*, An incision made parallel to skin tension lines tends to gape minimally. (After Borges, A. F.: Elective Incisions and Scar Revision. Boston, Little, Brown and Co., 1975, p. 14.)

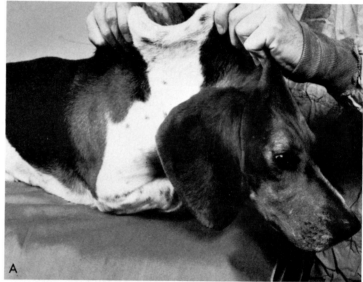

A

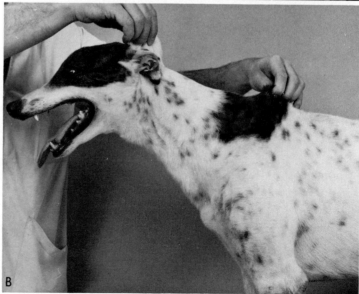

B

Figure 7–5: Tension line–incision line relationships are not as critical when there is an abundance of skin, *A*, as when there is not a great abundance of skin, *B*.

Based on studies that were performed on humans, there appear to be two factors involved in skin lines: (1) tension lines and (2) wrinkle lines of the skin. The term *tension line* seems to be more applicable for the veterinary surgeon in that dogs have few, if any, wrinkles as they are thought of in humans.[13] Gravity and muscle activity also have some effect on the dog's skin. Since the cutaneous muscles are better developed in dogs than they are in humans, they exert a greater physical action than does gravity.[13]

Knowledge of the general pattern of tension lines may be beneficial to the veterinary surgeon in that incisions that are made in these lines gape minimally, and, when closed, the wounds heal better and faster and with more aesthetic results. Incisions that are made across tension lines tend to gape widely, are subject to greater tension, require more sutures for coaptation, and are inclined to result in wider scars (Fig. 7–4).[5, 13] In addition, the veterinary surgeon must bear in mind that breed, age, sex, muscle mass, and adiposity are going to greatly influence the relationship between tension lines and incision lines. For example, the tension line–incision line relationship would be more critical in a greyhound, in which skin is not in great abundance, than in a basset hound, in which skin is quite abundant (Figs. 7–5A and B).

ADVANCING SKIN INTO PLACE

After a wound has been excised and the surrounding skin has been undermined, it is necessary to move the tissues into place over the lesion. Various types of tension sutures have been described and discussed in Chapter 6.

ECHELON SUTURES

This type of suture has been advocated for wound closure because it decreases the incidence of wound disruption, promotes faster healing, and reduces the occurrence of herniation through abdominal wounds.[21] It is possible that this type of suture could be modified for use in large open wounds to distribute tension and to advance tissue toward the center of the wound. To appose fasciae (or the deeper structures in a large wound), vertical mattress sutures are placed to form outer and inner echelons. If there is a distinct fascial layer within the wound, the edges of the fascia may be closed with simple interrupted sutures. A second set of outer- and inner-echelon sutures is placed through the skin and subcutaneous tissues to draw the wound edges closer together, and the final closure is accomplished by placing simple interrupted sutures to approximate the wound edges (Fig. 7–6). Stainless steel wire has been described for such sutures, utilizing heavier gauge wire for the echelon sutures and finer gauge wire for the simple interrupted sutures.[21] The more superficially placed echelon and simple interrupted sutures would be removed when wound healing is complete. However, the deeper echelon and simple interrupted sutures would remain in situ.

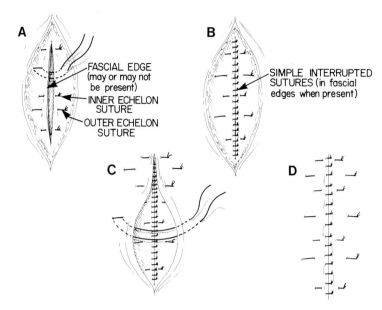

A —FASCIAL EDGE (may or may not be present)
—INNER ECHELON SUTURE
—OUTER ECHELON SUTURE

B —SIMPLE INTERRUPTED SUTURES (in fascial edges when present)

C

D

Figure 7–6: Placement of outer and inner echelon sutures and apposition sutures to close gaping, deep wounds. *A*, Placement of echelon sutures in a deep fascial layer. *B*, Placement of simple interrupted sutures in a deep fascial layer. *C*, Placement of echelon sutures in the skin. *D*, Completed skin suturing with echelon and simple interrupted sutures. (After Smithcors, J. F.: New methods of wound closure. Mod. Vet. Pract. *47*:123, 1966.)

"WALKING" SUTURES

A "walking" suture technique has recently been described as a means of moving skin over a defect.[26] This technique (1) provides a means of moving skin from the area around a wound to cover the wound, (2) obliterates dead space, and (3) evenly distributes tension to the tissues around the wound. The movement of skin to cover a defect is advantageous from the standpoint of reducing the time and special care that are needed for treating large open wounds by skin grafting or for allowing them to heal by wound contraction. The obliteration of dead space helps to reduce the possibility of hematoma formation. The even distribution of tension to the tissues around a wound rather than the concentration of tension by placing tension sutures within a few centimeters of the wound's edge may also be advantageous in helping to prevent wound disruption. If the surgeon so desires, any of the previously described tension suture techniques may be used in conjunction with the walking suture technique.

The principle of the walking suture technique is to move skin from peripheral areas toward the center or toward one side of the wound. The skin around the wound is undermined. Using absorbable suture material (2–0 or 3–0 chromic catgut or polyglycolic acid sutures*) with a swaged needle, the surgeon starts on one side of the wound near the junction of the skin with the underlying tissue. A bite is taken in the deepest portion of the dermis with the needle. By observing the deep portion of the dermis, the incorporation of large blood vessels into the suture can be avoided, thus assuring an adequate blood supply to the skin. This suture does not penetrate the full thickness of the skin. Instead of taking the second bite directly below the first one, the suture is easily advanced toward the center of the wound (Figs. 7–7*B* and 7–8). The elasticity of the skin is utilized in tying the suture, and the skin is

---

*Dexon is available from Davis and Geck (Lederle-Cyanamid), Pearl River, NY 10965.

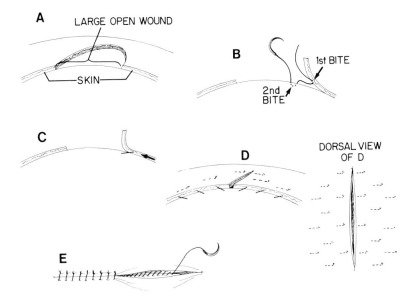

Figure 7-7: *A*, A large open wound. *B*, Placement of a walking suture in the deep layer of the dermis and underlying fascia. The first bite of the suture does not penetrate the full thickness of the skin. *C*, Slight advancement of skin over the wound as the suture is tied. *D*, Almost complete closure of the wound after placement of walking sutures. (Broken lines indicate sutures are under the skin and not seen). *E*, Placement of a simple continuous intradermal suture and simple interrupted skin sutures. (After Swaim, S. F.: A "walking" suture technique for closure of large skin defects in the dog and cat. Am. Anim. Hosp. Assoc. *12*:598, 1976.)

moved slightly toward the center or, if only one side is to be advanced, toward the other side of the wound (Fig. 7–7*C*). The surgeon continues to place walking sutures across the wound, thereby "walking" the surrounding skin over the defect. If the wound is to be closed from two sides, the same procedure is repeated on the opposite side of the wound, resulting in almost complete closure (Figs. 7–7*D*, 7–9, and 7–10).

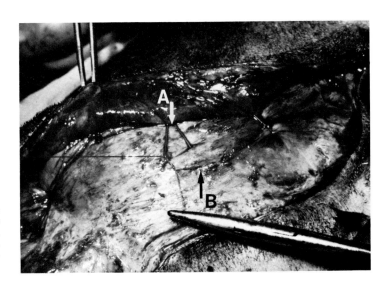

Figure 7-8: Placement of a walking suture. *A*, The first bite is in the deeper dermis. *B*, The second bite is in the underlying fascia toward the center of the wound.

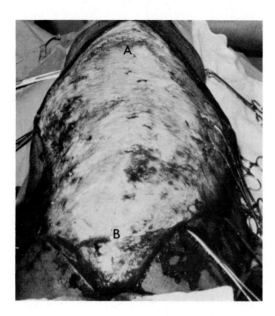

Figure 7–9: Large open wound on a dog's back. *A*, Area between the scapulae. *B*, Area between the ilial wings.

A simple continuous intradermal or subcuticular suture is placed along the wound's edge to close any dead space in this area and to more closely approximate the wound edges. Final closure of the skin for a cosmetic result is accomplished with simple interrupted nonabsorbable sutures that are placed close to the skin's edges. There is no tension on these sutures (Fig. 7–7E). Walking sutures may also be used to move advancement and transposition flaps into place.[26] A similar type of suture that is called the

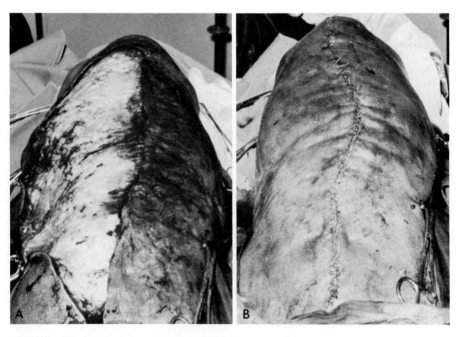

Figure 7–10: *A*, Skin from one side has been walked halfway across the lesion. *B*, Skin from the opposite side has been walked halfway across the lesion.

creeping advancement suture has been described for moving skin flaps into place in humans.[7]

CORRECTION OF VARIOUS-SHAPED DEFECTS

After excising a lesion to prepare the site for accepting skin from the surrounding area, the skin may contract in such a way as to leave a defect with a specific geometrical shape or one that can easily be converted to such a shape. In some instances (usually with smaller lesions), the surgeon may elect to initially excise the lesion in a manner that will create a geometrical shape. A discussion of the various techniques that are available to the surgeon for correcting certain geometrically shaped lesions follows.

FUSIFORM DEFECTS

As a point of geometrical interest, the configuration that is commonly referred to in the surgical literature as an ellipse is actually a lenticular configuration (i.e., shaped like a biconvex lens). A true ellipse is oval.[5, 15] Another term for lenticular is fusiform.[5] For the sake of accuracy, the term fusiform will be used in this text.

A large majority of skin lesions, both large and small, can be corrected by fusiform excision. This shape lends itself well to cosmetic closure, since it readily adapts to a straight line.[28] The technique for fusiform excision has been described in varying detail by several authors.[3, 8, 11, 12, 16, 21, 28]

When planning a fusiform excision in an area where the direction of the tension lines is uncertain, it would be wise to use a circular excision. Then, by noting the long axis of the defect that is created by the adjacent tension lines, the long axis of the fusiform excision can be determined and the wound may be remodeled as needed to create the desired fusiform shape (Fig. 7–11).[12] In excising two nearby lesions, the surgeon should not attempt to include both lesions in one fusiform excision, unless they are close together or unless they both follow the same skin tension line.[4]

To accomplish closure of a fusiform defect with cosmetic results, the length-width ratio must be taken into account. Various length-width ratios have been stated in the literature, including from 2.5 to 3:1, 3:1, and 4:1

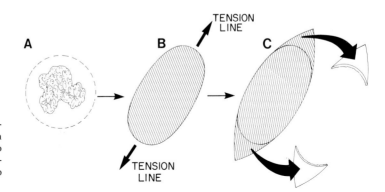

Figure 7–11: *A*, Circular excision of a lesion. *B*, Skin tension lines tend to pull the circle into an ellipse. *C*, The ellipse is converted into a fusiform shape to facilitate wound closure.

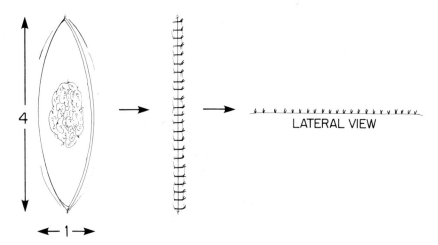

Figure 7–12: A 4:1 length-width ratio on a fusiform defect results in a smooth closure without dog-ears. (After Swaim, S. F.: Management and reconstruction of traumatized skin. Vet. Audio Review. Pacific Palisades, Calif. Vol. 7, 1978.)

Figure 7–13: A 2:1 length-width ratio on a fusiform defect results in dog-ears when closed. (After Swaim, S. F.: Management and reconstruction of traumatized skin, in Vet. Audio Review. Pacific Palisades, Calif., Vol. 7, 1978.)

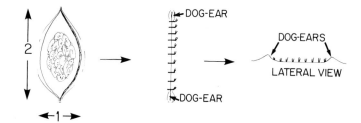

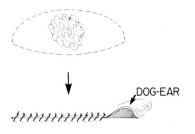

Figure 7–14: Dog-ear resulting from one side of a fusiform lesion being longer than the other. (After Grabb, W. C., and Smith, J. W.: Basic techniques of Plastic Surgery, in Plastic Surgery: A Concise Guide to Clinical Practice. Boston, Little, Brown and Co., 1968, p. 8.)

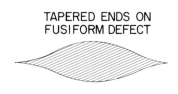

Figure 7–15: Prevention of dog-ears by tapering the ends of a fusiform defect. (After Stashak, T. S.: Reconstruction surgery in the horse. Am. Vet. Med. Assoc. 170:144, 1977.)

(Fig. 7–12).[11, 12, 28] The ratio will vary, depending on the part of the body that is involved. It is best to remember that if the long axis becomes too short, its sides form too great an angle with one another, and excess bunching of the skin results when the defect is sutured. This bunching of skin is called a "dog-ear" (Fig. 7–13). A dog-ear can also result if one side of the fusiform defect is much longer than the other (i.e., one side of the fusiform defect approaches a semicircle and the other side is a straight line) (Fig. 7–14). Dog-ears tend to flatten over a period of several months, but they can be eliminated through excision at the time of surgery.[12] In addition to maintaining an adequate length-width ratio, dog-ears may be prevented by tapering the ends of the fusiform defect when excising the lesion (Fig. 7–15).[6, 24] To help prevent dog-ears at the ends of long incisions, the middle of the proposed incision may be marked perpendicular to its long axis with a slight scratch of a scalpel blade or with marking ink. When closing the incision, the marked area is sutured first, and closure progresses toward the ends of the incision from this point.

The ideal technique for performing a fusiform excision begins by outlining the ellipse with methylene blue.[12] This is especially helpful if a large lesion is to be excised because it helps to assure that the sides of the fusiform defect will be symmetrical. The incision sites may also be marked by scratching the skin's surface with the back of a scalpel blade.[11] Before beginning the excision, tension should be exerted on the surrounding skin to stretch it. This prevents false cuts and aids the surgeon in following the lines of excision more accurately.[12, 23] Incising the midportion of both incisions before incising the ends also aids in making accurate cuts. The tissues are firm at the beginning of the procedure and thus facilitate a clean perpendicular cut. If one side were to be cut completely before the other side, the latter could become flaccid and difficult to incise properly.[5] However, one side may be completely incised and then supported by instrument traction while the opposite side is cut.[23] A No. 15 blade is used to cut through the skin at right angles to its surface so that vertical margins can be approximated in the closure. For a meticulous excision, a No. 11 blade may be used to cut the ends of the fusiform defect. This helps to prevent "X"-shaped "over cuts" at the ends of the defect.[12, 28] Another way to prevent over cuts is to incise from, not toward, the ends of the fusiform defect.[23] One end of the tissue that is to be removed is then elevated, along with a layer of subcutaneous adipose tissue ranging from 3 to 4 mm. in thickness. This tissue is then dissected away from its bed (Figs. 7–16A and B).[12, 28] The same technique is used for scar tissue removal except for the dissection, which is described in Chapter 6.

If undermining of the surrounding tissue is necessary to facilitate closure, the skin on either side of the fusiform defect should be undermined for a distance that is at least equal to the transverse measurement of the defect. This is followed by a two-layered closure of the wound (Figs. 7–16C and D).[12] Closing a large defect may require walking sutures in addition to the subcuticular and skin approximation sutures. If a fusiform excision is perpendicular to skin tension lines, the defect will gape more than if the excision is parallel to the tension lines. If the excision is oblique to the tension lines, it will assume an "S"-shaped curve.[5]

A modification of the fusiform excision has been described for correcting fusiform depressions. This technique, known as Poulard's technique, entails making a fusiform incision around a depressed scar, removing the

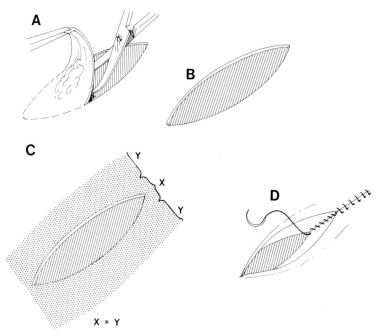

Figure 7–16: Removal of a fusiform lesion followed by closure. *A,* Scissors remove skin and a layer of subcutaneous adipose tissue from 3 to 4 mm. thick. *B,* Fusiform defect. *C,* Undermining on either side of defect equal to the width of the defect. (X indicates the width of the defect, and Y, the width of undermining on either side of the defect.) *D,* Wound closure.

epithelium from the scar tissue, and closing the skin's edges over the remaining dermal scar. This creates a buttress effect to prevent recurrence of the depression.[5]

Correction of Dog-Ears

Dog-ears are not an uncommon phenomenon in reconstructive surgery of the skin. Not only do they occur at the ends of fusiform defects, but they also occur when other geometrically shaped defects are closed and when various types of flaps are moved into position. It is important for the surgeon to be familiar with the various techniques for correcting them.

Wounds are generally sutured until the elevations of a dog-ear become pronounced; then one of several means may be used to correct the dog-ear. One method includes extending the original incision through the dog-ear. The two triangles of skin thus created are excised to produce a flat incision line that can be closed cosmetically (Fig. 7–17). Another technique entails incising the dog-ear along one side of its base, defining the large triangle of skin that is produced, and cutting it off. This results in a flat closure that is slightly curved.[19, 24] If this type of correction is used on both ends of a defect, the shape of the scar will be governed by the direction in which the curves are made. By curving the incisions in opposite directions, an "S"-shaped scar results. Curving the incisions in the same direction creates a "C"-shaped scar (Fig. 7–18).[28] The presence of a curve at the end of an

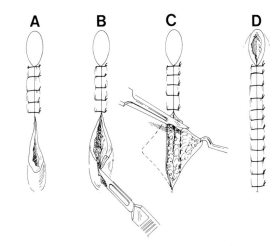

Figure 7–17: *A*, Dog-ear at the end of a defect. *B*, Extending the original incision through the dog-ear. *C*, Excision of the resultant triangles of skin. One triangle has already been excised (*dotted line*). *D*, Smooth closure of the area. The second dog-ear is removed in the same fashion. (After Swaim, S. F.: Management and reconstruction of traumatized skin, in Vet. Audio Review. Pacific Palisades, Calif. Vol. 7, 1978.)

incision and the direction of that curve could be important when that end of the defect lies close to another structure (e.g., eye, nose, ear, anus) (Fig. 7–19*A*). It is wise to suture from one end of a wide excision so that only one dog-ear will result.[11] This is particularly important in defects in which one end lies close to one of the aforementioned structures. In this situation, the defect should be closed by starting near the structure and suturing away from it. Thus, the dog-ear that develops is at a distance from the structure and can be removed without affecting that structure (Fig. 7–19*B*).

Other methods of correcting dog-ears include extending the fusiform defect[11, 12, 28] or removing a "V" of skin from one side of the dog-ear.[11] An arrowhead-shaped section of skin may also be removed in the area of a dog-ear, which will result in a "Y"-shaped closure (Fig. 7–20*A*, *B*, and *C*).

In incisions in which a dog-ear results from one side of the incision being longer than the other, it can be corrected by making a short right-angle incision at the end of the fusiform defect. The excess skin that overlaps the wound edge can be trimmed away to permit wound closure in the shape of an "L" (Fig. 7–20*D*).[12]

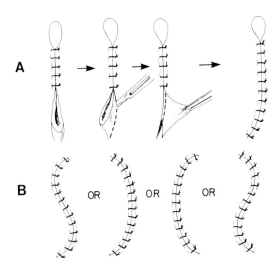

Figure 7–18: *A*, Incising a dog-ear along one side of its base, defining the large triangle of skin that is produced, cutting it off, and closing the wound smoothly. *B*, The various-shaped scars that can be created by removing dog-ears by this technique. (After McGregor, I. A.: Fundamental Techniques of Plastic Surgery, ed. 5. Edinburgh, Churchill Livingstone, 1972, p. 26.)

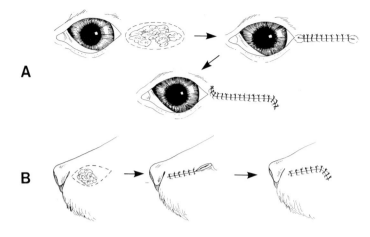

A

B

Figure 7–19: *A*, Fusiform removal of a lesion near the lateral canthus of an eye, with dog-ear removal in such a manner as to prevent invasion of the lateral canthus. *B*, Fusiform removal of a lesion near the nose, with closure beginning near the nose and dog-ear correction beginning away from the nose.

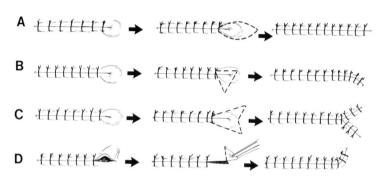

Figure 7–20: Techniques for removing dog-ears at the ends of wounds. *A*, Extension of the fusiform defect. *B*, Removal of a "V" of skin from one side of the dog-ear. *C*, Removal of an arrowhead-shaped section of skin from the area of the dog-ear. *D*, Right-angle incision at the end of the wound, and removal of excess skin when one side of the wound is longer than the other. (*B*, After Epstein, E.: Skin Surgery. Philadelphia, Lea & Febiger, 1962, p. 62. *A*, *C*, and *D*, After Grabb, W. C., and Smith, J. W.: Basic techniques of plastic surgery, in Plastic Surgery: A Concise Guide to Clinical Practice. Boston, Little, Brown and Co., 1968, p. 8.)

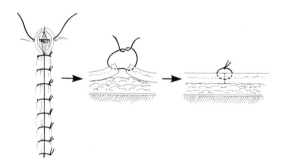

Figure 7–21: Technique for correcting *small* dog-ears. The suture is passed through the upper half of the skin. When tied, the dog-ear flattens. (After Archibald, J., and Blakely, C. L.: Sutures, in Archibald, J. (ed.): Canine Surgery, ed. 2. Santa Barbara, Calif., American Veterinary Publications, Inc., 1974, p. 47.)

Figure 7–22: Closure of a square defect from the corners to the center, resulting in an "X"-shaped scar. (After Cawley, A. J., and Archibald, J.: Plastic Surgery, in Archibald, J. (ed.): Canine Surgery, ed. 2. Santa Barbara, Calif., American Veterinary Publications, Inc., 1974, p. 146.)

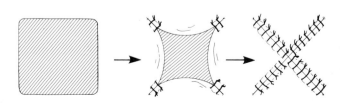

A technique that does not require excision for correcting small dog-ears entails passing a suture through the upper half of the skin that is involved in the dog-ear. As the suture is tied, the dog-ear is flattened.[2] This technique, of course, would be used only if the dog-ear were small (Fig. 7–21).

SQUARE DEFECTS

Square defects may be closed in one of two ways. One technique involves closing the defect from its corners toward its center by the alternate placement of simple interrupted sutures. This results in an "X"-shaped scar (Fig. 7–22).[8, 16, 21] Slight skin elevations at the ends of the "X" usually accompany such a closure; however, these are not large enough to be called dog-ears and will usually disappear in time. The second method of closure involves moving two single pedicle advancement flaps over the lesion in an H-plasty technique, which is discussed in Chapter 8.

RECTANGULAR DEFECTS

Several techniques have been described for the closure of rectangular wounds.[3, 8, 16, 21, 22] The two techniques that have been described for the closure of square wounds are applicable to rectangular wounds also. However, when a rectangular wound is closed from the corners, a double "Y"-shaped scar results. Other techniques for closing rectangular wounds entail converting the lesion to other related shapes before closure is begun (Fig. 7–23).[3]

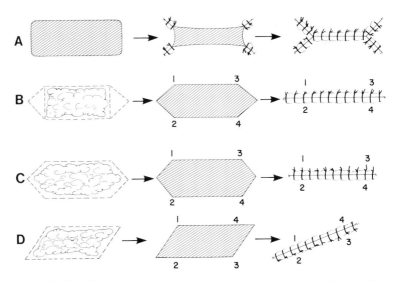

Figure 7–23: Various means of closing rectangular defects. A, Closure from the corners toward the center results in a double "Y" shaped scar. B, C, and D, Other techniques for closure of rectangular wounds convert the lesion to other related shapes. Numbers indicate points that are sutured together (1 to 2 and 3 to 4). (A, After Crawley, A. J., and Archibald, J.: Plastic Surgery, in Archibald, J. (ed.): Canine Surgery, ed. 2. Santa Barbara, Calif., American Veterinary Publications, Inc., 1974, p. 146. B, C, and D, After Berson, M. I.: Atlas of Plastic Surgery, ed. 2. New York, Grune & Stratton, Inc., 1963, pp. 9 and 12.)

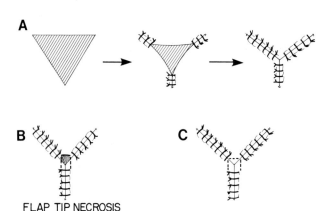

Figure 7–24: *A,* Closure of a triangular defect from the corners to the centers will result in a "Y"-shaped scar. *B,* An interrupted horizontal mattress suture at the tip of the flap may result in flap tip necrosis. *C,* A modified three-point suture (half-buried horizontal mattress) may be used to prevent flap tip necrosis. (*A,* After Cawley, A. J., and Archibald, J.: Plastic surgery, in Archibald, J. (ed.): Canine Surgery, ed. 2. Santa Barbara, Calif., American Veterinary Publications, Inc., 1974, p. 144. *C,* After McGregor, I. A.: Fundamental Techniques in Plastic Surgery, ed. 5. Edinburgh, Churchill Livingstone, 1972, p. 25.)

TRIANGULAR AND WEDGE-SHAPED DEFECTS

When excision results in a triangular defect that is not near free margins, such as those of the lips and eyelids, the defect may be closed in a manner similar to that for the closure of square and rectangular wounds. Suturing begins at the angles of the triangle and progresses toward its center, resulting in a "Y"-shaped scar.[3, 8, 16, 21, 22] At the juncture of the suture lines, a modified three-point suture that is half buried may be used to prevent necrosis of the skin in the center of the "Y" (Fig. 7–24).[5, 19] As with square and rectangular closures, this technique results in slight elevations of skin at the ends of the "Y" that usually disappear with time. Triangular lesions may also be closed by various forms of advancement flaps, as described in Chapter 8.

Numerous techniques have been described for the reconstruction of eyelids and lips; however, the following material deals with the use of wedge excisions in correcting lesions that are on or adjacent to the free margins of skin, such as those of the lips and eyelids. The technique that is used to excise and suture such lesions will depend upon whether the lesion fully penetrates the structure.

One technique for the excision of a lesion that does not fully penetrate the eyelid involves splitting the lid along a line just rostral to the meibomian glands with a No. 15 scalpel blade. The depth of splitting is dependent upon the size of the lesion, but it should be approximately even with the most ventral portion of the lesion. After the lid has been split, the le-

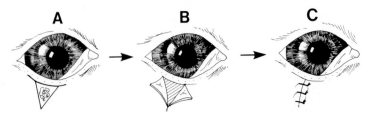

Figure 7–25: *A,* Triangular excision of a lesion that is on but does not fully penetrate the eyelid. The lid is split just rostral to the meibomian glands, and a triangle is designed on the lid that includes the lesion. *B,* The lesion is removed in the triangle of skin, and the skin edges are undermined. *C,* The wound edges are closed with simple interrupted sutures of fine silk. (After Wilder, D. T., and Albert, R. A.: Excision of tumors of the eyelids. Auburn Vet. *31*:53 and 54, 1975.)

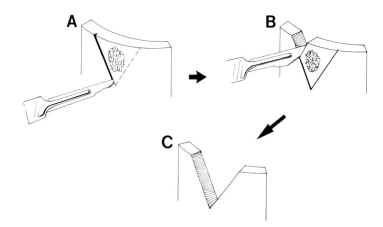

Figure 7–26: Wedge excision of a full-thickness lesion on a surface with a free margin. *A,* The wedge is outlined and *only* the skin is incised with a No. 15 blade. *B,* A No. 11 blade is used to cut through the remaining tissue with a sawing motion. *C,* A wedge-shaped defect results.

sion (tumor) is removed in a triangle of skin, with the apex pointing away from the lid margin. The remaining wound edges are undermined to provide elasticity, and the skin edges are approximated with simple interrupted sutures of fine silk (Fig. 7–25).[27]

One technique that has been described for the removal of full-thickness wedges from areas with free margins begins by outlining the wedge with methylene blue. A No. 15 scalpel blade is then used to incise through the skin surface only. The tissue is held firmly on either side of the wedge so that the point of a No. 11 blade can be passed completely through the tissues, which are then cut with a sawing motion (Fig. 7–26).[12] The initial outlining incision helps to prevent distortion of the skin, which might occur if the wedge were excised with a full-thickness excision. Such distortion could result in a less than cosmetic skin closure.

Lesions on the lips lend themselves to wedge excision. It has been stated that as much as one third of the lower lip[12, 19] and one fourth of the upper lip[12] in humans can be removed (not simultaneously) and the wound can still be closed primarily. Because of the anatomy of the dog, the upper lip lends itself more readily to wedge excision than the lower lip. Full-thickness excision of the lip can be accomplished in the manner previously described.

Closure of full-thickness wedge excisions is done in layers. A technique that has been described for lip closure involves closing the mucomuscular layer with vertical mattress sutures and tying the knots on the mucosal surface. The skin is closed with simple interrupted sutures (Fig. 7–27).[19] Three-layered closures have also been described.[1, 12] When using this type of layered closure on lips, the author prefers that the deepest layer not penetrate

Figure 7–27: A technique for closure of full-thickness wedge excisions of the upper lip. *A,* Interrupted vertical mattress sutures in the mucomuscular layer with the knots on the mucosal surface. *B,* Simple interrupted sutures in the skin. (After McGregor, I. A.: Fundamental Techniques in Plastic Surgery, ed. 5. Edinburgh, Churchill Livingstone, 1972, p. 167.)

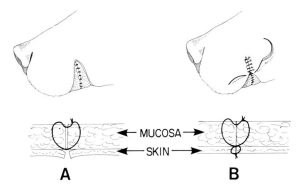

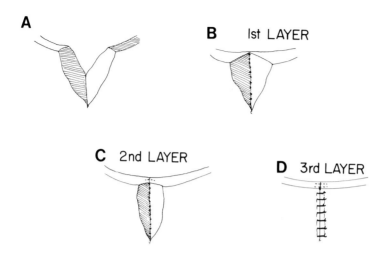

Figure 7–28: *A*, A full-thickness wedge defect of an eyelid. *B* and *C*, Layered closure of the eyelid with simple interrupted 5–0 catgut sutures in the conjunctiva, tarsal plate, and orbicular muscle layers, *D*, Simple interrupted 5–0 to 6–0 silk skin sutures. (After Albert, R. A., and Wilder, D. T.: Repair of lacerations of the eyelids. Auburn Vet., *31*:11 and 30, 1974.)

the mucosa and go only as deep as the submucosa. One technique for eyelid closure in the dog requires closure of the conjunctiva with simple interrupted sutures of 5–0 catgut. The sutures are placed so that the knots are contained within the tissues of the eyelid and are not against the cornea. In larger dogs or dogs with thicker lids, a second layer of simple interrupted catgut sutures is used to approximate the tarsal plate and orbicular muscle area. Skin approximation is accomplished with simple interrupted sutures of 5–0 or 6–0 silk (Fig. 7–28).[1] Blepharoplasty is discussed in detail in Chapter 11. The technique can also be used for closure of wedge excisions on the lips, using 2–0 or 3–0 beige, polyglycolic acid sutures in the submucosa — muscular layers and 4–0 polypropylene sutures in the skin.

CHEVRON-SHAPED DEFECTS

It is not uncommon to encounter "V"-shaped wounds, and in some of these wounds part of the flap may have been lost or will have to be trimmed off as a result of necrosis. The resulting chevron-shaped lesion may be closed in the form of a "Y." The flap is usually free and does not require undermining. The skin on each side of the chevron should be undermined. Starting at the point of the chevron, the two sides are drawn together to form the stem of the "Y." Suturing is continued as far as possible without causing too much tension. The remainder of the lesion is closed to form the arms of the "Y."[10] The suture at the junction of the three lines should be a modified three-point suture that is half buried (Fig. 7–29).[19]

In the case of a long, narrow, "V"-shaped wound, it may be wise to amputate the entire flap of skin, transform the wound to an elliptical shape, and close it accordingly. An alternative would be to amputate the flap and to close the defect that remains in the form of a "Y" (Fig. 7–30).[20]

When dealing with a loose flap of skin, the size and position of the flap as well as the length of time since injury may be important factors with regard to the flap's blood supply. A large ventrally based flap that has folded back on itself as a result of gravity may have an impaired circulation owing to the kinking of blood vessels at its base, especially if the flap has been present for any length of time (Fig. 7–31). The surgeon should evalu-

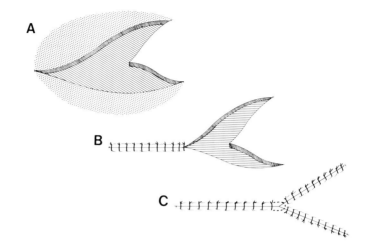

Figure 7–29: Closure of a chevron-shaped lesion. *A,* The skin edges are undermined. *B,* Suturing the two sides from the base of the chevron. *C,* Completed closure of the two arms of the "Y" and a modified three-point suture (half-buried horizontal mattress) at the junction of the three lines. (*A* and *C,* After Dixon, A. C.: The secondary closure of wounds. Vet. Rec. 75:1140, 1963.)

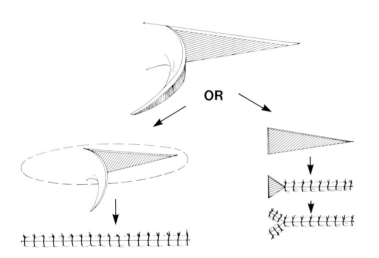

Figure 7–30: Long, narrow "V"-shaped flaps may be amputated with conversion of the defect into an elliptical defect (*dotted line*) for closure or amputated and closed in the form of a "Y." (After Pullen, C. M.: Reconstruction of the skin, in Bojrab, M. J. (ed.): *Current Techniques in Small Animal Surgery.* Philadelphia, Lea & Febiger, 1975, p. 283.)

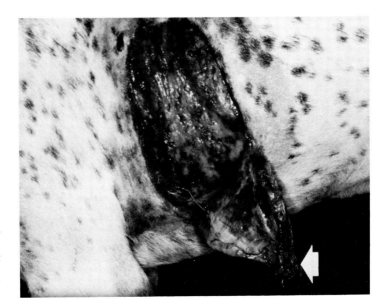

Figure 7–31: A large, ventrally based flap of some duration showing avascular changes at the tip of the flap (*arrow*). Such flaps must be evaluated and reshaped prior to wound closure.

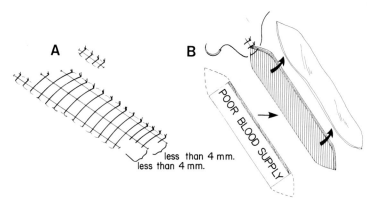

Figure 7–32: *A*, Parallel skin lacerations that are less than 4 mm. apart may be repaired with interrupted sutures that approximate the two most distant borders. *B*, A long, narrow strip of skin between parallel lacerations may be removed because of poor blood supply. The defect is reshaped and closed as a fusiform defect. (*A*, After Borges, A. F.: Elective Incisions and Scar Revision. Boston, Little, Brown and Co., 1975, p. 86.)

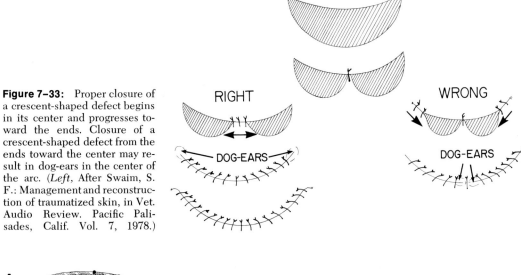

Figure 7–33: Proper closure of a crescent-shaped defect begins in its center and progresses toward the ends. Closure of a crescent-shaped defect from the ends toward the center may result in dog-ears in the center of the arc. (*Left,* After Swaim, S. F.: Management and reconstruction of traumatized skin, in Vet. Audio Review. Pacific Palisades, Calif. Vol. 7, 1978.)

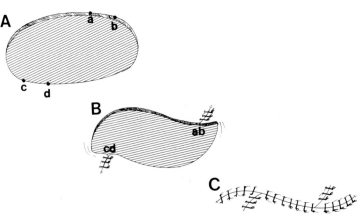

Figure 7–34: Closure of an oval defect. *A*, Selection of points (*a, b, c,* and *d*) along the defect to be sutured together. *B*, Suturing of the points (*a* to *b* and *c* to *d*) and the resultant tracts that are formed. *C*, Closure of the remainder of the wound. (After Dixon, A. C.: The secondary closure of wounds. Vet. Rec. 75:1139, 1963.)

ate such a flap carefully before deciding on the technique for reconstruction. A small dorsally based flap of short duration has a better prognosis than that of the previously described flap.

PARALLEL DEFECTS

Parallel defects that are very close to each other (less than 4 mm.) may be repaired with interrupted sutures that approximate the two most distant borders. This method encloses the intermediate strip or strips of skin.[5] If parallel defects are long and have a narrow strip of skin between them, this strip may be in danger of necrosis from an inadequate blood supply. In such a case, it might be wise to remove the strip and appose the remaining skin edges (Fig. 7–32).

CRESCENT-SHAPED LESIONS

A crescent-shaped lesion is closed in the shape of an arc.[8] When closing such a lesion, it is wise to place one suture in the center of the crescent and then to suture laterally on each side from this point toward the ends of the crescent. In this way, any dog-ears that form can be easily removed at the ends of the incision. Suturing from the ends toward the center may result in two dog-ears in the center of the arc that would be difficult to remove (Fig. 7–33). When suturing a crescent-shaped lesion, it should be kept in mind that the inner edge of the lesion is shorter than the outer edge. In such instances, placing sutures so that they are closer together on the short side of the wound and farther apart on the long side will help to overcome this discrepancy in length.[19]

OVAL DEFECTS

As mentioned earlier, oval defects are true elliptical defects. The shape of large oval wounds may be altered to facilitate closure. Two points are selected near one end of the oval, and they are drawn together with a suture. Two more points are selected on the other side of the oval, and they are treated in the same way. The short side tracts that are created are closed with simple interrupted sutures. Dog-ears may result at the ends of these tracts that will require correction. The effect of the side tracts is to make the wound smaller and thus easier to close in the usual manner.[10, 21] The scar of a wound that is closed in this manner is usually curved considerably (Fig. 7–34). This technique works best in areas where the skin is thin, and it is seldom applicable for thick skin, such as the backs of small animals.[10] Oval defects may also be converted to fusiform defects for closure.

CIRCULAR DEFECTS

Several techniques have been described to close circular wounds. One technique involves the excision of two triangle-like pieces of skin on opposite sides of the circle, with the base of the triangles incorporated into the

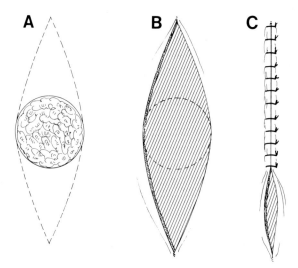

Figure 7–35: *A*, Correction of a circular defect by outlining triangle-like pieces of skin adjacent to the defect. *B*, Removal of the pieces of skin. *C*, Closure of the resultant fusiform defect. (After Swaim, S. F., and Votau, K.: Prevention and treatment of decubital ulcers in the dog. Vet. Med. Small Anim. Clin. *70*:1073, 1975.)

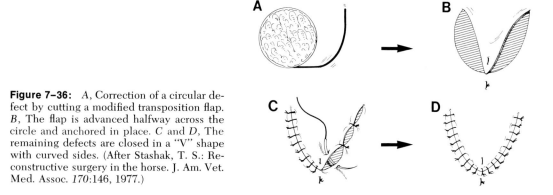

Figure 7–36: *A*, Correction of a circular defect by cutting a modified transposition flap. *B*, The flap is advanced halfway across the circle and anchored in place. *C* and *D*, The remaining defects are closed in a "V" shape with curved sides. (After Stashak, T. S.: Reconstructive surgery in the horse. J. Am. Vet. Med. Assoc. *170*:146, 1977.)

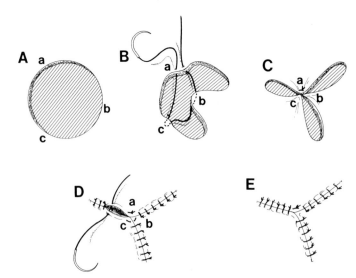

Figure 7–37: *A*, Closure of a circular defect by selecting three points (*a*, *b*, and *c*) around the circle. *B* and *C*, Placement and tying of an intradermal suture. *D* and *E*, Final closure of the resulting limbs in a "Y" shape. (After Dixon, A. C.: The secondary closure of wounds. Vet. Rec. 75:1139, 1963.)

edge of the circle. The resultant fusiform defect is closed in the manner previously described (Fig. 7–35).[3, 25] In lieu of this, two triangular subcutaneous pedicle flaps may be used to close a circular defect, as described in Chapter 8.

Another technique utilizes a modified transposition flap to close a circular defect.[24] The technique involves cutting a flap of skin at one side of the defect. This flap is advanced halfway across the circular defect and anchored there. The two remaining defects are then sutured to form a "V"-shaped incision with curved sides (Fig. 7–36).

Small circular defects may be closed by converting them to a "Y"- or "X"-shaped defect. Three or four points are selected along the circumference of the circle, and they are drawn together with one suture. To place this suture, the needle is passed into the skin at one of the selected points, but the needle does not go through the skin. It is turned so that it emerges on the edge of the cut surface. The second site is grasped and drawn well across the wound so that it comes to a point. The needle is passed through this point in the same plane as that of the skin. This is repeated on the third point for "Y"-shaped closure and a fourth point, if necessary for "X"-shaped closure. The needle is finally passed into the thickness of the skin near the starting point and up to the surface, where the suture is tied. The three of four short arms that result from placing this suture are closed with simple interrupted sutures.[10, 21] Dog-ears are corrected as needed to produce a flat surface (Fig. 7–37).

REFERENCES

1. Albert, R. A., and Wilder, D. T.: Repair of lacerations of the eyelids. Auburn Vet. *31*:10, 1974.
2. Archibald, J., and Blakely, C. L.: Sutures, in Archibald, J. (ed.): Canine Surgery, ed. 2. Santa Barbara, Calif., American Veterinary Publications, Inc., 1974.
3. Berson, M. I.: Atlas of Plastic Surgery, ed. 2. New York, Grune & Stratton, Inc., 1963.
4. Borges, A. F., and Alexander, J. E.: Relaxed skin tension lines, Z-plasties on scars, and fusiform excision of lesions. Br. J. Plast. Surg. *15*:242, 1962.
5. Borges, A. F.: Elective Incisions and Scar Revision. Boston, Little, Brown and Co., 1975.
6. Buntine, J. A.: "Elliptical" excision and suture. Med. J. Aust. 2:449, 1969.
7. Campbell, R. M.: The surgical management of pressure sores. Surg. Clin. North Am. *3a*:509, 1959.
8. Cawley, A. J., and Archibald, J.: Plastic surgery, in Archibald, J. (ed.): Canine Surgery, ed. 2. Santa Barbara, Calif., American Veterinary Publications, Inc., 1974.
9. Cox, H. T.: The cleavage lines of the skin. Br. J. Surg. 29:234, 1941.
10. Dixon, A. C.: The secondary closure of wounds. Vet. Rec. 75:1133, 1963.
11. Epstein, E.: Skin Surgery. Philadelphia, Lea & Febiger, 1962.
12. Grabb, W. C., and Smith, J. W.: Basic techniques of plastic surgery, in Grabb, W. C., and Smith, J. W. (eds.): Plastic Surgery: A Concise Guide to Clinical Practice. Boston, Little, Brown and Co., 1968.
13. Irwin, D. H. G.: Tension lines in the skin of the dog. J. Small Anim. Pract. 7:593, 1966.
14. Jensen, E. C.: Canine autogenous skin grafting. Am. J. Vet. Res. 20:898, 1959.
15. Jobe, R.: When an "ellipse" is not an ellipse. Plas. Reconstr. Surg. 46:295, 1970.
16. Johnston, D. E.: Wound healing and reconstructive surgery. J. Am. Anim. Hosp. Assoc. Sci. Proc. 2:383, 1975.
17. Knowles, R. P.: Repair of small animal skin defects. J. Am. Vet. Med. Assoc. *154*:1111, 1969.
18. Kraissl, C. J.: The selection of appropriate lines for elective surgical incisions. Plast. Reconstr. Surg. 6:1, 1951.
19. McGregor, I. A.: Fundamental Techniques of Plastic Surgery, ed. 5. Edinburgh, Churchill Livingstone, 1972.
20. Pullen, C. M.: Reconstruction of the skin, in Bojrab, M. J. (ed.): Current Techniques in Small Animal Surgery. Philadelphia, Lea & Febiger, 1975.
21. Smithcors, J. F.: New methods of wound closure. Mod. Vet. Pract. *47*:118, 1966.

22. Spreull, J. S. A.: The principles of transplanting skin in the dog. J. Am. Anim. Hosp. Assoc. 4:71, 1968.
23. Stark, R. B.: Plastic Surgery. New York, Harper & Row Publishers, Inc., 1962.
24. Stashak, T. S.: Reconstructive surgery in the horse. J. Am. Vet. Med. Assoc. 170:143, 1977.
25. Swaim, S. F., and Votau, K.: Prevention and treatment of decubital ulcers in the dog. Vet. Med. Small Anim. Clin. 70:1069, 1975.
26. Swaim, S. F.: A "walking" suture technique for closure of large skin defects in the dog and cat. J. Am. Anim. Hosp. Assoc. 12:597, 1976.
27. Wilder, D. T., and Albert, R. A.: Excision of tumors of the eyelid. Auburn Vet. 31:52, 1975.
28. Zovickian, A.: Closure of soft tissue surface wounds, surgical and traumatic, in Cooper, P. (ed.): The Craft of Surgery. ed. 2. Boston, Little, Brown and Co., 1971, vol. 1.

8

SKIN FLAPS

INTRODUCTION

A skin flap is a piece of skin that retains at least one vascular attachment to the donor site at all times during its transfer. Since this attachment is an essential part of the flap, most flaps include both skin and underlying subcutaneous tissue. The terms skin flap and pedicle flap can be considered synonymous.[1, 11, 29, 38, 41, 48, 49, 61, 66]

The indications for flaps as a means of skin reconstruction include the following:

1. Skin flaps may be used for the reconstruction of a severely scarred area such as that following a burn.[54]
2. Flaps are useful in covering exposed bone, cartilage, tendon, and nerve tissue, since these structures will not have sufficient circulation to support a skin graft unless they are covered by a vascular envelope.[14, 29, 49, 54, 56]
3. Flaps may be used in the reconstruction of depressed areas of the body where skin, as well as underlying fat and possible muscle, can be used to fill the defect.[14, 54, 56]
4. The reconstruction of structures around the face (e.g., eyelids, ears, lips) often requires flaps.[24, 29, 54, 66, 77]
5. Skin flaps are used to cover an area so that surgery can be performed at a later time on underlying structures.[29, 56]
6. The reconstruction of decubital ulcers can be accomplished with flaps.[9, 55, 56, 68, 75]

The skin of the dog lends itself readily to reconstruction by means of flaps, since the trunk is covered with skin that can move freely owing to its loose attachment to the subcutaneous connective tissue. This, coupled with the skin's natural elasticity, permits a flap to be mobilized by undercutting the subcutaneous tissue and sliding the flap to cover the defect.[11, 66] The trunk, neck, head, proximal aspects of the limbs, and tail of the dog are areas where the skin is sufficiently mobile to allow for flap construction. Because of the paucity of free skin, flaps cannot always be constructed on the peripheral parts of the limbs (Fig. 8–1).[48, 66] However, they can be transposed to such sites provided that both their construction and the fixation of the limb can be accomplished.[66]

When a defect can be repaired readily by a short direct flap, this method is preferable to the use of free grafts in the dog. Flaps are more easily constructed and hardier; as a result, they are more able to withstand the trauma involved in transfer to the recipient site and the subsequent trauma to which wounds in animals are subjected.[66]

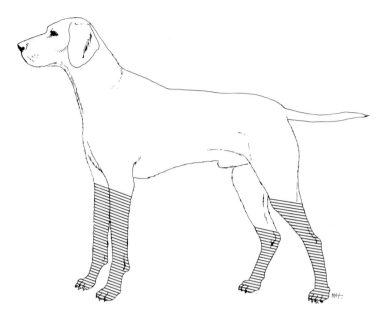

Figure 8–1: Shaded areas on the distal aspects of the limbs do not readily lend themselves to flap construction.

The main advantage of skin flaps over free grafts is the retention of a blood supply at all times. Because of this, flaps may actually improve the circulation in an area where it has been deficient.[79] Flaps also have a fairly high resistance to infection.[56]

Flaps have been classified as local or distant with regard to their relationship to the recipient site. Each of these types has its advantages and disadvantages. A distant flap is more versatile in its mobility (e.g., the potential movements of a tubed pedicle flap), and it is possible to obtain more tissue with this type than with a local flap.[23] The primary disadvantages are that tissue resemblance in the recipient area is not as good and that multiple operations are needed to complete the transfer.

Local flaps are advantageous in that the skin that is immediately adjacent to the defect is usually similar in texture, thickness, color, and hair type; therefore, tissue resemblance is much better. This type of flap is also advantageous in that it is placed in the defect in a one-stage operation (Table 8–1).[23, 27, 38, 48, 49] However, its use in the treatment of defects of the lower portion of the extremities is limited, since there is a scarcity of available skin in this area, and it is frequently scarred from the primary disease or trauma, thus rendering it inelastic.[69]

GENERAL FACTORS IN DESIGNING A SKIN FLAP

There are two distinct considerations in planning a flap: (1) deciding on the type of flap, and (2) planning the actual transfer.[48] Both of these are dependent upon the location, size, and nature of the recipient defect, the characteristics of the various flaps being considered, the ease of application, patient comfort, the availability of skin, and cosmesis.[48, 79] Two other factors of major importance are the financial status of the pet owner and his willingness to cooperate if a multistaged procedure is indicated.

TABLE 8–1   DISTANT AND LOCAL FLAPS

	Advantages	Disadvantages
Distant Flaps	Mobility More tissue	Less tissue resemblance Multiple operations
Local Flaps	Greater tissue resemblance One-stage operation	Less mobility Less tissue

Planning a flap should be done prior to the operation, when all possible sites and orientations of the flap can be considered adequately.[29] The animal should not be anesthetized, and the planning should be done with the animal in a normal standing position and again in a normal recumbent position. This practice will help to avoid a flap that will put undue stress on the animal and on the flap itself. No flap should be designed that will require the animal to be in an uncomfortable body position to maintain the flap. Neither should a flap be designed that will result in kinking, torsion, or tension as the animal assumes normal body postures. Following anesthesia, the stages of flap transfer should be checked again prior to taking the dog to the operating room.

Skin showing radiation damage or fibrotic and atrophic changes associated with old scarring is not good surgical material and should be regarded as part of the defect to be removed in order to reach the normal skin beyond it.[48] After surgically preparing the wound, the defect that is to be covered by the flap is outlined on a suitable material (clear developed x-ray film, sterile paper, or cloth toweling) (Figs. 8–2, 8–3, and 8–4).[29, 41, 48, 74] Flaps should be designed slightly larger than the defect to allow for primary contraction of the skin, and they should be designed to include any pedicle associated with them. It is easy to trim a flap but difficult to add to it once surgery is under way.[29, 32, 41, 48] Sharp angles at the corners of flaps should be avoided if possible, since these are subject to ischemic necrosis. It is advisable, therefore, to design a flap with slightly rounded corners.[23]

With this pattern representing the flap, the surgical procedure is carried out from the end result backward through the stage(s) of the transfer process until the pattern is placed on the skin area from which the flap will be taken ("planning in reverse") (Figs. 8–5 and 8–6).[29, 48] Each time the

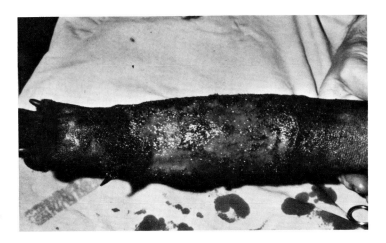

Figure 8–2: Large fibrotic lesion on the forelimb of a dog.

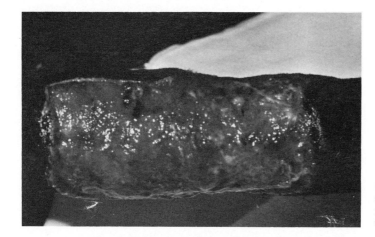

Figure 8–3: Forelimb lesion after the fibrotic lesion has been removed and a healthy granulation tissue bed has been established.

pattern is shifted in reverse, the base should be held in a fixed position and should not be allowed to shift with the flap.[29] The final pattern can be sterilized for use in the operating room. The veterinary surgeon must bear in mind the direction of hair growth when placing flaps or free grafts; it is important in planning a flap to be certain that the hair growth of the flap in its final position will correspond to that of the surrounding area.[41, 77]

An alternative technique for designing a flap is to measure with a ruler the skin defect while the animal is in a resting, undisturbed position. A pattern is made from this measurement that is used to create the flap.[58] This pattern, in combination with the plan in reverse technique, helps to insure an accurately designed flap.

The allowable length-width ratio for a flap depends upon the type of flap and the surgeon. The length-width ratio will also vary from one area of the body to another.[38] A flap with a narrow base is freer to move to another area, but its blood supply may be in jeopardy. Conversely, a broad-based flap has a good blood supply, but its mobility is limited.[38] The surgeon is faced with finding a compromise between these extremes. In general, the length-width ratio of a single pedicle flap is less than that for a bipedicle

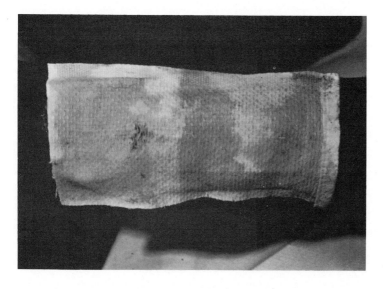

Figure 8–4: Cloth toweling has been laid over the forelimb lesion to make a pattern of the lesion that will be used in reverse to plan the flap.

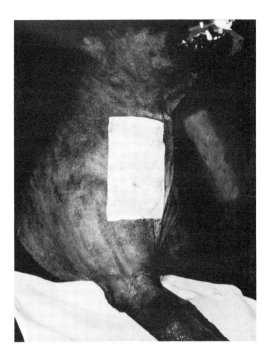

Figure 8–5: The pattern from the lesion has been used in reverse and is resting on the area where the flap will originate.

flap (e.g., a bipedicle tubed flap). A length-width ratio of 1:1 for a single pedicle flap is generally accepted;[20*, 29, 64*, 77*] however, ratios of 1.5:1,[5, 23] 2:1,[38*, 41*] 2.5:1,[9, 25*] and 3:1[38*, 56] have been reported. The most accepted length-width ratio for bipedicle flaps is 2.5:1[7, 29, 48] but ratios of 2:1[11*] and 3:1[49, 54, 61*] have been reported. The length-width ratio of a flap may be increased when (1) there are large blood vessels passing into the base along its axis, (2) the flap is located in an area of greater vascularity, or (3) the flap has been delayed.[29] In the opinion of the author, a set length-width ratio for different types of flaps does not exist for the dog and cat. The length

---

*These reports are from the veterinary literature or involve studies on dogs.

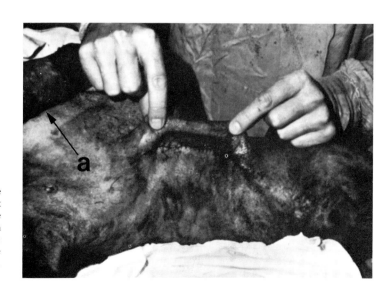

Figure 8–6: A tubed pedicle has been created on the neck that will be used to cover the forelimb lesion (*a*). (From Swaim, S. F., and Bushby, P. A.: Principles of bipedicle tube grafting in the dog. J. Am. Anim. Hosp. Assoc., *12*:601, 1976.)

may be longer in these species than would comply with the ratios previously stated. The surgeon must use discretion when planning a flap. There is a need for a controlled study on the acceptable length-width ratios of various types of flaps in the dog and cat.

After planning a flap, the next step is to prepare the recipient bed and the flap, if the flap is not going to be surgically delayed. The recipient site should be a healthy, clean, fresh wound or a healthy granulating surface.[41, 66] When placing a flap on the final recipient bed, the author prefers to remove all granulation tissue and surrounding unhaired epithelium so that there will be an edge-to-edge apposition of the normal skin around the lesion with the skin of the flap.

Hemostasis is very important, both on the underside of the flap and in the recipient bed, since a hematoma beneath the flap may result in tension on the flap, circulatory embarrassment, and finally necrosis of the flap. In addition, hematomas prevent early union of the flap with the recipient area.[49, 56] Hemostasis can be accomplished by an atraumatic technique, ligation or diathermy of bleeding vessels, and the use of fine catgut sutures to attach the underside of the flap to its bed.[29, 41, 54, 77] Such sutures must be placed carefully so that circulation to the end of the flap will not be altered. Hemostasis has also be accomplished by the application of a 1:10,000 solution of epinephrine or a 1 per cent solution of phenylephrine (Neosynephrine) hydrochloride. This is followed by an application of topical thrombin when nearly all oozing hemorrhage has stopped.[32] Additional measures to prevent hematomas include the installation of a drain under the flap[29, 49, 58] and the application of a bandage that exerts little or no pressure.[49, 54] Pressure on a flap could impair its circulation.

Placement of a simple continuous subcuticular suture with fine (3–0) catgut or other absorbable suture material helps to bring the wound edges into apposition and assures that there will be no tension on the skin sutures. The skin sutures, which consist of simple interrupted sutures of fine (4–0) monofilament nylon or polypropylene,* are placed with a swaged needle close to the wound edge for cosmesis (Fig. 8–7). An alternative to this technique is to place a few tension sutures at strategic positions to bring the flap edges into

---

*Prolene is manufactured by Ethicon, Inc., Somerville, NJ 08876.

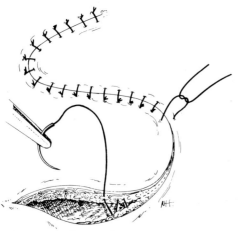

Figure 8–7: Suturing a flap into place. Fine absorbable suture material (polyglycolic acid [Dexon, available from Davis and Geck, American Cyanamid, Pearl River, NY] or chromic catgut) with a swaged needle is used in a simple continuous pattern for subcuticular closure. Fine monofilament polypropylene (Prolene, available from Ethicon, Inc., Somerville, NJ) with a swaged needle is used in a simple interrupted pattern for skin closure.

apposition with the wound edges of the recipient site. The remaining sutures are placed evenly between the tension sutures.[58] It has been stated that skin with a good blood supply can withstand high tension without necrosis.[52]

It is essential to maintain a flap in situ until it is safely established and to assure a satisfactory vascular circulation between the flap and its attachment to the donor site.[66] For these reasons it is important to confine the animal to a cage or a run for 96 hours following the procedure to minimize movement at the surgical site. Physical restraints are used when needed to prevent the animal from disturbing the surgical area.[58]

Since infection can be detrimental to the outcome of a flap, measures should be taken to prevent it.[79] In addition to a dry dressing of gauze that conforms to the wound, the animal should be given appropriate antibiotics for five days. If a drain has been installed, it should be removed after two or three days, and the skin sutures should be removed after ten to 14 days.[58] Possible fecal contamination of a bandage or a wound is something the veterinarian must be aware of and take measures to prevent, especially if the animal is confined to a cage or a run following surgery. Bandages should be changed as needed to help prevent wound infection. Dressing changes may be performed as frequently as every second day for ten days.[41]

DELAYING TECHNIQUES

A skin flap may be delayed either to improve its vascularity or to condition the tissues to ischemia, allowing it to survive on less blood flow than is normally needed.[51] These factors help to insure a flap's survival when it is transferred to its recipient bed. A flap should be delayed when its viability is in question, and this may be done by either surgical or physiological means.

Developing a flap in multiple surgical stages allows greater length-width ratios for both the single and the bipedicle flaps than could be obtained safely by a single operation.[29, 48] The type of surgical delay that is chosen by the surgeon will depend on the vascularity of the skin and the type and size of flap to be used. Some of the surgical delaying techniques that have been described include the following:

1. The skin and subcutaneous tissue are incised along three sides of the flap, and severed blood vessels are ligated as necessary. This cuts off all blood supply to the flap except for that entering the pedicle and deep surface of the flap. The wound is resutured and allowed to heal. In seven to ten days the flap is reincised and transferred (Fig. 8–8).[29, 48, 49]

2. The surgical technique is the same as that previously described, except that varying portions of the flap (one third, one half, or all) are undermined. This renders the flap dependent, to varying degrees, upon the blood vessels entering the pedicle. The extent of undermining depends upon the rapidity with which capillaries at the end of the flap, when blanched by digital pressure, will refill. The capillary fill should be approximately as rapid as that in an adjacent area that has not been operated on. The flap is reincised and transferred between seven and ten days (Figs. 8–9 and 8–10).[5, 11, 23, 29, 48, 49, 56]

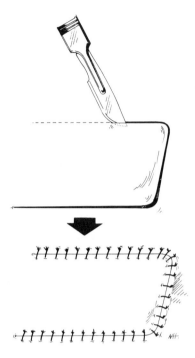

Figure 8–8: A technique for delaying a flap. The skin and the subcutaneous tissue are incised on three sides. The incisions are sutured, and the flap will be transferred at a later date.

3. Two parallel incisions are made, and the skin between the incisions is undermined; between seven and 14 days later an incision is begun along the third side and it is completed in two or three stages, each of which is separated by two or three days (Fig. 8–11).[29, 56]
4. Longer flaps can be created by making two parallel incisions, one

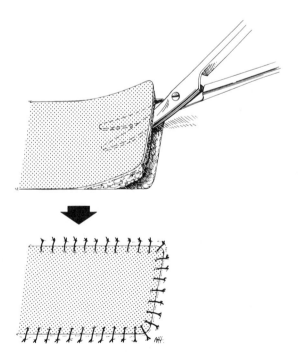

Figure 8–9: A technique for delaying a flap. The skin and the subcutaneous tissue are incised on three sides. The flap is undermined partially (one third or one half) or totally. The flap is returned to its bed and sutured in place until it is raised again for transfer at a later date.

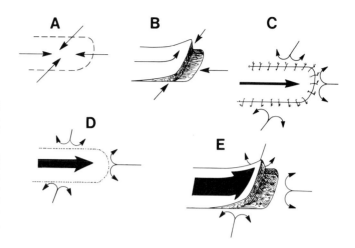

Figure 8–10: Diagrammatic representation of the effects of surgical delay on the blood supply of a flap. *A*, The flap is outlined, with blood supply coming from all directions. *B*, The flap is raised, cutting off all blood supply except that through the base. *C* and *D*, The flap is sutured back into position and left for a period of time to allow the efficiency of the blood supply to increase through the base. *E*, The flap is raised for transposition. (From McGregor, I.A.: Fundamental Techniques of Plastic Surgery, ed. 5. Edinburgh, Churchill Livingstone, 1972, p. 111.)

of which has a central bridge of skin that is preserved intact in the middle of the incision. The flap is completely undermined during the initial surgery. The intact skin at one end of the flap and the central bridge are divided in three or four stages after two weeks (Fig. 8–12).[29]

5. Staged incision and undermining one end of a tubed pedicle help to insure the tube's reliance on the blood vessels that are entering from the other end of the tube (Fig. 8–13).[29, 49]

The surgeon must realize that surgically delaying a flap has some dis-

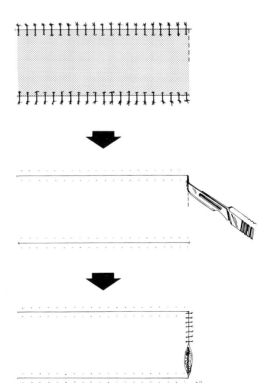

Figure 8–11: A technique for delaying a long flap. Two parallel incisions are made and the skin is undermined. The skin is sutured. At a later date (from seven to 14 days), two or three incisions are made across one end of the flap at two- to three-day intervals to complete outlining the flap.

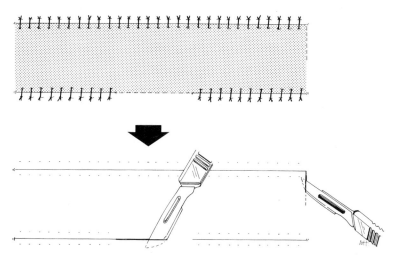

Figure 8–12: A technique for delaying a long flap. Two parallel incisions are made; however, one incision has a bridge in it. The skin is undermined and sutured back in place. After two to three weeks, the skin at one end of the flap and in the central bridge is divided in three or four stages to complete outlining the flap.

advantages as well as advantages. The primary advantage is the avoidance of flap necrosis, which could result from an inadequate blood supply. Related to this is the fact that a longer flap (a greater length-width ratio) can be created by using the delaying technique.[23] The disadvantages of surgically delaying a flap are that (1) it increases the length of time necessary to effect a repair; (2) it subjects the patient to additional operations; and (3) additional scar tissue is formed in the area of the flap when it is delayed. The scar tissue is formed not only in the bed to which the flap is returned but also on the underside of the flap. A hematoma in the area adds to the scar tissue reaction and should be prevented. Scar tissue can reduce the flexibility of the flap and possibly, through its constrictive effect, restrict the blood supply of the flap. When the flap is raised for its final transfer, the scar tissue can be removed and thus some of the flap's flexibility will be restored.[23, 48] However, the surgeon must use discretion in deciding whether the flexibility that would be gained by removing the scar tissue warrants the risk of damaging the blood supply to the flap. The author has not found the formation of scar tissue to be a problem in delaying flaps on dogs.

Physiological delay is used mainly in tubed pedicle grafts and is a means of "training" a tube to rely on its vascular support from one end

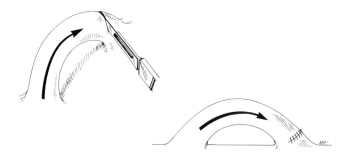

Figure 8–13: A delaying technique for tubed pedicle flaps. One end of the tube (the end to be moved) is incised partially through and then resutured. This helps to insure the tube's reliance on blood vessels from the other end.

alone.[48] This is performed by constricting the blood flow into one end of the tube (the end to be transferred) by means of sphygmomanometer cuff, a rubber-padded intestinal clamp, or a tourniquet fashioned from Penrose drain tubing (Fig. 8–14). Compression is applied initially for short periods, followed by increasingly longer periods. Temporary clamping produces a temporary reactive hyperemia.[29, 48] The feasibility of this technique in veterinary surgery depends upon the willingness of the animal's owner or the veterinarian or both to apply the necessary compression regularly.

Several theories have been stated regarding the benefits of delaying a skin flap. These include the following:

1. During the delay of a flap, there is axial reorientation of large blood vessels in the flap and an increase in the number and caliber of blood vessels.[5, 23, 25, 48, 49, 54, 56]

2. There is an increased blood flow into the flap, with resultant hyperemia a few days after the flap has been prepared.[11]

3. The delaying procedure conditions the flap tissues so that they will survive better in the hypoxic state that occurs after the flap is transferred to the recipient site.[23, 29, 47]

4. The circulation to the delayed flap is increased by a reduction in resistance to venous outflow, which results from an increase in the size of the channels of the dermal venous plexus.[8]

5. Surgical delay results in cutting off the sympathetic nerve control of blood vessels in the flap. Blood flow in the flap is thus improved as blood moves from an area of higher pressure to an area of lower pressure, forcing it into and out of the flap.[34]

6. The surgical incision of a flap denervates the blood vessels, thus opening arteriovenous shunts that are normally closed under sympathetic stimulation. During the time the flap is delayed, the blood vessels become increasingly responsive to circulating catecholamines, and the shunts gradually close, causing capillary circulation to resume in the flap.[59]

Studies of dogs in which rates of radioactive sodium (^{22}Na) clearance were measured in delayed flaps to determine circulatory efficiency have

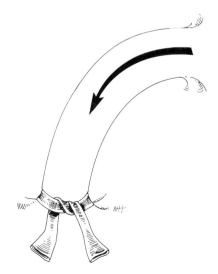

Figure 8–14: A technique for physiological delay. The blood vessels at one end of the tubed pedicle are temporarily occluded for progressively longer periods each day to "train" the tube to rely on blood vessels from the other end. A section of Penrose drain is being used as a tourniquet.

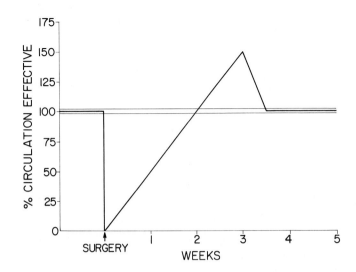

Figure 8–15: The circulatory efficiency of a surgically delayed flap that has been incised on three sides. Circulatory efficiency drops at the time of surgery and increases to greater than normal over the next few weeks. After reaching a peak, circulatory efficiency drops back to normal. (Based on data reported by Hoffmeister, Plast. Reconstr. Surg., 1957. After Grabb, W.C., and Smith, J.W.: Plastic Surgery: A Concise Guide to Clinical Practice. Little, Brown and Co., Boston, 1968, p. 56.)

shown that after a delaying procedure, the circulatory efficiency in a flap falls to zero in most instances. It then rises slowly during the next two to four weeks until it reaches values between 126 and 175 per cent of normal. The circulatory efficiency then drops to normal values (100 per cent) between two and seven days after its peak (Fig. 8–15).[29, 31] In these studies it was also found that the circulatory enhancement of the flaps that were created by making two parallel incisions was inadequate. However, surgically delaying a flap by incising three sides resulted in increased circulatory efficiency that ranged from 4 to 138 per cent of that of the control animals. In order to derive maximum clinical benefit from this enhanced circulation, transfer would have to be synchronized with the circulatory peak following surgical delay. This time will vary from animal to animal, and it would be clinically impractical to try to establish when this peak occurs. However, it was found that when a standardized time of three weeks had been allowed for delaying a flap, there was a significant circulatory enhancement in the flaps. The study revealed that a delay of one week was not sufficient to allow for the reestablishment of an adequate blood flow in a flap and that transfer at this time would be hazardous to the flap.[29, 31] The results of this study indicate that circulatory enhancement does follow surgical delay procedures in the dog.

Therefore, the veterinary surgeon should be familiar with the technique, since it may be necessary to use surgical delay on a flap with a questionable blood supply to avoid having to start the reconstructive procedure a second time as a result of losing the flap to ischemia. In general, the rate of skin flap survival in dogs and cats is good, and the veterinarian will have to decide whether the benefit that is gained from delaying a flap will be worth the time and effort involved.

EVALUATION OF THE BLOOD SUPPLY IN A FLAP

Numerous methods have been devised to ascertain the quality and quantity of circulation in a skin flap. Some of these techniques are practical for the veterinary surgeon, but others are more involved and require special materials and equipment. The following are some of the methods that have been used.

Skin Temperature Test. The temperature of a skin flap has been used to evaluate the circulation in the flap. One technique that has been used in dogs consists of (1) recording the temperature of a tubed pedicle at the end of the tube that was to be divided and transplanted; (2) applying a tourniquet to that same end of the tube; and (3) monitoring the temperature of the skin at that point on the pedicle for a ten-minute period while the tourniquet was in place. A sharp drop in skin temperature was interpreted as evidence of insufficient circulation. A slight drop (1 to 2° C) or no drop in temperature was viewed as evidence that circulation was adequate.[15] The skin temperature test for circulatory evaluation of flaps is not believed to be reliable.[15, 29, 80] Determining the temperature of a flap by thermography using an infrared scanner in a controlled environment has also been described.[29] This test requires sophisticated equipment, as does the previous test, and would probably not be practical for the veterinary practitioner.

Blood Pressure Test. After creating a tubed pedicle, the blood pressure within the tube dropped to 25 per cent of normal.[48] This pressure then reached 90 to 95 per cent of the normal pulse pressure by six to eight weeks following surgery.[21, 48] The miniature cuffs and thermocouple needles that are required for such recordings make this test impractical for the veterinary surgeon.

Radioisotope Test. The injection of radioisotopes into a flap has been used to evaluate circulation.[29, 31, 48] The rate of disappearance of the isotope from the flap is compared with that from a control area on the opposite side of the body.[31] This test also requires special equipment and material.

Hair Growth Evaluation. It has been observed in dogs that hair growth on a tubed pedicle flap is only slightly retarded in comparison with that on adjacent areas of the abdominal skin from which the flap was taken. However, the rate of hair growth on single pedicle tubed flaps is definitely retarded during the first 12 days after surgery, and by one month the rate of growth is still somewhat slower than that on the adjacent skin.[21]

Dermal Bleeding Test. The quality and quantity of blood from the cut edge of the flap have been used to evaluate a flap's circulation.[13] An adequate vascular supply is usually assured when well-oxygenated blood oozes from the cut edges of a flap. A lack of uniform bleeding along the incision or areas of dark bleeding suggest decreased perfusion. When one end of a tubed pedicle is cut free, an adequate backflow of blood from the cut end of the tube is a good sign.[2] This test may be helpful to the veterinary surgeon.

Color Test. A less sophisticated but commonly used test involves blanching the critical end of a flap by applying pressure and then observing the speed with which color returns. This provides an index of blood flow that can be compared with that of a control area on the opposite side of the body. If the release of pressure is followed by the prompt return of a reddish or bluish color, the flap will probably survive.[29] Observing the color of a flap and noting whether it is cyanotic or anemic will yield some information about the flap's circulation. Cyanosis implies venous inadequacy and stagnation of blood, whereas pallor, an ominous sign, indicates arterial and venous insufficiency.[23, 29]

A combination of compression and dermal bleeding has been described as a test to evaluate flaps.[56] If the flap remains pink after compression, it is viable. If the flap is white after compression and a slight incision results in red blood, it is usually viable. However, if the flap is blue in color after compression and a slight incision produces dark blood, the flap is in danger. A pinkish flap that blanches when pressure is applied and then returns to pink within five to seven seconds will usually survive. A bluish flap that returns to its original color slowly after blanching may be lost.[56] Though these principles are described for use in humans, the veterinarian should keep them in mind when evaluating flap circulation.

Saline Wheal Test.   A tuberculin syringe and a small-gauge needle have been used to inject 0.2 ml. of 0.8 per cent saline solution intradermally as a means of evaluating circulation in a skin flap.[71] The wheal thus created should disappear within 60 minutes if circulation is normal. Any delay in absorption indicates impaired circulation. Disappearance of the wheal should be judged by the sense of touch rather than by sight, since vasomotor changes that are produced by injection often render visual judgment inaccurate.[71] In addition to requiring one hour to perform, the test is disadvantageous in that it has an indistinct end point, since the exact time at which the wheal disappears is difficult to determine.[29] Performing this test on a tubed pedicle entails placing a tourniquet at the end of the tube to be tested and conducting the saline wheal test near the tourniquet. This technique needs further evaluation to determine the normal absorption times in dogs and cats; however, if the wheal on the flap or pedicle disappears at the same rate as that of a wheal on a control area of the body, the flap could probably be divided safely.

Histamine Wheal Test.   Application of the acid phosphate salt of histamine (1:1000) to small scarified areas on tubed pedicles and flaps has been used to evaluate circulation.[16] The area in question is compared with a control area on the opposite side of the body to give an index of circulatory efficiency. If a wheal develops in less than eight minutes on the distal end of the pedicle or flap, the flap will withstand transplantation successfully. The factors associated with the performance of this test on tubed pedicles in dogs and cats and its interpretation are the same as those for the saline wheal test.

Fluorescein Test.   A dependable test for circulation in the flaps of both dogs and humans is the intravenous injection of fluorescein.[19, 29, 56] A slow (10 ml./min.) intravenous injection of 10 ml. of 20 per cent sodium fluorescein is given and the flap is observed under an ultraviolet light.[19] Areas where blood is circulating become bright yellow-green within 15 to 20 seconds after injection. Using this test it is possible not only to determine whether blood circulates through a given section but also to determine the relative amount that is reaching that area by observing the varying intensities of the yellow-green color (Figs. 8–16 through 8–21).[19] The fluorescein test has the advantages of being quick, simple, accurate, and nontoxic. It does not cause discomfort to the patient and the fluorescein is readily detected at very high dilutions when observed under ultraviolet light. In addition, the test can be used when two pedicles are being evaluated, and it may be repeated daily.[36] Disadvantages of the test are that it does require an ultraviolet light,[36] and if given too rapidly, it may cause nausea.[16, 19] A combination of the fluorescein and histamine wheal tests has been described for evaluating the blood supply to a tubed pedicle.[36, 48]

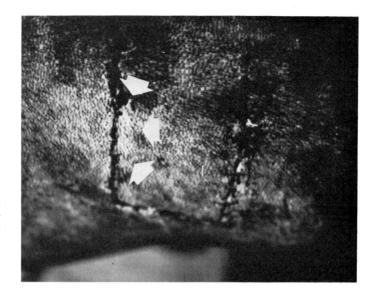

Figure 8–16: Fluorescein test was performed on a 3-day-old undermined single pedicle flap. Note small area of fluorescence within flap (*area between arrows and suture line*). The photograph was taken under ultraviolet light.

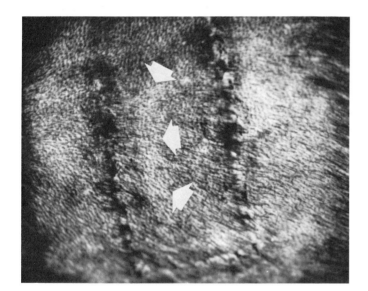

Figure 8–17: Fluorescein test was performed on the undermined single pedicle flap (Fig. 8–16) six days after surgery. Note fluorescence of flap compared with that three days previously (*area between arrows and suture line*). The photograph was taken under ultraviolet light.

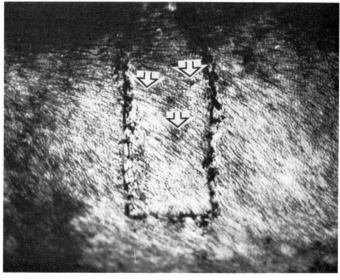

Figure 8–18: Fluorescein test was performed on the undermined single pedicle flap (Fig. 8–16) 14 days after surgery. Note the amount of fluorescence at the tip of the flap is greater than that of the previous two tests (*area between arrows and suture lines*). The photograph was taken under ultraviolet light.

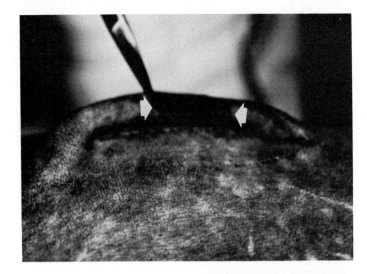

Figure 8–19: Fluorescein test was performed on a 3-day-old tubed pedicle flap. Note the lack of fluorescence in the center of the flap (*between arrows*), indicating poor circulation. The photograph was taken under ultraviolet light.

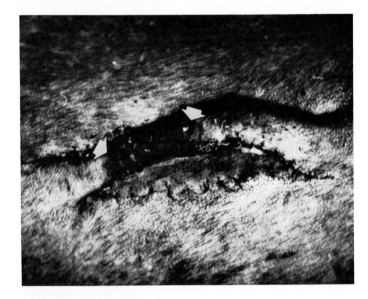

Figure 8–20: Fluorescein test was performed on the tubed pedicle flap six days following surgery. Note that the fluorescence is still not present in the center of the tube (*between arrows*). The photograph was taken under ultraviolet light.

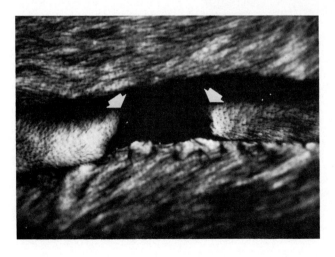

Figure 8–21: Fluorescein test was performed on the tubed pedicle flap 14 days following surgery. The center of the tube sloughed (*between arrows*). The photograph was taken under ultraviolet light.

Atropine Absorption Test.   Another test that has been used to evaluate flap circulation is the atropine absorption test.[29, 33, 36, 48] To evaluate the circulation of the tubed pedicle in humans, the end of the pedicle to be transferred is occluded with an intestinal clamp, and after ten minutes from 1/25 to 1/50 gm. of atropine that has been dissolved in 0.2 ml. of water is injected into the fat of the pedicle 1 cm. from the clamp. The absorption of atropine into the general circulation is detected by tachycardia, dryness of the mouth, the loss of visual accommodation, and pupillary dilation.[36] This test has the advantages of being simple, giving a more precise quantitative and qualitative measurement of blood supply, and evaluating both the arterial and venous supply to a flap.[33, 36] It needs to be further evaluated for its application in veterinary surgery.

In summary, the tests that appear to be most useful to the veterinarian are the fluorescein test, the dermal bleeding test, the color test, and possibly the atropine absorption test. However, these tests should not take the place of sound clinical judgment; if a test indicates that a flap is ready for transfer but the surgeon does not agree, his judgment should prevail.

TREATMENT OF FLAPS WITH POOR CIRCULATION

There are several factors that can cause necrosis of a skin flap, and all of these do so by impairing the blood flow within the flap. There are differing opinions as to what the ultimate cause of flap necrosis is. Some believe that flaps have an adequate arterial supply but that venous insufficiency causes necrosis. In other words, flaps die more often from congestion than from anemia.[10, 48] Another viewpoint is that flaps necrose as a result of combined arterial and venous insufficiency, with the arterial component being the more important factor.[52]

Regardless of whether it is arterial insufficiency or venous insufficiency or both that cause flap necrosis, there are several known reasons for vascular insufficiency. The surgeon should be aware of these and measures should be taken to prevent them.

Tension may develop in a local flap if it is stretched too tightly in order to reach the farthest extent of the wound. Blanching of the skin along the line of greatest tension (the line between the pivot point and the most distant part of the flap) may be observed in rotation, transposition, and interpolation flaps if they are stretched too tightly. A tubed pedicle that is being transferred from one point to another may place tension on its point of insertion if its weight is great enough to pull it away from this point. Measures should be taken to prevent tension on a flap by (1) designing the flap so that it does not have to be sutured under tension, (2) making a short back-cut at the base of the flap, or (3) supporting the flap (tubed pedicle) to prevent its weight from pulling on the insertion point.[29, 48]

When arterial pressure is higher than venous pressure, kinking of the flap impairs venous drainage, which results in a congested flap. This is more common in tubed pedicles (Fig. 8–22). Repositioning and immobilization can prevent kinking.[10, 29, 48]

Tension and kinking result in edema of the flap, which in itself is detrimental to circulation, since it may further obstruct venous outflow. Edema

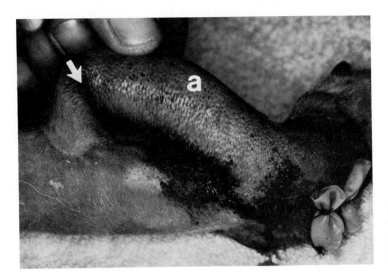

Figure 8–22: A kinked (*arrow*) tubed pedicle flap that has been tumbled is showing signs of impaired circulation in its distal aspect (*a*).

is usually more noticeable in tubed pedicles than in other types of flaps. The surgeon should be aware that some transient edema is common even in a flap that is progressing favorably. This edema increases between the first 24 and 36 hours and remains for two or three more days before it starts to subside.[48]

Pressure is a cause of impaired circulation and may be either external or internal in origin. External pressure usually results from a bandage or a cast that is too tight or from the patient's body position. Internal pressure is seen in tubed pedicles in which too much subcutaneous fat has been included. It is also seen in flaps where a hematoma is compressing blood vessels. Changing the wound dressing or changing the patient's position, when possible, may help to alleviate the causes of external pressure. If a hematoma is contributing to flap necrosis, it should be removed under aseptic conditions and hemostasis should be accomplished.[48] However, relief of internal pressure in a tubed pedicle with too much fat may be more difficult.[29, 48] This may require the removal of a few sutures in the tube in an attempt to relieve some of the internal pressure.

Infection in a skin flap in the early postoperative period may result in circulatory embarrassment. Because of its decreased circulation, a recently elevated flap is capable of supplying or supporting only its basic metabolic needs, and it will not be able to provide the increased blood flow that is necessary for an inflammatory reaction. As a result, an infection that might be of little consequence in normal tissue can easily destroy the poorly vascularized tissues of a skin flap. When an inflammatory reaction does occur, it adds to the tension on the tissues, which further impairs circulation and results in increased necrosis.[29, 48]

Numerous measures can be taken to preserve the viability of a skin flap with vascular insufficiency. These measures are aimed at increasing the blood flow in the flap, or increasing the oxygen dissociation into a flap, or decreasing the metabolic requirements of the flap tissues.

Vasodilators. Phenoxybenzamine has been injected directly into flaps with beneficial results in rats; however, it was not effective in the flaps of rabbits and pigs.[51] The topical application of phenoxybenzamine in dimethyl sulfoxide (DMSO) has also been reported as a means of improving vascularity in flaps.[49]

Dextran. The intraveous injection of dextran 40 has not proved to be an effective way of augmenting circulation in flaps;[28, 29, 51] however, some success has been reported in rabbits.[51]

Induced Anemia. In an experimental study it was found that induced anemia, i.e., bleeding followed by the infusion of saline or Ringer's lactated solution, improved the microcirculation in dogs. It was also found that the survival time for standardized skin flaps was consistently and significantly greater in dogs in which anemia had been induced than in normal dogs and dogs in which polycythemia had been induced.[22] The clinical application of this technique is questionable.

Gravity and Pressure. Placing a body structure on which a tubed pedicle has been created in such a position that gravity aids in alternately emptying and filling the pedicle has been described.[29, 34, 35] In addition, pressure cuffs that are applied on or around tubed pedicles have been used to force blood in and out of the flap.[29, 35] Of interest is a recent study on pigs and rabbits that showed that gravity had no effect on either the blood supply or the survival rate of tubed pedicles.[53] The positioning of a body structure and flap to take advantage of gravity and the application of pressure as methods of increasing blood flow in a flap are rather impractical in clinical veterinary situations.

Massage. Massage has been described as a means of eliminating edema from a flap.[70] However, more recent information states that this measure can be detrimental to a flap in that it may produce a local hyperemia in the area that would be undesirable.[48] The surgeon should consider this when contemplating massage as a means of treating a flap with circulatory problems.

Surgery. If a flap appears cyanotic at its distal end or has scattered small areas of cyanosis, the release of a few sutures in the adjacent areas may be sufficient to relieve the problem.[9] It has been reported[9] and the author concurs that superficial cyanosis may sometimes occur at the end a flap and may lead to necrosis and desquamation of the skin's edge. If this area is not too extensive and if it is confined to the skin, it will epithelialize, which will result in a delay but not failure of the flap. When a segment of a flap is undoubtedly dying, the surgeon may decide to remove that portion in the hopes that removal of the necrotic focus will give the flap a fresh start. When excising a dying segment, the surgeon should rely on the color and quantity of dermal bleeding to determine the limits of excision.

DMSO. Studies on gas levels in the tissues of skin flaps of rats, rabbits, and pigs before and after the application of DMSO and a DMSO–hydrogen peroxide mixture showed that the PCO_2 levels rose and the PO_2 levels fell after preparing the flaps. However, the application of DMSO resulted in a fall in the PCO_2 levels in rabbits and rats. The application of DMSO and hydrogen peroxide raised the PO_2 levels in the rabbit only. The drugs produced no consistent results in the blood gas levels in the skin flaps of the pig.[51] Further studies are needed on this method of treating the endangered flap, since variable results have been reported.[51]

Hyperbaric Oxygen. Hyperbaric oxygen therapy has been shown to have a marginal effect on the survival of skin and subcutaneous tissue in which circulation has ceased.[29, 40] This form of therapy does work in reversing anoxic changes in a flap, but it requires early and regular treatment by qualified persons.[57] The clinical application of this type of therapy is quite involved and of questionable benefit at best.

Hypothermia. It has been found in experimental skin flaps that cooling the flap to a surface temperature of between 0° and 20° C reduces the severity of necrosis but does not prevent it. Such extreme cooling has not been adopted clinically, although fans have been used in an attempt to decrease the metabolic needs of a flap.[29, 39]

Various methods have been used to increase the blood supply to a flap or to reduce a flap's metabolic needs. In general, these methods (1) need further investigation; (2) are of questionable clinical value; (3) require special equipment and training; or (4) all of the preceding. It can be concluded that the proper design, creation, and care of a flap are important to its survival.

CLASSIFICATION OF FLAPS

Skin flaps have been classified in many different ways.[23, 27, 29, 48, 68] The classification that is presented here will be a modification of a current system.[27] The primary factors of classification are the blood supply and whether a flap is local or distant in nature.

Blood Supply

I. Random pattern flaps

A random pattern blood supply in a flap denotes a blood supply that is provided by many smaller vessels rather than by one major or specific vessel.

The majority of flaps are designed with a random blood supply on which the delaying procedure may be performed to enhance vascular efficiency.

A. Single pedicle random peninsular flaps

These are flaps in which the pedicle is composed of a full thickness of skin and subcutaneous tissue and their associated vascular structures (e.g., rotation flaps, transposition flaps, interpolation flaps, single pedicle advancement flaps, and single pedicle direct flaps) (Fig. 8–23).

B. Double pedicle random peninsular flaps

These flaps have the same type of pedicle as that of the single pedicle peninsular flap except that they have two such pedicles (e.g., bipedicle advancement flaps, tubed pedicle flaps, and pouch flaps) (Fig. 8–24).

C. Pedicle random island flaps

These are flaps in which the pedicle is composed only of subcutaneous tissue and its associated vascular structures (e.g., subcutaneous pedicle flaps) (Fig. 8–25).

II. Axial pattern flaps

This type of flap is not used as often as the random pattern flap. These are flaps that have a distinct vascular component running along their long axis or radiating from a central point or points. As a result of their increased vascularity, they can be designed with a greater length-width ratio.

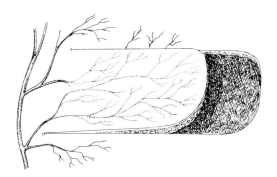

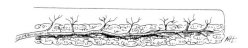

Figure 8–23: Single pedicle random peninsular flap. The pedicle of the flap is composed of skin and subcutaneous tissue, with their associated blood vessels. Note that no major vessel supplies the flap.

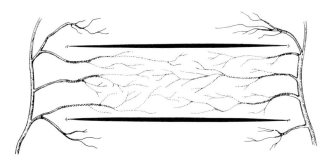

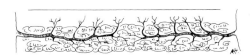

Figure 8–24: Double pedicle random peninsular flap. The pedicles of the flap contain skin, subcutaneous tissue, and blood vessels. Note that no major blood vessel supplies the flap.

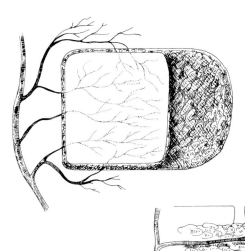

Figure 8–25: Pedicle random island flap. The pedicle is composed of only subcutaneous tissue and its associated blood vessels. Note that the skin has been completely incised, and there are no major vessels supplying the flap.

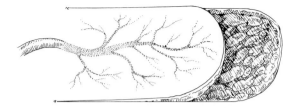

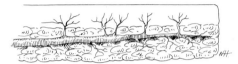

Figure 8–26: Single pedicle axial peninsular flap. Major vessel enters the flap through intact skin and subcutaneous tissue. Such flaps permit a greater length-width ratio.

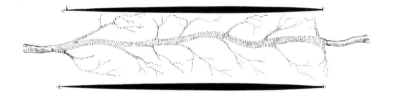

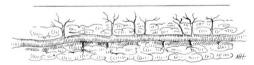

Figure 8–27: Double pedicle axial peninsular flap. A major blood vessel runs the length of the flap. Such flaps permit a greater length-width ratio.

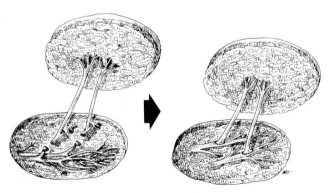

Figure 8–28: Pedicle axial island flap. A segment of skin with its subcutaneous tissue and major blood vessels is removed from one part of the body and placed in a defect some distance away. The major vessels are anastomosed to vessels in the recipient bed.

   A. Single pedicle axial peninsular flaps
     A major vessel or vessels enter the base of the flap through intact skin and subcutaneous tissue (e.g., rotation flaps, transposition flaps, interpolation flaps, single pedicle advancement flaps, and single pedicle direct flaps) (Fig. 8–26).
   B. Double pedicle axial peninsular flaps
     A major vessel or vessels enter the bases of this type of flap through intact skin and subcutaneous tissue (e.g., bipedicle advancement flaps, pouch flaps, tubed pedicle flaps) (Fig. 8–27).
   C. Single pedicle axial island flaps
     This type of flap is completely removed from one part of the body, along with the artery and the vein that supply it, and is moved to the recipient area, where the vessels are anastomosed to an artery and a vein (Fig. 8–28).

Distance of Flaps

Flaps are classified according to whether they are local or distant, and each category has subclassifications according to the following arrangement.

  I. Local Flaps
   A. Flaps that rotate about a pivot point
     1. Rotation flaps
     2. Transposition flaps (either single lobed or bilobed)
     3. Interpolation flaps
   B. Flaps that do not rotate about a pivot point
     1. Single pedicle advancement flaps
     2. Bipedicle advancement flaps
  II. Distant Flaps
   A. Indirect flaps transferred from a distance
     1. Tubed pedicle flaps
     2. Axial island flaps
   B. Direct flaps transferred from a distance
     1. Pouch flaps
     2. Single pedicle direct flaps

Local Flaps

Flaps that Rotate About a Pivot Point

Rotation Flaps. A rotation flap is a semicircular or three-fourths circular flap of skin and subcutaneous tissue that rotates about a pivot point into the defect to be closed. The donor site is usually closed by direct suture of the wound; however, skin grafting can be used.[27, 29, 48, 49] This type of flap is economical to construct and is of particular value for closing defects in areas where skin is available only on one side of the lesion (e.g., lesions around the eye, ear, or anus).[66, 77] The technique is also indicated in areas where obtaining skin from one side of the lesion would result in distortion of the structures that are covered by that skin (e.g., the prepuce, scrotum, or ear). Rotation flaps have been described for use around the cheek, scalp, thigh, and sacral areas (Fig. 8–29).[66]

The skin incision that is made to create a rotation flap should be four times longer than the space through which the skin is to be rotated (Fig.

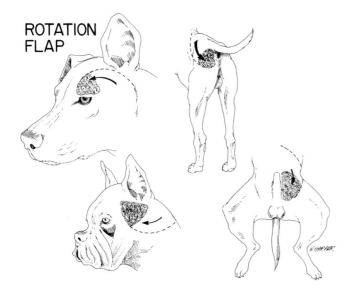

ROTATION FLAP

Figure 8–29: Areas where rotation flaps would be indicated. Such flaps are indicated in areas where skin for closure is available only on one side of the lesion (e.g., eyes, ears, or anus) or where obtaining skin from one side of the lesion would result in distortion of structures in the area (e.g., scrotum, prepuce). (After Swaim, S.F.: Management and reconstruction of traumatized skin. Vet. Audio Rev., Vol. 7, 1978.)

8–30)[56, 68] However, it has been the author's experience that the 4:1 length-rotation ratio is not a rigid rule in dogs and cats owing to the inherent elasticity of the skin. Generally speaking, the longer the incision, the easier it is to distribute the secondary defect along the incision (Fig. 8–31).[48] If the incision is too short (one-fourth circle), the flap becomes more of an advancement flap that is dependent upon stretching rather than upon rotation to move it into place.[49] When a flap is rotated without a back-cut, redundant skin begins to appear along the outer side of the suture line as suturing progresses. Eventually, a dog-ear develops that must be removed for the two sides to be of equal length (Fig. 8–32).[29, 48]

A pure rotation flap has no secondary defect, but often, depending on the laxity of the tissues and the degree of rotation that is required, the primary defect cannot be closed by the redistribution of tension along the suture line.[48] In such instances, a short back-cut is necessary to help relieve tension. This back-cut is made along the diameter line of the circle at the end of the incision that is opposite the lesion.[23, 27, 29, 48] This allows the flap to move by a combination of rotation and transposition. The pivot point of the flap is now located halfway between the end of the back-cut and the apex of the lesion

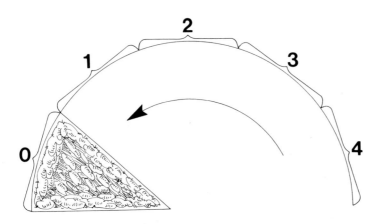

Figure 8–30: The skin incision for a flap should be four times longer than the space through which the skin is to be moved. (After Stark, R.B.: Plastic Surgery. New York, Harper & Row, Publishers, Inc., 1962, p. 60.)

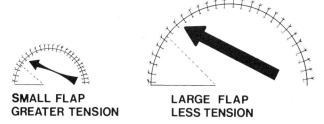

Figure 8–31: Larger flaps result in less tension. This is important around the eye, where tension could distort the palpebra.

SMALL FLAP
GREATER TENSION

LARGE FLAP
LESS TENSION

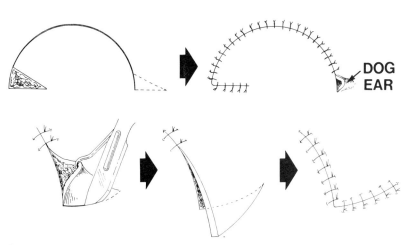

DOG EAR

Figure 8–32: When a rotation flap is rotated without a back-cut, redundant skin will remain along the outer side of the suture line to form a dog-ear. This skin is defined and excised, and a smooth closure is made. (After McGregor, I.A.: Fundamental Techniques of Plastic Surgery, ed. 5. Edinburgh, Churchill Livingstone, 1972, p. 127.)

Figure 8–33: Small back-cut is made along the diameter line of the circle at the end of the incision opposite the lesion. This helps to relieve tension by allowing the flap to move by transposition and rotation. This also reduces the vascular area at the base of the flap.

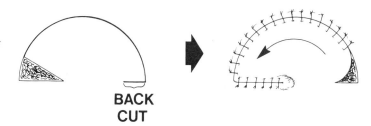

BACK CUT

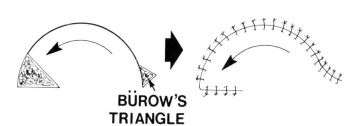

BÜROW'S TRIANGLE

Figure 8–34: Bürow's triangle is a triangle of skin removed tangent to the rotation incision at its base. This is designed to relieve tension but is not as effective as a back-cut. (From Grabb, W.C., and Smith, J.W.: Basic techniques of plastic surgery, in Plastic Surgery: A Concise Guide to Clinical Practice. Boston, Little, Brown and Co., 1968, p. 61.)

(Fig. 8–33).[48] The surgeon should be aware that the back-cut also reduces the vascular area at the base of the flap.[29, 48] In some instances it is possible to cut only those tissues that are responsible for the tension without cutting the blood supply to the flap.[29] In other words, the skin would be incised, but the subcutaneous tissue and its blood vessels would remain intact at the back-cut.

To avoid cutting back into the pedicle of a rotation flap with a back-cut, a small triangle of skin may be removed at the same end of the incision where a back-cut would be made; the triangle (Bürow's triangle) is outside the semicircle and tangent to it.[27, 29, 56] This is of limited benefit in decreasing tension along the radius of the flap (Fig. 8–34).[29]

A modified double rotation flap technique has been described for closing rectangular wounds.[20] As illustrated in Figure 8–35, a curving incision is made starting at one corner of the rectangle (b) and extending to a point level with the base of the lesion (e). The skin between the end of the incision and the base of the lesion forms the pedicle for the flap (ec). The length of this pedicle (ec) should be greater than the width of the lesion (dc). A small triangle of skin (efg) is removed lateral and tangent to the base of the flap incision. The length of the base of the triangle (ef) should be equal to the width of the lesion (ab). The flap is undermined, and the corner of the flap (b) is rotated to meet the corner of the lesion (a). As the flap rotates, the triangle (efg) is obliterated, and the skin edges are sutured together. This closes one half of the rectangle. The

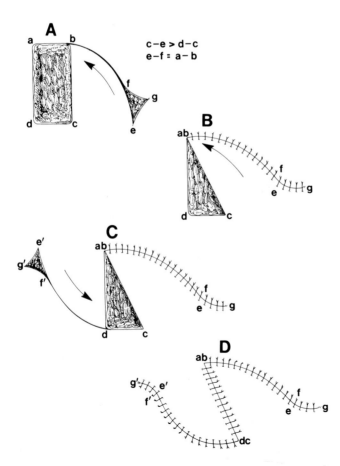

Figure 8–35: A modified double rotation flap for closing large rectangular wounds. Flap *cbe* is rotated to cover one half of the rectangular lesion *abcd*. A triangle of skin, *efg*, is removed at the base of the flap to relieve tension. Note that distance *ce* is greater than distance *dc* and distance *ef* equals distance *ab*. *A*, Designing half of the flap. *B*, Creating half of the flap. *C*, Designing second half of the flap. *D*, Creating second half of the flap. (After Dixon, A.C.: The secondary closure of wounds. Vet. Rec. 75:1141, 1963.)

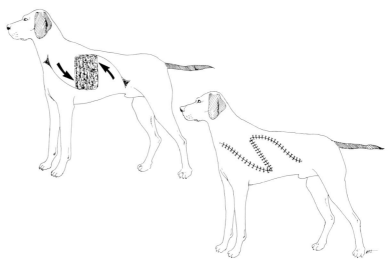

Figure 8–36: Closure of a large rectangular lesion on the trunk of a dog using the modified double rotation flap. The same technique could be used if the lesion were on the dog's back by rotating skin up from the dog's sides.

other half is closed in the same fashion by a flap that is based along the other end of the lesion. This type of rotation flap would be useful for closing large rectangular wounds or wounds that could be converted to a rectangular shape on the trunk of an animal (Fig. 8–36).

Transposition Flaps.   A transposition flap has been described in various ways, but it consists basically of a piece of skin and subcutaneous tissue that is generally rectangular and is turned on a pivot point to reach the adjacent defect that is to be closed. The defect is on a different axis from that of the flap; it is usually, but not necessarily, at a right angle to the axis of the

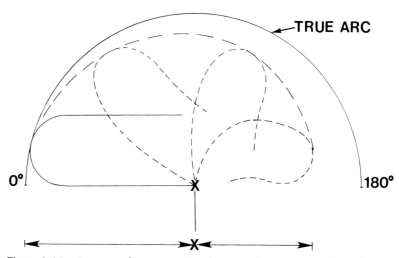

Figure 8–37:   Rotation of a transposition flap around a pivot point (X) results in a loss of effective length the farther the flap is rotated. (From Grabb, W.C.: Classification of skin flaps, in Grabb, W.C., and Myers, M.B. (eds.): Skin Flaps. Boston, Little, Brown and Co., 1975, p. 149.)

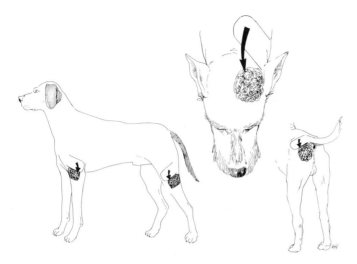

Figure 8–38: Areas where transposition flaps would be indicated. Such flaps could be used in some of the same areas where rotation flaps are used. (After Swaim, S.F.: Management and reconstruction of traumatized skin. Vet. Audio Rev., Vol. 7, 1978.)

flap.[7, 11, 27, 29, 38, 48, 49, 61] A transposition flap becomes shorter in effective length the farther it is rotated (Fig. 8–37).[27] A flap of this kind is used when the recipient area is adjacent to an area covered by loose skin. The proximal antebrachial area and crural regions may be reconstructed with flaps from the brachial and femoral areas, respectively.[11] This type of flap could also be used in many of the same areas in which a rotation flap is used (i.e., around the eye, anus, or ear) (Figs. 8–38 — 8–42). It has been described for the closure of wounds (decubital ulcers) over the pelvic area[75] and of lesions on the distal portions of the limbs.[63] However, it may be difficult to obtain enough skin on the limbs of most dogs for this type of flap.

A piece of cloth may be cut to the shape of the lesion and used as a pattern for designing a transposition flap. The flap of appropriately shaped skin is then incised and transposed from an adjacent area of abundant skin that is 45 to 90 degrees from the recipient site.[41, 58, 61] It is desirable for the flap to be from a different plane from that of the lesion (e.g., a horizontal defect should

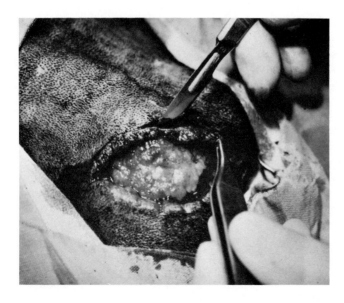

Figure 8–39: A decubital ulcer over the lateral epicondyle of the humerus. Skin edges are being excised.

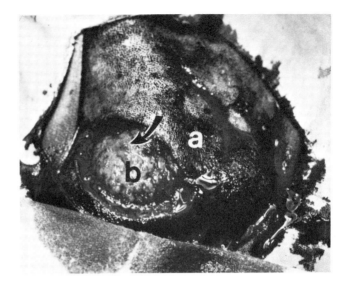

Figure 8–40: A transposition flap (*a*) has been created dorsal and adjacent to the decubital ulcer (*b*). The flap will rotate as indicated by the arrow to cover the lesion.

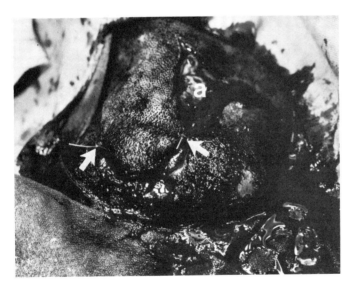

Figure 8–41: The transposition flap has been moved over the lesion and anchored by two sutures (*arrows*). Donor site (*a*).

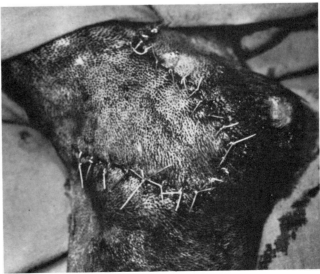

Figure 8–42: The transposition flap is sutured into place.

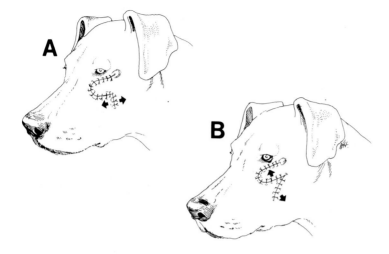

Figure 8–43: *A*, A transposition flap that is taken 90 degrees from the recipient site results in tension away from the recipient site when the donor area is closed. *B*, Tension on the recipient area could result from a flap that is taken at less then 90 degrees to the lesion.

be closed with a vertical flap). When the flap is taken from a different plane, closure of the donor site by undermining and suturing is possible without disturbing the recipient site, since the tension of the approximating sutures is in a different direction from that of the defect. The greater the angle at which the flap is taken, the less the tension will be on the primary area of repair (Fig. 8–43).[23]

The proper design of a transposition flap will prevent undue tension. When a flap is designed, the pivot point should not be adjacent to the lesion but at the other side of the flap's base. If the flap is to close the defect without tension, the diagonal distance from the pivot point to the far point of the lesion must equal the diagonal distance of the flap as measured from the pivot point. It can be seen that the flap must be made longer than the defect to be effective (Figs. 8–44 — 8–50).[48] This will help to compensate for the loss of effective length as the flap is rotated. Before any incision is made, the pivot point of the

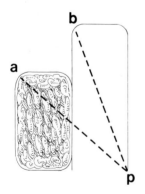

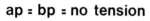

ap = bp = no tension

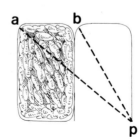

bp < ap = tension

Figure 8–44: To prevent undue tension on a flap, the diagonal distance from the pivot point to the far point of the lesion (*ap*) should be equal to the diagonal of the flap measured from the pivot point (*bp*) (*ap* = *bp*). When *bp* is less than *ap*, there is increased tension across the flap.

flap should be clearly defined, and the diagonal distance from the pivot point across the flap should be compared with that from the pivot to the farthest point of the lesion. If the diagonal distance of the flap is shorter than from the pivot point across the lesion, there will be a line of tension across the flap (Figs. 8–44 and 8–50).[48]

To design a flap that will transpose at a 90-degree angle with no tension, three things should be kept in mind: (1) One edge of the defect should be incorporated into one edge of the flap. (2) The width of the base of the flap should be at least equal to the width of the defect. (3) The edge of the flap that has incorporated the edge of the defect should be at least twice as long as the width of the base of the flap,[27, 79] and it should preferably be long enough to provide a diagonal measurement that closely approaches, if not equals, the diagonal distance from the pivot point to the farthest point of the lesion (Fig. 8–45A and B).

A flap that is designed according to these specifications will have no tension across it but will have a sizable dog-ear (Fig. 8–47A and B). A flap that is

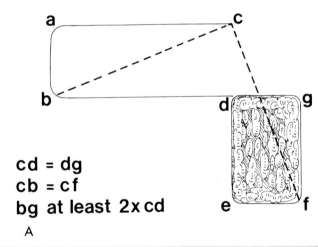

cd = dg
cb = cf
bg at least 2x cd

A

Figure 8–45: *A,* Three factors in designing a nontension flap 90 degrees from the lesion (lower case letters are used as reference points): (1) One edge of the defect (*dg*) should incorporate one edge of the flap (*bdg*). (2) The width of the base of the flap should at least equal the width of the defect (*cd* = *dg*). (3) The edge of the flap that incorporates one edge of the lesion (*bdg*) should be at least twice as long as the base of the flap (*cd*) and should preferably be long enough to provide a diagonal measurement (*cb*) that closely approaches, if not equals, the diagonal distance from the pivot point (*c*) to the farthest point of the lesion (*cf*). *B,* Incision of an actual nontension flap.

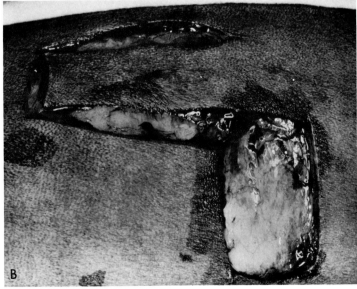

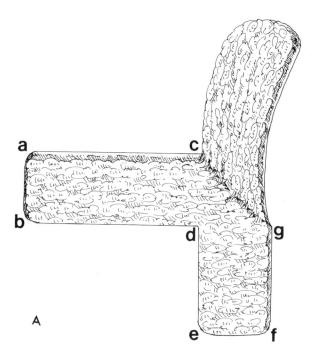

A

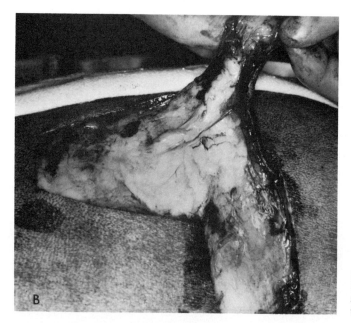

B

Figure 8–46: *A*, The transposition flap has been reflected (lower-case letters are used as reference points). *B*, Reflection of an actual nontension flap.

designed with shorter dimensions will have a line of tension across it after transposition (Fig. 8–50*A* ad *B*).

The main disadvantage of a 90-degree transposition flap is the large dog-ear that is formed. Excising this dog-ear without jeopardizing the blood supply presents a challenge to the surgeon (Fig. 8–49).

Since the skin of the dog and the cat is relatively elastic and mobile, the veterinary surgeon may be able to get by without strict adherence to the rules of flap length. However, it is wise to keep the principles in mind when designing any flap and especially when there is the potential for tension on the flap. If they are going to develop, vascular problems and wound dehiscence most commonly occur at the far corner of a transposition flap (Fig. 8–50).

If a flap is to be designed at less than 90 degrees from the lesion, the surgeon should consider the intervening skin that will be left between the edge of the defect and the defect that is created by the flap. If this peninsula of skin is too long and narrow, it may be subject to necrosis owing to an insufficient blood supply (Fig. 8–51).

After a flap is transposed into a freshened defect, fine chromic catgut sutures are used to join the deep surface of the flap with the recipient bed tissue. This helps to eliminate dead space in which blood and tissue fluid can accumulate to interfere with vascularization of the flap.[54] A procedure has been described in which "walking" sutures or "creeping advancement" sutures have been used to move a flap onto its recipient bed.[9, 72] The technique for performing this procedure has already been described in Chapter 7. This procedure is advantageous in that it moves the flap over the defect, obliterates dead space, and more evenly distributes any tension that may be on the flap.[72]

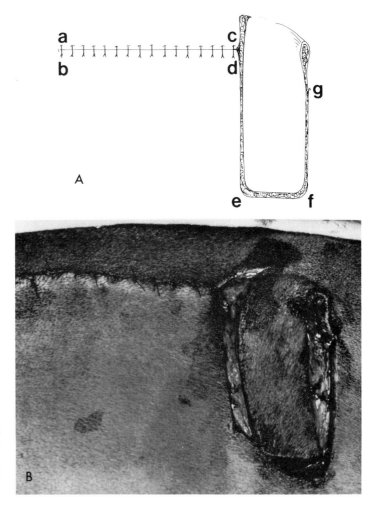

Figure 8–47: A, The transposition flap has been transposed with no tension across the flap. Note dog-ear near point g (lower-case letters are used as reference points). B, Transposition of an actual nontension flap.

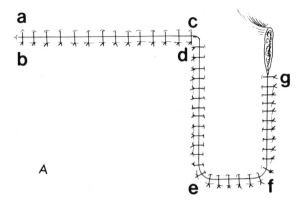

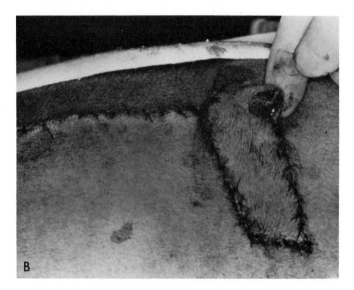

Figure 8–48: *A*, The transposition flap has been sutured into place. A dog-ear is created at the corner of the flap (*g*) (lower-case letters are used as reference points). *B*, Suturing of an actual nontension flap.

After moving a transposition flap into position, the dog-ears will have to be removed from the areas of abundant skin at the base of the flap. If removal of this skin will result in narrowing the base of the flap and jeopardizing its blood supply, it would be wise to close all of the raw edges and leave the dog-ears. After the flap's circulation has been reestablished in its new bed (from 14 to 21 days), the dog-ears may be removed.

Two types of double transposition flaps have been described (Fig. 8–52),[7] and a modification of one of these has been used to reconstruct the perianal area.[11] The technique, which is illustrated in Figure 8–53, requires amputation of the tail and utilization of its skin as flaps. Following removal of the anal sacs and debridement of the perianal area, the tail is amputated in such a manner as to leave a dorsal (*a*) and a ventral (*b*) flap of skin. The ventral flap is divided on the midline to form two flaps (b_1 and b_2), which are transposed over the lateral and ventral areas of the perianal defect. The dorsal perianal defect is covered by the skin of the dorsal flap (*a*). The skin of the tail can also be used to reconstruct injuries in the gluteal area.[11] The use of the tail as a source of skin flaps is dependent upon the breed of dog, the length of the tail, and the desires of the pet owner as to amputation of the dog's tail.

Bilobed Transposition Flaps.   The bilobed flap is a double transposition flap.[49] This type of flap is indicated for use around the face, since a large rotation flap may cause some facial asymmetry and distortion. Long incisions, combined with large areas of undermining, can lead to the development of hematomas and scars. Single transposition flaps are often used for facial closures, but they are frequently complicated by dog-ears and distortion.[50] By using a bilobed flap and shifting the tissues at more than one angle, there may be fewer problems involved in the closure of the donor site, with less distortion and asymmetry and less tension on the suture lines.[50] A bilobed flap allows the surgeon to utilize the laxity of tissue along the axes of both lobes, with the greater laxity being along the secondary lobe.[18] This type of flap also uses the skin adjacent to the defect, resulting in a more cosmetic appearance.[18, 50]

When designing a bilobed flap, one must first be sure that the primary lobe is adequate to cover the defect without undue tension or distortion. After designing the primary lobe the secondary lobe must be placed along an axis

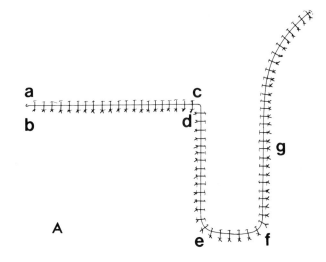

A

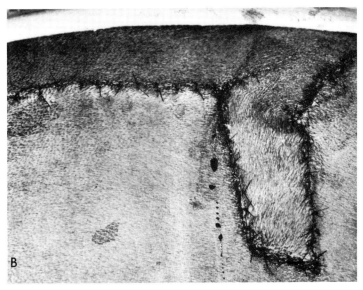

B

Figure 8–49: *A*, The correction of dog-ears on a transposition flap should be done without cutting back into the base of the flap. If this is not possible, the skin should be sutured as it is, and the dog-ear should be corrected at a later date when circulation has been reestablished in the flap (lower-case letters are used as reference points). *B*, Actual nontension flap following correction of the dog-ear.

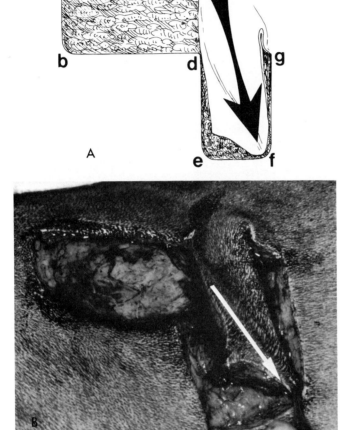

Figure 8–50: *A,* A transposition flap that is designed too short will have tension across it when it is transposed 90 degrees (*arrow*) (lower-case letters are used as reference points). *B,* Transposition of an actual flap that is too short with resultant tension line across the flap (*arrow*). When tension lines develop, vascular problems and wound dehiscence most commonly occur at the far corner of a transposition flap (*tip of arrow*).

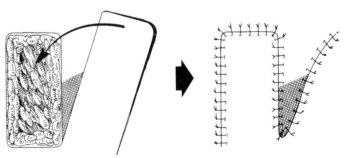

Figure 8–51: When a flap is designed at less than a 90-degree angle to the lesion, if the angle is long and narrow there is the possibility of necrosis of the angle of skin between the flap and the lesion.

▨ = POTENTIAL NECROSIS

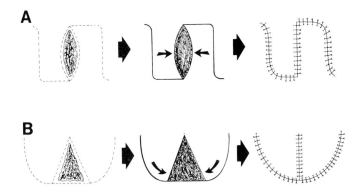

Figure 8–52: Two types of double transposition flaps. *A*, Double transposition flaps that pivot from opposite ends of a lesion. *B*, Double transposition flaps that pivot from the same end of a lesion. (From Berson, M.I.: Atlas of Plastic Surgery, ed. 2. New York, Grune & Stratton, Inc., 1963, pp. 7–8.)

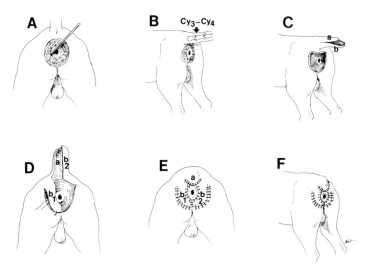

Figure 8–53: A modified double transposition flap to correct a perianal defect. *A*, The anal sacs are removed. *B*, The tail is amputated between Cy_3 and Cy_4. *C*, The skin incisions for tail amputation are designed to leave two flaps (*a* and *b*). The lesion is débrided. *D*, The ventral flap (*b*) is incised on the midline to make two flaps (*b₁* and *b₂*), which are, *E*, sutured over the ventrolateral aspects of the lesion. *F*, The dorsal flap (*a*) is trimmed and sutured over the dorsal aspect of the lesion. (Based on work by W. B. Singleton. After Cawley, A.J., and Archibald, J.: Plastic surgery, in Canine Surgery, ed. 2. Santa Barbara, Calif., American Veterinary Publications, Inc., 1974, p. 150.)

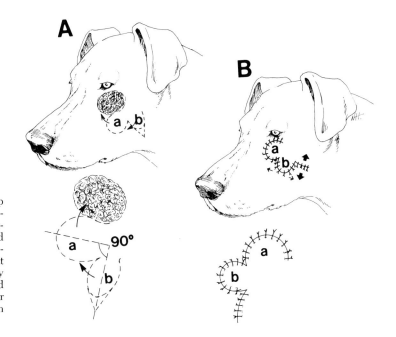

Figure 8–54: *A*, A bilobed flap has been designed with the primary lobe (*a*) as large as, or a little smaller than, the lesion and adjacent to the lesion. The secondary lobe (*b*) is smaller and at a 90-degree angle to the primary lobe. *B*, After the flap is rotated into place, closure of the donor site results in tension away from the area of the defect (*arrows*).

that will allow closure of the secondary lobe defect under the least amount of tension with the least deformity in the area of the secondary lobe defect.[18] The conventional bilobed flap has an angle of 90 degrees between the two lobes.[18, 50] As shown in Figure 8–54, the larger lobe *(a)* is adjacent to the lesion and is the same size as or slightly smaller than the defect. The secondary lobe *(b)* is smaller and may be at an angle of 30 to 120 degrees from the larger lobe.[18, 29, 50] Angles of 45 to 180 degrees have also been reported; however, the larger the angle between the lobes, the larger is the resultant dog-ear at the point of rotation.[18] When designing a bilobed flap, it is important to have a pedicle that is wide enough to insure an adequate blood supply to the lobes. In addition, adequate undermining of the base, the pivot point, and the margins of the defect is necessary for proper approximation.[50]

In summary, a bilobed flap may be considered a refined transposition flap. This type of flap is preferred in reconstruction around an animal's eyes, since a transposition flap that is rotated 90 degrees might necessitate excision of a relatively large dog-ear, and a transposition flap that is rotated less than 90 degrees could still result in tension lines in a direction that would distort the palpebrae (Figs. 8–43 and 8–54).

Interpolation Flaps.   A third type of flap that rotates about a pivot point is the interpolation flap. This flap consists of skin and subcutaneous tissue that are rotated in an arc about a pivot point into a nearby, but not immediately adjacent, defect. The pedicle of the flap passes over or under the intervening tissue (Fig. 8–55).[27, 29, 68] The primary disadvantage of this type of flap when it is passed over intact skin is the exposed undersurface of the pedicle, which presents a problem with drainage and possible infection. If the pedicle were long enough, it could be sutured into a tube to help prevent these problems. This type of flap is not used often in veterinary surgery.

Flaps That Do Not Rotate About a Pivot Point

Single Pedicle Advancement Flaps.   A single pedicle advancement flap (French flap) is a flap of skin that is mobilized by undermining and is ad-

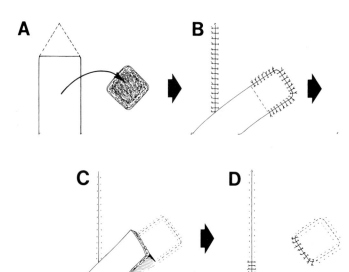

Figure 8–55: *A,* Designing an interpolation flap. *B,* The flap is rotated into position. *C,* The pedicle is excised. *D,* Final closure. (After Grabb, W.C., and Smith, J.W.: Basic techniques of plastic surgery, in Plastic Surgery: A Concise Guide to Clinical Practice. Boston, Little, Brown and Co., 1968, p. 29.)

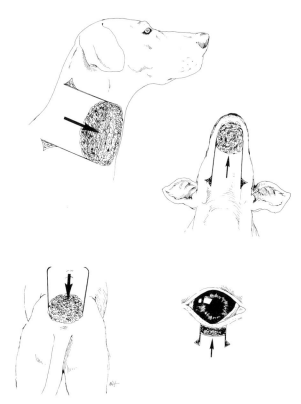

Figure 8–56: Areas where single pedicle advancement flaps would be indicated. (After Swaim, S.F.: Management and reconstruction of traumatized skin. Vet. Audio Rev., Vol. 7, 1978.)

vanced into a defect without altering the plane of the pedicle.[23, 27, 29, 54, 56, 58] This type of flap is of value in defects around which the skin is loose and abundant (e.g., the eyelids, lips, cheeks, and neck).[23] It has also been described for use over the sacral area of a dog (Figs. 8–56 — 8–60).[72]

The surgeon utilizes the elasticity of the skin with this type of flap to move it over a defect.[27, 29] It has been stated that advancing the skin too far will

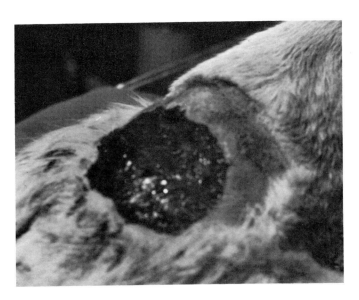

Figure 8–57: A large, nonhealing lesion over a dog's sacrum.

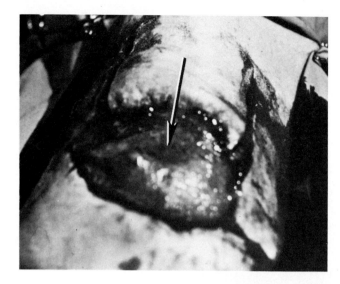

Figure 8–58: Granulation tissue has been removed from the sacral lesion, and a single pedicle advancement flap has been incised cranial to the lesion. The flap will be advanced over the lesion (*arrow*). (From Swaim, S.F.: "Walking" suture technique for closure of large skin defects. J. Am. Anim. Hosp. Assoc., *12*:599, 1976.)

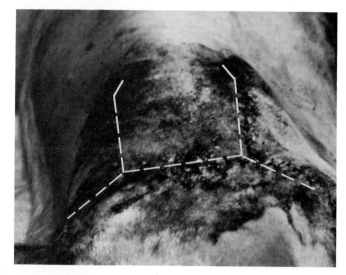

Figure 8–59: The flap has been moved back over the lesion and sutured into place. (From Swaim, S.F.: "Walking" suture technique for closure of large skin defects. J. Am. Anim. Hosp. Assoc., *12*:599, 1976.)

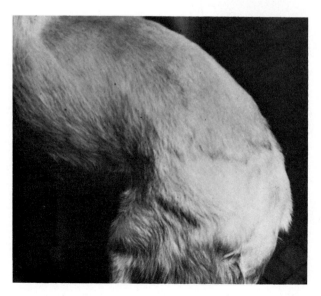

Figure 8–60: Complete healing of the single pedicle advancement skin flap over the sacral area. (From Swaim, S.F.: "Walking" suture technique for closure of large skin defects. J. Am. Anim. Hosp. Assoc., *12*:599, 1976.)

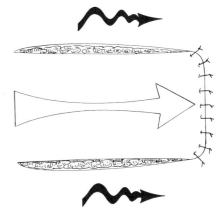

Figure 8–61: When a single pedicle advancement flap is sutured into place, there is tension on the flap but laxity of the skin lateral to the flap.

result in occlusion of the blood vessels by stretching and eventual necrosis of the end of the flap.[67] Contrary to this, a more recent review has stated that a flap with an adequate blood supply will withstand great tension without necrosis.[52] When suturing the flap into place, the surgeon is faced with the problem of suturing the margins of the flap, which are stretched and shorter, to the relaxed lateral margins of the wound, which are longer (Fig. 8–61).[67]

Measures have been taken to overcome the problem of tension on a single pedicle advancement flap. To help equalize the length between the sides of the flap and the adjacent wound margins, triangles (Bürow's triangles) may be excised lateral to the base of the flap (Fig. 8–62).[7, 23, 27, 29, 58, 67] Pantographic expansion also aids in relieving tension on a single pedicle flap. It has been found that if incisions are made perpendicularly into both sides of the base of the pedicle, they will open into a "V" as the flap is advanced. This tends to elongate the shorter sides of the flap as the "V" approaches a straight line and helps to relieve tension on the flap. This technique is similar to the back-cut that is used to relieve tension in rotation flaps; therefore, it presents the same problem. Back-cutting may transect blood vessels that are vital to the distal tip of the flap. To circumvent this problem, the base of the flap may be cut wider

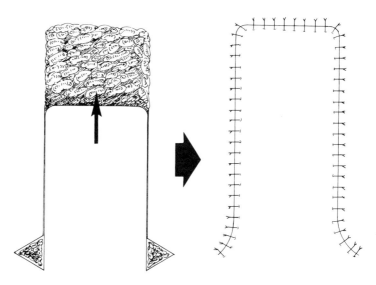

Figure 8–62: Bürow's triangles may be removed lateral to the base of the flap to help equalize the length between the sides of the flap and the adjacent wound margins. (After Grabb, W. C., and Smith, J. W.: Plastic Surgery: A Concise Guide to Clinical Practice. Boston, Little, Brown and Co., 1968, p. 67.)

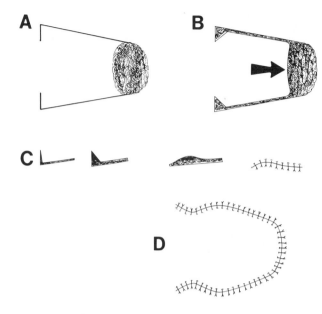

Figure 8–63: *A*, Back-cuts may be made at the base of the flap to help elongate the sides of the flap. *B* through *D*, The cuts open into a "V" and approach a straight line as the flap is advanced. Since back-cuts impinge upon the blood supply entering the base of the flap, the base of the flap is made wider as a compensatory measure. (From Stark, R. B.: The pantographic expansion principle as applied to the advancement flap. Plast. Reconstr. Surg. *15*:223, 1955.)

so that the pedicle remains sufficiently wide to assure a blood supply to the tip of the flap (Fig. 8–63).[23, 27, 29, 67, 68] The addition of small incisions that are made perpendicular to the flap incision in the tissue that is lateral to the flap creates modified Z-plasties, which help to relieve tension (Fig. 8–64).[68] Another way to overcome tension or to distribute it more evenly over the entire flap is to use walking sutures to move the flap into position.[72]

Many modifications have been described for the pedicle advancement flap. The surgeon should consider the shape and location of the wound to be reconstructed and then decide whether a rotation, transposition, advancement, or tubed pedicle flap would best correct the defect. The surgeon has several designs at his disposal if an advancement flap is decided upon (Fig. 8–65).[7, 11, 20, 38, 58]

Subcutaneous Pedicle Flaps.   A subcutaneous pedicle flap is essentially the transposition of an island of skin on a pedicle of subcutaneous tissue. It is unnecessary to include an artery in the design of the pedicle; however, if one is present, it may be included. The vascularity of the flap is dependent upon an adequate subdermal anastomotic network.[3]

This type of flap is useful when primary closure might result in excessive tension on the skin or the distortion of adjacent structures. It has been found to be useful on the trunk, especially in the abdominal wall, and on the lower portion of the leg in humans.[65] The flap has been described for closing circular

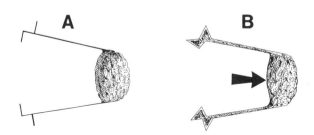

Figure 8–64: *A*, Small incisions are made on the lateral sides of the flap incision near its base. *B*, These create a modified Z-plasty as a tension-relieving technique. (After Stark, R. B.: Plastic Surgery. New York, Harper & Row, Publishers, Inc., 1962, p. 104.)

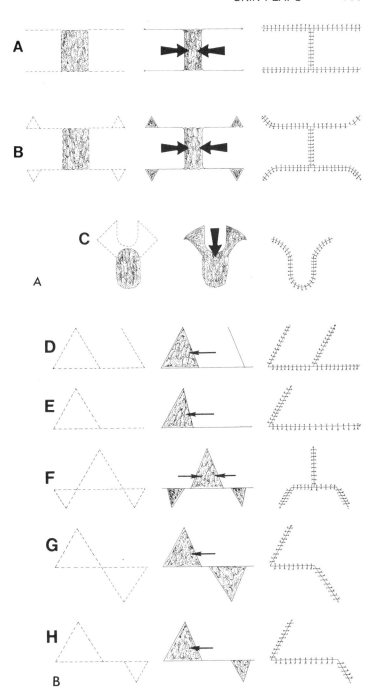

Figure 8–65: Modifications of single pedicle advancement flaps that are used to close square and rectangular lesions, A through C, and triangular lesions, D through H.[7, 11, 20, 38, 58]

wounds and has the advantage of not requiring the removal of significant amounts of skin to correct dog-ears (Fig. 8–66).[76]

Subcutaneous pedicle flaps are effective for resurfacing small defects after tumor excision or trauma and for use in areas where *dermal* pedicle flaps might distort or disfigure the anatomy.[65] The main function of the skin in the pedicle of other types of flaps is to protect the vital structures of the pedicle (e.g., blood vessels). The skin of the pedicle could place an extra metabolic

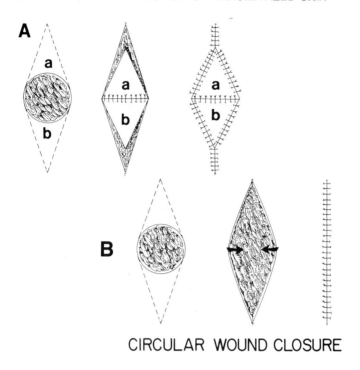

CIRCULAR WOUND CLOSURE

Figure 8-66: *A*, Subcutaneous pedicle flaps (*a* and *b*) are advanced on their pedicles of subcutaneous tissue to close a circular defect. (After Swaim, S. F., and Votau, K.: Prevention and treatment of decubital ulcer in the dog. Vet. Med. Small Anim. Clin. *10*:1073, 1975.) *B*, Closure of the same wound without flaps would require removal of the skin that is used for pedicles (*a* and *b*).

requirement on the flap,[3] and elimination of the skin in a pedicle and retention of the blood vessels could result in a more mobile flap that has a good blood supply.[3] The replacement of eyelids with this type of flap depends on the thickness of the flap. If the flap along with its subcutaneous tissue is too thick, it might not give a good cosmetic result.[44]

When this technique is used to close a circular defect, the skin that would normally form dog-ears is incised, leaving the subcutaneous tissue intact. The area is undermined judiciously so that the blood vessels in the underlying subcutaneous tissue are not damaged. The flaps are then moved into position

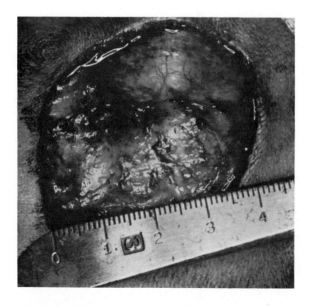

Figure 8-67: A freshened lesion that will be closed by a subcutaneous pedicle flap.

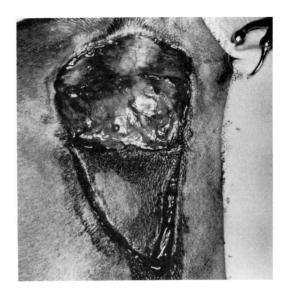

Figure 8–68: A subcutaneous pedicle flap was created by incising the skin only, leaving the subcutaneous tissue intact. Skin lateral and ventral to the flap was undermined. (*The flap itself is not undermined.*)

and sutured. The placement of 4–0 catgut sutures in the subcutaneous tissue at the wound edges and fine nylon sutures in the skin has been described.[44] The placement of subcutaneous sutures could be hazardous if any of the blood vessels in this tissue are occluded by sutures. Although it is particularly useful in circular lesions, this type of flap can be used to close lesions of other shapes (Figs. 8–67 through 8–69).

The movement of subcuticular pedicle flaps under the skin between the donor site and the defect has been described in humans.[3, 29, 49] This may also be considered a form of interpolation flap.[29]

Bipedicle Advancement Flaps. A bipedicle advancement flap can be constructed by making an incision parallel to the long axis of the defect. The skin between the incision and the defect is undermined and advanced into the defect.[7, 23, 27, 29, 38, 68] Closure of the donor site by skin grafts has been described,[27, 29] although undermining and primary closure of the donor site

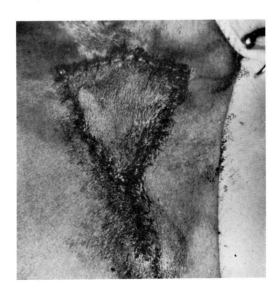

Figure 8–69: After the flap shown in Figure 8–68 was advanced into place, a simple continuous subcuticular suture of 4–0 chromic catgut was used to hold the flap in place. Simple interrupted nylon sutures have been used to suture the skin and to close the ventral defect.

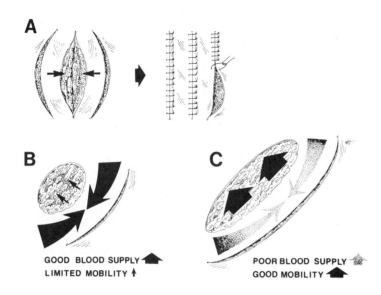

Figure 8–70: *A,* Bilateral bipedicle advancement flaps that advance to cover a central lesion. *B,* A short, wide flap has a good blood supply but limited mobility. *C,* A long, narrow flap has good mobility but poor blood supply.

are usually possible in small animals owing to the elasticity of their skin. This is especially true if the initial incision to create the flap has been in an area of loose skin. This type of flap may be unilateral or bilateral in relation to the lesion. The advancement of a bipedicle flap is facilitated by curving the relaxing incision so that its concave side is toward the lesion (Figs. 8–70 through 8–75).[27, 29]

A bipedicle advancement flap is actually a form of relaxing incision, and care should be taken in making the incision. A short, wide flap has an adequate blood supply but limited mobility. A long, narrow flap has good mobility, but its blood supply may be endangered, which could lead to necrosis of the center of the flap (Fig. 8–70). A bipedicle flap that is two to three times as long as it is wide has been described.[68] The surgeon should bear in mind the stated length-width ratios for bipedicle flaps in order to design a flap that has

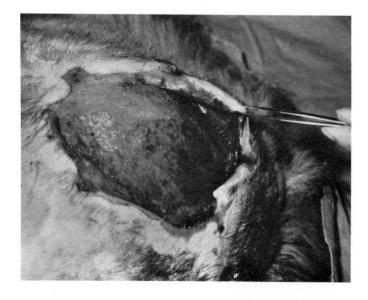

Figure 8–71: A large nonhealing skin lesion over the gluteal area of a collie.

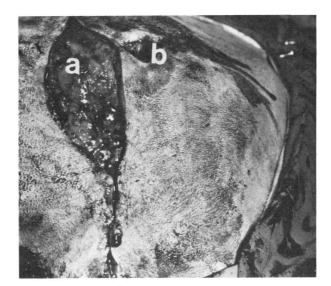

Figure 8–72: The gluteal lesion has been closed with the exception of its center (*a*). Note the lesion over the trochanter major (*b*).

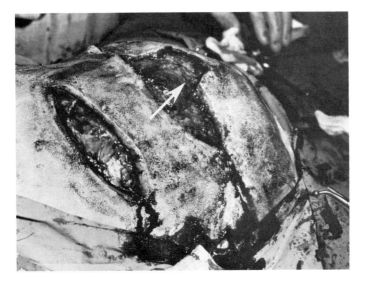

Figure 8–73: A bipedicle advancement flap has been created from the lateral abdominal skin for advancement over the lesion (*arrow*).

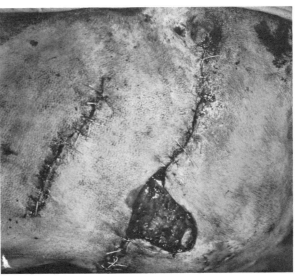

Figure 8–74: The bipedicle advancement flap has been sutured into position. The lesion over the trochanter was corrected at a later date.

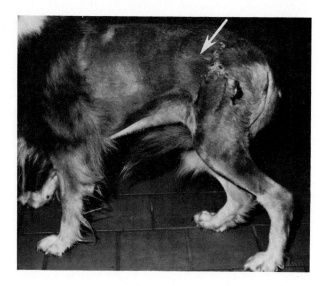

Figure 8–75: Healed bipedicle advancement flap over the gluteal area (*arrow*).

an adequate blood supply and yet is sufficiently mobile to accomplish its purpose.

Distant Flaps

Indirect Flaps Transferred From a Distance

Tubed Pedicle Flaps. In 1916 and 1917 three surgeons recognized independently the value of closing the parallel edges of open pedicle flaps by suturing them together to form tubes. These men were V. P. Filatov of Russia, Hugo Ganzer of Germany, and Harold Delf Gillies of England. Filatov is generally credited with the first use of the tubed pedicle flap. He constructed tubed pedicles experimentally on rabbits prior to using the technique to reconstruct a man's eyelid.[74, 78]

A tubed pedicle skin flap is essentially a bipedicle flap, the edges of which have been sutured together to form a tube resembling a suitcase handle. The skin beneath the flap is closed by a skin graft or by undermining and primary suture. The tubed pedicle is initially attached at both ends, but it is moved one end at a time at about 14-day intervals from the donor to the recipient site.

It has been stated that tubed pedicles should be used only as a last resort for reconstruction in animals.[12, 74] This procedure requires multistaged operations and a longer time period to complete the surgery. Between operations, careful bandaging and close observation are necessary to prevent the animal from mutilating the flap and to protect against other sources of damage to the flap. For these reasons, it is necessary to have both a cooperative owner and animal when using this form of flap.

When the skin that is needed to cover a defect is not available in the immediate area, as on the distal parts of the limbs, it can be moved to these areas by means of a tubed pedicle flap that is created from another area where skin is abundant.[11, 12] It has been stated that lesions on the distal aspect of the pelvic limbs lend themselves best to the use of this type of flap. A flap can be formed on the medial aspect of the tibial and femoral region, thus lessening the chances of a conspicuous scar.[37, 61] However, flaps have been formed on the lateral aspect of the pelvic limb without difficulty (Fig. 8–76).

Designing Tubed Pedicles.   To design a tubed pedicle that is viable, the surgeon must adhere to the stated length-width ratios. The most accepted length-width ratio for tubed pedicle flaps is 2.5:1,[7, 48, 56] but ratios of 2:1[11] and 3:1[49, 54, 61] have also been reported. It has been stated that a tubed pedicle may slough in the middle because of an inadequate blood supply if the width is considerably less than one third of the length.[54] As mentioned earlier, there is a need for a controlled study to determine the length-width ratios for single and bipedicle flaps in the dog and the cat.

When designing a tubed pedicle, it is wise to use the plan in reverse technique, making a pattern of the lesion and "walking" this in reverse through the stage(s) of the surgery back to the origin of the skin flap (Figs. 8–4 through 8–6). The surgeon should consider the direction of hair growth on the flap and determinte how this direction will change each time the flap is moved. The flap should be designed so that when the last transfer is made, the direction of hair growth on the flap will be the same as that of the hair growth on the surrounding area.

Creating Tubed Pedicle Flaps.   After deciding upon the size and the location of the flap, it is helpful to make four small stab incisions at the corners of the pedicle to serve as guideposts for making the parallel incisions. The two parallel skin incisions are made through the full thickness of the skin. It has been suggested that the flap be cut slightly larger than is needed, since it will atrophy some in both length and width during stages of transference.[56] The amount of subcutaneous fat will vary with the patient, but no matter how much fat there is, the pedicle should be raised initially in the plane between the layers of superficial fascia and muscle, leaving no fat on the resulting raw area (Fig. 8–77 *A, B,* and *C*).[48] When the flap and subcutaneous fat are raised in this manner, the flap should be elevated along its full length or even a little beyond and then thinned uniformly until it forms a tube that exerts no tension on the skin edges as they are sutured together.[48] Others have advocated dissecting the fat from the skin as the flap is raised.[54]

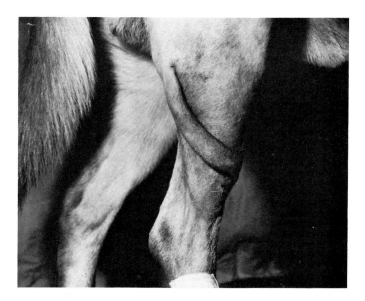

Figure 8–76: A tubed pedicle flap has been created over the lateral aspect of a dog's leg.

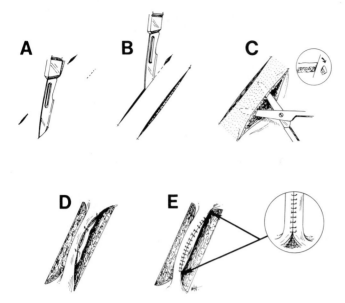

Figure 8–77: The technique for creating a bipedicle tubed flap. *A*, Stab incisions are made at the extremities of the tube. *B*, The stab incisions are connected by parallel incisions. *C*, The flap of skin is undermined, and lifted, and subcutaneous tissue and fat are removed from the undersurface. *Insert*, Fat is trimmed from the edges of the flap. *D*, The flap is sutured into a tube. *E*, Tubing is stopped near the ends of the tube (*arrows*) when tension develops.

Thinning is important because if too much fat is left in the tube, tension results that will interfere with the circulation and may lead to venous congestion and necrosis.[29, 54] It is crucial that thinning be uniform; otherwise the tension on the suture line will vary at different points along the completed tube. This may cause overdistention of the tube at some points and may leave adjoining dead spaces in which blood and serum can accumulate.[54] The hand that holds the flap should be used to judge the amount of thinning that is necessary, since touch and sight give a much more accurate measure than sight alone.[48] The fat along the margins of the skin should be trimmed to prevent small protrusions between the sutures when the flap is tubed (Fig. 8–77C and insert).[48, 54] In an obese patient in which trimming too much fat may lead to major blood vessel damage, the alternatives to thinning are (1) making the flap shorter or (2) developing a wider flap that can be made into a tube without excising the fat.[29]

Hemostasis is of the utmost importance when making a tubed pedicle. If this is not attained, a hematoma may develop within the tube that will not only interfere with circulation but will also provide a focus for the growth of microorganisms. If a blood clot should form in a tube and cause signs of venous congestion, the sutures in the tube should be removed in that area, along with the clot.[54]

A few preliminary interrupted sutures may be used to start tubing the flap (Fig. 8–77D and E). The tubing may then be completed with a simple continuous suture pattern.[48] Simple interrupted sutures may also be used to tube the entire flap, but stainless steel sutures should not be used in such cases, since the tags on these sutures could result in irritation to the underlying skin and suture line.[74] The author prefers 3–0 to 4–0 monofilament nylon or polypropylene for tubing a flap. As each end of the flap is approached, the tension increases, and the tubing should be stopped as soon as there is any suggestion of difficulty in bringing the skin's edges together (Fig. 8–77E).[48]

The area from which the tube was taken must be closed, either by direct suturing[1, 29, 48, 49, 54, 56, 61] or by a skin graft.[29, 48, 49, 54, 56] Owing to the relative elasticity and mobility of the skin of the dog and cat the surgeon is usually able to undermine the surrounding skin and suture the wound edges together. If some tension is present, walking sutures may be used to advance the skin edges together (Fig. 8–78A).

Closure at the junction of the two axial suture lines (suture line of the flap and suture line of the donor area) may present some minor difficulties in that the area of junction that is formed may undergo a small amount of separation or even sloughing.[54] Closure may then be accomplished by a modified three-point suture technique (Fig. 8–78B).[48]

Modifications in Design. Modifications in the design of a tubed pedicle flap have been described. One alteration entails staggering the parallel incisions.[7, 17, 29, 54, 56, 68] This facilitates closure of the extremities of the tube without constricting the pedicle[7] and circumvents the problems that are encountered at the junction of two axial suture lines.[54] There is also less tendency for this type of tube to shorten.[56] The disadvantage of this type of pedicle is that it produces a linear scar beyond the end of the tube that could interfere with the designing of a flap of skin ("pancake") on the end of the tube (Fig. 8–79).[54]

Another modification of the tubed pedicle technique is called the Bunnell method. One of the parallel incisions is converted into an advancement flap, which results in closure of the donor site at a point slightly lateral to the tube and a three-way closure at the junction of the tube with the underlying tissue (Fig. 8–80).[4, 68]

The Vasculature of Tubed Pedicles. A classic study on dogs has shown that the blood vessels in tubed pedicles that have been designed with a random blood vessel pattern undergo significant changes during the first seven days after they have been formed. Immediately after preparation, blood vessels have been found to cross tubes at right angles to their long axis, with no vessels running parallel to the long axis of the tube. One day after the formation of tubes, a few blood vessels have been shown to run almost the entire length of the tubes. By the fourth postoperative day, vessels running parallel to the long axis of the flaps were more marked, and by the seventh day the tubes revealed a well-developed blood supply, with vessels running the entire length of the tube. From the seventh to the 14th day there appeared to be little change in the number, size, or character of vessels in the tubes.[25]

Various times have been proposed as to when the vasculature of a tubed pedicle is sufficiently developed to allow one end of the tube to be transferred

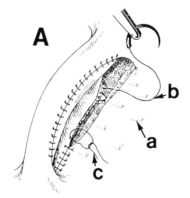
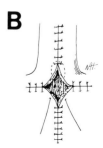

Figure 8–78: *A,* The skin under the tube is closed with walking sutures *(a),* continuous subcuticular sutures *(b),* and simple interrupted skin sutures *(c). B,* The junction of the two axial suture lines is closed by a modified three-point suture.

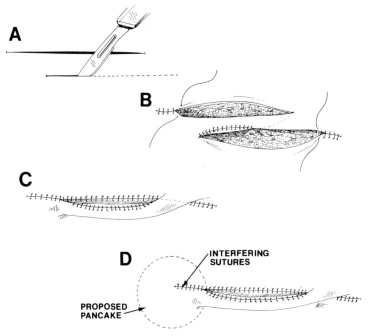

Figure 8-79: *A*, The use of staggered incisions to make a tubed pedicle flap. *B* and *C*, The junction of the two axial suture lines closes more easily with this technique. *D*, The suture line extending beyond the end of the flap could interfere with placing a pancake on the end of the tube.

without endangering the tube. Based on the results of the study just mentioned,[25] as well as those of another study on dogs in which the ends of tubed pedicles were transferred successfully at seven-day intervals,[21] it would appear that seven days is sufficient for the vasculature to reestablish itself in a tubed pedicle. Another study on abdominal tube pedicles in dogs also bears out the seven-day theory.[19] However, most authors in the veterinary literature

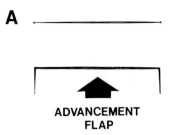

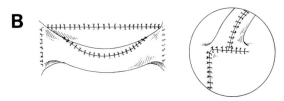

Figure 8-80: Bunnell's technique for making a tubed pedicle. *A*, One of the parallel incisions is transformed to an advancement flap. *B* and *insert*, Closure of the donor site is slightly lateral to the tube, and a three-way closure results at the junction of the tube and the underlying skin. (After Stark, R. B.: Plastic Surgery. New York, Harper & Row Publishers, Inc., 1962.)

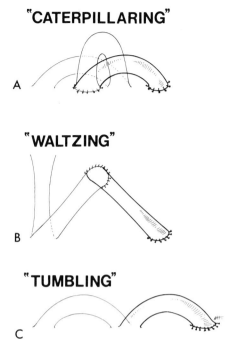

"CATERPILLARING"

A

"WALTZING"

B

"TUMBLING"

C

Figure 8–81: The techniques for moving a tubed pedicle flap: *A*, caterpillaring, *B*, waltzing, and *C*, tumbling. (After Grabb, W. C.: Classification of skin flaps, in Skin Flaps. Boston, Little Brown and Co., 1975, p. 153.)

suggest waiting two weeks before transferring the end of a tube.[1, 11, 58, 61] Other times that have been reported are from 12 to 40 days,[37] from 2½ to three weeks,[49] three weeks,[68] and six weeks.[48] Research on dogs has shown that the blood supply in tubed pedicles that were transferred immediately after being formed was not as good as that in delayed tubed pedicles. All tubes that were transferred immediately progressed through color changes similar to those that are seen in free full-thickness grafts. No 100 per cent takes were achieved in flaps that were transferred in this way.[37]

Techniques for Transferring Pedicles.   Three techniques have been described for transferring the ends of tubed pedicle flaps. These are "caterpillaring,"[4, 27, 29, 74] "waltzing,"[4, 27, 29, 48, 54, 74] and "tumbling" (Fig. 8–81).[27, 29, 74] Caterpillaring involves moving one end of the tube close to the other end so that the flap is doubled on itself in the first stage. Following this stage the other end of the tube is moved away from the first end as far as possible. The movement is analogous to that of an inchworm or caterpillar (Figs. 8–82, 8–83, and 8–84). This type of movement is advantageous in that the direction of hair growth is the same at all times; however, it takes longer to move the flap to the recipient site than if tumbling were used.[74]

Waltzing entails alternate movement of the ends of the tube laterally from the donor to the recipient site (Fig. 8–85). Each time the tube is moved, the direction of hair growth is changed, and it may take longer to move a flap to the recipient site than it would if tumbling were used.

When a tube is tumbled, one end is cut free and moved up and over the attached end to a new site (i.e., the flap is moved in the same way that an athlete tumbles head over heels). This technique requires less time to move a tubed pedicle to the recipient site; however, with this type of movement the possibility of kinking the blood vessels of the tube is greater, and the direction of hair growth changes each time the tube is moved (Fig. 8–22). With

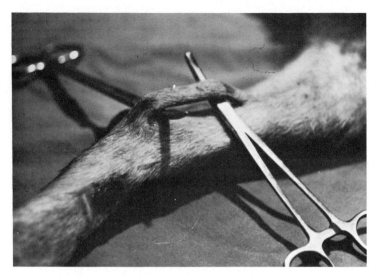

Figure 8–82: A tubed pedicle flap has been created on a dog's leg.

regard to the direction of hair growth on a tubed pedicle, it can be seen why it is especially important to plan the flap in reverse if waltzing or tumbling is to be used as a transfer method.

When one end of a tubed pedicle is to be transferred to an intermediate site prior to moving the other end of the tube, a "trap door" technique may be used to affix the end of the tube to the intermediate site.[4, 29, 48, 54] The end of the tube is moved to the intermediate site and a blood-stained imprint is made with the cut end of the tube.[48] This determines the size of the trap door to be made. A semicircular incision is made around the imprint. Undermining this semicircular incision creates a flap of skin. When this flap is turned back like a trap door, a rounded, raw surface is exposed. The end of the tube is placed over this surface.[54] Fine chromic catgut sutures are used to attach the raw surface on the end of the tube to the prepared bed, and fine silk sutures may be used to approximate the skin (Fig. 8–86).[54] The author prefers 3–0 catgut for attaching the raw surface on the end of the tube to the bed and 4–0 mono-

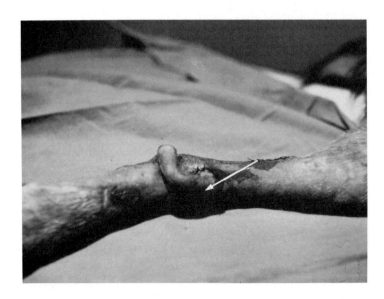

Figure 8–83: The proximal end of the tube has been moved near the distal end (arrow) in the first stage of caterpillaring a tube.

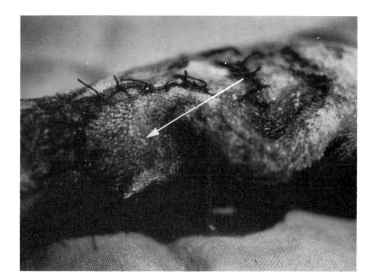

Figure 8–84: The distal end of the tube has been moved away from the proximal end *(arrow)* and opened over the lesion in the second stage of caterpillaring.

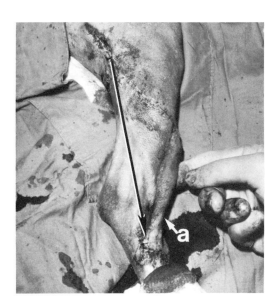

Figure 8–85: A tubed pedicle *(a)* has been waltzed laterally down a dog's leg. The proximal end of the tube was detached from a point indicated by the base of the arrow and reimplanted in the area indicated by the point of the arrow.

Figure 8–86: The trap door technique for attaching a tubed pedicle to an intermediate site. *A*, The cut end of the tube makes a bloody imprint on the intermediate site. *B*, A semicircular incision is made around the imprint site, with undermining of the semicircular flap. *C*, The semicircular trap door is reflected back, and the end of the tube is attached to the raw areas with simple interrupted catgut sutures. *D*, Skin closure is accomplished with simple interrupted sutures. *E*, Completed implantation of the end of a tubed pedicle.

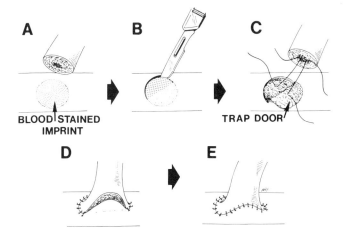

filament nylon or polypropylene for suturing the skin. As with the transplantation of a simple open flap, it is important to eliminate dead space at the site of attachment of the tube. The accumulation of blood or tissue fluids in such a space interferes with the peripheral vascularization of the flap; it is imperative that hemostasis be complete in both the tube and the recipient bed,[54] and if a clot does form, it should be evacuated.[48]

Revascularization Following Transference. A study on rabbits has yielded some insight into the revascularization of a tubed pedicle after one end has been transferred.[6] This study revealed that vascular connections appeared uniformly on the fourth or fifth day following transfer and that the vasculature developed from these.

Based on the assumption that blood vessels within a flap are sympathectomized and toneless, a theory has been presented to explain how the vasculature within the flap develops from the transferred end of a tubed pedicle. When the cut end of a tube is inset at an intermediate site, new capillaries cross the inset within five to six days to join the vessels at the intermediate site with those in the end of the tube. The vessels at the intermediate site, which are feeding the capillaries, are normal and contain blood at a normal blood pressure. The vessels at the end of the tube are denervated and therefore contain blood at a very low pressure. Blood is therefore driven from the vessels at the intermediate site, through the capillaries at the inset, and into the dilated vessels at the end of the tube. As more capillaries grow across the inset each day, more blood enters the tube and is driven farther along it. Finally, when the second attachment of the tube is divided, all of the vessels in the tube are denervated. The blood that is entering from the intermediate site does not encounter any peripheral resistance and is easily driven from one end of the tube to the other by the blood pressure of the vessels in the intermediate site.[34]

Covering the Recipient Site. To cover a recipient site, a tubed pedicle may be "untubed,"[48, 54, 58, 74, 78] or a flap (pancake)[2, 29, 48, 56, 70] of tissue may be transported on the end of the tube to cover the recipient site. When the

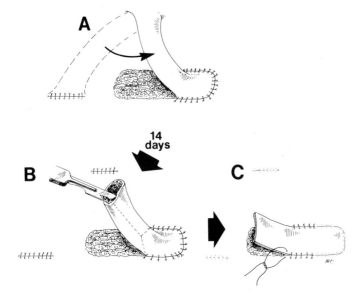

Figure 8–87: *A,* One end of a tubed pedicle is detached, untubed, and affixed to one end of the recipient bed, leaving the other end attached. *B,* Fourteen days later the other end is detached and untubed and (*C*) then affixed to the remainder of the recipient site.

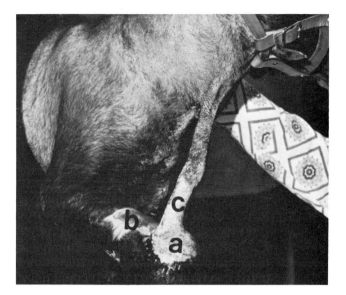

Figure 8–88: One end of a tubed pedicle has been attached to part of a lesion (a). The remainder of the lesion (b) will be covered with the adjacent part of the tube (c). (From Swaim, S. F., and Bushby, P. A.: Principles of bipedicle tube grafting in the dog. J. Am. Anim. Hosp. Assoc. *12*:602, 1976.)

untubing of a pedicle is to be used for covering a defect, the surgeon may perform the procedure in one of two ways, depending upon the size of the lesion.

For large lesions the aim is to untube one end and attach that end to a suitable segment of the defect in such a manner that a vascular linkup will be established, and this vascular linkup will be sufficient to support the remainder of the tube when it is detached, untubed, and placed over the remainder of the defect. After a three-week delay, the other end of the tube is cut free, untubed, and attached to the recipient site[48, 74] (Figs. 8–87 through 8–89).

With small lesions the detached end of the tube is untubed so that it covers the entire recipient site. After waiting from ten days to two weeks, the remaining portion of the tube is excised at its attachment to the untubed

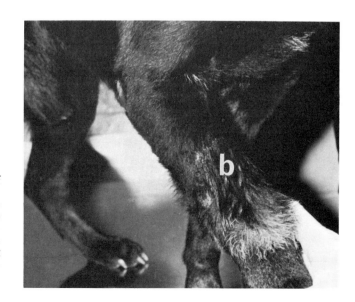

Figure 8–89: The remaining end of the tubed pedicle has been detached. The portion of the tube adjacent to the lesion has been untubed and affixed to the lesion (b). Healing is complete. (After Swaim, S. F., and Bushby, P. A.: Principles of bipedicle tube grafting in the dog. J. Am. Anim. Hosp. Assoc. *12*:602, 1976.)

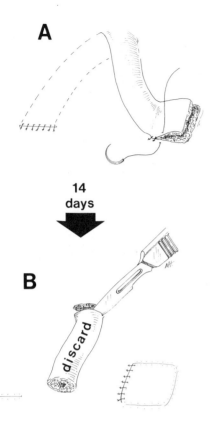

A

14 days

B

discard

Figure 8–90: *A*, One end of a tubed pedicle has been detached and untubed and is being affixed to the entire lesion. *B*, At the end of 14 days the remainder of the tube is detached and discarded.

portion and at its other attachment and is discarded (Figs. 8–90 through 8–92).[58, 74, 78]

When a tubed pedicle is untubed, the incision should be made along the longitudinal scar on its undersurface. This incision should extend to the core of the tube so that it can be unrolled to form a flat flap.[54] When the tube is opened, it may be found that an axial line of scarring has developed along its

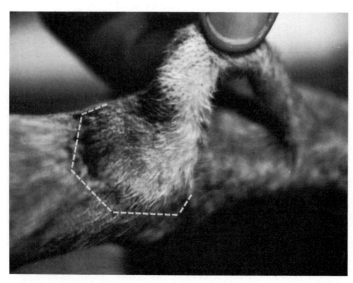

Figure 8–91: One end of a tubed pedicle has been untubed and applied to a lesion.

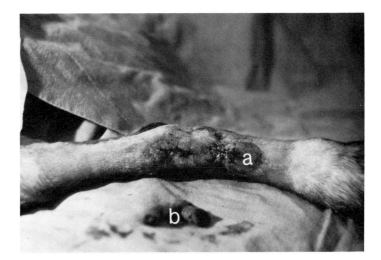

Figure 8–92: The untubing and transfer of a tubed pedicle have been completed (*a*). The remainder of the pedicle (*b*) has been detached.

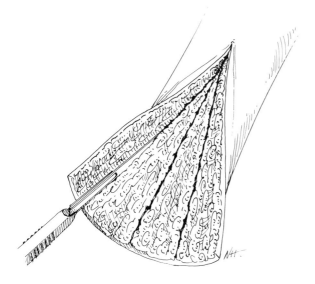

Figure 8–93: An incision is made along the longitudinal scar on the undersurface of a tube. A central core of scar tissue is removed when necessary, and longitudinal scoring of the flap is performed. These procedures should be done judiciously, since extensive scar removal and longitudinal scoring may result in damage to the nutrient vessels supplying the skin.

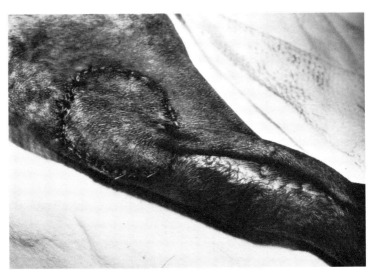

Figure 8–94: A pancake has been delayed on the end of a tubed pedicle.

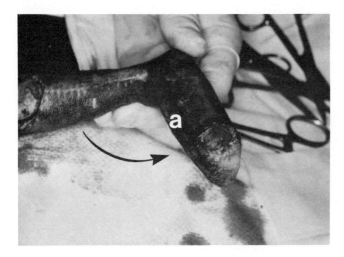

Figure 8–95: The pancake has been raised and rotated *(arrow)* on the tubed pedicle *(a)* to cover the lesion on the distal aspect of the limb.

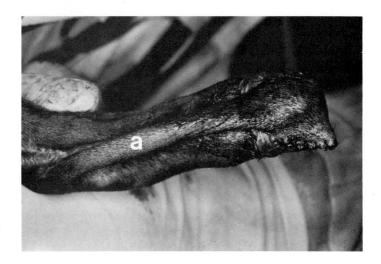

Figure 8–96: The pancake has been sutured in place over the lesion. Note the tubed pedicle *(a)*.

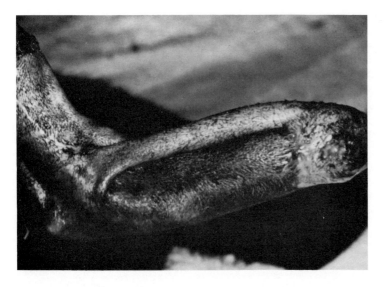

Figure 8–97: The pancake has healed over the lesion.

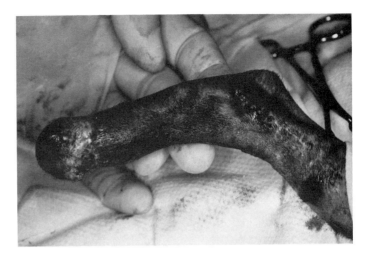

Figure 8–98: The tubed pedicle has been removed.

center, which may prevent the untubing. The excision of this scar tissue or longitudinal scoring may be indicated to permit the tube to unroll fully (Fig. 8–93).[48] However, the removal of scar tissue or the longitudinal scoring of the tube should be done judiciously, since these procedures may result in damage to vital blood vessels in the end of the tube.[74]

The second method of covering a recipient site is with a flap (pancake) of skin that is transferred on the end of a tubed pedicle.[2, 48, 56, 70, 74] The pancake should be prepared two or more weeks after the tubed pedicle has been made (Fig. 8–94).[56] Delaying the pancake on the end of the tube is advisable if there is any question about the blood supply to it.[2, 48, 56] This technique offers additional tissue to cover a defect, as well as the mobility provided by the tube to get the tissue to the defect (figs. 8–95 through 8–98).

Lengthening Tubed Pedicles. When it is desirable to create a long tubed pedicle that will reach directly to a defect without the use of multistaged operations, a "bridging" technique may be used.[54] To create such a tube, two

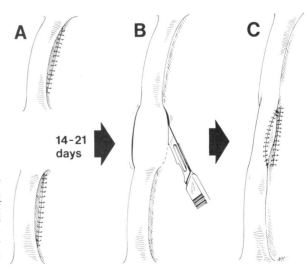

14-21 days

Figure 8–99: *A,* A long tubed pedicle may be created by making two shorter tubes with a connecting bridge. *B,* After a period of delay, the connecting bridge is incised and *C,* tubed to form one long tubed pedicle. (After Swaim, S. F., and Bushby, P. A.: Principles of bipedicle tube grafting in the dog. J. Am. Anim. Hosp. Assoc. *12*:601, 1976.)

tubes of standard length and a connecting bridge are constructed. After a delay period, the bridge is cut and tubed, thus forming one long tube (Fig. 8–99).[7, 48, 54, 56, 68, 74, 78] The surgeon may desire to cut the bridge in stages if there is any question about the blood supply to the tube.[48] With this technique it is possible to create an even longer tube by using more than one bridge.[56] Flaps that are created in this fashion have the advantage of allowing the donor site to be at a greater distance from the defect that is to be covered; however, they have the disadvantage of requiring more time for their construction.[74]

A second technique that has been described for lengthening a tubed pedicle requires making two parallel incisions at one extremity of the tube. A flap is created by undermining the skin and subcutaneous tissue between these incisions. The flap is sutured back into its original bed in a delaying procedure and a tube is formed after two weeks (Fig. 8–100).[54]

Advantages and Disadvantages.   The main advantage of a tubed pedicle is that it maintains a blood supply at all times while being transferred.[58, 74, 78] It also has the advantages of being more mobile,[56, 78] allowing more skin to be obtained for closure of a defect,[56] and resisting infection.[78] The disadvantages of a tubed pedicle flap are the additional time that is required to establish a good blood supply in the tube following each movement, the multiple operations, and the care that is needed to prevent injury to the tube between operations.[58, 61] It is necessary to check a recently attached tube frequently, since kinking, torsion, and gravity may have a deleterious effect on the circulation of the tube as a result of impaired venous drainage.[7, 48, 56] Venous congestion may interfere sufficiently with the blood supply to cause sloughing of the tissue.[54] If a small area of slough does develop along a tube, this area may be removed and the ends of the tube may be sutured together again (Fig. 8–101). After healing, the tube is treated as if no complication had occurred. If one end of a tube should slough prior to migration, the necrotic area should be excised if possible, and its new end should be implanted in an adjacent area. If this end takes, the procedure may then be continued in the normal fashion; however, it may be necessary to lengthen the affected end of the tube to regain any length that was lost owing to the slough (Fig. 8–101*B*).[4]

Aftercare.   The proper bandaging and aftercare of a tubed pedicle are essential to its survival. Positioning and supporting the tube are often necessary to prevent kinking and torsion. When a tube is dependent, it is important that it be supported to prevent the weight of the tube from pulling the sutures out of their bed.[7] One way to position and support a tube is by means of gauze pads that are placed along the full length of the tube on both sides. Strips of

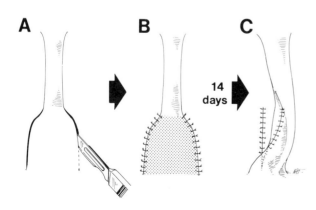

Figure 8–100: *A,* To lengthen a tubed pedicle, two parallel incisions are made at one extremity of the tube, and the tissue is undermined. *B,* The skin is sutured back into its original position as a delaying technique. *C,* At a later date the skin is reincised and sutured into a tube. (After New, G.B., and Erich, J.B.: The Use of Pedicle Flaps of Skin in Plastic Surgery of the Head and Neck. Springfield, Ill., Charles C Thomas, Publisher, 1950, p. 28.)

A   B   C

14 days

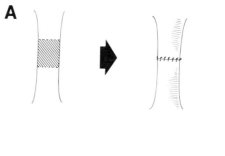

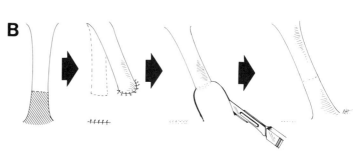

Figure 8–101: *A*, If a small area of slough develops in the center of a tube, it may be excised and the tube resutured. *B*, If a slough develops at one end of the tube, it may be excised. The end of the tube is reimplanted and, if necessary, may be lengthened (see Fig. 8–100) at a later date. (After Barsky, A.J., Kuhn, S., and Simon, B. E.: Principles and Practice of Plastic Surgery, ed. 2. New York, McGraw-Hill Book Co., 1964, p. 81.)

adhesive tape running parallel to the long axis of the tube are used to hold the padding in position (Fig. 8–102). Wrapping and tape are then applied over the flap and the tube.[54] Dressings must be applied so that no pressure is exerted on the tube, and any strips of tape that are placed at right angles to the tube should be loose.[7, 54]

The tubed pedicle is a unique and interesting type of skin flap, and, as with all other surgical techniques, it has advantages and disadvantages that must be taken into consideration before deciding on such a flap. The author reserves the use of tubed pedicles as a last resort for skin reconstruction because of the time involved in performing the multistaged operations of tube transfer. If the veterinarian decides to use this type of flap for reconstruction, both a cooperative animal and owner are necessary. For economical reasons, it would be worth the veterinarian's time to instruct the pet owner on how to

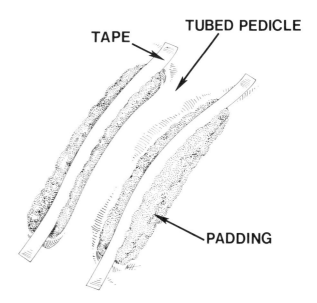

Figure 8–102: A tubed pedicle is bandaged to prevent kinking and torsion. Support padding is placed on both sides of the tube and held in place by strips of tape. The tube is covered by additional wrapping.

change bandages to protect a tubed pedicle during the stages of its transfer. In this way the animal could be treated as an outpatient between surgical procedures.

Axial Island Flaps.   The axial pattern island flap is a relatively new type of flap when compared with the other types that have been discussed. The basic procedure is the complete removal of a piece of skin, leaving its subcutaneous tissue and vascular supply intact. The major vessels supplying the flap of skin and subcutaneous tissue are anastomosed to vessels in the recipient bed. The piece of skin thus qualifies as a flap, since it has a pedicle supplying its circulatory needs (Fig. 8–28).

A technique for creating island flaps in dogs has been described. In this experimental study a section of abdominal skin was removed along with the superficial epigastric vessels supplying it. The vessels were then anastomosed to vessels in a cervical recipient area, and the flap was sutured onto the overlying defect.[42]

Modifications of this technique in which muscle has been included in the flap have been described.[30, 62] In one study a section of gracilis muscle with its intact blood supply, which also supplied the overlying skin, was used as a flap.[30] In another study a piece of gracilis muscle, along with the branches of the femoral artery and vein supplying it, was sutured to the undersurface of a section of skin that was later to be used as a flap. After vascular connections had been established between the muscle and the skin, these tissues and the blood vessels supplying them were removed and placed in the cervical area, where these vessels were anastomosed to recipient vessels.[62] In both studies, the results were relatively successful.

The use of this type of flap in dogs has, for the most part, been experimental. The technique has the advantage of requiring only one operation to transfer the flap to the recipient site. However, the disadvantages associated with the procedure make it of limited value to the practitioner. They include (1) the need for an operating microscope to anastomose the small vessels involved; (2) the possibility of not having suitable blood vessels in the recipient area to anastomose with the donor vessels; and (3) the possibility that the skin from the abdominal area that is supplied by the superficial epigastric vessels may be cosmetically unacceptable as a flap (especially in the female) because of the mammary structures. Likewise, skin from the proximal-medial aspect of the pelvic limb, which is supplied by branches of the femoral vessels, may not have sufficient hair to provide a cosmetically acceptable repair elsewhere on the body. The transfer of island flaps on a pedicle containing their original nerve and vessel supply has been described for the correction of trophic metacarpal pad ulcers in dogs.[26a]

Direct Flaps Transferred From a Distance

Pouch Flaps.   A pouch flap is a direct flap that is transferred from a distance.[27] The pouch flap is an open type of flap and is used to reconstruct defects on an extremity.[10, 27, 38, 38a, 58, 61, 81] Therefore, the mobility of the extremity must be considered in the construction of this type of flap. A pouch flap is actually a bipedicle advancement flap in which the lesion is advanced to the flap rather than the flap being moved to the lesion. Such flaps are usually constructed in one stage and transferred in a second stage.

When the direction of hair growth on a limb will affect cosmesis (e.g., on a short-haired dog), a pouch flap would be indicated more often for front limb lesions than for hind limb lesions. The direction of hair growth along the lateral aspect of the thorax and on the forelimb is usually similar, but the direction of

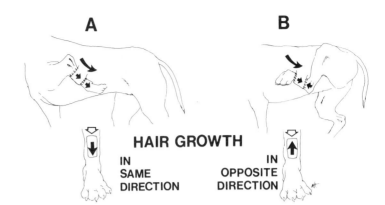

Figure 8–103: *A*, The direction of hair growth on the lateral thoracic area and the forelimb is usually similar in dogs. *B*, The direction of hair growth on the distal aspect of the hind limb is usually dissimilar to that on the lateral thoracic and abdominal area.

hair growth on the distal aspect of the pelvic limb and along the lateral abdominal and thoracic areas is dissimilar (Fig. 8–103). However, it must be borne in mind that hair growth directions will vary on individual animals. Other factors to be considered when using a pouch flap are the color, texture, and length of the hair on the donor site as compared with those characteristics of the hair in the area of the lesion.

The size and temperament of an animal must be considered when a pouch flap is contemplated. For example, a cat or a small dog will more readily tolerate a limb being bandaged up along its side than a Saint Bernard or a Great Dane.

When preparing a pouch flap, particular attention should be given to the aseptic preparation of the limb on which the pouch flap will be used, since a portion of the limb or paw will be in contact with an area of subcutaneous tissue on the thorax or abdomen. The scar tissue surrounding the lesion should be removed when preparing the recipient site for a flap of this type. In addition, some normal tissue should be removed to insure a good attachment for the flap (Fig. 8–104).[10] As with other types of flaps, it is wise to plan a pouch flap in reverse. It is thus possible to arrive at the correct origin of the flap (Fig. 8–105).[26] After determining the size and origin of the flap, two parallel dorsoventral incisions are made on the lateral aspect of the thorax or abdomen. The distance

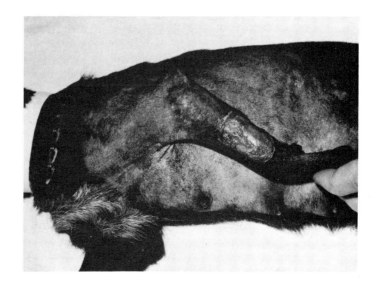

Figure 8–104: The edges of a forelimb lesion have been trimmed and the wound has been prepared for a pouch flap.

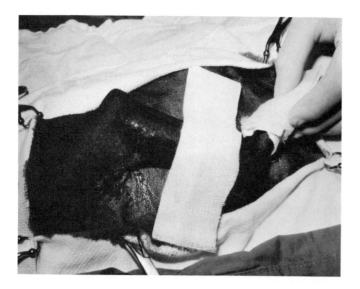

Figure 8-105: A pouch flap was planned in reverse using a piece of sterile surgical sponge. The surgical sponge is the same width as the lesion. Two parallel incisions this width will be made in the skin on the dog's thorax.

between these incisions is equal to the dorsoventral dimension of the defect. The flap thus created is undermined and freed from the subcutaneous fat and fascia, and the injured extremity is placed through the flap so that the lesion lies under the flap (Fig. 8-106). Simple interrupted sutures are used to join the edges of the flap with the edges of the wound (Fig. 8-107).[58, 61] With flaps of this type, the surgeon should try to get as much of the flap as possible in contact with the defect during this initial procedure. A good rule is to construct the flap so that any movement pulls the flap onto the defect rather than away from it. In essence, an attempt should be made to wrap the flap around the limb (Fig. 8-108).[48] Tacking sutures (two or three) may be used to help immobilize the flap over the lesion. A small Penrose drain may be installed at the base of the flap to drain off any fluids that may accumulate in the tissues under the flap and the limb. The drain is usually removed after a few days if there is no drainage (Fig. 8-109).

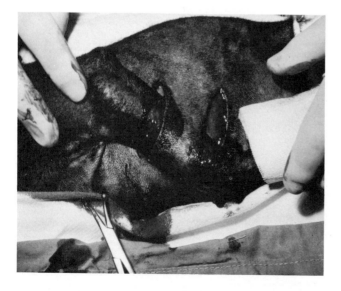

Figure 8-106: The limb was placed through the pouch flap so that the flap lies over the lesion.

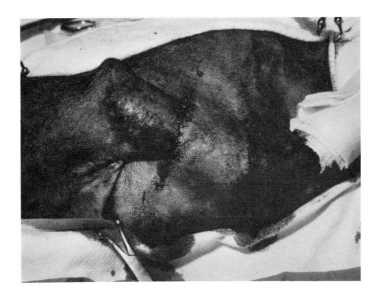

Figure 8–107: Simple interrupted sutures were used to join the edges of the flap with the edges of the wound.

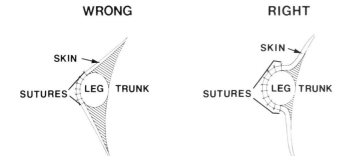

WRONG   **RIGHT**

Figure 8–108: A pouch flap should be sutured in as close contact to the lesion as possible in an attempt to wrap the flap around the limb.

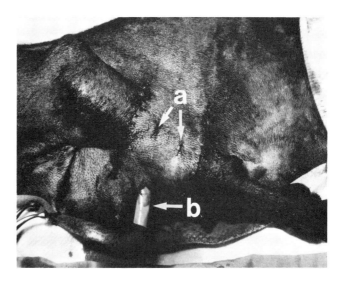

Figure 8–109: Tacking sutures (*a*) may be used to help immobilize the flap against its bed. A Penrose drain (*b*) may be placed at the base of the flap to drain any tissue fluids that might accumulate.

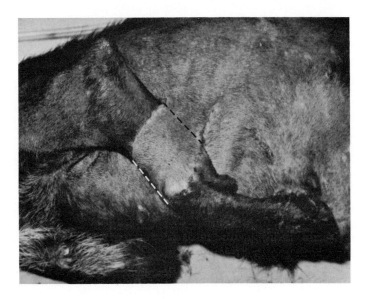

Figure 8–110: The pouch flap two weeks after its construction. The flap was severed at the dotted lines and sutured to the remaining edges of the lesion.

Complete immobilization is necessary for 14 days, at which time the attachments of the flap to the donor site are excised, trimmed, and sutured to the adjacent wound margins of the defect.[58, 61] Owing to the mobility of the skin over the thoracic and abdominal area, the defect that remains at the donor site is usually closed by undermining and moving the skin edges together (Figs. 8–110 and 8–111).

If there is doubt as to the adequacy of the blood supply that has developed in the flap during the 14-day postoperative period, the flap may be separated from the donor area in stages as a surgical delaying technique. A delaying technique may also be effective in increasing the size of the flap so that surfaces that were not accessible during the primary procedure may be covered. If a flap appears edematous and the circulation is in question, all surgery should be postponed a few days.[10]

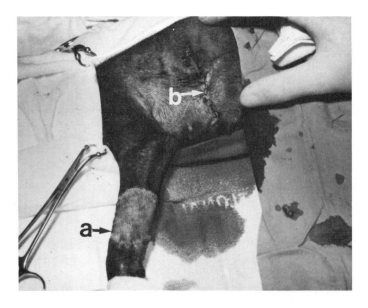

Figure 8–111: The completed transfer of the pouch flap (a) to the forelimb, with closure of the thoracic defect by primary suturing (b).

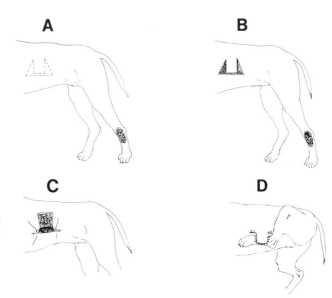

A   **B**

C   **D**

Figure 8–112: *A*, A single pedicle direct flap is designed along the lateral thoracic area. *B*, The flap is created, and *C*, undermined. *D*, the flap is sutured in place over the lesion. (After Spreull, J.S.: The principles of transplanting skin in the dog. J. Am. Anim. Hosp. Assoc. 4:77, 1968.)

Single Pedicle Direct Flaps. A modification of the pouch flap is the single pedicle flap in which the limb lesion is advanced toward the flap (Fig. 8–112).[11, 38, 79] The principles and techniques for constructing this type of flap are basically the same as those for a pouch flap.

The aftercare of a pouch flap or of its single pedicle modification entails immobilization of the limb in a body bandage or cast. If there is any drainage from the surgical area, the dressings will have to be changed periodically to help prevent infection. Topical antibiotics, systemic antibiotics, or antibiotic flushes under the flap may be used to control any infection that might develop. Caution should be exercised in flushing the area so that neither too much nor too caustic a solution is used, since either of these would damage the delicate vascular linkage between the underside of the flap and its bed. Such irrigation should be used only if infection is definitely present.

The advantage of a pouch flap or a single pedicle flap over a tubed pedicle flap is that it reduces the number of essential operations to two, and yet the blood supply to the flap is still maintained.[26] The primary disadvantage of these flaps is the immobilization of a limb in a body bandage for a period of time[11, 58] and the resultant joint stiffness that often accompanies this.[48, 69] To help prevent the stiffening of joints during the time of immobilization, the joints that are not covered by a dressing may be massaged. In addition, tranquilizers may help to make the period of immobilization more tolerable for the patient.[69]

ADAPTATION OF A FLAP TO ITS BED

Revascularization

After transferring a flap to a new bed, the divided blood vessels in the flap and in the walls of the recipient site are thrombosed. Small buds of protoplasm from the nearest capillaries in the approximated surfaces of the flap and the defect soon appear. As these buds grow, solid projections are formed that eventually unite with one another. Later, protoplasmic threads, which extend from the flap to the recipient bed, undergo a physiological process of canalization that permits blood to flow through them. These new capillaries are soon lined by endothelium and are strengthened by connective tissue that is produced by fibroblasts.[54]

Reinnervation

Studies that have been performed on humans have shown that flaps reinnervate from the periphery toward the center[45] and from the recipient bed.[29] A study has shown there to be a marginal zone of sensation that equals that of the surrounding skin. This zone encloses an inner area that begins with a band of hyperesthesia along the outer edge and passes through various bands with differing degrees of sensation into anesthesia in the very center. This is true in larger flaps. In small flaps the anesthetic zone diminishes rapidly or cannot be found at all, since reinnervation reaches the center of the flap relatively soon.[45] It may take from six weeks to three years for sensation to reappear.[29, 45] Though these studies were done on humans, the areas of hyperesthesia may also exist in the dog and may account for a dog's licking and chewing a flap or a graft after it is placed on its bed. A tingling sensation (Tinel's sign) has been described with nerve regeneration in humans,[46] and other bizarre sensations have been reported to precede the return of true sensation.[43] The presence of such sensation has been postulated in dogs also.[73] The reinnervation of skin in the dog warrants further study. The reader is referred to Chapter 10 for information on the reinnervation of skin grafts.

Hair Growth and Sebaceous Secretion

Hair growth and sebaceous secretion have the same characteristics in a skin flap as they would have had at their site of origin.[29]

EFFECTS OF ANESTHESIA ON FLAPS

Studies have been conducted to determine what effect, if any, various anesthetics have on skin flaps. A review of the studies has stated the following concerning various anesthetic agents:[60]

Halothane

In studies on rats, more flap necrosis occurred in animals that were anesthetized with halothane than in those that were anesthetized with methoxyflurane. The operative times, acid-base values, and central venous pressures were similar in both groups of animals. Such findings warrant further investigation. Another factor to consider when using halothane as an anesthetic is the potential hepatic damage that it can cause. Since it is believed that multiple exposures to this agent are contraindicated, its use in multistaged reconstructive procedures should be avoided.

Ketamine

In humans, this drug produces analgesia and amnesia and is used for short procedures involving somatic pain. Ketamine has a cardiovascular-stimulating action that results in tachycardia and blood pressure elevations; however, it is unlikely that the hypertension would have any beneficial effect on flap survival. If the hypertension causes increased hemorrhage, it could possibly be detrimental to flap survival.

This drug has been authorized for use in cats but not in dogs. When multi-staged flap transfer is being performed in a cat, the surgeon may want to consider using ketamine during one or more of the stages to avoid any problems that might be associated with the repeated use of halothane.

Spinal Anesthesia

Spinal anesthesia paralyzes the sympathetic nervous system, with a resultant loss of tone in the peripheral blood vessels. The pooling of blood in the periphery that is caused by arterial and venous dilation can produce a moderate degree of hypotension, which is detrimental to flap survival.

Local Anesthesia

There is a hesitancy to use local anesthesia in flap surgery because it is believed that vasoconstriction, needle puncture, and fluid infiltration are deleterious to flap survival. The use of epinephrine in flaps with a questionable blood supply is also believed to be contraindicated because it results in ischemia and masks bleeding from the distal end of the flap, which is considered by some to be a valuable clinical sign of future tissue viability. However, it has been found in studies on pigs that infiltration anesthesia, even with epinephrine in a concentration of 1:200,000, has no harmful effect on the survival of primarily raised skin flaps. Epinephrine in concentrations of 1:100,000 or greater may be harmful to flap survival. Delayed flaps are very sensitive to vasoconstriction, which is caused by epinephrine.

REFERENCES

1. Archibald, J.: Procedures in plastic surgery. J. Am. Vet. Med. Assoc. *147*:1461, 1965.
2. Arnall, L.: Repair of an extensive brachial skin slough by a cervical pedicle flap graft. J. Small Anim. Pract. *1*:286, 1961.
3. Barron, J.N.: Subcutaneous pedicle flaps, in Grabb, W.C., and Myers, M.B.(eds.): Skin Flaps. Boston, Little, Brown and Co., 1975.
4. Barsky, A.J., Kahn, S., Simon, B. E., et al.: Principles and Practice of Plastic Surgery, ed. 2. New York, McGraw-Hill Book Co., 1964.
5. Beasley, R.W.: Principles and techniques of resurfacing operations for hand surgery. Surg. Clin. North Am. *47*:389, 1967.
6. Bellman, S., and Velander, E.: Vascular transformation in experimental tubed pedicles. Br. J. Plast. Surg. *12*:1, 1959.
7. Berson, M.I.: Atlas of Plastic Surgery, ed. 2. New York, Grune & Stratton, Inc., 1963.
7a. Blanchard, G.L., and Keller, W.F.: The rhomboid graft-flap for the repair of extensive ocular adnexal defects. J. Am. Anim. Hosp. Assoc. *12*:576, 1976.

8. Braithwaite, F.: Some observations on the vascular channels in tubed pedicles: II. Br. J. Plast. Surg. *4*:28, 1952.

9. Campbell, R.M.: The surgical management of pressure sores. Surg. Clin. North Am. 39:509, 1959.

10. Cannon, B., and Trott, A.: Expeditious use of direct flaps in extremity repairs. Plast. Reconstr. Surg. *4*:415, 1949.

11. Cawley, A.J., and Archibald, J.: Plastic surgery, in Archibald, J. (ed.): Canine Surgery, ed. 2. Santa Barbara, Calif., American Veterinary Publications, Inc., 1974.

12. Cawley, A.J. and Francis, S.M.: Pedicle graft in a dog: Case report. Cornell Vet. *48*:12, 1958.

13. Climo, S.: Dermal bleeding and the delay operation. Plast. Reconstr. Surg. 8:59, 1951.

14. Conway, H.: Skin grafting, in Cooper, P. (ed.): The Craft of Surgery, ed. 2. Boston, Little, Brown and Co., 1971, vol. 1.

15. Conway, H., Stark, R.B., and Docktor, J.P.: Vascularization of tubed pedicles. Plast. Reconstr. Surg. *4*:133, 1949.

16. Conway, H., Stark, R.B., and Joslin, D.: Cutaneous histamine reaction as a test of circulatory efficiency of tubed pedicles and flaps. Surg. Gynecol. Obstet. *93*:185, 1951.

17. Davis, J.S., and Kitlowski, E.A.: A method of tubed pedicle formation. South. Med. J. *29*:1169, 1936.

18. Dean, R.K., Kelleher, J.C., Sullivan, J.G., et al.: Bilobed flaps, in Grabb, W.C., and Myers, M.B. (eds.): Skin Flaps. Boston, Little, Brown and Co., 1975.

19. Dingwall, J.A., and Lord, J.W.: The fluorescein test in the management of tubed (pedicle) flaps. Bull. Johns Hopkins Hosp. *73*:129, 1943.

20. Dixon, A.C.: The secondary closure of wounds. Vet. Rec. *75*:1133, 1963.

21. Douglas, B., and Buchholz, R.R.: The blood circulation in pedicle flaps: An accurate test for determining its efficiency. Ann. Surg. *117*:692, 1943.

22. Earle, A.S., Fratianne, R.B., and Nunez, F.D.: The relationship of hematocrit levels to skin flap survival in the dog. Plast. Reconstr. Surg. *54*:341, 1974.

23. Epstein, E.: Skin Surgery. Philadelphia, Lea & Febiger, 1962.

24. Gelatt, K.N.: Blepharoplastic procedures in horses. J. Am. Vet. Med. Assoc. *151*:27, 1967.

25. German, F., Finesilver, E.M., and Davis, J.S.: Establishment of circulation in tubed skin flaps: An experimental study. Arch. Surg. *26*:27, 1933.

26. Gillies, H.I.: The design of direct pedicle flaps. Br. Med. J. *2*:1008, 1932.

26a. Gourley, I.M.: Neurovascular island flap for treatment of trophic metacarpal pad ulcer in the dog. J. Am. Anim. Hosp. Assoc. *14*:119, 1978.

26b. Gourley, I.M., and Snyder, C.C.: Microsurgery. J. Am. Anim. Hosp. Assoc. *12*:604, 1976.

27. Grabb, W.C.: Classification of skin flaps, in Grabb, W.C., and Myers, M.B. (eds.): Skin Flaps. Boston, Little, Brown and Co., 1975.

28. Grabb, W.C. and Oneal, R.: The effect of low molecular weight dextran on the survival of experimental skin flaps. Plast. Reconstr. Surg. *30*:649, 1966.

29. Grabb, W.C. and Smith, J.W.: Basic techniques of plastic surgery, in Plastic Surgery: A Concise Guide to Clinical Practice. Boston, Little, Brown and Co., 1968.

30. Harii, K., Ohmori, K., and Sekiguchi, J.: The free musculocutaneous flap. Plast. Reconstr. Surg. *57*:294, 1976.

31. Hoffmeister, F.S.: Studies on timing of tissue transfer in reconstructive surgery: I. Effect of delay on circulation in flaps. Plast. Reconstr. Surg. *19*:283, 1957.

32. Hogle, R., Kingrey, B., and Jensen, E.C.: Skin grafting in the horse. J. Am. Vet. Med. Assoc. *35*:165, 1959.

32a. Howard, D.R., Lammerding, J.J., and Bloomberg, M.S.: Principles of pedicle flaps and grafting technique. J. Am. Anim. Hosp. Assoc. *12*:573, 1976.

33. Hynes, W.: A simple method of estimating blood flow with special reference to the circulation in pedicled skin flaps and tubes. Br. J. Plast. Surg. *1*:159, 1948.

34. Hynes, W.: The blood vessels in skin tubes and flaps. Br. J. Plast. Surg. *3*:165, 1950.

35. Hynes, W.: The "blue flap": A method of treatment. Br. J. Plast. Surg. *4*:166, 1951.

36. Hynes, W., and MacGregor, A.G.: The use of fluorescein in estimating the blood flow in pedicled skin flaps and tubes. Br. J. Plast. Surg. *2*:4, 1949.

37. Jensen, E.L.: Canine autogenous skin grafting. Am. J. Vet. Res. *20*:898, 1959.

38. Johnston, D.: Wound healing and reconstructive surgery. Am. Anim. Hosp. Assoc. Sci. Proc. 2:383, 1975.

38a. Johnston, D.E.: The repair of skin loss on the foot by means of a double-pedicle abdominal flap. J. Am. Anim. Hosp. Assoc. *12*:593, 1976.

39. Keihn, C., and Des Prez, J.: Effects of local hypothermia on pedicle flap tissue: I. Enhancement of survival of experimental pedicles. Plast. Reconstr. Surg. *25*:349, 1960.

40. Kernahan, D.A., Zingg, W., and Kay, C.W.: The effect of hyperbaric oxygen on the survival of experimental skin flaps. Plast. Reconstr. Surg. *36*:19, 1965.

41. Krahwinkel, D.J., and Howard, D.R.: Reconstructive surgery. Am. Anim. Hosp. Assoc. Sci. Proc. 2:439, 1975.

42. Krizek, T.J., Tani, T., Des Prez, J.D., et al.: Experimental transplantation of composite grafts by microsurgical vascular anastomosis. Plast. Reconstr. Surg. *36*:538, 1965.

43. Larsen, R.D., and Posch, J.L.: Nerve injuries in the upper extremity. Arch. Surg. 77:469, 1958.
44. Lejour, M.: Cheek sliding flap. Chir. Maxillofac. Plast. 2:247, 1974.
45. Maris, F., Jurkovic, I., Kohut, P., et al.: Reinnervation of free and flap skin grafts. Acta Chir. Plast. 5:57, 1963.
46. Marmor, L.: Peripheral Nerve Regeneration Using Nerve Grafts. Springfield, Ill., Charles C Thomas Publisher, 1967.
47. McFarlane, R.M., Heagy, F.C., Radin, S., et al.: A study of the delay phenomenon in experimental pedicle flaps. Plast. Reconstr. Surg. 35:245, 1965.
48. McGregor, I.A.: Fundamental Techniques of Plastic Surgery, ed. 5. Edinburgh, Churchill Livingstone, 1972.
49. Millard, D.R.: Pedicle flaps, In Cooper, P. (ed.): The Craft of Surgery, ed. 2. Boston, Little, Brown and Co., 1971, vol. 1.
50. Morgan, B.L., Samiian, M., and Reza, M.: Advantages of the bilobed flap for closure of small defects of the face. Plast. Reconstr. Surg. 52:35, 1973.
51. Myers, M.B.: Attempts to augment survival in skin flaps: Mechanism of the delay phenomenon, in Grabb, W.C., and Myers, M.B. (eds.): Skin Flaps. Boston, Little, Brown and Co., 1975.
52. Myers, M.B.: Investigation of skin flap necrosis, in Grabb, W.B., and Myers, M.B. (eds.): Skin Flaps. Boston, Little, Brown and Co., 1975.
53. Myers, M.B., Cherry, G., and Bombet, R.: On lack of any effect of gravity on the survival of tubed flaps: An experimental study in rabbits and pigs. Plast. Reconstr. Surg. 51:428, 1973.
54. New, G.B., and Erich, J.B.: Pedicle Flaps in Plastic Surgery of the Head and Neck. Springfield, Ill., Charles C Thomas Publisher, 1950.
55. Olivari, N., Schrudde, J., and Wahle, H.: The surgical treatment of bedsores in paraplegics. Plast. Reconstr. Surg. 50:477, 1972.
56. Padgett, E.C., and Stephenson, K.L.: Plastic and Reconstructive Surgery. Springfield, Ill., Charles C Thomas Publisher, 1948.
57. Perrins, J.D.: The effect of hyperbaric oxygen on ischemic skin flaps, in Grabb, W.C., and Myers, M.B. (eds.): Skin Flaps. Boston, Little, Brown and Co., 1975.
58. Pullen, C.M.: Reconstruction of the skin, in Current Techniques in Small Animal Surgery. Philadelphia, Lea & Febiger, 1975.
59. Reinisch, J.F.: The pathophysiology of skin flap circulation: The delay phenomenon. Plast. Reconstr. Surg. 54:585, 1974.
60. Reinisch, J.F.: The effects of anesthetic agents on skin flap survival, in Grabb, W.C., and Myers, M.B. (eds.): Skin Flaps. Boston, Little, Brown and Co., 1975.
61. Ross, G.E.: Clinical canine skin grafting. J. Am. Vet. Med. Assoc. 153:1759, 1968.
62. Schechter, G.L., Biller, H.F., and Ogura, J.H.: Revascularized skin flaps: A new concept in transfer of skin flaps. Laryngoscope 79:1647, 1969.
63. Schiller, A.G., and Helper, L.C.: Pedicle graft accelerates healing. Mod. Vet. Pract. 45:68, 1964.
64. Smithcors, J.F.: New methods of wound closure. Mod. Vet. Pract. 47:118, 1966.
65. Spira, M., Gerow, F.J., and Hardy, S.B.: Subcutaneous pedicle flaps on the face. Br. J. Plast. Surg. 27:258, 1974.
66. Spreull, J.S.: The principles of transplanting skin in the dog. J. Am. Anim. Hosp. Assoc. 4:71, 1968.
67. Stark, R.B.: The pantographic expansion principle as applied to the advancement flap. Plast. Reconstr. Surg. 15:222, 1955.
68. Stark, R.B.: Plastic Surgery. New York, Harper & Row Publishers, Inc., 1962.
69. Stark, R.B., and Kernahan, D.A.: Reconstructive surgery of the leg and foot. Surg. Clin. North Am. 39:469, 1959.
70. Steiss, C.F.: Utilization of the tube pedicle in the reconstruction of facial defects. Plast. Reconstr. Surg. 4:545, 1949.
71. Stern, W.G., and Cohen, M.B.: The intracutaneous salt solution wheal test. J.A.M.A. 87:1355, 1926.
72. Swaim, S.F.: A "walking" suture technique for closure of large skin defects in the dog and cat. J. Am. Anim. Hosp. Assoc. 12:597, 1976.
73. Swaim, S.F.: Peripheral Nerve Surgery in the Dog, Master's thesis. Auburn University, Auburn, Ala., 1971.
74. Swaim, S.F., and Bushby, P.A.: Principles of bipedicle tube grafting in the dog. J. Am. Anim. Hosp. Assoc. 12:600, 1976.
75. Swaim, S.F., and Votau, K.: Prevention and treatment of decubital ulcers in the dog. Vet. Med. Small Anim. Clin. 70:1069, 1975.
76. Trevaskis, A.E., Rempel, J., Okunski, W., et al.: Sliding subcutaneous pedicle flaps to close a circular defect. Plast. Reconstr. Surg. 46:155, 1970.
77. Twaddle, A.A.: Rotation flap skin graft. N.Z. Vet. J. 17:178, 1969.
78. Webster, J.P.: The early history of the tubed pedicle flap. Surg. Clin. North Am. 39:261, 1959.

79. White, W.L.: Flap grafts to the upper extremity. Surg. Clin. North Am. *40*:389, 1960.
80. Winsten, J., Manalo, P.D., and Barsky, A.J.: Studies on the circulation of tubed flaps. Plast. Reconstr. Surg. 28:619, 1961.
81. Yturraspe, D.J., Creed, J.E., and Schwach, R.P.: Thoracic pedicle skin flap for repair of lower limb wounds in dogs and cats. J. Am. Anim. Hosp. Assoc. *12*::581, 1976.

9

Z-, V-Y, AND W-PLASTIES

SINGLE Z-PLASTY

Of the procedures used for reconstructive surgery, the Z-plasty is probably one of the most intriguing. Although the surgeon knows from practice that the Z-plasty will produce a certain result, it is not always obvious why it does so.[26]

By definition, the Z-plasty involves the transposition of two interdigitating triangular flaps.[27] Geometrically, it consists of a central limb and two arms that are positioned in the shape of the letter "Z." The two arms of the "Z" are equal in length to the central limb and are at an angle that can vary from 30 to 90 degrees (Figs. 9–1 and 9–2).[18]

INDICATIONS

A Z-plasty is indicated in the following instances:

1. To release the tension along linear cicatricial contractures that have formed web-, bridle-, or bowstring-type scars across flexion or concave surfaces. Such scars tend to limit extension (Fig. 9–3).[1, 2, 9-11, 13, 14, 16, 18, 20, 26-28, 31, 32, 34-36]

2. To change the direction and appearance of a scar[5, 6, 8, 10, 16, 18, 25-28] or to change the direction of an incision or excision (Figs. 9–4 and 9–5).[3, 37]

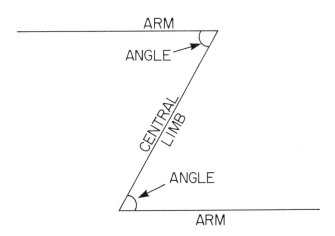

Figure 9–1: Components of a Z-plasty.

CENTRAL LIMB LENGTH = ARM LENGTH
ANGLES = FROM 30°-90° (60° is most common)

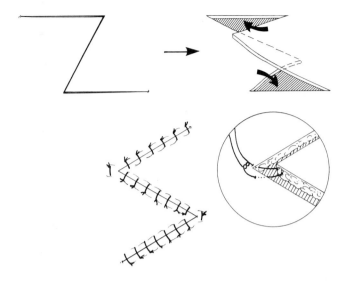

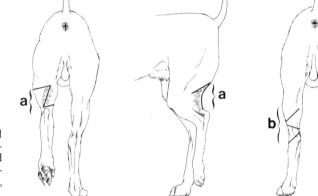

Figure 9–2: Dynamics of a Z-plasty. *Insert,* Modified three-point suture (half-buried horizontal mattress) for anchoring the tips of Z-plasty flaps.

Figure 9–3: *A,* A linear cicatricial contracture (*a*) across a flexion surface. A Z-plasty has been designed over the contracture. *B,* After transposition of the Z-plasty flaps (*b*), the contracture is released.

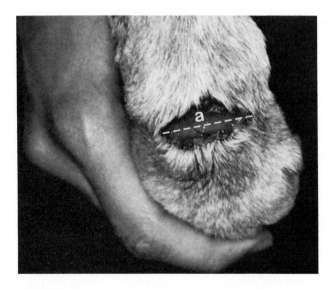

Figure 9–4: A horizontal, nonhealing wound over the extensor surface of the carpus (*a*). (Courtesy of M. J. Bojrab.)

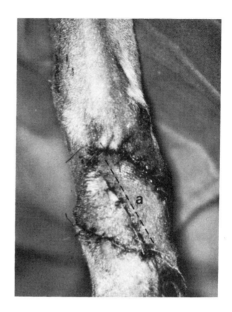

Figure 9–5: Following Z-plasty, the direction of the non-healing wound is changed (*a*) to allow for better healing. (Courtesy of M. J. Bojrab.)

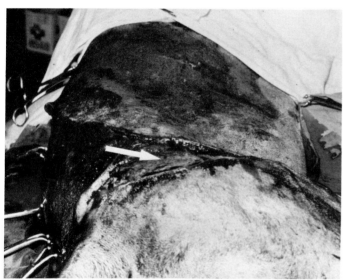

Figure 9–6: Open wound over the gluteal region (*arrow*). (The dog's tail is in the lower left portion of the picture.)

Figure 9–7: Two Z-plasties adjacent to the skin lesion. The Z-plasties will be used as relaxing incisions. Central limbs of the "Z's" are perpendicular to the long axis of the wound. The flaps of the Z-plasty under the most tension, *A*, have tended to transpose themselves. (The dog's tail is in the lower left portion of the picture.)

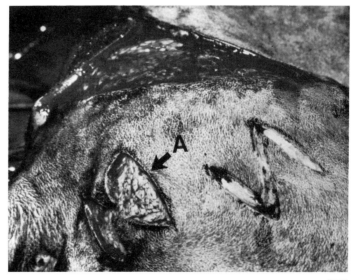

397

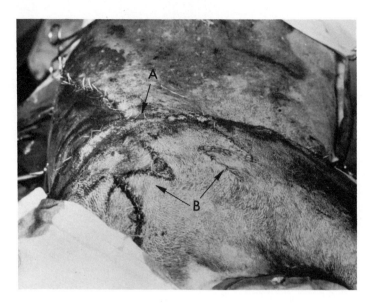

Figure 9–8: Skin lesion, A, and Z-plasties, B, are closed (in that order). Note that the central limbs of the "Z's" are now parallel to the long axis of the wound.

3. As a relaxing incision to allow the closure of large wounds (Figs. 9–6 through 9–9).[6, 21, 35]
4. To realign tissues in a normal position that have healed out of line (e.g., the lateral canthus of the eye) (Fig. 9–10).[6, 11, 16, 18]
5. To relieve the constriction that is caused by circular scars[5, 16, 18, 26] and to increase the circumference of an orifice (e.g., the anus) (Figs. 9–11, 9–12, and 9–13).[18, 20]

CHARACTERISTICS

Transposing the flaps of a Z-plasty has several effects. Two of these have special relevance and will be discussed in more detail than the others. They are related to the first two indications previously listed.

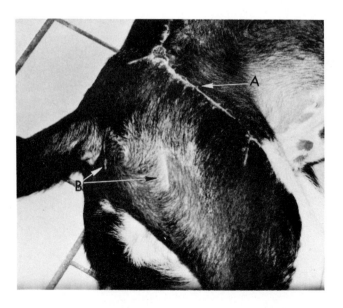

Figure 9–9: Healed skin lesion, A, and Z-plasties, B, two weeks postoperatively.

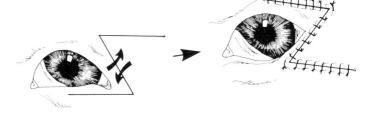

Figure 9–10: Relocation of the lateral canthus of an eye using a Z-plasty. (After Borges, A. F.: Elective Incisions and Scar Revisions. Boston, Little, Brown and Co., 1975, p. 47.)

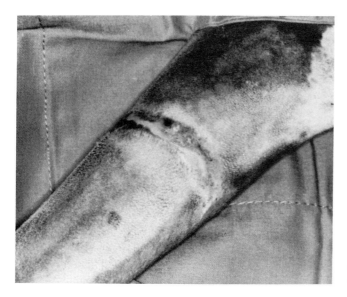

Figure 9–11: Circumferential constricting scar around a dog's forelimb.

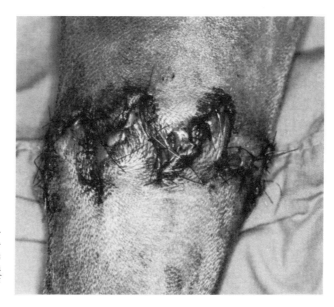

Figure 9–12: Correction of a constricting circumferential scar by multiple Z-plasties. Note that the tissue appears bulkier in the area of the Z-plasties as a result of increasing the circumference of the leg through surgery.

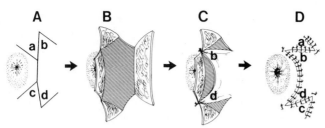

Figure 9–13: Use of two Z-plasties to enlarge a stenotic anal orifice. *A*, Design of the two Z's (*a, b* and *c, d*). *B*, Lines of the Z-plasties have been incised and the resulting flaps have been reflected. *C*, Transposition of one flap of each of the Z-plasties (*b* and *d*). *D*, Transposition of the remaining flap of each of the Z-plasties (*a* and *c*), with completed suturing of all of the skin's edges. (After Converse, J. M.: Introduction to plastic surgery, in Reconstructive Plastic Surgery: Principles and Procedures in Correction, Reconstruction and Transplantation, ed. 2. Philadelphia, W. B. Saunders Co., 1977, vol. 1, p. 60.)

1. There is a gain in length along the direction of the central limb of the "Z" (Fig. 9–14).
2. The central limb of the "Z" changes direction when the flaps are transposed (Fig. 9–14).[27]

By exploiting these changes the surgeon can use the Z-plasty to accomplish the reconstruction of an area where these effects are required.

INCREASING LENGTH BY Z-PLASTY

Theory and Dynamics of Gaining Length

The most valuable characteristic of a Z-plasty is that it allows the lengthening or shortening of an area as desired.[26] To understand the sequence of events when a Z-plasty is used to lengthen an area of linear contracture, it is essential to know the basic method of designing a Z-plasty. The central limb of the "Z" is placed along the line of contracture

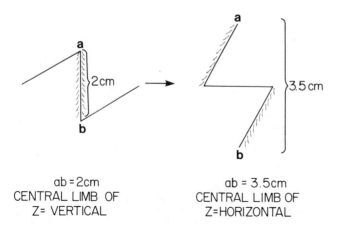

ab = 2cm
CENTRAL LIMB OF
Z = VERTICAL

ab = 3.5 cm
CENTRAL LIMB OF
Z = HORIZONTAL

Figure 9–14: Two basic characteristics of Z-plasties: (1) a gain in length in the direction of the original central limb (after flap transposition is completed, the distance between point *a* and point *b* is increased) and (2) a change in direction of the central limb.

that is to be lengthened. Since the skin flaps must fit together after being transposed, the arms must be equal in length to the central limb. These arms are designed on either end of the central limb on opposite sides. The angles of the "Z" are also usually equal, with the most common angle measure being 60 degrees (a compromise figure that has been reached by experience) (Fig. 9–1). If the figure were completed by drawing lines across the bases of the triangles that are formed by the "Z," a parallelogram would be formed. The central limb of the "Z" is the short diagonal of the parallelogram and is called the contractural diagonal. The line connecting the ends of the arms is the long diagonal and is called the transverse diagonal (Fig. 9–15).[5, 6, 10, 11, 16, 18, 26, 27]

In some instances it may be necessary to make one limb of the "Z" longer than the other. This is done when one limb is to be made in thick, rigid, scarred skin. By making this limb longer, greater mobility is given to the flap for transposition.[10]

When the "Z" is incised, the ends spring apart as the fibrous tissue band along the linear contracture (contractural diagonal) is divided at the time the flaps are raised. As the contracture springs apart, it changes the shape of the parallelogram and transposes the flaps. The contractural diagonal lengthens and the transverse diagonal shortens (Figs. 9–14 and 9–15).[27] Because of the tension along the contractural diagonal, the surgeon does not have to actively transpose the "Z" flaps when the procedure is performed. Flap transposition follows naturally as a result of the change in the shape of the parallelogram.[27]

The changes in length are such that the length of the contractural diagonal *after* transposition is equal to that of the transverse diagonal *before* transposition. In other words, the difference between the two diagonal lengths will be the length that is gained along the contractural diagonal after the flaps have been transposed. The increase in length in the contractural diagonal is achieved at the expense of the transverse diagonal, since the skin that has been donated for lengthening the contracture has been taken from either side of the contracture (Fig. 9–15).[6, 11, 16, 18, 26, 27, 35]

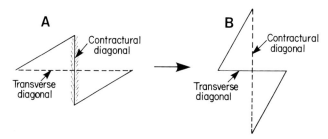

TRANSVERSE DIAGONAL OF **A** = CONTRACTURAL DIAGONAL OF **B**
CONTRACTURAL DIAGONAL OF **A** = TRANSVERSE DIAGONAL OF **B**
TRANSVERSE DIAGONAL MINUS CONTRACTURAL DIAGONAL
= LENGTH GAIN IN NEW CONTRACTURAL DIAGONAL.

Figure 9–15: The diagonals of a Z-plasty showing how the original contractural diagonal lengthens and the original transverse diagonal shortens. *A*, Original Z-plasty design with its two diagonals. *B*, Z-plasty after flap transposition showing the change in diagonal lengths. (After McGregor, I. A.: Fundamental Techniques of Plastic Surgery, ed. 5. Edinburgh, Churchill Livingstone, 1972, p. 37.)

Effect of Angle Measure on Length Gain

Equal Angles. It has been found that the wider the angles of the triangular flaps of a Z-plasty, the greater is the difference between the lengths of the long and the short diagonals. As a result of this, the lengthening effect of the Z-plasty increases as the measure of the angle increases. When 75-degree angles are used to construct a Z-plasty, the increase in length along the contractural diagonal is 100 per cent of the length of the central limb. Using 60-degree angles the increase in length is 75 per cent; with 45-degree angles the increase is 50 per cent; and with 30-degree angles the increase is only 25 per cent (Fig. 9–16).[16, 18, 27]

It should be remembered that it is *percentage* increase in length that is controlled by the angle measure. These increases are theoretical and cannot be applied clinically with strict accuracy. Factors such as skin extensibility and the amount of scarring in an area will affect the length that is gained by a Z-plasty. The actual lengthening is usually a little less than that predicted by theoretical calculations.[27]

Sixty-degree angles are the most commonly used angles for Z-plasties.[5, 10, 11, 16-18, 27] Increasing the angle width much beyond 60 degrees increases the lengthening effect of the Z-plasty; however, this lengthening would be accompanied by an equal amount of transverse shortening, and this tissue is seldom available in unlimited quantities. As a result, angles that are wider than 60 degrees produce greater tension on the surrounding tissues when they are transposed, thus making the transposition difficult.[5, 17, 27] A four-flap Z-plasty has been described as a means of overcoming the difficulties of transposition that are associated with the wide-angle Z-plasty. Each wide-angle flap is divided into two separate flaps to convert the usual Z-plasty into a four-flap Z-plasty. This technique permits a maximum gain in length and still allows narrower flaps to be moved with ease (Fig. 9–17).[10, 15, 36]

At the other end of the scale, a reduction in the measure of the angle much below 60 degrees tends to defeat the object of the Z-plasty, since the narrower angles produce less gain in length. It must also be remembered

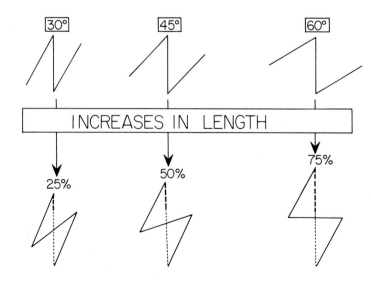

Figure 9–16: Percentage increase in length with various angle sizes. (After Grabb, W. C., and Smith, J. W.: Basic techniques of plastic surgery, in Plastic Surgery: A Concise Guide to Clinical Practice. Boston, Little, Brown and Co., 1968, p. 78.)

Figure 9–17: Dynamics of transposing a four-flap Z-plasty. *A,* A four-flap (*a, b, c,* and *d*) Z-plasty is designed. The first flaps to be transposed are *a* and *b. B,* After this transposition, the flaps are again transposed (*a* and *d* transpose and *b* and *c* transpose). *C,* The flap transposition is completed. Such a technique has the advantage of transposing narrower flaps while gaining the length associated with larger angles.

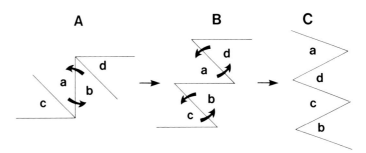

that narrowing the flap reduces its blood supply, and a flap that is too narrow could degenerate owing to an inadequate blood supply.[27]

Unequal Angles. Most Z-plasties have two equal angles; however, this is not mandatory. Occasionally, scarring in an area will limit the angle of one flap, and dissimilar angles may have to be used. In these cases, the three component limbs of the "Z" must remain equal in length in order to make the transposition practical.[11, 27] The length that is attained in these cases is the average of the length to be expected from each angle alone. If the two other sides of the "Z" were drawn along with the contractural and transverse diagonals, the transverse diagonal would still indicate the actual length to be expected when the flaps are transposed, just as it does with equal-angle Z-plasties.[27] As would be expected, the tension needed to transpose the narrower flap is less than that required for the wider flap.[17]

The technique for a "half-Z," which is a form of unequal-angle Z-plasty, has been described. One angle is acute, and the other is 90 degrees. When the flaps are transposed, the acute-angle flap is inserted into the horizontal incision of the 90-degree flap, resulting in greater elongation along one side of the surgical field than along the other side (Fig. 9–18).[10]

Effect of Limb Length on Length Gain

Limb Length. It has already been stated that the angle measure controls the *percentage* increase in length that is gained in a Z-plasty. The *actual* increase in length is governed by the length of the limbs of the "Z." Longer limbs result in a greater increase in length for a particular angle measure. When the limb length increases, the amount of tissue that is brought in from the sides is increased (Fig. 9–19). Since 60 degrees has

Figure 9–18: Technique for a "half-Z." *A,* Design of a half-Z along a contracture. *B,* Transposition of the 60-degree angle flap above the 90-degree angle flap. *C,* Completed half-Z for elongation of skin along a contracture. (After Converse, J. M.: Introduction to plastic surgery, in Reconstructive Plastic Surgery: Principles and Procedures in Correction, Reconstruction and Transplantation, ed. 2. Philadelphia, W. B. Saunders Co., 1977, vol. 1, p. 58.)

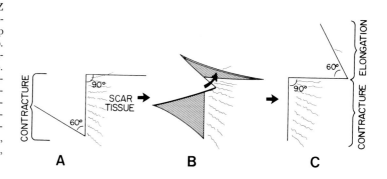

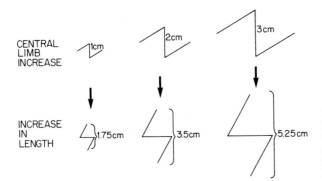

Figure 9–19: Actual gain in length with various central limb lengths. (After Grabb, W. C., and Smith, J. W.: Basic techniques of plastic surgery, in Plastic Surgery: A Concise Guide to Clinical Practice. Boston, Little, Brown and Co., 1968, p. 78.)

been established as the most workable angle for Z-plasties, the major variant is the limb length; however, this has its limits also. The nature (scarred or normal) and the amount of tissue lateral to a contracture govern the limb length that can be used and thus the amount of tissue that can be brought in from the lateral aspects of the area. Large amounts of unscarred tissue will allow a large Z-plasty; conversely, a small amount of normal tissue limits the size of the "Z."[27]

Large and small Z-plasties have different effects on the surrounding tissues that may or may not be deleterious. The distorting effect of small Z-plasties is dispersed within the immediate surrounding skin, and the stress effects of large Z-plasties are dispersed over larger areas. The large flaps may therefore encounter anatomical obstacles, such as areas of attachment to limbs and limitations of body circumference, and these may significantly affect the mechanics of flap transposition. As with wider angles, longer limbs have the effect of increasing the tension on the surrounding tissues during transposition of the flaps.[17]

DESIGN

The basic factors involved in designing a Z-plasty have already been discussed in the section on "Theory and Dynamics of Gaining Length." At this point, some of the other factors involved in Z-plasty design will be discussed. In planning a Z-plasty, the measure of the angle that is created by the central limb and each arm and the actual length of the central limb

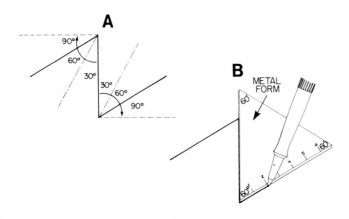

Figure 9–20: Designing the angles of a 60-degree Z-plasty. A, Sighting a 90-degree angle and dividing it into thirds to establish a 60-degree angle. B, Using a metal equilateral triangle form with linear gradations to draw a "Z." (After Grabb, W. C., and Smith, J. W.: Basic techniques of plastic surgery, in Plastic Surgery: A Concise Guide to Clinical Practice. Boston, Little, Brown and Co., 1968, p. 76.)

are the only two factors that are variable.[18, 27] It is important to reemphasize that the length of the arms of the "Z" should always be equal to the length of the central limb (Fig. 9–1).[5, 6, 11, 16, 18, 26, 27]

After drawing the central limb along the line of contracture, the arms are drawn at the desired angle from either end of the central limb. If a 60-degree angle is to be used, it can be drawn by first making a 90-degree angle and then dividing it by sight into thirds. Two of the thirds make a 60-degree angle.[18] A precut 60-degree pattern in the form of a piece of thin metal with its edges marked in inches or centimeters can be included in a surgical pack to make the measurement of angles and limbs more accurate (Fig. 9–20).[11, 18] The author prefers a form made from a piece of developed x-ray film. To check the accuracy of a 60-degree Z-plasty design, a straight line is drawn to connect the free ends of the arms. This line should be perpendicular to and pass through the center of the central limb.[18]

Designing a Z-plasty depends not only on geometry but also on the surgeon's intuition and judgment. The biomechanical properties of the tissues in the proposed area of surgery have a definite effect on the surgical outcome and are important in planning Z-plasties.[17] Skin that is scarred has lost much of its normal elasticity and this can affect the planning of the Z-plasty flaps. A flap of scarred skin should initially be made a little longer than its counterpart in normal skin.[27] Situating the central limb of the "Z" is usually no problem; however, it may be difficult to decide where the flaps should be located in relation to it. A good method for selecting the sites for the flaps is to draw an equilateral triangle on either side of the central limb and to choose the more suitable of the two sets of limbs from the resulting parallelogram. Factors that should be considered in deciding which set of limbs to use in constructing a Z-plasty include the following:

1. Lines should be avoided that will create triangular flaps with scar tissue across their base. The flap with the better blood supply is preferable (Fig. 9–21).[11, 27]

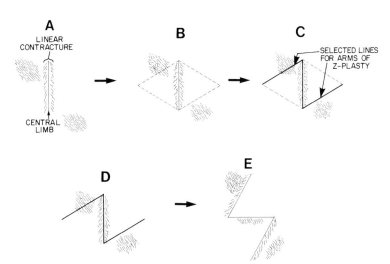

Figure 9–21:   Selection of arms for a Z-plasty. *A*, Central limb is plotted on the linear contracture. *B*, Arm possibilities are drawn in as a parallelogram. *C*, Arms are selected for a Z-plasty that will create two flaps that will not have scar tissue across their base. *D*, Z-plasty is incised, and *E*, the flaps are transposed.

2. Lines should be chosen so that the triangular flaps that are produced will result in a scar that falls into a better line cosmetically.[11, 27]

3. Lines should be selected so that triangular flaps will be produced that will rotate more readily into their transposed position.[27]

One set of lines may have no particular advantage over the other set, in which case either set may be used to construct the Z-plasty.[27] In general, when healthy tissue surrounds a linear contracture, longer side arms may be employed on the "Z."[9]

SURGICAL TECHNIQUE

After a Z-plasty has been designed, incisions are made along the predetermined lines with a scalpel blade. The scar tissue underlying the central limb of the "Z" can be excised in a fusiform shape if it is not too wide (Fig. 9–22).[18] Another technique for eliminating a thick, rigid scar that has poor circulation involves removing an elliptical piece of tissue that includes the scar along the area of linear contracture. The edges of the skin are then apposed with a few temporary sutures. This sutured wound is used as the central limb of the "Z" and the arms are marked in the usual way (Fig. 9–23).[11] If the scar is reasonably thin and flexible or composed of partially infiltrated skin, it is split with the central limb incision and utilized as part of the flaps.[11] The triangular flaps that have been created are completely undermined at a uniform thickness to include the subcutaneous tissue.[2, 11, 18, 37]

When these procedures have been performed, the ends of the central limb incision are drawn away from each other. The central limb becomes longer, and the angles become blunt. The flaps are transposed so that their outer margins approximate and the tip of each flap touches the outer corner of the base of the opposite flap.[11] Closure of the deeper tissues is of value; however, nothing is gained by interdigitating the borders of the deep layers, and this could add to fibrosis.[25] A few deep sutures to immobilize large, thick flaps that are composed of fairly normal tissue have been advocated.[11] Simple interrupted sutures of fine nonabsorbable suture material are used to appose the skin edges.[2, 11, 18] Half-buried horizontal mattress sutures are used to hold the tips of the flaps in position (Fig. 9–2, insert).[18] It is not uncommon for two dog-ears to form as the flaps are rotated into

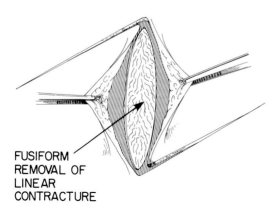

FUSIFORM
REMOVAL OF
LINEAR
CONTRACTURE

Figure 9–22: Scar tissue that underlies the central limb of the "Z" may be removed in a fusiform fashion before transposing the flaps of the "Z."

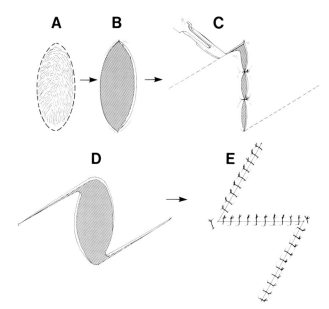

Figure 9–23: Removal of a thick, rigid linear contracture. *A* and *B*, Removal of an elongated ellipse of the scar tissue. *C*, Apposition of the wound edges with temporary sutures and design of the Z-plasty. *D*, Removal of the temporary sutures. *E*, Transposition and fixation of the Z-plasty flaps.

their new position.[16] These can be dealt with surgically by one of the techniques described in Chapter 7. The sutured wound is also in the shape of a "Z"; however, the "Z" is turned approximately 90 degrees if 60-degree angles were used to construct the Z-plasty. The new "Z" is elongated, and the central limb now lies transversely across the area where the linear contracture was situated.[2, 11]

PREVENTING VASCULAR PROBLEMS

The most common complication of the Z-plasty is necrosis of the tips of the flap, especially when there has been much scarring of the skin. Three things can be done to help prevent this:

Provide for Maximum Vascular Capacity of the Flaps. This may be accomplished by designing flaps that are wide at the tip. The tip of a flap can be broadened without affecting the measure of the angle by gently curving the arms of the "Z" (Fig. 9–24).[11, 18, 27] This has also been called an S-plasty, since the flaps take this configuration.[10] Delaying the flaps of a Z-plasty in tissue that has a poor blood supply has also been advocated.[33] See Chapter 8 for information on delaying flaps. Avoiding flaps that have scar tissue across their base[27] and preparing flaps as thick as possible also help to provide a good blood supply to Z-plasty flaps.[11, 27]

Figure 9–24: Modification of the Z-plasty by curving the arms away from the central limb to allow for maximum vascular capacity. (After McGregor, I. A.: Fundamental Techniques of Plastic Surgery, ed. 5. Edinburgh, Churchill Livingstone, 1972, p. 47.)

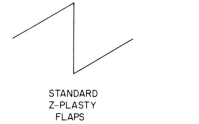

STANDARD
Z-PLASTY
FLAPS

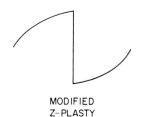

MODIFIED
Z-PLASTY
FLAPS

Avoidance of Undue Tension.   Tension can be a difficult problem, especially in borderline cases in which the contracture may be treated either by a Z-plasty or by skin grafting. As mentioned earlier, larger Z-plasties tend to have more tension associated with transposition of their flaps. Multiple small Z-plasties may be considered in such cases to help diffuse the tension. Multiple Z-plasties are discussed later in this chapter. When possible, an area on which a Z-plasty has been performed should be bandaged in a position that provides for the relaxation of tissues in all directions.[27]

Meticulous Hemostasis.   In addition to interfering with the circulation in a flap and thereby causing necrosis, hematomas provide a good medium for bacterial growth, which may lead to infection and flap necrosis.[27]

CHANGING DIRECTION BY Z-PLASTY

Occasionally it is necessary to change the direction of a scar or a defect that has been caused by incision or excision. The Z-plasty has been described for accomplishing this change (Figs. 9–4 and 9–5).[5, 6, 8, 10, 16, 18, 25, 26-28, 37]

It has been stated that a scar that lies perpendicular to the lines of tension is parallel to the direction of muscle pull and is situated in a plane that has changing tensions. This stress and pull result in a thickened scar.[25] The same theory has been stated without relating the tension lines to the underlying muscle activity. In other words, the hypertrophy of the scar is

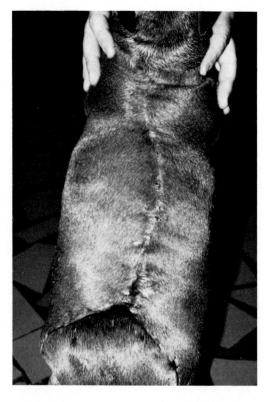

Figure 9–25: Widened scar resulting from a large wound that was closed under tension. (Courtesy of R. A. Lefebvre.)

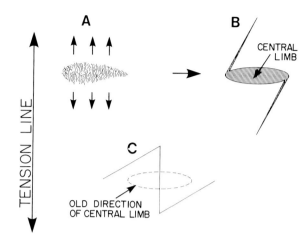

Figure 9–26: *A,* A short, widened scar resulting from tension. *B,* Removal of the scar tissue and design of a Z-plasty. *C,* Transposition of Z-plasty flaps, resulting in a change of direction of the central limb (lesion).

related to the tension that is exerted upon it by the skin tension lines only; this tension is most marked when the scar is perpendicular to these lines.[6]

Because of the overlying hair coat and looseness of the skin, the problem of widened or hypertrophic scars is not as prevalent in dogs and cats as it is in humans. However, an unsightly widened scar can occasionally be a problem in a short-haired animal that has undergone closure of a wound upon which sufficient tension has been exerted to change the tension lines in the area. A scar results that is oriented perpendicular to the newly formed tension lines; this scar may hypertrophy and produce an unaesthetic result (Fig. 9–25). In other cases, the scar may be oriented against the normal skin tension lines, resulting in a widened scar. The Z-plasty is beneficial in correcting such widened scars from the standpoint of lengthening, but of more importance, it changes the direction of the scar tissue and thereby alleviates the tension on the scar by aligning it more parallel to the skin tension lines (Fig. 9–26).[25]

In the case of a long, widened scar, the scar may be broken up by several small Z-plasties that tend to redistribute tension in such a fashion that much of it is borne as a shearing strain by the new common limbs of the Z-plasties. It appears that shearing strains cause much less stretching of the scar than does straight tension (Fig. 9–27).[6, 10, 27]

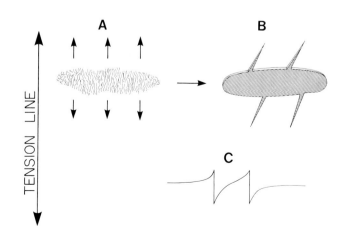

Figure 9–27: *A,* A long widened scar resulting from tension. *B,* Removal of scar tissue and design of two Z-plasties. *C,* Transposition of Z-plasty flaps, resulting in breaking up of the original scar to redistribute tension and cause less stretching of the scar. (After McGregor, I. A.: Fundamental Techniques of Plastic Surgery, ed. 5. Edinburgh, Churchill Livingstone, 1972, p. 51.)

When the direction of the entire length of a scar or a defect that has been produced by incision or excision is to be changed, it is wise to keep in mind the preoperative and postoperative positions of the central limb of the "Z" when various angles are used to design the Z-plasty. Most important is the central limb's change in direction when a 60-degree Z-plasty is used. If the central limb is initially situated between the 6-o'clock and 12-o'clock positions, the central limb's final direction will be between the 3-o'clock and 9-o'clock positions.[16] In other words, a 60-degree angle Z-plasty produces a 90-degree rotation of the central limb.[16, 26] Through the use of this type of Z-plasty, the direction of a hypertrophic scar lying perpendicular to the tension lines of the skin can be changed so that the scar will be parallel to the tension lines (Fig. 9–26).

A technique for designing a Z-plasty that would rotate a linear lesion 90 degrees entails using the linear lesion as the central limb of the Z-plasty and constructing the two arms on the opposite sides and opposite ends of the lesion. These arms would be constructed at 60-degree angles and would be equal in length to the central limb (linear lesion). Transposition of the flaps would result in a 90-degree rotation of the lesion so that it lies along skin tension lines.

This technique was used to change the direction of a nonhealing linear wound that ran horizontally across the dorsum of a dog's carpus.[3] The wound would not heal because of constant disruption when the carpus was flexed. Using a Z-plasty with the wound as the central limb, the wound was rotated perpendicular to the line of flexion and it healed (Figs. 9–4 and 9–5).

If the surgeon does not have a form or a protractor with which to measure the 60-degree angles for a 90-degree rotation Z-plasty, such a Z-plasty can be constructed by drawing a perpendicular line through the center of the lesion and extending it on both sides of the lesion. A second line whose length is equal to that of the lesion is plotted, beginning at one end of the lesion and ending on the first line that was drawn. A third line is

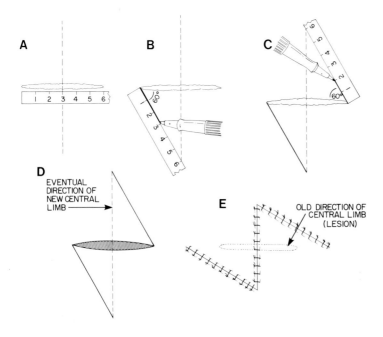

Figure 9–28: Designing a 60-degree equal-angle Z-plasty without a protractor or triangle form. *A,* Measuring the central limb (lesion) and bisecting it with a perpendicular line. *B* and *C,* Plotting the arms from the ends of the central limb (lesion) with a gradated measure. Note that the arms equal the central limb length. *D,* Original position of the "Z," and *E,* final position of the "Z" with central limb direction rotated 90 degrees.

drawn in like manner from the opposite end and on the opposite side of the lesion. The linear lesion and the two lines that are drawn from its ends constitute the Z-plasty incisions. The first line that lies between the ends of the arms of the "Z" denotes the direction of the new central limb of the Z-plasty after the Z-plasty flaps have been transposed (Figs. 9–28).

TENSION RELIEF BY Z-PLASTY

Many times difficulty is encountered in closing a fusiform excision in an area where the mobility or quantity of the skin or both are limited around the excision. In such cases a Z-plasty may be performed lateral to the excision on one or both sides to help alleviate the tension that is encountered when closing the excision.[6, 21] This method has been called an adjacent Z-plasty adjunct procedure. Such a procedure tends to add tissue in the direction of skin closure; this relaxes the suture line and makes closure of the excision easier, with minimal distortion of the neighboring landmarks (Figs. 9–6 through 9–9).[6]

With this procedure the central limb is made perpendicular to the long axis of the fusiform excision, and its arms are constructed at 60-degree angles from the central limb (Fig. 9–7).[6, 21] The flaps of the "Z" are undermined and left in their original position while the incision is closed. As closure proceeds the "Z"-shaped incision becomes more elongated, and the skin flaps are transposed automatically. The flaps are sutured into their new position with simple interrupted sutures (Fig. 9–8).[21]

The advantage of Z-plasty as a relaxing incision is that it can be used in areas where there is little excess skin.[21] However, it has the disadvantage of the added scarring that results from the incisions.[6] Because of the hair coat of animals, this is of minimal cosmetic concern.

STRUCTURE RELOCATION BY Z-PLASTY

The Z-plasty may be used to realign structures that have been distorted owing to traumatic scarring or congenital malalignment.[6, 11, 18] For example, tissues that have healed out of line around the lateral canthus of the eye may be relocated by Z-plasty. In this procedure, the malaligned structure is included in one of the Z-plasty flaps, and as the flaps are transposed the structure is moved back into position (Fig. 9–10).

MULTIPLE Z-PLASTIES

DEFINITION AND INDICATIONS

In multiple Z-plasties a linear contracture is divided into several segments, on each of which a small "Z" is constructed.[27] The multiple Z-plasty technique has some specific indications:

1. The technique may be used to break up long linear contractures that have formed.[2, 9, 10, 14, 16, 27]
2. Related to the first indication is the use of the Z-plasty to gain length in areas where the anatomy or pathology of the region or

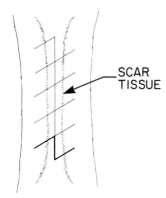

SCAR
TISSUE

Figure 9–29: Long contracture on a limb where skin is not available for two large flaps of a single Z-plasty. The linear contracture is divided into several segments with a small "Z" constructed on each segment.

both limit the size of the skin flap.[9, 27] When the central limb of the Z-plasty extends the full length of a long contracture, a correspondingly large quantity of tissue must be brought in from the sides, and this tissue may not be available. This is particularly so on a limb on which the available tissue is spread out along its length (Fig. 9–29).[27]

3. Multiple Z-plasties are indicated for enlarging the circumference of a circular or constricting scar.[2, 14, 26] Such cases include traumatic scars or congenital strictures that encircle a limb (Figs. 9–11 and 9–12) or the fibrous constriction of a body orifice (e.g., the anus) (Fig. 9–13).

DESIGN

Multiple Z-plasties may be constructed in a parallel or a skew pattern. With either of these patterns, the Z-plasties may be continuous or interrupted.[2, 11, 16, 27]

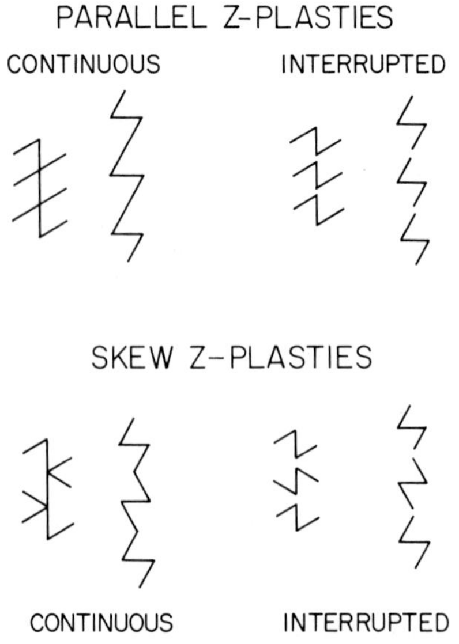

PARALLEL Z-PLASTIES

CONTINUOUS   INTERRUPTED

SKEW Z-PLASTIES

CONTINUOUS   INTERRUPTED

Figure 9–30: Various types of multiple Z-plasties. (After McGregor, I. A.: Fundamental Techniques of Plastic Surgery, ed. 5. Edinburgh, Churchill Livingstone, 1972, p. 45.)

In continuous parallel Z-plasties there is one long central limb, off which parallel arms are constructed at 60-degree angles at various points. All flaps of the Z-plasties rotate in the same direction. Interrupted parallel Z-plasties are the same as continuous parallel Z-plasties, with the exception that the long central limb is interrupted along its length (Fig. 9–30).[2, 16, 27]

Continuous skew Z-plasties have one long central limb, off which side arms project in a nonparallel fashion at various points. In other words, the small Z-plasties along the central limb alternate in the direction of rotation as the flaps are transposed (i.e., clockwise — counterclockwise). Interrupted skew Z-plasties are similar to continuous skew Z-plasties, with the exception that the long central limb is interrupted (Fig. 9–30).[2, 16, 27]

Parallel multiple Z-plasties allow all flaps to rotate in the same way, thereby maintaining broad bases. Skew multiple Z-plasties are indicated in areas along the central limb where scarring dictates that the flaps of each "Z" rotate in various directions. Such flaps are more subject to vascular problems, since they have a broad tip and a narrow base.[27]

ADVANTAGES AND DISADVANTAGES

The diffusion of lateral tension is the primary advantage of multiple Z-plasties over a single Z-plasty. In a single Z-plasty, all of the lateral tension is concentrated along the single transverse limb of the "Z." With multiple Z-plasties, the tension is diffused over several transverse limbs (Fig. 9–31).[5, 27] In both the single and multiple Z-plasty techniques, the amount of lengthening that is achieved is the same, but the amount of shortening is greatly reduced with the multiple Z-plasties. The lengthening in multiple plasties is done in a series and the result is additive, but the shortening is accomplished in a parallel manner, and the amount of shortening remains the same for each small "Z."[27]

In contradiction to the previous findings, a study on dogs comparing the single Z-plasty with the multiple Z-plasty technique revealed that the gain in length from one large Z-plasty was greater than the gain from several small Z-plasties that were designed theoretically to produce the same

SINGLE Z-PLASTY = LATERAL TENSION CONCENTRATED

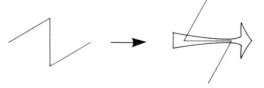

MULTIPLE Z-PLASTY=LATERAL TENSION DIFFUSED

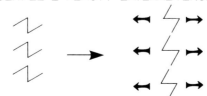

Figure 9–31: Tension differences with single and multiple Z-plasties.

gain in length. The gain in length for a single 8-cm. Z-plasty was nearly twice that for a series of eight 1-cm. Z-plasties. This study also showed that the axillary web of a dog was totally (100 per cent) effaced by a single Z-plasty and only partially (70 per cent) effaced by a series of three Z-plasties. However, the force that was required to transpose the single Z-plasty flaps was considerably more than that required for multiple Z-plasties.[17]

APPLICATIONS OF MULTIPLE Z-PLASTIES

Lengthening Long Contractures

As has already been stated under the indications for multiple Z-plasties, they have a primary application in relieving tension along long linear contractures.[2, 9, 14, 16, 27] In such instances any one of the types of multiple Z-plasties may be used, depending on the case and the surgeon's discretion (Fig. 9–30).

Enlarging the Circumference of a Circular or a Constricting Scar

When the circumference of a constricting scar is enlarged, the circumference is increased (lengthened) at the expense (shortening) of the tissue on either side of the stricture. A circular incision is made at the depth of the stricture to serve as the central limb of the "Z," and multiple arms are constructed off this line to form multiple Z-plasties. Transposition of the Z-plasty flaps results in increasing the circumference of the area (Figs. 9–11, 9–12, and 9–32).[2, 26]

Enlarging the circumference of an orifice that is constricted by fibrous scar tissue may be accomplished by means of Z-plasties. Double opposing Z-plasties have been described[10, 29] and would be applicable in such instances. Such a procedure would be indicated when fibrosis has constricted the anus following surgery for perianal fistulae; however, this condition may be more prevalent following the cryosurgical treatment of perianal fistulae (Fig. 9–13).[7, 23, 24]

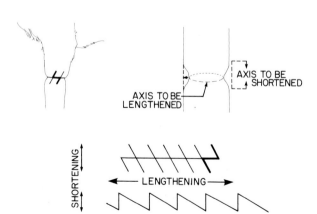

Figure 9–32: Designing multiple Z-plasties to enlarge the circumference of a constricting scar. (After McGregor, I. A.: The Z-plasty. Br. J. Plast. Surg. *19*:86, 1966.)

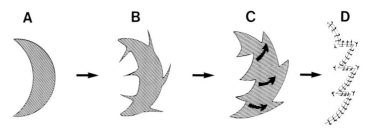

Figure 9–33: The use of multiple Z-plasties to close a crescent-shaped defect. *A*, Crescent-shaped wound. *B*, Incision of Z-plasty arms off the edges of the wound. *C*, Movement of the flaps to close the lesion. *D*, Completed closure of the crescent-shaped wound utilizing Z-plasties. (After McGregor, I. A.: Fundamental Techniques of Plastic Surgery, ed. 5. Edinburgh, Churchill Livingstone, 1972, p. 54.)

Closure of Crescent-Shaped Wounds

The unequal lengths of the sides of a crescent-shaped wound can make closure difficult. Placing sutures closer together on the short side of the wound and farther apart on the long side of the wound as a corrective measure has already been described in Chapter 7. Multiple Z-plasties can be used to further reduce the discrepancy in lengths (Fig. 9–33).[27] Since dog-ears are inevitable in closing such wounds, Z-plasties may be considered as a means of eliminating them.

THEORY VS. PRACTICALITY

Although the Z-plasty is a fascinating and useful tool in reconstructive surgery, it does have its limitations. The theoretical gain in length can be readily calculated; however, the normal tissue tension in the surrounding area may prevent the attainment of the maximum increase in length. Consequently, this prevents the science of surgery from being quite as exact as the science of mathematics.[18] In addition to the limitations of normal tissues, the presence of scarring in the operative area has an influence on the efficiency of a Z-plasty. If sufficient slack skin is not available around an area of proposed Z-plasty, the procedure will not work, and a skin graft may have to be used for reconstruction.[27]

V-Y-PLASTY

INDICATIONS

The V-Y-plasty is a technique that is indicated when it is necessary to advance skin to cover a lesion. It may be considered a type of advancement flap; however, it does not use advancement in the same sense as a single pedicle advancement flap.[18, 19] The technique involves making a "V"-shaped incision in the skin, after which the skin on each side of the "V" is advanced. This permits the advancement of the flap that is situated between the branches of the "V" to help cover a lesion. The closure converts

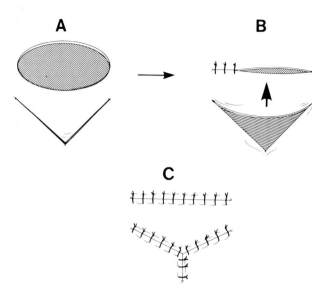

A

B

C

Figure 9–34: The V-Y-plasty technique is used to advance skin to cover a lesion. *A,* 'V''-shaped incision in the skin adjacent to a lesion. *B,* Advancement of the flap of skin between the branches of the "V" to close the lesion. *C,* Completed closure of the lesion and closure of the "V''-shaped incision in a "Y''-shape.

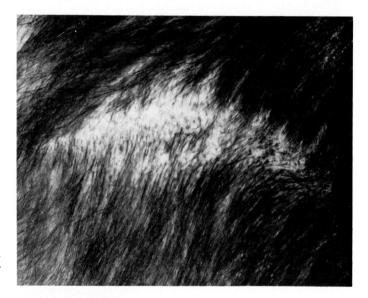

Figure 9–35: Widened scar resulting from wound closure under tension.

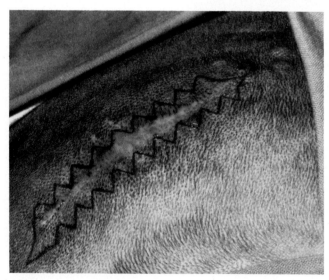

Figure 9–36: W-plasty designed for scar removal.

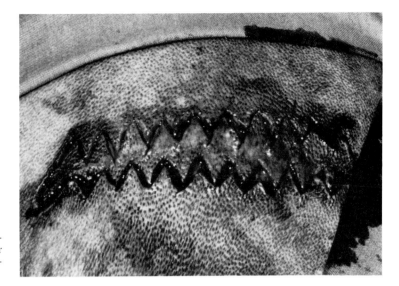

Figure 9–37: Completed incision of the W-plasty. Scar tissue between the two incisions will be removed.

the "V" to a "Y," and the easing of tension and the amount of movement of the flap are proportional to the length of the leg that converts the "V" to a "Y" (Fig. 9–34).[2, 14, 18, 19, 34] It is useful in the revision of scars of the palpebra and as a relaxing procedure for closing fusiform defects.[35]

W-PLASTY

DEFINITION, INDICATIONS, AND CONTRAINDICATIONS

The W-plasty technique is used for revision of a straight or a curved scar, which is usually hypertrophic owing to its orientation against skin tension lines. Such scars are converted to a zigzag pattern without the rotation of tissue (Figs. 9–35 through 9–39).[6, 10, 18, 22] The ideal scar on which to use

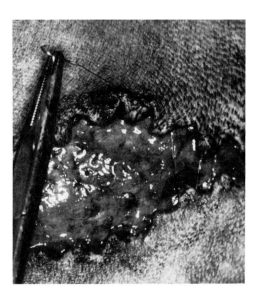

Figure 9–38: Placement of a continuous intradermal suture of 4–0 polypropylene to interdigitate the triangles of the W-plasty.

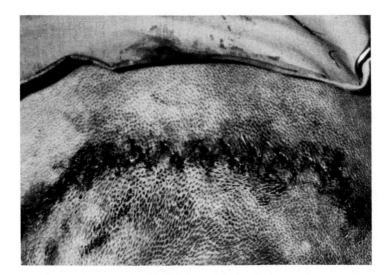

Figure 9–39: Simple interrupted skin sutures of 4–0 polypropylene are placed at the tip of each triangle to complete the W-plasty closure.

this technique is the linear scar that is not depressed or raised above the surrounding skin but that crosses the lines of skin tension. The technique is contraindicated if the scar follows the lines of skin tension or if it has contracted to form a linear bridle, web, groove, or circular constriction. Single or multiple Z-plasties are indicated in such instances. The technique should not be used in areas where the skin is very taut, since a W-plasty requires the presence of lax tissue on each side of the scar to be effective.[4] The author has found that even in areas where the skin is taut on dogs, a W-plasty helps to prevent the widening of scars better than a conventional closure technique in which a simple continuous intradermal suture and simple interrupted skin sutures are used.

As mentioned with Z-plasties, hypertrophic scars are not usually a problem in veterinary surgery because of the overlying hair coat and the loose skin of dogs and cats. However, large wounds that are closed under tension in short-haired dogs may result in an unaesthetic scar (Fig. 9–25).

THEORY AND DESIGN

The W-plasty technique follows the premise that angled or broken-line scars that run, for the most part, against tension lines generally produce a better result in reconstructive surgery than linear scars that run against tension lines. The reason for this is that some components of angled or broken-line scars usually follow the skin tension lines, and such jagged scars have an accordion-like elasticity if placed under tension from their two most distant points.[6]

When designing a W-plasty, the measure of the angles, the length of the limbs of the "W," and the proper termination of the procedure must be considered. The angles of the running W-plasty may range from 60 to 90 degrees;[6] however, the most common angle is between 50 and 55 degrees.[22] Angles that are too wide result in a scar line that does not follow skin tension lines closely enough to accomplish the purpose of the W-plasty; such scars have less elasticity. Angles that are too narrow create too many triangles, which prolong the time required for surgery and which may have an inadequate blood supply.[4, 6, 22] The limbs of a W-plasty are from 4 to 7 mm. long, with 5.5 mm. being the most common length. Longer sides necessitate including more normal skin on either side of the scar and increasing the tension of closure.[6, 22] The W-plasty should be placed as close to the scar as possible so that the amount of normal skin that is sacrificed is minimal.[6] If the sides of the triangles are too short, the necessary accordion-like elasticity of the scar will be lost.[6, 22] The triangular flaps that are created by a W-plasty have been described as isosceles triangles; each is approximately 6 mm. at its base and 6.5 mm. in height and has two 65-degree angles and one 50-degree angle (Fig. 9–40).[4] The ends of a W-plasty are in the form of Ammon's triangles. This helps to prevent dog-ears at the ends when the W-plasty is closed (Fig. 9–40, insert).[6, 22]

The size of the triangular flaps of the W-plasty may be tapered toward the ends of the excision to allow them to blend into Ammon's triangles more easily.[6, 10, 22]

The triangular flaps of a W-plasty are designed so that they will interdigitate perfectly when the wound is closed.[4, 6, 16, 18, 22] The use of a special metal form with the pattern of the triangles (or "W's") cut into it has been described for designing a W-plasty.[4, 6, 18] A soft metal band that is bent into a series of 60-degree angles by hemostats has also been described.[10] However, freehand measuring and drawing may be used in designing the W-plasty.[6, 10] The author prefers to use a piece of developed x-ray film cut to the proper dimensions as a W-plasty form. Marking on the skin may be done with a sterile toothpick dipped in methylene blue.

SURGICAL TECHNIQUE

A No. 11 blade is used to incise one triangular flap on one side of the scar. This is followed by the incision of the corresponding triangle on the opposite side. The process is continued along the length of the scar until the entire area of the W-plasty has been incised (Fig. 9–37). This helps (1) to guarantee an equal number of triangles on each side of the incision, (2) to hold the skin firm while the incisions are being made, and (3) to keep apposing triangles equal in measure.[6, 10] Cutting should progress from the lowest point on the scar to the highest point. This helps to prevent blood from running down over any pattern lines that have been drawn and washing them away.

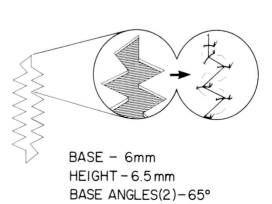

Figure 9–40: Design and proper dimensions for the triangles of a W-plasty. *Insert,* Ending a W-plasty with Ammon's triangles results in smooth closure of the ends. (After Borges, A. F.: Elective Incisions and Scar Revision. Boston, Little, Brown and Co., 1973, p. 185.)

BASE – 6mm
HEIGHT – 6.5 mm
BASE ANGLES(2) – 65°
TIP ANGLE – 50°

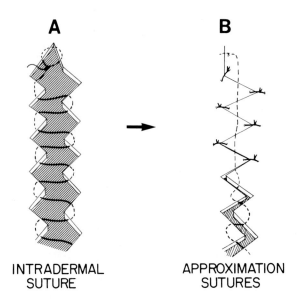

A   INTRADERMAL SUTURE

B   APPROXIMATION SUTURES

Figure 9–41: *A*, Proper placement of the continuous intradermal suture and *B*, the simple interrupted skin approximation sutures. (After Borges, A. F.: Elective Incisions and Scar Revision. Boston, Little, Brown and Co., 1973, p. 188.)

After removing the scar tissue, the triangular flaps are undermined so that they are thick enough to have a sufficient blood supply.[4, 6, 22] The serrated edges are then apposed with a continuous intradermal suture of 4–0 monofilament nylon. The suture is placed halfway between the tip and the base of each triangular flap to assure good interdigitation of the flaps as the suture is pulled tight (Figs. 9–38 and 9–41). This suture may be placed so that it ends beyond the ends of the W-plasty and can be removed at a later date. Final approximation of the skin edges is by means of fine simple interrupted nonabsorbable sutures that are placed at the tip of each flap (Figs. 9–39 and 9–41).[6, 10] The author prefers to place the simple continuous intradermal suture with 4–0 polypropylene, which remains buried (Fig. 9–41).

ADVANTAGES

Several advantages have been stated for the W-plasty in correcting hypertrophic scars that run against tension lines. However, the primary ad-

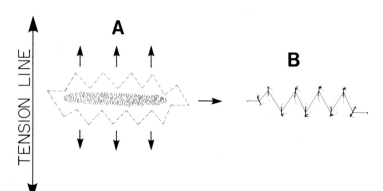

TENSION LINE

A

B

Figure 9–42: *A*, A scar that is oriented against tension lines tends to widen. *B*, Revision of the scar by W-plasty helps to break up the scar and to orient it more in line with tension lines and helps prevent scar widening.

vantage is that the scar is removed and the area is closed in a zigzag fashion so that the tension on the new scar is more in line with the skin tension lines, and these lines do not tend to widen the scar (Fig. 9–42).[6]

SUMMARY

In summary, the various plastic procedures that are referred to by letters of the alphabet are interesting and useful in reconstructive operations. To help understand the principles and dynamics of the various forms of the Z-plasty, it may be helpful to design and create the various Z-plasties on a piece of cloth or sheet rubber. As with all surgical procedures, these various forms of plastic surgery have their limitations (e.g., Z-plasty angles that are greater or less than certain measures work in theory but are not practical for actual use owing to the limitations of tissue flexibility). Each of these procedures has its indications, contraindications, advantages, and disadvantages, all of which the surgeon should be familiar with before attempting any one of the methods.

REFERENCES

1. Archibald, J. A.: Procedures in plastic surgery. J. Am. Vet. Med. Assoc. *147*:1461, 1965.
2. Berson, M. I.: Atlas of Plastic Surgery, ed. 2. New York, Grune & Stratton, Inc., 1963.
3. Bojrab, M. J.: Personal communication, 1976. College of Veterinary Medicine, Depart. of Veterinary Medicine and Surgery, University of Missouri, Columbia, MO 65201.
4. Borges, A. F.: Improvement of antitension-lines scar by the "W-plastic" operation. Br. J. Plast. Surg. *12*:29, 1959.
5. Borges, A. F., and Alexander, J. E.: Relaxed skin tension lines, Z-plasties on scars, and fusiform excision of lesions. Br. J. Plast. Surg. *15*:242, 1962.
6. Borges, A. F.: Elective Incisions and Scar Revision. Boston, Little, Brown and Co., 1973.
7. Bushby, P. A.: Cryosurgery: A Clinical and Pathological Study — Cryosurgical Treatment of Perianal Fistulae, Master of Science thesis. Auburn University, Auburn, AL 36830, 1976.
8. Cawley, A. J., and Archibald, J. A.: Plastic surgery, in Archibald, J. A. (ed.): Canine Surgery, ed. 2. Santa Barbara, Calif., American Veterinary Publications, Inc., 1974.
9. Converse, J. M.: Burn deformities of the face and neck: Reconstructive surgery and rehabilitation. Surg. Clin. North Am. *47*:323, 1967.
10. Converse, J. M.: Introduction to plastic surgery, in Converse, J. M. (ed.): Reconstructive Plastic Surgery: Principles and Procedures in Correction, Reconstruction, and Transplantation, ed. 2. Philadelphia, W.·B. Saunders Co., 1977, vol. 1.
11. Davis, J. S., and Kitlowski, E. A.: The theory and practical use of the Z-incision for relief of scar contractures. Ann. Surg. *109*:1001, 1939.
12. Dixon, A. C.: The secondary closure of wounds. Vet. Rec. *75*:1133, 1963.
13. Dowd, C. N.: Some details in the repair of cicatricial contractures of the neck. Surg. Gynecol. Obstet. *44*:396, 1927.
14. Epstein, E.: Skin Surgery. Philadelphia, Lea & Febiger, 1962.
15. Furnas, D. W.: The tetrahedral Z-plasty. Plast. Reconstr. Surg. *35*:291, 1965.
16. Furnas, D. W.: The four fundamental functions of the Z-plasty. Arch. Surg. *96*:458, 1968.
17. Furnas, D. W., and Fischer, G. W.: The Z-plasty: Biomechanics and mathematics. Br. J. Plast. Surg. *24*:144, 1971.
18. Grabb, W. C., and Smith, J. W.: Basic techniques of plastic surgery, in Grabb, W. C., and Smith, J. W. (eds.): Plastic Surgery: A Concise Guide to Clinical Practice. Boston, Little, Brown and Co., 1968.
19. Grabb, W. C.: Classification of flaps, in Grabb, W. C., and Myers, M. B. (eds.): Skin Flaps. Boston, Little, Brown and Co., 1975.
20. Johnston, D.E.: Wound healing and reconstructive surgery. Am. Anim. Hosp. Assoc. Sci. Proc. *2*:383, 1975.
21. Kirk, M. D.: Selective scar revision and elective incision techniques applicable to the legs of horses: I. Application of adjacent Z-plasty adjunct procedure in the repair of skin wounds on the lower legs of horses. Vet. Med. Small Anim. Clin. *71*:661, 1976.
22. Kirk, M. D.: Selective scar revision and elective incision techniques applicable to the legs

of horses: II. Application of modified W-plasty surgical techniques in scar revision on the lower legs of horses. Vet. Med. Small Anim. Clin. 71:801, 1976.

23. Lane, J. G., and Burch, D. G. S.: The cryosurgical treatment of canine anal furunculosis. J. Small Anim. Pract. 16:387, 1975.

24. Liska, W. D., Greiner, T. P., and Withrow, S. J.: Symposium on surgical techniques in small animal practice: Cryosurgery in the treatment of perianal fistulae. Vet. Clin. North Am. 5:449, 1975.

25. Marino, H.: The leveling effect of Z-plasties on lineal scars of the face. Br. J. Plast. Surg. 12:34, 1959.

26. McGregor, I. A.: The Z-plasty. Br. J. Plast. Surg. 19:82, 1966.

27. McGregor, I. A.: Fundamental techniques of plastic surgery, ed. 5. Edinburgh, Churchill Livingstone, 1972.

28. Millard, D. R.: Pedicle flaps, in Cooper, P. (ed.): The Craft of Surgery, ed. 2. Boston, Little, Brown and Co., 1971, vol. 1.

29. Mühlbauer, W. D.: Elongation of mouth in post-born microstomia by a double Z-plasty. Plast. Reconstr. Surg. 45:400, 1970.

30. Mulliken, J. B., and Hoopes, J. E.: W-epicanthoplasty. Plast. Reconstr. Surg. 55:435, 1975.

31. Padgett, E. C., and Stephenson, K. L.: Plastic and Reconstructive Surgery. Springfield, Ill., Charles C Thomas Publisher, 1948.

32. Pullen, C. M.: Reconstruction of the skin, in Bojrab, M. J. (ed.): Current Techniques in Small Animal Surgery. Philadelphia, Lea & Febiger, 1975.

33. Spina, V.: "Z" plasty. Rev. Paul. Med. 36:347, 1950.

34. Spreull, J. S. A.: The principles of transplanting skin in the dog. J. Am. Anim. Hosp. Assoc. 4:71, 1968.

35. Stashak, T. S.: Reconstructive surgery in the horse. J. Am. Vet. Med. Assoc 170:143, 1977.

36. Woolf, R. M., and Broadbent, T. R.: The four-flap Z-plasty. Plast. Reconstr. Surg. 49:48, 1972.

37. Zovickian, A.: Closure of soft tissue surface wounds, surgical and traumatic, in Cooper, P. (ed.): The Craft of Surgery, ed. 2. Boston, Little, Brown and Co., 1971, vol. 1.

10

SKIN GRAFTS

A free skin graft is a segment of epidermis and dermis that is completely detached from the body and transferred to a recipient site.[15, 18, 32, 52, 65, 74] At this site its survival is dependent upon the absorption of tissue fluid[15] and the development of a new blood supply.[18, 52, 65]

CLASSIFICATION OF GRAFTS

Skin grafts are classified according to their donor-host relationship and their thickness. The following terms categorize grafts by their donor-host relationship: (1) autograft (autogenous graft), which is a graft that is transferred from a donor site to a recipient site on the same animal; (2) allograft (homograft), which is a graft that is transferred between genetically different individuals of the same species; and (3) xenograft (heterograft), which is a graft that is transferred between individuals of different species.[16, 18, 32, 41, 70] An isograft is an allograft between highly inbred (genetically pure) strains of animals.[16, 18] Clinically, autografts are the most successful type of graft, since the graft and the host are antigenically identical.[3] The majority of this chapter will deal with this type of graft.

When classified according to thickness, grafts may be either full thickness (composed of epidermis and all of the dermis)[16, 32, 80] or split thickness. Split-thickness grafts may be (1) thin split-thickness (Thiersch's grafts), (2) intermediate split-thickness, or (3) thick split-thickness grafts (Fig. 10–1).[18, 32]

INDICATIONS FOR SKIN GRAFTS

Skin grafts are indicated when there has been a loss of skin, either as the result of trauma or of other factors that cause skin defects. In the dog, skin grafting is primarily indicated for facial lesions[40] and injuries to the skin of the extremities.[40, 85] The author has found that grafting is most needed on lesions of the distal aspect of the limb, where skin immobility precludes tissue shifting and the construction of local flaps for repair.

FACTORS TO CONSIDER

Before attempting a skin grafting procedure, the general condition of the patient should be considered. Graft "takes" are generally more successful in young individuals; however, the difference in outcome between the young

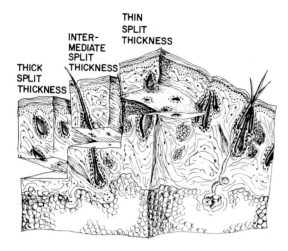

GRAFT THICKNESS

Figure 10–1: Various thicknesses of split-thickness skin grafts.

and the aged is not marked. Debilitated individuals with chronic disease have a greater tendency to infection.[62] Deficiencies should be corrected prior to grafting, particularly blood deficiencies such as anemia. A low hemoglobin level has been associated with an unsuccessful skin graft. If immediate surgery is necessary, the hemoglobin level can be raised by a whole blood transfusion.[3]

Local factors, including the nature of the tissue lost and the type and condition of the graft bed, should be considered.[62] Since transplanted skin will maintain most of its original characteristics,[32] the skin that is selected for a graft should match the adjacent integument as closely as possible.[21]

The decision to apply a graft to a lesion should be made after considering (1) the animal's value, (2) the cosmetic effect desired, (3) the wound's location, (4) the age of the wound, and (5) the wound's size.[35] Skin grafting techniques that are successful in humans are also applicable in dogs; however, bandaging and postoperative care differ markedly. Restraint, effective bandaging, and the possibility of contamination are major problems in the dog.[40] In the dog, as in the horse,[9, 10] a graft over the cranial tarsal area may take poorly unless the joint is adequately immobilized. This is attributable to the wrinkling of the graft during tarsal flexion, which prevents the continuity of apposition between the graft and the bed.

GRAFT BEDS

WHERE GRAFTS WILL TAKE

A graft "take" may be defined as a graft that has established arterial connections and in which venous drainage is adequate.[63] Certain factors are necessary for a graft to take.

A skin graft should be placed either on healthy granulation tissue or on a fresh surface that is vascular enough to produce granulation tissue.[32, 44, 51, 52, 54, 84, 85] The latter type of surface may be a surgically created raw surface or a surgically clean surface.[52] Such surfaces include the deep fascia, muscle and deepithelialized scar tissue.[18, 32, 44] A lightly contaminated wound that is seen early may be cleaned, irrigated, and débrided, and a graft may be applied at the same time,[62] with the main function of the débridement being the production of a richly vascularized graft bed.[51] A graft should not be applied to an infected wound until the infection has been controlled and a healthy granulation base has been established.[62, 80] Preference for a fresh, well-vascularized graft bed that is free of granulation tissue has been stated in the veterinary literature.[54, 66, 71, 85] One study in dogs indicated that grafts revascularized faster when placed on a fresh, non-granulating surface than when placed on granulation tissue.[40]

WHERE GRAFTS WILL NOT TAKE

None of the body's stratified squamous epithelial surfaces will support the growth of a skin graft.[32] A graft will not take over cortical bone that is not covered by periosteum, tendon that is bared of paratenon, cartilage that is denuded of perichondrium, or nerve that is not surrounded by perineurium.[14, 18, 32, 44, 52, 80, 85] An exception to the previous statement is the bridging phenomenon in which a small area of a graft over an avascular surface will survive as a result of the vessels from the vascularized part of the graft linking together in the portion of the graft over the avascular surface.[32, 52] Bridging can occur from any one margin over a gap of 0.5 cm. Thus, a graft may be applied to an avascular area 1 cm. in diameter and can be expected to survive if the surrounding graft bed is good (Fig. 10–2).[13, 14, 32] By using a prepared graft on a prepared bed or a fresh graft on a prepared bed, a larger avascular area might be bridged[31] (see the section on preparation of grafts and beds).

Heavily irradiated tissues, fat, long-standing granulation tissue, and the exposed surfaces of chronic ulcers are also relatively poor recipient beds for skin grafts.[32]

If a graft bed is not level, the graft may not take. Unless the bed is shallow, irregularities can cause "tenting" of the graft across the depressions (Fig. 10–3A and B).[52] Measures to obtain contact between the graft and the bed on a concave surface include (1) cutting the graft so that it is large enough to cover the depths of the wound and using a tie-over bandage (Fig. 10–4),[32] (2) cutting a pie-shaped triangle of tissue from the graft and closing the triangle to form a cone,[32] and (3) suturing the graft to the concave base (Fig. 10–5).[14, 62] Smooth convex immobile graft beds provide for good graft and bed contact.[62]

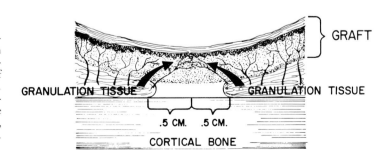

Figure 10–2: Bridging phenomenon. Blood vessels can grow into a skin graft over a nonvascular area for a distance of 0.5 cm. from a vascular edge. (After McGregor, I. A.: Fundamental Techniques of Plastic Surgery, ed. 6. Edinburgh, Churchill Livingstone, 1975, p. 63.)

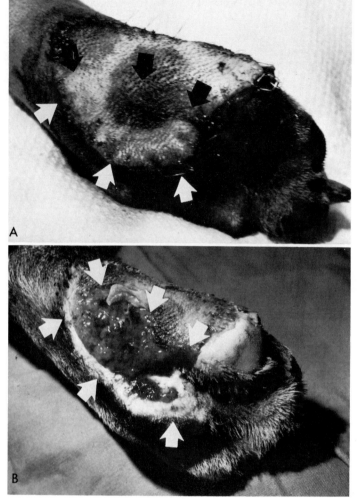

Figure 10–3: Free full-thickness graft on a dog's foot. *A*, Area where graft was over an irregular surface (*arrows*). *B*, Area where graft did not take owing to poor contact with the irregular surface (*arrows*). See color plate III–F, p. 570.

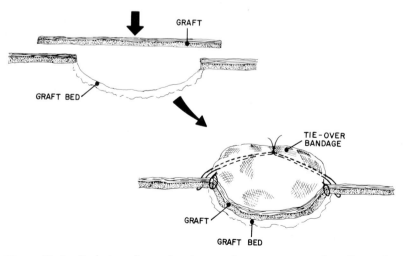

Figure 10–4: Technique for conforming a graft to a concave surface. Cut graft large enough to fit into concavity, suture graft edges, and place a tie-over bandage over the graft to hold it against the bed.

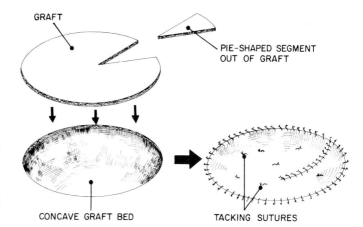

GRAFT

PIE-SHAPED SEGMENT OUT OF GRAFT

CONCAVE GRAFT BED

TACKING SUTURES

Figure 10–5: Technique for conforming a graft to a concave surface. Remove a pie-shaped segment from the graft. Suture the graft to the bed using apposition sutures to close the wedge-shaped defect in the graft, apposition sutures along the graft's edge, and tacking sutures to hold the graft against the bed.

FACTORS INFLUENCING THE TAKE OR LOSS OF A GRAFT

GRAFT TAKE

The conditions that are necessary for a good skin graft take include (1) a graft bed that is free of infection; (2) a richly vascularized graft bed; (3) hemostasis of the graft bed; (4) proper preparation of a granulation tissue bed; (5) the proper tension for suturing a graft; and (6) adequate immobilization of and contact (pressure) between the graft and the bed to permit rapid serum imbibition and revascularization of the graft.[18, 32, 52, 53, 62]

Adherence of Graft to Bed

The initial adherence of a graft to its bed is by a fibrin network. This network is later invaded by fibroblasts, leukocytes, and phagocytes and converted to a fibrous tissue attachment between the graft and the bed.[15, 16, 22, 32, 37, 41, 44, 52, 62] The adherence between the graft and the bed gains the greatest strength in the first eight hours and continues to gain strength more slowly for up to four days.[64] By ten days the union is complete and firm.[16, 62] The amount of collagen in the graft-bed area then increases; the collagen matures over days and weeks and is responsible for graft contraction.[16]

Considerable research has been performed and many articles have been written dealing with the maintenance and revascularization of skin grafts. The following section summarizes the basic facts.

Maintenance: Plasmatic Imbibition

Immediately following the removal of a skin graft from the donor area, its blood vessels undergo spasm and expel most of the formed hemic elements from the severed ends of the vessels.[6, 38] After the graft is placed on the

A. PLASMATIC IMBIBITION

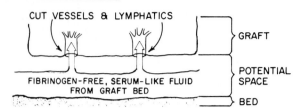

B. INOSCULATION

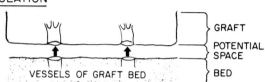

Figure 10–6: Stages of maintenance and revascularization of skin grafts: *A*, plasmatic imbibition. *B*, inosculation, and *C*, ingrowth of vessels.

C. INGROWTH OF VESSELS

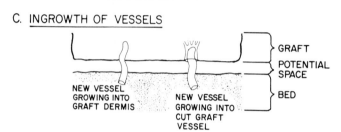

recipient bed, these vessels, as well as the lymphatics of the dermis of the graft, act as a sponge and absorb a fibrinogen-free serum-like fluid containing erythrocytes and other cellular elements from the graft bed.[6, 17, 18, 22, 32, 33, 70] The fluid does not circulate but rather has a to-and-fro movement, which serves to keep the vessels open for easy revascularization of the graft (Fig. 10–6A).[6, 18, 20, 70] The absorption of fluid and cells into the graft occurs primarily within the first 48 hours[32, 38, 62] and reaches its maximum at 72 hours,[6] resulting in a clinically edematous graft. This edema may persist for as long as five days.[65] It then subsides as the newly established blood and lymphatic flow carry the absorbed fluid from the graft.[17, 18, 32] This stage of plasmatic imbibition serves to maintain the graft until it is revascularized, and the surgeon should not become distressed at the blue edematous appearance of a graft within the first few days after grafting.

Others have stated that graft survival during the first three or four days is dependent upon the development of a semipermeable membrane effect between the graft's undersurface and its bed. Gases and nutrients are then able to diffuse across the membrane to support the graft.[63]

Revascularization

Inosculation. Revascularization of a graft begins with the formation of anastomoses between the vessels of the bed and the existing vessels within the graft (Fig. 10–6B).[7, 17-19, 22, 32, 33, 52, 62, 87] The formation of such anastomoses may begin as early as 24 hours postoperatively, but it starts more commonly at 48 hours.[18, 19, 22, 32] Many vessels may make contact and anastomose, but only a few survive and develop, as shown by studies that were conducted between five and six days after transplantation.[19] Preexisting vessels within the graft may also actively proliferate[6, 41] and establish host and graft connections.[55]

Ingrowth of Vessels.   A graft is also revascularized by the ingrowth of new vessels from the bed into the dermis of the graft.[7, 18, 19, 22, 32, 52, 56] Studies in dogs have shown that most of the revascularization of a free full-thickness graft is accomplished in this way,[22, 56] whereas a thin split-thickness graft is revascularized primarily by inosculation.[56] The stimulus for vessel growth from the bed into the graft may be a diffusible substance from the dead or damaged cells in the graft, or, more probably, it is hypoxia of the area.[87] The vessels of the graft bed may also grow into the graft by invading the open end of a cut vessel in the graft and growing along the path of least resistance (Fig. 10–6C).[18, 22, 89] Although most vascularization comes from the graft bed, vessels can also invade the graft from the surrounding skin margins.[69]

The growth of vessel sprouts is faster in grafts of young tissue than in those of older tissue.[55] Vessel invasion of the graft *may* start as early as between six and 12 hours after transplantation.[19] The circulation may be completely reestablished anywhere from four[19] to 12[15, 22] days after transplantation.

Delayed Grafting and Preparation Phenomena

If hemorrhage persists when a bed is being prepared to receive a graft, it is best to apply a nonadherent pressure bandage to the bed and wait for one or two days before grafting. This provides hemostasis and allows the graft bed to improve (form granulations).[15, 18, 32, 62, 80]

A study in rats has shown that this delayed grafting results in a "prepared" bed. In other words, the reparative process (formation of capillary sprouts) has already started when the graft is placed at a later date (48 hours). The time for plasmatic imbibition was reduced by half and there was better revascularization in the graft. In one part of this study, it was found that the revascularization of a fresh skin graft on a prepared bed begins most commonly between the 18th and 20th hours after transplantation.[76]

Another study in rats has shown that grafts themselves can be prepared to enhance revascularization. After removal, a graft may go through a stage of anaerobic metabolism, during which graft cells may release proteinaceous vasoactive metabolites. These metabolites are thought to stimulate vessel growth in both the bed and the graft. In one part of this study it was determined that a prepared graft on a prepared bed began revascularization as early as between the fifth and eighth hours after transplantation. A technique for preparing a skin graft is to cut the graft and replace it on its original site for a period of about 12 to 15 hours to allow the biochemical changes to occur within it before placing it on the graft bed.[77]

By the use of a fresh graft on a prepared bed or a prepared graft on a prepared bed, the amount of the graft that survives over avascular defects can be increased.[31] In other words, the effect of the bridging phenomenon can be increased.

GRAFT LOSS

The three main factors that are responsible for graft loss are (1) the accumulation of fluid (blood and serum) beneath the graft; (2) the improper immobilization of the graft and the bed; and (3) bacterial infection.[21, 32, 43, 52, 54, 71, 80]

Hematomas and Seromas

A hematoma under a graft is a barrier to capillary growth from the graft bed, and this interferes with revascularization[15, 18, 22, 44, 52] and plasmatic imbibition (Fig. 10–7).[15, 80] A clot that is 5 mm. thick will retard the revascularization of a graft for five days as the vessels grow through the clot, and the graft will not take. However, a clot that is 0.5 mm. thick delays revascularization by only about 12 hours, and this graft will probably take.[32] A seroma may form under a graft that tents across concavities and is not held against the bed after the pressure bandage has been removed.[52] Such a graft survives only by plasmatic imbibition and will not revascularize until the graft contacts the bed.[21] The following techniques can be used to prevent hematomas and seromas:

1. Prepare the graft bed first and then harvest the graft to allow time for hemostasis to occur in the bed before the graft is applied.[14, 32, 52]
2. Apply gentle pressure on the bed with saline solution–soaked sponges,[3, 14, 15, 66, 71] and exert continual digital pressure on the graft while suturing.[54]
3. Clamp bleeding vessels.[37, 66]
4. Ligate vessels with fine ligatures.[3, 14, 15, 52, 80]
5. Cauterize bleeding vessels.[32, 52]
6. Inject or apply topically epinephrine or norepinephrine to the graft bed.[14, 37, 52] Norepinephrine is a weaker vasoconstrictor, but it is less likely to cause central effects if it is absorbed. A concentration of 1 part to 200,000 parts of saline solution is considered safe.[52] Others have reported using a 1:10,000 epinephrine solution, or a 1 per cent solution of phenylephrine hydrochloride.[37]
7. Apply thrombin topically to the bed.[5, 80]
8. Make "pie crust" or stab incisions in a graft prior to its placement on the bed to prevent fluid accumulation.[28, 66, 71, 80]
9. Apply a tourniquet prior to preparation of the graft bed. It should be released before the graft is applied.[32] Wrapping a limb snugly with an elastic bandage may produce good hemostasis.
10. Place graft-anchoring sutures so that they ligate marginal bleeders as well as anchor the graft.[52]

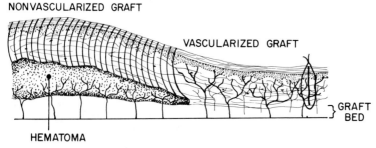

NONVASCULARIZED GRAFT

VASCULARIZED GRAFT

GRAFT BED

HEMATOMA

Figure 10–7:   Hematoma under a portion of a graft is a barrier to capillary growth from the graft bed, thus interfering with revascularization. (After McGregor, I. A.: Fundamental Techniques of Plastic Surgery, ed. 6. Edinburgh, Churchill Livingstone, 1975, p. 62.)

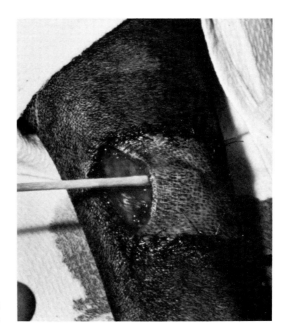

Figure 10–8: A cotton-tipped applicator stick is used to gently remove a blood clot from under a graft.

If a hematoma or a seroma develops under a graft during application or during the early postoperative period, it may be removed in one of the following ways:

1. Prior to placing the last anchor sutures or after removing a few anchor sutures, the area under the graft should be flushed with a saline or a thrombin solution.[14, 18, 32, 52, 80] Other methods for removing hematomas are to gently swirl a cotton-tipped applicator between the graft and the bed (Fig. 10–8)[18, 32, 52] or to roll gauze lightly over the graft.[44, 62] An alternative is to remove any clotted blood with a moist gauze sponge.[32]
2. A graft may be incised and the underlying contents may be evacuated by gentle pressure,[14, 32, 52, 80] or by the use of a sterile eyedropper[18] or a cotton-tipped applicator.[32, 52] When incisions are made in a graft that is on its bed, care should be taken to raise the graft above the bed before incising it to prevent damaging the graft bed and causing more hemorrhage.[32]

A graft should be inspected daily after a seroma or a hematoma has been removed from beneath it.[18, 32] A safety precaution that is employed by the author is to omit two or three sutures at the most dependent portion of the graft. This allows serum drainage and leaves an opening through which hematomas can be expressed or removed by a sterile cotton-tipped applicator. The result of healing in this small area is cosmetic.

Infection

Sepsis will slow the migration of cells into a wound and thereby delay revascularization of a graft. Bacteria cause cell death in both the graft and the recipient bed as well as destruction of the fibrin film that holds the graft to its bed.[15] In light of this, it follows that skin grafting should not be undertaken until wound infection has been controlled.[3, 79] Mechanical cleanliness of the wound, which can be accomplished by débridement of necrotic tissue and frequent moist saline soaks, is essential for wound care.[32] Techniques have been devised to make a quantitative bacterial analysis of a wound to determine its suitability for primary closure or grafting. The reader is referred to Chapter 4 for more information on the subject.

The signs of infection after a graft has been placed include a low-grade fever, odor, and redness around the graft margins between the second and the fourth postoperative day.[32] Culture and sensitivity studies should be performed to aid in selecting the proper antibiotic for topical and systemic administration.[3, 32]

B-hemolytic streptococci (*Streptococcus pyogenes*) are detrimental to skin grafts and may cause complete graft dissolution by interfering with the normal fibrin attachment of the graft to its bed.[21, 32, 52, 79] When these organisms are present, grafting should be postponed while one of the penicillins or the penicillin derivatives is given systemically along with the topical application of penicillin.[21, 32, 52]

Pseudomonas aeruginosa is less damaging to a graft[32] but may cause partial loss of the graft as the extensive exudate floats the graft off its bed.[21, 32] In large wounds, such as burns, the organism may sometimes be controlled by dressings of 0.5 per cent silver nitrate, by topically applied 10 per cent mafenide (Sulfamylon) acetate, or by the application of 0.5 per cent acetic acid to change the wound pH.[32] Topically applied polymyxin B sulfate has also been found to be beneficial.[21, 32]

The treatment of a β-hemolytic streptococcal infection with topically applied penicillin may result in the elimination of this organism but the overgrowth of *Pseudomonas aeruginosa* or *Proteus vulgaris*. Alternate applications of penicillin and polymyxin B may prevent this problem.[21]

Research by Eade and associates, as reported by Grabb and Smith, has shown that topically applied antibiotics have little effect in decreasing the bacterial count of organisms other than streptococci in granulating wounds, whereas systemically administered antibiotics are effective in reducing the number of bacteria. The mechanical cleansing of wounds by frequent dressing changes has a definite effect on controlling infection.[32]

Other organisms that may cause infection but rarely result in loss of the graft are *Staphylococcus aureus*, *Escherichia coli*, and *Proteus vulgaris*.[32, 52] The last two organisms are usually found in combination with *Pseudomonas aeruginosa* and give the wound a foul-smelling discharge.[32] *Pseudomonas*, *Escherichia coli*, and *Proteus* infections have caused the most problems for the author, and the topical application of 0.1 per cent gentamicin sulfate ointment* has been quite effective in their treatment.

Grabb and Smith have reported on a study in which skin grafts were immersed for 15 minutes in an antibiotic solution prior to applying them to the granulation tissue of a burn wound. In a series of patients, grafts that were soaked in 5 per cent neomycin sulfate solution had a mean take of 71 per cent compared with that of 47 per cent in untreated grafts.[32] It is interesting to note that just the application of grafts to infected wounds has been reported to reduce the bacterial count in the wound.[21, 32]

---

*Garamycin Ointment is available from Schering Corp., Kenilworth, NJ 07033.

Mobility

One of the main reasons that grafts do not take is the inadequate immobilization of the graft against its bed. This immobilization is necessary to allow revascularization of the graft to take place from the bed. Until the graft adheres firmly to the bed and the vascular connections are adequately established, movement between the graft and the bed breaks down the developing vascular connections (e.g., inosculating vessels and ingrowing vessels). Techniques for immobilizing a graft on its bed will be covered in detail in the section on bandaging grafts.

PREPARATION OF GRANULATION TISSUE BEDS

In the presence of a good blood supply, open wounds develop a granulation tissue covering between seven and ten days, that serves as a mechanical barrier to and physiological filter for invading organisms. The phagocytes in the tissue have antibacterial properties that limit the invasion of the body by organisms. Healthy granulations are firm, flat, and red. Epithelialization of a bed's edges is evidence that it will support a graft. Chronic granulations are edematous, grayish red, gelatinous, and covered by a relatively tenacious exudate.[32] They are more fibrotic and less vascular and do not provide a good graft bed.[32, 52]

Wounds with chronic granulation tissue should be radically excised to allow new granulations to form before grafting.[54] This may include complete excision to the level of healthy underlying fascia; excision to the level of the dense yellow base has also been described.[9, 10, 14] With less chronic granulations, the top 2 to 3 mm. of the surface may be removed.[41] The goal is a level granulation tissue bed that is free of exuberant granulation tissue,[21, 84] along with the removal of the epithelium covering the periphery of the tissue.[14] The undesirable granulation tissue may be shaved off with a skin graft knife, a straight razor, or a scalpel blade.[13–15, 21, 32, 35] Scraping the area with a knife handle[32] will also remove the granulations. By rapidly scraping excess granulation tissue down to a fibrous tissue bed but not incising through the dense connective tissue, 20 to 30 per cent of the body surface can be made ready for grafting within a few minutes. The application of a compression dressing within seconds after the removal of granulation tissue makes it possible to perform such an extensive procedure with minimal blood loss. In large wounds, the dressings can be removed in ten to 15 minutes and grafting can be performed.[63] Brisk rubbing with a gauze sponge may be used when granulations are not exuberant.[35] The removal of granulation tissue should be done within 24 to 48 hours prior to grafting.[41, 84] This permits hemostasis. The enzymatic débridement of granulation tissue has been described,[21, 52] but it has little advantage over established methods.[52]

After removing the chronic granulation tissue, the bed may be covered with sterile petroleum jelly or with an ointment applied to gauze.[13, 41] However, none of the petroleum jelly or ointment should remain on the new granulation tissue when the graft is placed on the bed two days later. The removal of ointment by ether or by other solvents has been described.[13] However, the author believes that this may be rather harsh on the new granulation tissue and has not found ointment retention to be a problem.

When it is necessary to stimulate granulation tissue growth, dressings of povidone-iodine* may be utilized. A small amount of a solution containing 10 ml. of povidone-iodine whirlpool concentrate in 1 liter of physiological saline solution is applied to the wound dressing three times a day. The dressing is changed every other day for three weeks.[2, 36] Since anemic individuals produce poor granulation tissue, a transfusion may be indicated in such cases.[62]

---

*Betadine Whirlpool Concentrate is available from The Purdue Frederick Co., Norwalk, CT 06856.

The appearance of the granulating surface can be used as an index to determine the appropriate time for grafting. The bed should be free of exudate and should appear firm, flat, and red, with evidence of epithelialization at the edges.[32, 62, 76]

GRAFT STORAGE

If a graft has been cut and for some reason will not be placed immediately on the wound or if it is to be prepared as previously described, it may be stored. If it is to be prepared, the deep surface of the graft may remain in contact with the donor site until the graft is transferred.[77, 79] Grafts may be stored in sterile saline solution–moistened gauze sponges at 4° C. Grafts so stored grow well on new granulation tissue.[15] They have been found to take better than grafts that have been immersed in saline solution, which washes out the endothelial spaces.[62]

TYPES OF SKIN GRAFTS

FREE FULL-THICKNESS GRAFTS (WOLFE'S GRAFTS)

Definition and Characteristics

This type of graft is composed of epidermis and the full thickness of dermis.[5, 32, 52] These grafts closely resemble normal skin in color, texture, elasticity, and hair growth.[32, 52, 79] They undergo minimal to no contraction after transplantation, provide a good weight-bearing surface to tolerate friction, and tend to maintain sebaceous and sweat secretion functions better than split-thickness grafts do.[32, 52] However, these grafts do not take well in the presence of infection[52] and require optimal conditions (i.e., immobilization and a good blood supply) for a take, since they revascularize more slowly than split-thickness grafts do.[18]

Indications

From the standpoint of cosmesis, free full-thickness grafts are often indicated in veterinary surgery because of their ability to support hair growth. The physician does not have to be as concerned about hair growth on grafts as does the veterinarian who is dealing with a completely hirsute (haired) patient. Specific indications for free full-thickness grafting include the closure of lesions on flexion surfaces to prevent contraction; lesions on the face and legs following removal of a tumor, in which cases shifting of the tissues cannot cover the defect; and areas over pressure points.[32, 40] These grafts would also be indicated for lesions on the distal aspect of the limb resulting from various types of trauma (e.g., degloving injuries, sloughs following perivascular injections, snakebite and so on). These grafts are relatively successful over lesions that are free from infection and that do not have excessive granulation tissue.[40]

Donor Sites

A free full-thickness graft should be taken from an area where the skin is loose and abundant and the hair is of the same texture, color, and thickness as that of the recipient area.[15, 44, 66] A common donor site is the lateral thoracic wall.[66, 71, 79, 85] When avulsed skin is available and relatively normal, it may be worthwhile to remove the subcutaneous fat and reapply it. Skin from a pure degloving injury may be viable and quite successful as a free graft.[51] The surgeon has nothing to lose and everything to gain by reapplying viable skin. However, the degree of contamination of the piece of skin should be considered before reapplying it to the wound.

Patterns for Grafts

A pattern of the area to be grafted can be made before or after the recipient area has been excised and prepared.[52] However, it is preferable to make the pattern after the area has been excised. This allows a true measurement of the final lesion, since the excision of malignancies may be more extensive than originally expected,[32] and the excision of old scar tissue results in retraction of the wound's edge, which enlarges the wound.[18, 32]

A sterile gauze sponge, a piece of sterile towel, a piece of sterile disposable drape, the sterile inner wrapping of a disposable surgical glove, and a piece of developed x-ray film are the items from which the author prefers to cut patterns. After excising the lesion (Figs. 10–9A and B), the absorbent material is laid over it, and the pattern is cut to fit the lesion based on the bloody imprint that is left on the material (Fig. 10–10). If x-ray film is used, the lesion is traced on the film under direct vision using methylene blue and a sterile toothpick.

If the lesion is irregular, it is best to maintain both the pattern and the graft in the proper orientation to the defect by marking each of them with corresponding symbols or dots. It is also wise to mark which side of the pattern corresponds to the epidermal side of the graft; otherwise the pattern could be placed on the donor site in such a way as to get a useless mirror image of the defect.[32]

A graft pattern helps to assure an accurate fit of the graft in the defect. A graft that is too small will be stretched when it is sutured into place. It may then act as a drumhead, in which case it will not dip into the recesses of the bed. A graft that is too large may wrinkle and thus will not contact the bed properly. Poor graft-bed contact will result in poor revascularization of the graft. In addition, improper tension of the graft may distort the openings of the

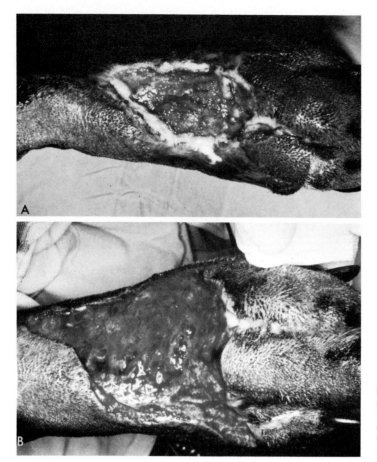

Figure 10–9: *A,* Chronic lesion on the dorsum of a dog's foot prior to excision. *B,* The lesion after excision of the chronic granulation tissue and epithelium. See color plate IV–A, p. 571.

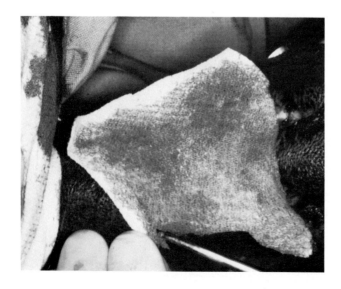

Figure 10–10: A piece of sterile toweling has been laid over the excised lesion, and scissors are being used to trim around the bloody imprint left by the lesion.

blood vessels of the graft and thereby interfere with the reestablishment of circulation.[21, 22, 32, 80]

Cutting and Elevating Grafts

The pattern is placed on the donor area so that the direction of hair growth on the graft is the same as that of hair growth surrounding the recipient area. A pen that is designed for skin marking or some other marking device (e.g., a sterile toothpick and methylene blue) may be used to trace around the pattern. When the pattern is removed, the skin is held taut by an assistant and the graft is cut. Another technique, and one preferred by the author, is to use a No. 15 blade to lightly incise around the pattern, making sure that no tension is exerted on the skin. Only enough pressure as is necessary is used to incise the epidermis. If desired, this incision may be made from 1 to 2 mm. larger than the pattern to allow for primary contraction. Pressure during this outlining incision should be avoided, since this can distort the skin and result in a misshapen graft. Incising through the remaining skin thickness completes the graft cutting (Fig. 10–11).[14, 15, 18, 66, 71, 79]

Since this type of graft should contain only dermis and epidermis, it is necessary to remove all fat from the dermis because it would block revascularization of the graft. An edge of the graft may be elevated by stay sutures, by skin hooks, or by forceps while dissection of the graft between the dermis and subcuticular fat is begun using a sharp blade in a cutting (not scraping) action (Fig. 10–12). The graft may be rolled over a finger or over a gauze roll for further elevation as it is dissected free (Fig. 10–13).[3, 5, 15, 16, 32, 52, 62, 71, 79, 80, 85]

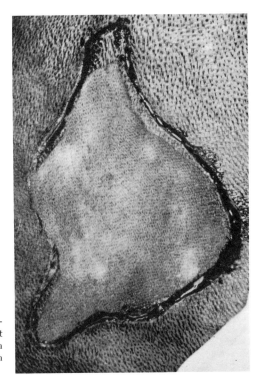

Figure 10–11: The cloth pattern of the defect (Fig. 10–10) has been placed on the donor site and arranged so that the direction of hair growth on the graft will be like that on the foot where it will be placed. An incision has been made around the pattern.

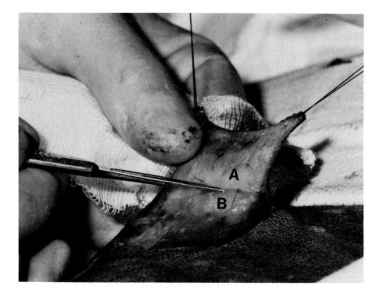

Figure 10–12: Stay sutures are used to elevate the graft as a sharp scalpel blade is used to cut (not scrape) the graft between, *A*, the dermis and, *B*, the subcuticular fat.

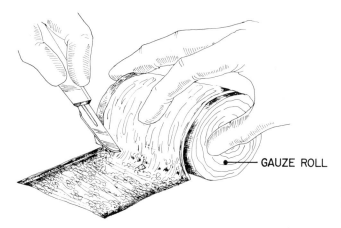

Figure 10–13: A gauze roll is being used to elevate a full-thickness graft as it is cut from the donor site.

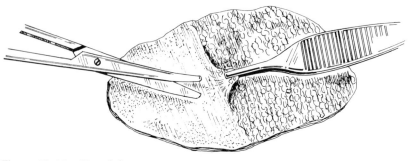

Figure 10–14: Use of sharp scissors to remove subcuticular fat from the undersurface of a full-thickness graft.

Dissection may be tedious, and it may be difficult to determine where the subcuticular fat and the dermis divide. Visualization of the bases of the hair follicles will indicate the base of the dermis.[15, 79] However, some follicles extend into the subcuticular area and will be damaged during dissection, resulting in poor hair growth on the graft.[32, 40] An injection beneath the dermis of saline solution or of a solution containing procaine and epinephrine may cause the area to balloon, which will assist in separating the fat from the dermis.[18, 32, 52] Hair growth may be maintained on a graft by leaving fat on the dermis; however, the graft must be narrow to allow revascularization from the sides.[16] This is the case with strip grafts.

A second technique for graft elevation entails elevating the graft in total but leaving the subcuticular fat on the dermis and removing it later with sharp scissors (Fig. 10–14).[9, 10, 16, 18, 32, 52] However, the scissors may crush the ends of the dermal vessels and thus interfere with plasmatic imbibition.[22, 80]

The development of a technique for harvesting skin grafts that have a full complement of hair follicles and that revascularize rapidly would be of particular benefit to veterinary reconstructive surgery.

Application of Grafts

It is important that a graft not be allowed to dry. One way to prevent drying is to place the graft on the defect and then to close the donor site.[32, 79] A moist gauze sponge laid over the donor site will prevent it from drying while the graft is being placed.

The graft is placed on the defect so that the direction of hair growth is the same as that of the hair growth of the surrounding area;[9, 10, 53, 71, 79, 85] it is then anchored in place by a few nonabsorbable stay sutures at key points (Fig. 10–15). Definitive suturing is performed by placing simple interrupted sutures from 3 to 4 mm. apart between the stay sutures[66] or by placing a simple continuous suture pattern.[32, 62] The author prefers to use 4–0 polypropylene suture material on a swaged cutting needle to place simple interrupted sutures (Fig. 10–16). Ideally, sutures are placed through the graft first and then through the wound's edge. If this order of placement is followed, the graft will not be lifted off its bed as the suture is placed.[28, 79, 80] Long ends may be left on interrupted sutures to secure a tie-over bandage.

A three-point suture has been described in which the needle passes through the graft between 4 and 5 mm. from its edge, into and out of the subcuticular tissue at the wound's margin, and finally through the skin, where it is tied (Fig. 10–17).[16, 32] If the edge of the defect is thick, the suture is passed through the dermis of the marginal skin as the second step rather than through

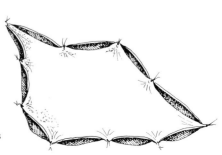

Figure 10–15: Anchor sutures have been placed at key points to anchor the graft to the edges of the bed.

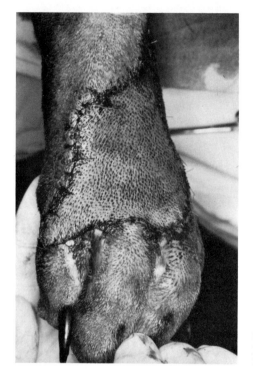

Figure 10–16: Simple interrupted sutures of 4–0 polypropylene have been used to complete the suturing of the graft into place.

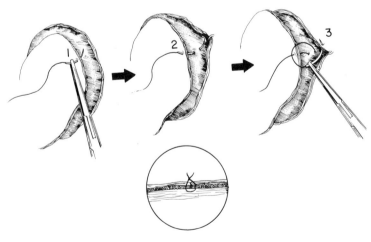

Figure 10–17: Three-point suture technique for suturing a graft into place. *1*, The needle passes through the graft (4 to 5 mm. from the edge). *2*, The needle then passes through the subcuticular tissue near the wound margin. *3*, The needle's final passage is through the skin at the wound's edge before it is tied. (From Converse, J. M., Plastic Surgery and Transplantation of skin, in SKIN SURGERY, 4th Ed., 1977, p. 186. Courtesy of Charles C Thomas, Publisher, Springfield, Illinois.)

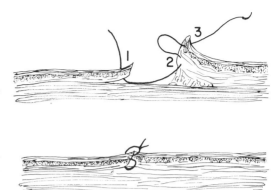

Figure 10–18: Three-point suture technique for suturing a graft to a thickened wound edge. *1*, The needle passes through the graft. *2*, The needle then passes through the base of the dermis at the wound's edge. *3*, The needle finally passes through the skin's surface. (From Converse, J. M., Plastic Surgery and Transplantation of Skin, in SKIN SURGERY, 4th Ed., 1977, p. 186. Courtesy of Charles C Thomas, Publisher, Springfield, Illinois.)

the subcutaneous tissue. This obliterates the dead space that results from tenting the graft over the groove along the edge of the defect (Fig. 10–18).[16]

Before tying the last sutures, it is important to remove all blood clots from under the graft as previously described.

Closure of the Donor Site

The donor site is usually closed by undermining the surrounding skin and closing the defect with deeply and superficially placed sutures. It may be helpful to convert the defect to a fusiform shape for closure. In some instances in which large grafts have been taken, other reconstructive techniques (e.g., a split-thickness graft) may be necessary to close the donor site. Owing to the mobility of the skin on the trunk of the dog and of the cat, this would rarely be necessary.[3, 5, 15, 32, 62, 79]

Advantages and Disadvantages of Free Full-Thickness Grafts

These grafts, along with skin flaps, are the most useful type of graft in canine wound repair.[3, 66, 71] They are also very useful in the cat and take well because of their thinness.[41] Their advantages include the following:

1. They appear more nearly like normal skin both soon and at a later time after transplantation.[10, 14, 40, 62, 71, 79]
2. The amount of postoperative contraction is minimal.[14, 18, 62]
3. The grafts are tough and provide good protection for the grafted area.[18, 62, 71]
4. No expensive equipment or technical help is needed for the procedure.[3, 79]

The following are disadvantages of these grafts:

1. Preparing the pattern, cutting the graft, and removing the fat from the dermis are more time-consuming.[21]
2. The take is not as good as with a split-thickness graft.[40, 41, 44, 62]
3. There is a decrease in hair growth when compared with that of skin flaps; however, this is less of a problem than with split-thickness grafts.

FREE SPLIT-THICKNESS GRAFTS

Definition and Characteristics

This type of graft is composed of the epidermis and a variable quantity of dermis. The graft may be thin, intermediate in thickness, or thick, depending upon how much dermis is included (Fig. 10–1).[18, 32, 52] The term split graft comes from the operation of a leather-splitting machine in a harness shop.[14] The properties of a split-thickness skin graft depend upon how much dermis is left on the graft. The thicker the dermis, the closer the properties approach those of a full-thickness graft.[52]

Indications

The primary indication for this type of graft in the dog would be reconstruction of the skin following severe burns in which extensive areas of integument have been destroyed.[40]

Donor Sites

The donor sites for split-thickness skin grafts in the dog include the ventral thoracic wall and the lateral aspect of the thigh.[79] In cachectic individuals, the area over the thoracic cage may still be used as a graft donor site by ballooning the subcuticular tissues in the intercostal area with injections of saline solution to provide a smooth surface from which to cut the graft.[21] The use of a Pitkin syringe and an 18-gauge needle has been described for the subcutaneous injections of saline solution in small laboratory animals. The injection of saline solution greatly enhances the reproducibility as to size, thickness, and uniformity of split-thickness grafts.[67]

Cutting Grafts

Three basic types of instruments have been designed for cutting split-thickness grafts: (1) the freehand instruments, (2) the drum-type dermatome, and (3) the electric and pneumatic dermatomes. The action of each instrument is that of a sharp blade moving back and forth to cut a piece of skin whose thickness is controlled by a calibrated setting on the instrument or by the surgeon.[32] The donor area must be flat, held under tension, and immobile.[62]

Freehand Cutting   Dermatomes are expensive and may be difficult to use in the dog,[41] in addition to increasing operative time.[21] Skin graft knives for freehand cutting have been developed (Blair and Ferris-Smith), along with modifications by others to allow for some form of depth control on the knife (Humby, Bodenham, Braithwaite, Marcks, and Caltagirone) (Fig. 10–19).[18, 32, 80] When using one of these instruments, certain preoperative procedures should be followed. The knife should be sterilized by immersing it for 30 minutes in 95 per cent alcohol,[14] by immersing it in boiling water, by placing it in a hot air oven,[79] or by gas autoclaving. It is advisable to use a freehand cutting knife on a cadaver first to get a feel for how it cuts.[79] It can be difficult to obtain a good split-thickness graft with a freehand cutting knife.

The donor area is prepared for aseptic surgery and lubricated with miner-

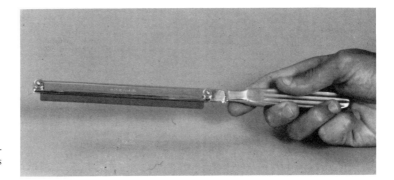

Figure 10–19: Knife for free-hand cutting of split-thickness skin graft.

al oil or petrolatum. The area is held under tension by wooden boards, tongue depressors, or some other flat instrument. More elaborate suction boxes have been described for this but would probably be less practical. Using one of the aforementioned items or the finger tips, the assistant surgeon pulls the skin in one direction while the surgeon does the same in the opposite direction. With the remaining free hand, the surgeon lays the knife against the skin and angles it at about 30 degrees for the first few strokes in a back-and-forth motion. After the skin is invaded, the blade is placed at a more acute angle (almost parallel to the skin surface or at 15 degrees). Most grafts in dogs are 1 mm. in thickness. The blade is moved to and fro with short strokes at about 1 to 2 in. behind the board that is creating tension as it is advanced. One method for successful cutting is to concentrate on the to-and-fro knife movement rather than on the advancement of the blade (Fig. 10–20).[14, 16, 18, 32, 52, 62, 79, 80]

The graft may stick to the blade as it is cut. To prevent this, the blade may be lubricated with sterile mineral oil or with liquid petrolatum. If it does stick, the assistant may flick the graft off the blade with hemostats. Ideally, the graft should slide smoothly back and forth across the blade and the graft should not be kept taut.[14, 52, 80]

The shims and rollers on some knives may be used to control the depth of the cut, or the surgeon may determine the depth by sight. It is always wise to

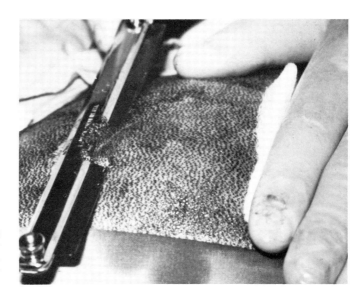

Figure 10–20: Technique for using a knife for freehand cutting of a split-thickness skin graft. Tension is held on the skin as the knife moves to and fro to cut the skin.

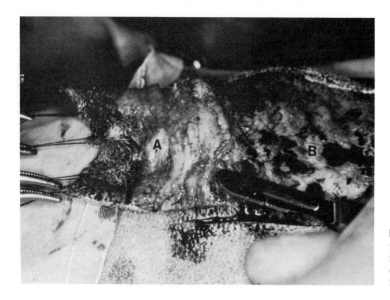

Figure 10–21: Scalpel blade is used to cut a split-thickness graft from the skin on the back of a dog. *A,* Graft. *B,* Underlying remaining dermis.

observe the graft and the bed, even if there is a depth control on the instrument.[32, 52]

Observation of the graft and of the bed may be used to gauge the depth of the cut. The surgeon will get a good indication of how thick the graft will be within the first 6 mm. of the cut, and adjustments can be made accordingly. A very thin graft will be somewhat translucent, i.e., the knife blade can be seen through the graft. Thicker grafts become increasingly opaque. With a thin graft there is a high density of small bleeding points on the donor site as opposed to the larger, more widely spaced bleeders that are seen with thicker grafts.[16, 32, 52]

Freehand cutting may also be done with a sharp razor[5] or with a scalpel blade.[41] The author has found the use of scalpel blades to be somewhat tedious, resulting in the dulling of several scalpel blades and the cutting of some holes in the graft. The procedure seems to work best on the thick skin over the back and the shoulder area (Fig. 10–21). An unmodified Shick injec-

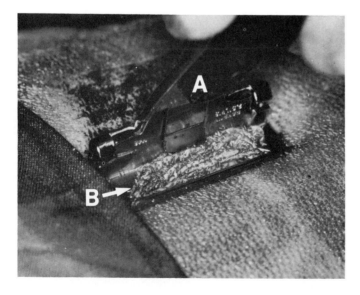

Figure 10–22: Injector razor, *A,* is used to cut a split-thickness graft, *B*.

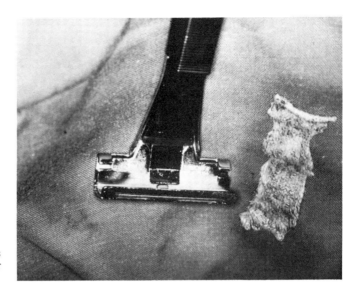

Figure 10–23: Strip of skin that has been cut with the adjacent injector razor.

tor razor and blade have been used to cut split-thickness skin grafts of 0.012 to 0.014 in. in thickness and 1.25 in. in width.[78] The author has found this to be a relatively easy and inexpensive means of obtaining grafts. The grafts may be cut in long strips or in small squares (Figs. 10–22 and 10–23). A Gillette safety razor that has been modified by filing out the central strut of the safety guard has been described for cutting split-thickness grafts. The thickness of the graft may be varied by inserting additional blades into the razor that have their cutting edges broken off. Three such shims give a graft that is 0.012 in. in thickness and 1.25 in. in width.[75]

The excision of a full-thickness graft and the removal of the subcutaneous tissue and part of the dermis with a scalpel have also been described.[54]

Dermatomes

Padgett-Hood Dermatome*. This instrument is shaped like a half-drum with a radial yoke, to which is affixed a disposable knife blade. The yoke and the blade can be adjusted by a calibrated dial so that a predetermined graft thickness may be cut. The skin of the donor area and the drum are spread with rubber cement and then pressed together at the forward edge of the drum; as the drum is rotated, the adherent skin is elevated. The blade is oscillated to and fro to cut a graft at a predetermined thickness (Fig. 10–24).[5, 14, 16, 18, 21, 32, 62, 80]

This dermatome cuts a graft of more uniform thickness than the freehand cutting knives and avoids some of the clumsiness of freehand cutting. However, it may be a more time-consuming technique when large areas are to be grafted.[18, 52]

Reese Dermatome.† This dermatome is similar to the Padgett-Hood dermatome; however, calibration is by means of shims, and adherence of the skin to the drum is by special tape. It is more solidly constructed than the Padgett-Hood instrument and more accurately calibrated.[18, 62, 80]

Electric Dermatome (Brown Dermatome).‡ An electric dermatome

---

*The Padgett-Hood dermatome is available from Kansas City Assemblage Co., 3953 Broadway, Kansas City, MO 64111.

†The Reese dermatome is available from Bard-Parker Co., Danbury, CT 06810.

‡The Brown dermatome is available from Zimmer Manufacturing, Warsaw, IN 46580.

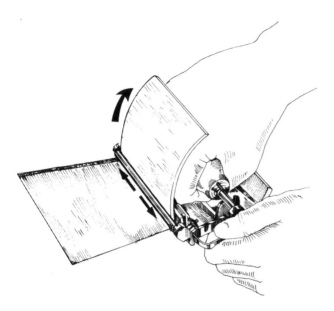

Figure 10–24: Padgett-Hood derma-tome. Half-drum is rolled back (*curved arrow*) while the knife blade moves to and fro (*straight arrows*) to cut the skin.

looks like a large hair clipper and operates similarly, with an electrically powered, rapidly oscillating cutting blade. The instrument allows the rapid removal of long strips of split-thickness skin without the use of adhesives, which cause difficulties and waste time. It is relatively simple to use and eliminates the need for much of the skill that is required for freehand graft cutting. One disadvantage is the instrument's delicacy; it is therefore more subject to breakdown and must be sent back to the manufacturer for repairs. Another disadvantage is the lack of fine calibration relative to that of the drum dermatomes. The surgeon's exerting pressure on the instrument may vary the graft's thickness.[16, 18, 32, 52, 80]

Pneumatic Dermatome.* This instrument is a modification of the Brown dermatome and is air (nitrogen) driven (Fig. 10–25).

Disposable Dermatome† This is a dermatome that cuts a graft of about 0.15 in. thickness and of 1.5 in. width. The disposable cutting head comes in a sterile plastic bag. The motor is an Oral B rechargeable toothbrush motor that can be placed in a plastic bag and sealed. The sterile cutting head is pushed through the bag onto the motor, thus keeping the unit sterile (Fig. 10–26).[18] The author has had limited success with this type of instrument.

Application of Grafts

The graft is laid on the bed, with the direction of hair growth being the same as that of hair growth of the surrounding area. The graft is smoothed into place so that it overlaps the skin at the wound's edges by about 0.25 to 0.50 in. Fine (3–0 to 5–0) monofilament suture material on a swaged needle or fine black silk may be used to suture grafts into place. Just enough simple inter-

---

*The pneumatic dermatomes are manufactured by Hall Instrument, Inc., Santa Barbara, CA 93102, Stryker Corp., Kalamazoo, MI 49001, and Zimmer Manufacturing, Warsaw, IN 46580.

†The disposable dermatome is available from Davol, Inc., Providence, RI 02901.

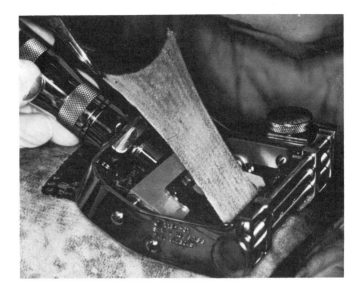

Figure 10–25: Pneumatic Brown dermatome. Dermatome is advanced as oscillating blade splits the skin.

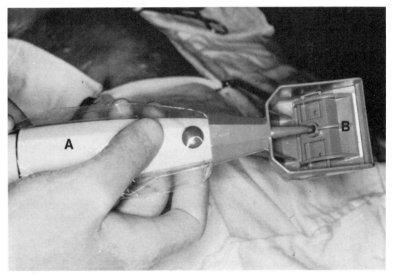

Figure 10–26: Disposable dermatome. *A*, Rechargeable handle. *B*, Disposable cutting head.

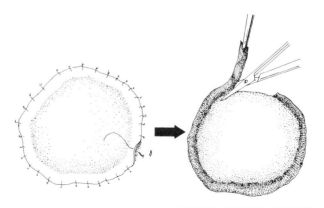

AFTER GRAFT TAKES

Figure 10–27: Split-thickness graft sutured over defect with 0.25- to 0.50-inch overlap. After graft takes, the necrotic overlapped edges are cut away.

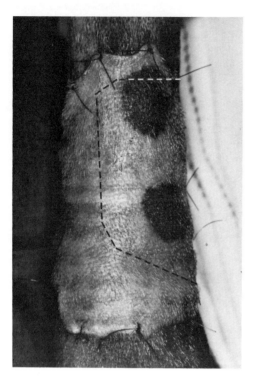

Figure 10–28: Split-thickness graft sutured into place. Note underlying wound edge (*dotted lines*).

rupted sutures are placed through the graft and through the skin surrounding the lesion to hold the graft in place. By overlapping the wound edges, the needle does not enter the skin's edge, and the formation of hemorrhage beneath the graft is prevented. The overlapped skin edges will necrose and can be excised later (Figs. 10–27, 10–28, and 10–29).[14, 16, 18, 40, 41, 43, 52-54]

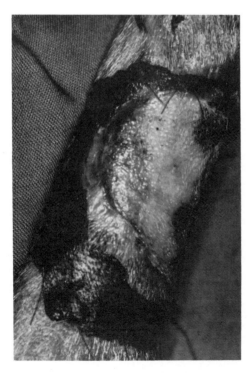

Figure 10–29: Overlapped skin edge has sloughed and remainder of the graft has taken over the lesion.

A graft may also be sutured to the defect in an edge-to-edge manner with no overlap.[18, 40, 84] However, the graft's edges may roll inward and produce an unaesthetic scar.[52] Basting or quilting sutures have been described to hold the graft against its bed.[14, 43]

Methyl 2-cyanoacrylate tissue adhesive can be spread on the skin around the recipient site. After drying the graft's undersurface, the graft is applied in an overlapping manner so that it adheres to the recipient site. Overlapped edges will be débrided later.[32]

Modern surgical staplers and clips have been used to fix skin grafts in place over large complex defects. Their advantages include a reduction in the time required for surgery and the elimination of suture tracts.[12]

Healing and Management of Donor Sites

When a split-thickness graft is removed, the epidermis is taken with it. Healing of the site occurs by reepithelialization of the denuded surface: epithelium spreads over the area from the cut surfaces of the hair follicles, of the sebaceous glands, and of the sweat glands that remain in the dermis as well as from the wound's edges.[13, 14, 16, 21, 32, 52-54] It follows that in a thin graft, more epithelializing elements will be left in the dermis and healing will occur faster.

Healing of the donor site in the dog takes from two to four weeks, and the site usually heals as a thin, hairless layer of epithelium (Fig. 10–30). For this reason, it is probably more cosmetic to excise the donor area and appose the cut edges.[15, 79] If the donor site is left to heal on its own, it should be bandaged with a nonadherent dressing. Either sterile gauze soaked in petroleum jelly or antibiotic ointment or a commercial nonadherent padding may be placed over the wound, followed by some absorbent bandaging material and tape.

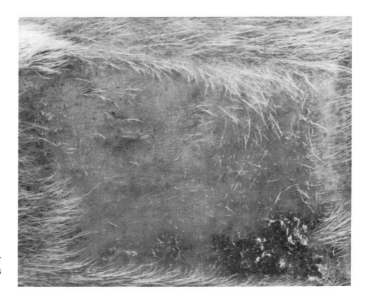

Figure 10–30: Thin, hairless layer of epithelium over split-thickness graft donor site.

SPLIT THICKNESS

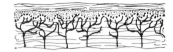

MORE EXPOSED VESSELS

FULL THICKNESS

FEWER EXPOSED VESSELS

Figure   10–31: Split-thickness grafts take better than full-thickness grafts because there are more exposed vessels on the underside of a split-thickness graft than on that of a full-thickness graft. There is a better chance of graft and graft bed capillaries meeting.

Advantages and Disadvantages of Free Split-Thickness Grafts

The primary advantage of free split-thickness grafts is that they take more successfully than free full-thickness grafts. This is because of the denser capillary network in the more superficial dermal layers. Thus, there is a better chance of the capillaries from the graft meeting with those of the graft bed (Fig. 10–31). With thinner grafts, ingrowing capillaries have a shorter distance to grow, and these grafts can survive longer on plasmatic imbibition until revascularization occurs.[15, 18, 32, 40, 52, 62]

The disadvantages of free split-thickness grafts are attributable to the fact that they lack some of the properties of normal skin. The disadvantages include the following:

1. The grafts are less durable and more subject to trauma, making their use questionable on the limbs of the dog.[40, 71, 85]
2. They are less cosmetic from the standpoint of hair growth: it is either absent or sparse. When hair is present, it may be shorter and a different color (Fig. 10–32).[9, 10, 21, 40, 41, 54, 79, 85]
3. If left to heal on its own, the graft donor site will have either a sparse hair coat or none at all (Fig. 10–30).[15, 37, 79]
4. The grafts may have a scaly appearance and lack sebaceous secretions[37, 40] or sweat glands.[9, 10, 18, 85]
5. The secretion of cut sebaceous glands under the graft causes delayed healing. Excoriation and graft loss may result if the gland secretions become infected.[13, 21]

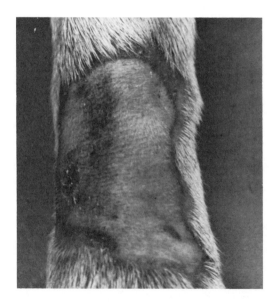

Figure 10–32: Less cosmetic (hairless) appearance of a split-thickness skin graft.

6. The grafts undergo considerable postoperative contraction.[9, 37, 40, 62, 85]

7. The undersurface of the graft may epithelialize from the cut surface of the hair follicles; this epithelium must be scraped off before the graft will attach to its bed.[15]

8. The grafts may require the use of special and sometimes expensive equipment that is designed primarily for use in humans.[40, 71]

9. There may be difficulty in finding a suitable donor area for the use of a dermatome, since a dog has very few flat areas of skin.[40] This would apply to the use of freehand cutting instruments also.

10. Because many more hair shafts are encountered on a dog than on a human, the removal of spit-thickness grafts entails cutting numerous hair shafts. This factor results in the rapid dulling of any blade that is used for cutting.

In the author's opinion, split-thickness skin grafting is useful in small animal reconstructive surgery in that the percentage of graft takes is better than that achieved with full-thickness grafting; however, the final cosmetic appearance may be inferior. Furthermore, there are a large number of potential disadvantages associated with split-thickness grafting. A major disadvantage is the expensive special equipment that is required. In addition, freehand cutting using knives and safety razors requires a skill that may be lacking if the surgeon has had limited experience with this procedure.

MESH GRAFTS

Definition

A mesh graft is a split-thickness skin graft in which multiple tiny slits have been cut to allow the graft to be stretched or expanded in two directions to many times its original size.[18]

Indications

The following are three indications for mesh grafting: (1) to cover large skin defects when there are inadequate donor sites, especially on extensively burned patients;[21, 48, 50] (2) to apply a graft to a somewhat less than ideal graft bed, e.g., one in which exudate, blood, or serum is present;[34, 50] and (3) to reconstruct irregular (i.e., concave or convex) surfaces that are difficult to immobilize.[34, 35, 50]

Cutting Grafts

Mesh grafts for animals may be made from split-thickness skin[35] or from full-thickness skin.[34] In the dog, split-thickness skin is cut from the ventrolateral thoracic area using a freehand cutting knife or an electric dermatome.[35] If full-thickness skin is used, a technique similar to that described for horses[34] and for humans[26] can be utilized. The skin is cut from the body in an elliptical shape that is about one third longer than the defect and between one third and one half of the width of the defect. This skin is fixed, with the dermal side up,

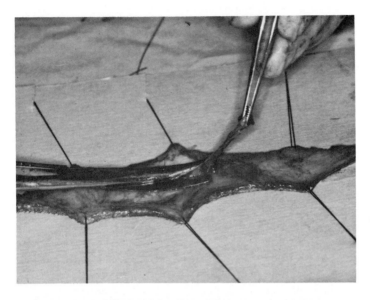

Figure 10–33: A full-thickness ellipse of skin has been fixed, dermal side up, to a piece of sterile cardboard. Thumb forceps and scissors are used to remove all subcutaneous fat from the dermis.

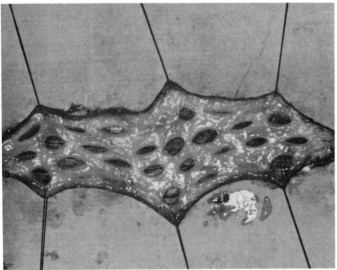

Figure 10–34: Numerous short incisions (1.0 to 1.5 cm. long) have been made in the skin with a No. 11 scalpel blade. The cuts are in parallel rows about 5 mm. apart, with the incisions of each row overlapping those in the adjacent row.

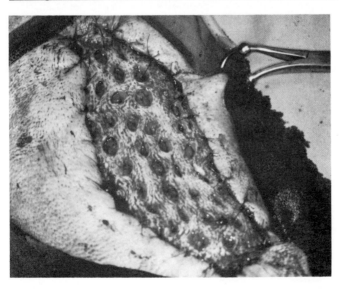

Figure 10–35: A full-thickness mesh graft is applied to a lesion on the medial aspect of a dog's pelvic limb.

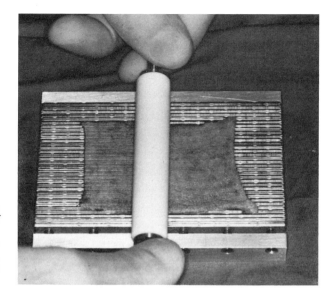

Figure 10–36: Aluminum block containing numerous staggered parallel rows of small cutting blades. The Teflon roller is rolled with moderate pressure over the split-thickness graft in the direction of the blades, which cut slits in the graft. The dermal side of the graft is against the blades.

to a cutting board by means of peripheral fixation. Fixing the graft to a piece of sterile cardboard by pulling peripheral stay sutures through slits in the edges of the cardboard is simple and economical. Thumb forceps and curved scissors are used to remove all subcutaneous fat from the skin (Fig. 10–33). Numerous short incisions (from 1.0 to 1.5 cm. long) are made in the skin with a No. 11 scalpel blade. The cuts are made in parallel rows that are about 2 to 5 mm. apart, with the incisions in each row overlapping those in the adjacent row. A lattice network of the skin is produced that will allow the graft to be expanded (Figs. 10–34 and 10–35).

Another technique for cutting a graft into a mesh, which is used on split-thickness grafts, is to employ a special mesh grafting instrument that cuts the slits in the graft. One such instrument* provides four variations of expansion ratios, ranging from 1.5:1 to 9:1.[18] This instrument is more expensive than a simpler one that is called a mesh graft dermatome.†[18, 35] After cutting the graft, it is laid on an aluminum block containing numerous staggered parallel rows of small cutting blades. The blades are 0.719 cm. long, with 0.127-cm. gaps between the blades within a row and 0.127-cm. gaps between the staggered rows. As a Teflon roller passes over the graft with moderate pressure in the direction of the blades, the blades cut slits in the graft (Fig. 10–36). A graft with an expansion ratio of 3:1 is produced that may be used to graft an area three times wider than the original width of the graft before it was meshed (Fig. 10–37).

Application of Grafts

When applying a graft to a granulation tissue bed, excess granulation tissue should be sharply excised to produce a good bed.[34, 35] If the tissue is not

---

*Meshgraft II Dermatome is available from Zimmer Manufacturing, Warsaw, IN 46580.

†Mesh-Skin Graft Expander, No. P-160, is available from Padgett Instruments, Kansas City, MO 64111.

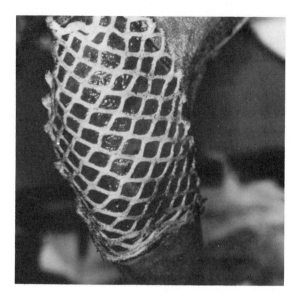

Figure 10–37: An expanded mesh graft has been placed over a lesion on the cranial aspect of a dog's stifle.

exuberant, it is necessary only to freshen the site by rubbing it briskly with a sponge. Hemorrhage can be controlled by applying gauze sponges and pressure.[35]

Three factors should be considered when placing a mesh graft on its bed: (1) When the cuts in the graft are placed parallel to the skin tension lines, the cosmetic results are improved.[32, 50] (2) The direction of hair growth on the graft should match that of hair growth of the surrounding area.[34] (3) The graft should be placed so that the mesh can be expanded to cover the wound.[34, 35] The last factor is the most important, since the main reason for using a mesh skin graft is to cover a large area with a small graft. This type of graft heals faster, is thicker, and resembles more closely the surrounding skin if it is not expanded to its full extent when placed on the bed.[34, 35]

Simple interrupted sutures are placed at the periphery of the graft to hold it in place. Size 2–0 and 4–0 medium chromic gut have been used for this.[34, 35, 82] The author prefers 4–0 polypropylene sutures (Fig. 10–38).

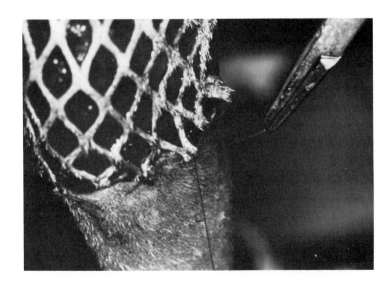

Figure 10–38: Simple interrupted sutures of 4–0 polypropylene are used to suture mesh graft to wound margins.

Growth of Grafts

Wounds in which grafts take successfully usually heal in a 12- to 18-day period.[35] One study has reported that grafts take at 14 days and that the skin appendages appear on grafts at 30 days in the dog.[82] The open areas in the mesh heal by epithelialization, which spreads from the edges of the ribbons of skin in the mesh. Epithelialization is rapid, since there is a nine-fold increase in the number of borders from which it can occur (Fig. 10–39).[15]

Advantages and Disadvantages

The advantages of mesh grafts include the following:
1. They can be applied to lesions with uneven edges and are flexible enough to conform nicely to concave and convex surfaces.[34, 35, 50, 81]
2. They can be applied to less than ideal graft beds (e.g., those with exudate, blood, or serum) since the openings of the graft allow for drainage.[4, 18, 24, 29, 32, 34, 35, 44, 50, 81, 82]
3. They can be used to reconstruct large defects when graft donor sites are scarce, such as on extensively burned patients.[21, 44, 48, 50, 81]
4. They increase the number of edges from which healing can occur, and thus graft contracture is prevented.[34, 81, 82]
5. They can be used on areas that are difficult to immobilize.[50]

The primary disadvantage of mesh grafts in veterinary surgery is the initial cosmetically undesirable appearance of the graft. The graft has a diamond-shaped pattern, especially when it is expanded to its maximum.[34, 35] It can be seen that when the graft is expanded widely, an increased healing time will be required for epithelialization to fill the interstices. There is also a wider dispersion of skin adnexa, and larger areas of scar epithelium result that could be predisposed to early breakdown if they are subjected to trauma.[81] The cosmetic problem is reduced when the graft is placed with the slits running parallel to the skin tension lines. As the graft matures, it tends to assume more of the characteristics of a standard split-thickness graft.[34, 35]

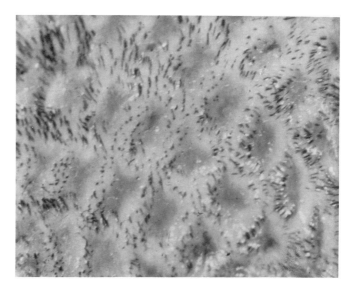

Figure 10–39: Healing mesh graft with epithelialization covering the open spaces that were left by the mesh.

SIEVE GRAFTS

With the sieve graft, a pattern of the wound is outlined on the donor skin and the graft is cut in full thickness. A steel die is used to cut small plugs of skin in the graft. The graft is lifted from the donor area in such a way as to leave the plugs of skin attached to the donor site. The graft, with its multiple holes for drainage, is placed on the recipient bed, and the plugs of skin that remain on the donor site are left to epithelialize and thereby heal the area in the fashion of a seed-type graft (Fig. 10–40).[14, 25, 62] A modification of this grafting technique has been described for horses. A split thickness of skin is cut and then evenly spaced holes of 5 mm. in diameter are cut in the graft with a skin punch prior to placing the graft on its bed.[28]

SEED-TYPE GRAFTS

Definition and History

In general, seed-type grafts are small pieces of skin that are placed in or on a granulating graft bed with some regular spacing between the pieces of skin. This type of graft has been known by many names — Reverdin's graft, small skin graft, small deep graft, pinch graft, pin graft, island graft, and seed graft. The term that will be used in this text is seed-type graft, unless specified otherwise. As originally described by Reverdin, these small grafts were composed of little more than epidermis, whereas Davis later described a cone-shaped small piece of skin that was almost full thickness in its center and thinner at the edges.[14, 62, 70]

Indications

The following are indications for seed-type grafts: (1) to repair granulating wounds, especially when they are large;[3, 71] (2) to reconstruct contaminated and infected wounds;[37, 71] and (3) to cover wounds that can be

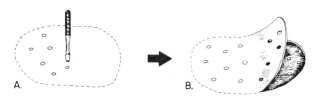

CUTTING AND ELEVATING SIEVE GRAFT

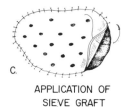

APPLICATION OF
SIEVE GRAFT

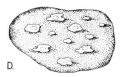

DONOR SITE HEALS FROM
SKIN PLUGS LEFT ON IT

Figure 10–40: Sieve graft. *A*, Cutting plugs of skin in the graft. *B*, Elevating the graft while leaving the skin plugs on the donor site. *C*, Applying the graft to the recipient bed. *D*, Leaving the donor site to heal by epithelialization from skin plugs that were left.

firmly bandaged for an indefinite period (e.g., wounds on the lower portion of the limbs).[58]

Donor Sites

In the dog and the cat, the recommended sites for cutting seed-type grafts are the ventral surface of the abdomen,[71] the inner surface of the thigh,[3, 40] and the flank.[2, 36] In general, the grafts should be taken from areas where a slight cosmetic defect will not be noticed.

Cutting Grafts

Each graft may be harvested by first elevating or tenting the skin with a straight hypodermic needle, a straight atraumatic intestinal needle, or a curved suture needle. Fine-toothed forceps (Addison's forceps) may also be used to elevate the skin. With a sharp scalpel, the tissue is cut at right angles to the tent (Fig. 10–41). The result is a small piece of skin that is approximately 2 to 4 mm. in diameter and that is full thickness in the center and thinner at the edges.[2, 36, 37, 40, 49, 62, 71, 74, 80]

Another technique is to cut the grafts from the donor site using a skin biopsy punch that is 5 mm. in diameter (Fig. 10–42).[2] Skin has also been taken as a split-thickness graft, and seed-type grafts have been cut from it using a 7-mm. biopsy punch.[11] Cutting a split-thickness graft into small pieces to serve as seed-type grafts has also been described.[15, 88]

Application of Grafts

Seed-type grafts may be placed *on* or *in* the granulation tissue surface. Various lengths (ranging from 3 mm. to 13 mm., or 0.5 in.) have been advocated for the distance between grafts. The author prefers to leave from 5 to 7 mm. between grafts.

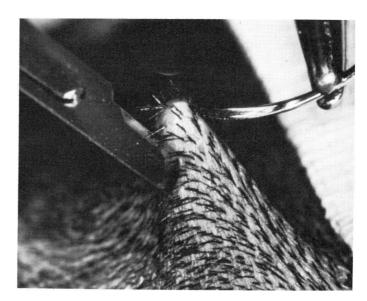

Figure 10–41: Cutting a plug of skin to be used as a seed-type graft. A suture needle elevates the skin while a No. 15 scalpel blade cuts it at a right angle.

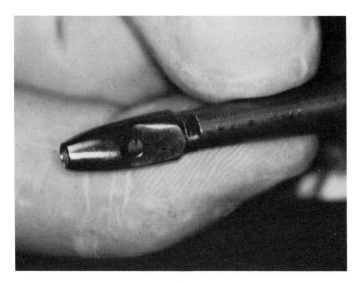

Figure 10–42: Skin biopsy punch (5 mm. in diameter) that can be used to cut seed-type grafts.

When placed *on* a granulation tissue bed, the grafts may be placed directly[9, 37] or may be placed after scarifying the surface.[74] Snug bandaging is necessary (Fig. 10–43).[37, 71]

Grafts may be placed *in* granulation tissue in several ways:

1. The grafts may be thrust into the granulation tissue with forceps, the blunt end of a needle, or a probe and left below the surface of the bed.[37, 58, 59, 62, 88]

2. A 5-mm. biopsy punch may be used to cut plugs from the granulation tissue; the grafts are placed in the plugholes after the clots are removed from them.[11]

3. Small pockets may be cut in the granulation tissue almost parallel to the wound's surface with the openings upward. The grafts are placed in these pockets (Fig. 10–44).[2, 36, 41, 49] A similar technique entails placing grafts into channels in the granulation tissue, followed by cauterization of the end of the channel.[73]

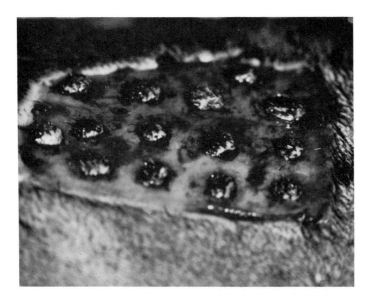

Figure 10–43: Placement of seed-type grafts *on* the graft bed after scarifying areas for their placement. Such placement requires snug bandaging.

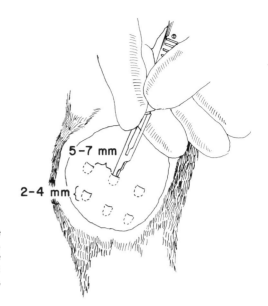

Figure 10–44: Creating pockets in the granulation tissue parallel to the wound's surface. Pockets are 2 to 4 mm. deep and 5 to 7 mm. apart. Each pocket will receive one seed-type graft. (After Hoffer, R. E., and Alexander, J. W.: Pinch grafting. J. Am. Anim. Hosp. Assoc. *12*:645 and 646, 1976.)

4. Small hollows can be made in the graft bed with a No. 15 blade, and the grafts are placed into them; however, this is not much different from placing the grafts on the bed.

The last two techniques seem to be the most practical in small animal surgery. When using pockets for the grafts, the pockets are made from 2 to 4 mm. deep and from 5 to 7 mm. apart. If hemorrhage floats the graft out of the pocket, the graft can be held in place with forceps for one to two minutes, or direct digital pressure can be applied on the outside of the pocket.[2, 36] A disadvantage of placing a graft in a hollow rather than in a pocket is the increased dependency on the bandage to hold the graft in place.

When placing seed-type grafts, the surgeon should always work from the distal area of the wound upward. This prevents hemorrhage from obscuring the operative field.[36, 49, 59]

Closure of Donor Sites

Seed-type graft donor sites may be bandaged and allowed to heal as open wounds. If a cosmetic appearance is of primary concern, the multiple

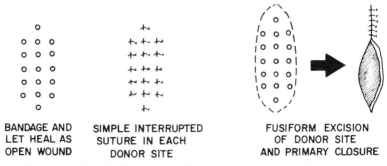

BANDAGE AND LET HEAL AS OPEN WOUND   SIMPLE INTERRUPTED SUTURE IN EACH DONOR SITE   FUSIFORM EXCISION OF DONOR SITE AND PRIMARY CLOSURE

Figure 10–45: Techniques for closing donor sites of seed-type grafts.

small perforations may be sutured by placing one suture in each in the direction of skin tension lines. Another method is to excise the perforated donor area in a fusiform shape and to suture the skin from edge to edge.[80] Taking the grafts from a small fusiform area would facilitate this type of closure (Fig. 10–45).[14]

Growth of Grafts

Seed-type grafts heal by the spreading of epithelium from the edges of each graft over the granulation tissue until the epithelial zones coalesce. Epithelialization also occurs from the wound's edges.[2, 14, 15, 36, 41, 59]

In the dog, grafts that are buried in pockets show evidence of healing by about the fifth to seventh day. The granulation tissue over the seed is gone, and the graft appears as a small whitish-pink spot. By the third week, the epithelial tissue will have coalesced over the wound.[2, 36] The author and others[2, 58, 88] have noticed that epithelialization from the wound's edges is stimulated by seed-type grafting (Fig. 10–46).

Advantages and Disadvantages

The advantages of seed-type grafts include the following:
1. They are resistant to infection.[15, 36, 62]
2. Grafts that are placed *in* granulation tissue (such as in pockets or in punched holes) can withstand some movement of the area without jeopardizing the grafts.[2, 11, 36, 58]
3. The technique is simple.[62]

The following are three disadvantages of seed-type grafts:
1. Their appearance (cobblestone-like) is not cosmetic (Fig. 10–47).[2, 14, 36, 40, 59, 63, 70, 71, 79]
2. The quality (thickness, elasticity, resistance to excoriation) of the skin is poor, and it has a tendency to crack and bleed.[28, 40, 71, 79]

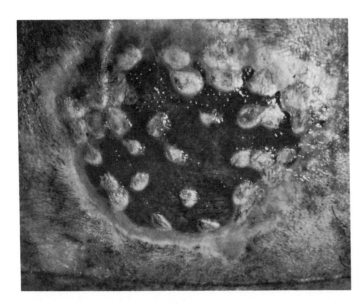

Figure 10–46: Seed-type grafting tends to stimulate epithelialization from the wound edges.

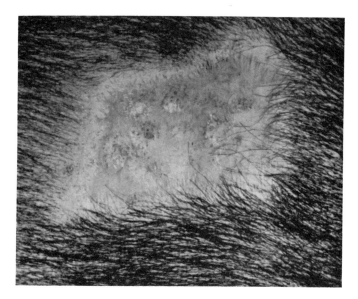

Figure 10-47: Uncosmetic "cobble-stone" appearance of healed seed-type grafts.

3. Grafts that are placed *on* granulation tissue are susceptible to movement and friction between the wound and the bandage.[2, 40, 88]

Even though they are protected, seed-type grafts that are placed in granulation tissue may still have problems; they may be squeezed out of the pocket by movement,[88] or they may be surrounded by blood in the pocket, which interferes with graft revascularization.[59]

STAMP GRAFTS

Stamp grafts (chessboard grafts) are based on the same principle as that of seed-type grafts. They are generally made from split-thickness skin that is cut into patches ranging from 5 sq. mm. to postage stamp size. They are placed on the bed with between 1 to 2 mm. and 1 cm. of space between grafts. This allows for drainage, and if infection occurs, only one or a few grafts are lost rather than all of the grafts. Healing between grafts is by epithelialization from the graft's edges. This epithelium is very delicate and unaesthetic at first; however, stability and cosmesis both improve with time. In addition, such grafts have a checkered appearance and are less resistant to pressure and rubbing than normal skin. Movement of the graft on the bed is a problem; however, this may be prevented to some extent by cutting the granulation tissue so that the graft fits into it.[28, 32, 52, 80, 84]

STRIP GRAFTS

These grafts are similar to stamp grafts. Strips of full-thickness skin from 1 to 2 mm. wide are placed in parallel linear grooves that have been cut in the granulation tissue.[41] The grooves in the granulation tissue are about 2 mm. deep and from 3 to 4 mm. apart. Because of the normal primary contraction of full-thickness skin, the author prefers to anchor the strips at each end of the groove with a simple interrupted suture (Fig. 10–48).

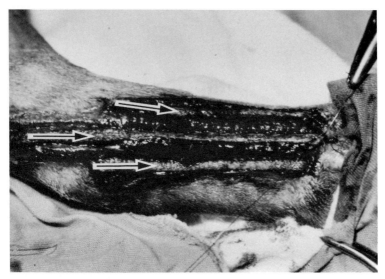

Figure 10–48: Anchoring strip grafts (*arrows*) at either end with a simple interrupted suture of 4–0 polypropylene.

The granulation tissue between strips is eventually covered by epithelium from the strip graft's edges (Fig. 10–49). Such grafts are unappealing, especially a short time after placement when the newly formed epithelium is very delicate; however, with time, the grafts become a little more cosmetic and durable.

TUNNEL GRAFTS

Tunnel grafts have been described in horses and in humans. They are a series of skin strips that have been threaded parallel to each other in tunnels through the granulation tissue bed. After a period of from five to ten days, the tunnel roof of the granulation tissue is removed over each skin strip and the grafts are allowed to heal in place.[8, 37, 60, 62] The author questions the applicability of such grafts in small animals.

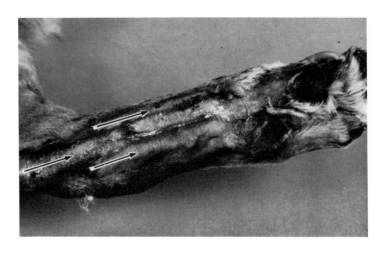

Figure 10–49: Healing strip grafts (*arrows*). Epithelium has covered the area between grafts. See color plate IV–B, p. 571.

ALLOGRAFTS AND XENOGRAFTS

It is generally accepted that allografts (homografts) and xenografts (heterografts) are utilized as biological dressings and temporary bandages in an attempt to prepare a wound for accepting a graft at a later time. Such dressings are indicated for (1) covering partial-thickness wounds to enhance re-epithelialization; (2) covering exposed tendons, nerves, and vessels; (3) preparing grossly contaminated wounds to receive a graft; (4) covering large burn wounds; (5) treating ulcers and large denuded areas; and (6) covering split-skin donor sites.[15, 21, 27, 39, 48, 70]

The function of biological dressings is basically to quickly reestablish the integrity of the skin's protective functions.[27] Specifically, they serve to (1) minimize fluid, electrolyte, protein, and red blood cell loss; (2) increase patient comfort and facilitate early movement; (3) decrease surface bacteria; and (4) clean the wound and promote the growth of granulation tissue.[15, 18, 21, 27, 39, 48, 61]

The blood vessels within grafts have been suggested to have an angiogenic property that stimulates neovascularization of the recipient bed.[61]

Allografts have been found to heal to a wound by six days, and they may survive for as long as two weeks in dogs.[3, 15] Graft survival time is longer if the host and the donor are related or if the volume of grafted tissue is small.[3] However, most allografts are changed at 2- or 3-day intervals.[18] When allografts are to be used, they are removed aseptically, wrapped in sterile gauze sponges that have been soaked in a 0.25 per cent neomycin solution, placed in a sterile glass jar, and refrigerated in an ordinary refrigerator for an average period of seven to ten days.[48]

Xenografts may be in the form of fetal calf skin or porcine skin.[18] Porcine skin* is available in several forms: (1) fresh porcine skin, which can be used for up to 14 days after harvesting if it is refrigerated at 4° C; (2) lyophilized porcine skin, which has an 18-month shelf life, requires no refrigeration, and can be reconstituted with sterile saline solution; (3) freshly frozen porcine skin, which can be stored for three months at or below the common freezer temperature ($-18°C$), and after it has been thawed, can be stored in a refrigerator for up to seven days; and (4) frozen irradiated porcine skin that can be stored indefinitely at $-78°C$ or for six months at freezer temperature ($-18°$ C). The lyophilized product† has the advantages of being easy to use, readily available commercially, and reasonably priced. It has been described for use in the dog[39] and would probably be the product of choice in most veterinary practices.

Prior to application, the wound should be surgically débrided of nonviable tissue. Cleansing with ether has been described to remove the gelatinous layer and enhance the adhesive properties of the recipient site.[27] Placement of the graft with[39] and without[27] sutures has been described. The graft is usually changed every three to five days, depending on the nature of the wound.[27, 39] If the wound is grossly contaminated, daily dressing changes may be necessary.[27] Bandage changes are continued until the wound is healthy enough to receive a graft or until the wound heals under the dressing.[39]

---

*Porcine skin is available from the Burn Treatment Skin Bank, Inc., Phoenix, AZ 85034.

†Lyophilized Porcine Cutaneous Dressing is available from the Burn Treatment Skin Bank, Inc., Phoenix, AZ 85034.

BANDAGING, CASTING, AND SPLINTING GRAFTS

Dressing a grafted area is probably the most important factor in having a graft take, with the possible exception of wound preparation.[14] A dressing should be nonadherent and protective, and, most importantly, should maintain immobilization of the area by means of sufficient, even (but not excessive) pressure. One to two weeks of bed rest have been prescribed to immobilize grafts on the lower extremities in human patients.[32] From this, it can be seen that the veterinarian is at a disadvantage.

INITIAL DRESSING

Various forms have been described for the initial dressing. These include the application of antibacterial ointments or gauze soaked in petrolatum to the grafted area, followed by the placement of nonadherent pads, fine mesh gauze, or conforming gauze.[14, 40, 54, 66] The fixation of the initial dressing has been accomplished by the placement of simple interrupted sutures through the corners of the pads and through the surrounding skin[28, 40] or by the application of collodion to glue the dressing to the surrounding skin.[21] Moist dressings in the form of saline solution–soaked gauze have also been reported.[14, 15, 37] The author prefers to apply an antibiotic ointment at the edges of the graft, followed by the placement of a nonadherent wound dressing pad, a tie-over bandage, and a protective, immobilizing bandage-splint combination.

PRESSURE AND IMMOBILIZATION

During the phase of revascularization, the graft and the bed must remain immobile with relation to each other. Movement, especially in the form of a shearing strain, will not allow a capillary linkup to occur between the graft and the bed. Theoretically, the immobilization must be continued until there is fibrous tissue anchorage strong enough to take such a strain without rupturing the capillaries.[52]

The purposes of a pressure bandage are to immobilize the area and to prevent the occurrence of a hematoma.[52] Immobilization is especially important so that contact is maintained between the graft and the host bed.[18] Firm, even pressure that is sufficient to immobilize the graft is all that is needed. Too much pressure can impede the normal blood flow and result in pressure (ischemia) necrosis.[15, 16, 63] One source has stated that there should be no pressure on bandages.[41]

Tie-Over Bandages

Tie-over dressings have been adequately described in the literature. They provide good local immobilization of a graft against its bed. The author prefers to suture the graft into place, to cut all of the sutures short, and to apply an initial dressing of antibiotic ointment and nonadherent pads. Several sutures of 2–0 or 3–0 monofilament nylon are placed in the host's tissue equidistant

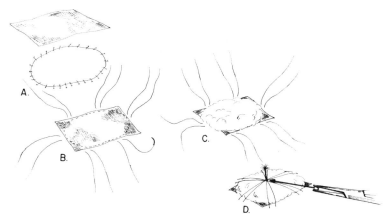

Figure 10–50:   Construction of a tie-over bandage. *A*, Applying a nonadherent pad over the graft. *B*, Preplacing tie-over sutures around the wound periphery. *C*, Placing cotton padding over the nonadherent pad. *D*, Pulling the tie-over sutures together, twisting them, and fixing them with a metal clip.

around the graft about 1 cm. from the graft margin. The ends of the sutures remain long. A bolus of sterile cotton or gauze is then placed over the initial dressing. All of the long ends of the preplaced sutures are drawn over the bolus and twisted until they pull the bolus gently but firmly down against the graft. One or two metal clips* are then used to fix the twisted sutures near the bolus, as described by Levin and Masters (Fig. 10–50).[47] The tie-over bandage may be modified according to the shape of the graft. Additional absorbent wrapping is placed over this bandage.

Other techniques and modifications for placing tie-over dressings include leaving the ends of the sutures that are used to place the graft long and tying them over the bolus,[14, 18, 21, 41, 52, 80] tying regular rubber bands into the graft fixation sutures and fixing these over the bolus,[68] cutting the initial dressing and bolus to the shape of the graft,[32, 80] or using foam rubber for the bolus.[80, 86]

---

*Versa-clips are manufactured by Ethicon, Inc., for Pitman Moore, Inc., Washington Crossing, NJ 08560.

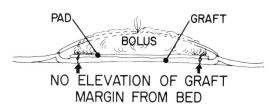

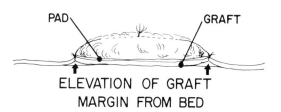

Figure 10–51:   Tie-over sutures placed away from the graft's edge do not tend to elevate the edge from the bed, but tie-over sutures that are part of the graft anchor sutures may do so.

By placing the tie-over sutures away from the graft margin, there is less tendency to elevate the graft margin when the sutures are tied over the bolus. This can occur if the graft fixation sutures themselves are tied over the bolus (Fig. 10–51).[32]

It has been stated that a cotton bolus becomes compacted quickly and thus the pressure effect is gone within 30 minutes, leaving the cotton to serve as a conformer. The elasticity or resilience of the skin is the pressure-inducing agent on the graft surface. As the long ends of the graft fixation sutures are tied, they tend to draw the skin edges up around the bolus. It is believed that the skin's elasticity acts continuously to transmit mild pressure on the graft's surface.[63]

The edges of the tie-over dressing should be inspected daily. If infection is evident under the graft, the dressing should be removed and cultures should be taken. If the graft margin remains dry and odorless, the tie-over dressing may be left for five to seven days.[32] However, the author usually removes them on the third or the fourth day.

Casts and Splints

The use of casts and splints for additional immobilization of a grafted area is advocated.[16, 18, 32, 41, 52, 66, 71, 79] Casts should remain in place for 14 days, and if the graft has been placed over a joint, a second cast may be necessary for a good graft take.[79] The goal is to immobilize the joints adjacent to the graft.[32] The author prefers a properly applied metal or plastic splint outside the tie-over and wrapping bandages. Plaster-type casts may be bulky, and if they become wet, they are ineffective. However, there are newer casting materials that are resistant to moisture. A bivalved cast of a polyester and cotton knitted fabric impregnated with water-activated polyurethane* has been found to be effective by the author. The bivalve design allows for periodic inspection of the graft.

DRESSING CHANGES

The appropriate time for changing the initial dressing over a graft is controversial. Times ranging from 24 hours to 14 days have been reported in the literature. Of primary concern is that the dressing change does not move a graft on its bed. The author has tried both extremes of time and has drawn the following conclusions:

1. It takes a cooperative dog to maintain a clean, dry dressing for 14 days.
2. The time for changing a dressing will differ with individual animals. A clean, dry graft requires fewer dressing changes than one with infection under it. Likewise, if an animal does not urinate and defecate on the dressing, fewer bandage changes will be required.
3. When dressings are changed early and frequently, the dog should be very cooperative or should be tranquilized. No graft benefits from an "acrobatic" dressing change.

---

*Cutter Cast 7 is manufactured by Cutter Biomedical, a Division of Cutter Laboratories, Inc., San Diego, CA 92111.

All attempts should be made to keep the dressing clean and dry (i.e., keep the animal out of wet grass, apply a plastic bag over the dressing, and so on). The initial dressing is changed two or three days postoperatively, with the animal sedated if it has *any* tendency to become excited during the procedure. The splint and wrappings are carefully removed, and the tie-over bandage is gently lifted along one edge for inspection. If all is well, the tie-over bandage may be left on for two or three more days. By fixing the tie-over sutures with a metal clip, it is possible to remove the clip, open the sutures, remove the bandage material, inspect the graft, and replace the tie-over bandage. If there appears to be moisture or exudate under the tie-over bandage, it is removed. Adhesions to the tie-over bandage can be released by soaking the area with sterile warm saline solution or by using a cotton-tipped applicator and hydrogen peroxide to gently work the bandage away from the wound. After the tie-over bandage is removed, antibiotic ointment, nonadherent pads, soft wrapping, and the splinting material are reapplied. The bandage is changed every two to three days or less frequently if all appears well. *It is essential that the graft not be moved on its bed during dressing changes.*

DRESSINGS OVER MESH GRAFTS

A dressing that has been described for mesh grafts includes an elastic bandage that holds a nonadherent pad over the graft. A pad that is 1.27 cm. thick is applied over this and held in place with more elastic adhesive bandage. The bandage is removed on the fourth postoperative day and the graft is cleaned with physiological saline solution and rebandaged with an appropriate antibiotic ointment. Bandages are changed subsequently every other day.[34, 35]

DRESSINGS OVER SEED-TYPE GRAFTS

The initial dressing will have to remain in place longer (from 10[74] to 14[71] days) when grafts have been placed *on* a graft bed. However, a dressing change on the fifth postoperative day has been described for such grafts.[40] When grafts are placed in pockets, they may be covered by gauze soaked in petroleum jelly and a modified Robert Jones' dressing that is changed every three to five days.[2, 36]

DEGENERATIVE CHANGES IN GRAFTS

Skin that is removed from its blood supply (i.e., skin graft) is subject to degeneration of both the dermis and the epidermis. Within the dermis there is degeneration of the connective tissue elements, including the blood vessels. Hair follicles and sebaceous glands show little degeneration. They are the most viable elements of the skin and are the last structures to disappear in a sloughing graft.[22]

The epidermis seems to suffer the most, and sloughing is common.[22] In thicker grafts, especially full-thickness grafts, blebs form, and areas of epithelium exfoliate, baring the underlying dermis. Areas of necrosis and ulceration may be present in the dermis, and these may easily become infected. Such areas may be situated over a blood clot, and they must be resurfaced by new epithelium before the graft is considered healed.[16] This phenomenon has been noted by the author on free full-thickness grafts in dogs.

A balance is usually reached by seven to eight days postoperatively, when proliferation of the surviving graft elements starts to exceed the degenerative process.[22]

POSTOPERATIVE APPEARANCE OF GRAFTS

Immediately after placing a graft on its bed, it appears white.[16, 18, 70] During the first three to four days after placement, it appears bluish, and by the seventh or eighth postoperative day, the graft takes on a red coloration (Fig. 10–52). It then becomes more normal in appearance over the next 14 days (Fig. 10–53).[40, 66, 71] Some have described grafts as changing from white to a pink coloration;[16, 18, 70] however, the bluish appearance seems to be the most common in the dog. The white appearance corresponds to a lack of hemic elements within the graft. The bluish color is due to hemic elements that have been absorbed into the graft from the bed (plasmatic imbibition), and the reddish hue is caused by new hemic elements entering the graft as it revascularizes.

A graft becomes edematous rapidly after placement. The edema reaches its maximum on the third postoperative day, and it regresses by the fifth to the seventh day.[7] During the first 24 hours, the epidermal cells undergo vacuolization and swelling, which gradually disappears as the damaged cells degenerate and new epithelial cells are formed.[37] Graft edema is related to plasmatic imbibition and disappears as revascularization carries the fluids from the graft.

Blue, pink, and red can be considered favorable colors for a graft, whereas the presence of a white or a black appearance of some duration is an unfavorable sign. A lack of drainage, firm adherence to the bed, and a pink coloration are signs of a take.

The surgeon should not lose faith when a graft takes on an unfavorable appearance. In veterinary skin grafting, the author and others have observed that when a graft fails, spontaneous epithelialization from the wound margins is

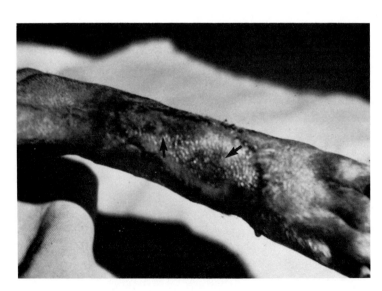

Figure 10–52: A free full-thickness graft eight days after surgery. The graft has a reddish coloration with a few remaining bluish areas (*arrows*). See color plate IV–C, p. 471.

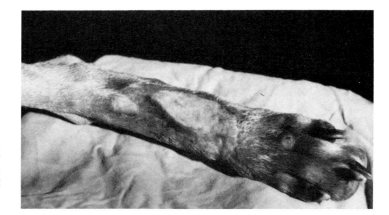

Figure 10–53: The graft shown in Figure 10–52 approximately 21 days after surgery. The skin appears normal, and hair has not started to grow on the graft yet. See color plate IV–D, p. 571.

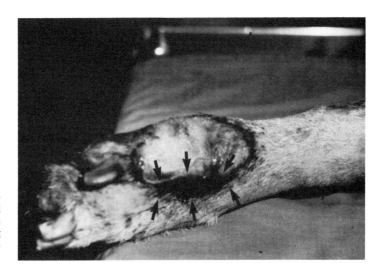

Figure 10–54: A free full-thickness graft with a dark, hardened area along one edge (*arrows*). This area was not tampered with during graft healing. See color plate IV–E, p. 571.

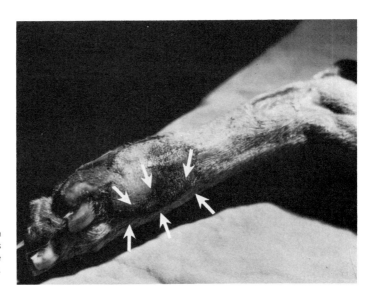

Figure 10–55: Healed graft from Figure 10–54 showing area that was under the dark, hardened tissue (*arrows*). See color plate IV–F, p. 571.

enhanced,[40] and islands of viable epithelium that may appear in the grafted area expand.[37] The author's philosophy on skin grafts is to place them, care for them, and let them undergo as much or as little healing as they will, leaving unfavorable-appearing areas alone and letting them heal or slough as they will. A surgeon can be pleasantly surprised at what has been going on under a dark, hardened, nonviable section of a graft after this dead tissue sloughs (Figs. 10–54 and 10–55).

GRAFT CONTRACTION

Primary graft contraction is shrinkage of the skin immediately after its removal from the donor site. It is caused by elastic tissue in the graft's dermis. The greater the number of elastic tissues, the greater the primary contraction will be; thus, primary contraction is greatest in full-thickness grafts (Fig. 10–56).[18, 32] This contraction is easily overcome by stretching the graft as it is sutured in place. Full-thickness grafts should be cut to fit exactly into the bed, since they undergo little, if any, secondary contraction.[32] An exact fit and proper skin tension on the graft are assured when a pattern of the lesion is used to cut the graft, as was discussed in an earlier section.

Secondary graft contraction is the shrinkage of the graft after it has been placed on the recipient bed and has revascularized. It is caused by biological changes in the host bed and not in the skin itself.[18] It is more marked in split-thickness grafts and is influenced by several factors:

1. There is less secondary contraction with thicker split-thickness grafts.[18, 32, 52]
2. There is less secondary contraction with more rigid recipient beds.[18, 32]
3. Grafts on convex surfaces undergo less secondary contraction than those on concave surfaces.[32]
4. There is less secondary contraction with a more complete take.[32]

Grafts have been noted to appear wrinkled and corrugated after healing. This may be due to continued wound contraction after grafts have been placed, resulting in wounds with a smaller circumference. Other grafts may appear smooth and tight, even though the wounds are reduced in size. This may be due

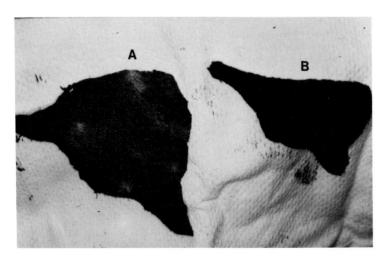

Figure 10–56: Primary contraction of a free full-thickness graft. A, Cloth pattern around which graft was cut. B, Contracted graft after removal from the donor site.

to collagenolytic activity exceeding collagen synthesis. It should be remembered that once wound contraction is started, it is not suddenly stopped by grafting; however, it is slowed.[63] This phenomenon has been noted by the author after the placement of full-thickness grafts on granulating wounds. To prevent further wound contraction and to prevent wound retraction when preparing the bed, the entire wound contents, including the granulation tissue, the scarred base, and a thin edge (1 mm.) of normal dermis, can be excised prior to grafting.[63] Since it is desirable for haired skin around a wound to be in contact with the haired skin of the graft in animals, a wider area is usually excised, and the wound retracts to its original size when prepared as described.

GRAFT REINNERVATION

Skin graft reinnervation has been the subject of considerable study, and it plays an important role in the success or failure of grafts in animals.

Grafts have no innervation immediately after transplantation, but in humans they usually begin to recover sensation anywhere between four and nine weeks.[18, 42] In small animals, reinnervation may begin by three weeks postoperatively and may take several months for completion, if it occurs at all.[41] Terui has described the progression of the reinnervation of skin grafts over a nine-month period, including reinnervation of the adnexal structures of the skin.[83]

The rate and amount of reinnervation depend on the type of transplant, its thickness, the presence and amount of scar tissue, and the state of adjacent peripheral nerves that have cutaneous branches in the area involved.[15, 23] Free grafts generally do not reinnervate well when placed on periosteum or muscle. Neither do they reinnervate well when placed on areas where there has been (1) deep tissue injury or destruction (e.g., full-thickness burn areas); (2) nerve damage in the surrounding skin; (3) infection; (4) a hematoma;[18] or (5) granulation tissue derived from bone.[18, 32]

The quality of reinnervation of skin flaps and of grafts is best in pedicle flaps, followed by full-thickness grafts and split-thickness grafts.[15, 18, 23, 45] The reason for this is that once nerves have penetrated the border of a flap, they grow unimpeded through the subcutaneous tissues and finally course superficially to their termination in the dermis and epidermis. In full-thickness grafts in which all of the subcutaneous tissue has been removed, the ingrowing nerves encounter fibrosis to some degree at all points where they penetrate the dermis. The fibrosis seems to be even greater with split-thickness grafts.[45]

Studies in pigs have shown that nerves enter a graft through the sides and the base by following the course of blood vessels or of suitably oriented collagen bundles. Once in the graft, 90 per cent of the nerves enter vacated neurilemmal sheaths, and the remainder follow blood vessels as unsheathed axis cylinders. Therefore, the pattern of reinnervation in a graft is reproduced and determined primarily by the disposition of neurilemmal cell pathways within the graft,[30] a finding that was suggested by an earlier investigation.[57]

A study on rabbit skin revealed similar findings, with some exceptions. Few axons penetrated the graft's periphery because of scar tissue, and of those that did, most had no neurilemmal sheath and terminated as free nerve endings. Few axons entered the existing Schwann tubes of the graft. Of the axons penetrating the base of the graft, some entered the existing Schwann tubes, and others ended as independent filaments before reaching the graft's surface. Thus, the reinnervation pattern roughly resembles that of the grafted skin, especially in the center of the graft, with a supplemental marginal fringe of abnormal nerve fibers that is made up of independent axons invading from the side and below.[1]

In 1952 a report by Napier described three types of reinnervation for skin grafts:[57]

Type I.   Around the perimeter there is an outer zone of fairly constant width where pain and touch sensibility have a normal or nearly normal threshold. Recovery may be limited to this area. However, this outer zone may give way to an inner zone where the threshold to both pain and touch is raised. In large grafts this zone may fade into one of complete anesthesia. In narrow grafts, the outer zones tend to merge in the center of the graft, leaving no inner zone. This was found to be the most common and the most efficient type of reinnervation in grafts.

Type II.   Sensation tends to recover patchily all over the graft, irrespective of its size.

Type III.   A peripheral neuroma develops close to the graft. It has a low-threshold abnormal response that is peripherally referred. The response to any type of stimulus that is applied to this area is a tingling or a pins-and-needles sensation that has been described as ranging from mildly pleasant to intensely uncomfortable. This type of nerve growth has been called neurotization rather than reinnervation of the skin. The area of skin exhibiting this phenomenon may vary, but it frequently extends for several centimeters on either side of the neuroma.

Pain is the first sensation to return to a skin graft,[18, 42, 45] followed by touch and then temperature discrimination.[18, 45] As stated by Converse and associates, several workers have reported that the stimuli for touch, heat, and cold may be experienced as painful, and there may be intense pain in the surrounding skin.[18] This hypersensitivity may be due to a greater number of nerve fibers than is normally present in grafts during reinnervation.[72] A study in humans has shown the presence of hyperalgesia in grafts. This protopathic pain was described as being like an electric shock that spread from the point of stimulation. Later this reaction began to disappear as tactile stimuli began to be recognized, and eventually it disappeared entirely.[23] This change from hyperalgesia to a normal state of sensibility over a period of months has been reported by others.[32]

The author has noted clinical signs in dogs that could be attributed to abnormal sensations in and around the area of the graft. These signs include the persistent licking and chewing of the grafted area, starting at approximately three to four weeks after grafting. This behavior may subside over a period of time, or it may persist. The nature of the sensation is unknown (i.e., whether it is a needles-and-pins sensation, a painful sensation, or some other abnormal sensation). The cause of the abnormal sensation is also unknown; it may be due to a type III innervation (neurotization) as described by Napier, an abnormally large number of nerve fibers in the graft, a marginal fringe of abnormal nerve fibers that is made up of independent axons invading the graft, or some other form of abnormal reinnervation. The reinnervation of skin grafts in the dog needs further study from the standpoints of what occurs and what can be done either to encourage normal reinnervation or to prevent abnormal reinnervation. It is discouraging to have a skin graft revascularize and take completely only to have the animal lick at it continually, thereby jeopardizing the graft.

Studies have shown the return of sympathetic innervation in grafts to occur late and to be of poor quality.[45, 46] Sympathetic nerve function did not return in split-thickness grafts but was regained to a slight degree in full-thickness grafts, as evidenced by sweating.[46]

The reinnervation of skin flaps is discussed in Chapter 8.

SEBACEOUS AND SWEAT SECRETIONS IN GRAFTS

Sebaceous and sweat secretions are less functional in split-thickness grafts than in full-thickness grafts or in skin flaps. In split-thickness grafts, the problem is attributable to the transection of the glands and their nerves when the graft is cut.[80] Split-thickness grafts rarely contain functioning sweat glands and almost never acquire the ability to sweat. The number of sweat glands and the ability to sweat increases in full-thickness grafts and to a greater degree in skin flaps. There is apparently a close relationship between the return of sensory innervation and the secretion of sweat.[18] In humans the sebaceous glands of a graft may not secrete for several months. Likewise, sweat glands may take from six months (full-thickness grafts and pedicle flaps) to a year (split-thickness grafts) to regain any function.[80]

Split-thickness grafts may have a scaly appearance owing to the lack of sebaceous secretions.[37, 40] Massaging the graft with cold cream, lanolin, or cocoa butter has been advocated until reactivation of the glands occurs.[14, 16, 80]

Another problem with split-thickness grafts is that the transected sebaceous glands may secrete under the graft, resulting in slow healing and possible excoriation and graft loss if they become infected.[13, 21]

GROWTH AND METAPLASIA OF GRAFTS

Skin grafts have been found to grow in proportion to the growth of a child.[32] This can also be expected with a young animal.

In some instances it would be desirable to transplant skin from one area and to have it undergo metaplasia at its new site so that it becomes like the surrounding skin. An example would be to place skin from the trunk into a defect of the foot pad in the hopes that skin will become like that of the foot pad. This type of metaplasia does not take place in humans; therefore, a sole or a palm cannot be fully restored to normal. These grafts or flaps may develop calluses but do not undergo metaplasia to become the true skin or subcutaneous tissue of the area. Transplanted hair will continue to grow, but it may be worn off.[13] The author has found these factors to be true in animals also.

MANAGEMENT OF BURN WOUNDS PRIOR TO GRAFTING

Management of the pain associated with burn wounds is a major concern in the treatment of human burn cases, as it should be in the treatment of burned animals. In children, ketamine hydrochloride has been the subject of clinical investigation in many surgical centers. It is a dissociative agent. The main advantage to using the drug in children is that the patient does not perceive pain, and therefore skin grafts may be removed, wounds may be débrided, and other usually painful procedures may be accomplished.[48] Currently this drug has *not* been approved for use in the dog, but it has been approved for use in the cat. A combination of ketamine and a phenothiazine-derivative tranquilizer* has also been authorized for use in the cat. Other drugs should be considered for pain management in the dog.

Firm, red, healthy-looking granulations should be present before a graft is applied to a burn wound. These usually appear between the fifth and the 15th day after thermal injury. The wound may look pale at this time, but it has been described as being literally hungry for skin grafts. The ideal time for grafting must be anticipated, recognized, and taken advantage of by applying a graft.[21] If a graft is not applied at the appropriate time, the granulation tissue may proliferate, become boggy and edematous, and bleed readily. Skin grafts do not take well on such surfaces. Scraping the granulation tissue has been described to prepare it to receive a graft; however, this may cause excessive hemorrhage that may interfere with a graft's taking. A firm compression bandage may be needed for 24 hours to stop the hemorrhage before the graft is applied.[48] Another possibility if a graft is not being applied to a burn wound is healing by contraction, in which case the scar tissue will become very thickened and fibrotic. If this type of healing occurs over a flexion surface, it can limit joint movement.

REFERENCES

1. Adeymo, C., and Wyburn, G. M.: Innervation of skin grafts. Transplant. Bull. 4:152, 1957.
2. Alexander, J. W., and Hoffer, R. E.: Pinch grafting in the dog. Canine Pract. 3:27, 1976.
3. Archibald, J.: Procedures in plastic surgery. J. Am. Vet. Med. Assoc. 147:1461, 1965.
4. Baksic, R. W., Wilber, M. C., Willett, C. U., et al.: The use of mesh skin graft in war wounds. J. Trauma 10:608, 1970.
5. Berson, M. I.: Atlas of Plastic Surgery, ed. 2. New York, Grune & Stratton, Inc., 1963.
6. Birch, J., and Branemark, P. I.: The vascularization of a free full thickness skin graft: I. A vital microscopic study. Scand. J. Plast. Reconstr. Surg. 3:1, 1969.
7. Birch, J., Branemark, P. I., and Lundskog, J.: The vascularization of a free full thickness skin graft: II. A microangiographic study. Scand. J. Plast. Reconstr. Surg. 3:11, 1969.
8. Björck, G., and Twisselman, K.: Tunnel skin grafting in the equine species. Proc. Ann. Conven. Am. Assoc. Equine Pract. 17:311, 1971.
9. Boyd, C. L.: Equine skin autotransplants for wound healing. J. Am. Vet. Med. Assoc. 151:1618, 1967.
10. Boyd, C. L.: Equine skin transplants. S.W. Vet. 20:265, 1967.
11. Boyd, C. L., and Hanselka, D. V.: A skin punch technique for equine skin grafting. J. Am. Vet. Med. Assoc. 158:82, 1971.
12. Brody, G. S., and Mackby, L. F.: Rapid application of skin grafts. Arch. Surg. 112:855, 1977.
13. Brown, J. B., and McDowell, F.: Epithelial healing and the transplantation of skin. Ann. Surg. 115:1166, 1942.
14. Brown, J. B., and McDowell, F.: Skin Grafting. ed. 2. Philadelphia, J. B. Lippincott Co., 1949.
15. Cawley, A. J., and Archibald, J.: Plastic surgery, in Archibald, J. (ed.): Canine Surgery, ed. 2. Santa Barbara, Calif., American Veterinary Publications, Inc., 1974.
16. Converse, J. M.: Plastic surgery and transplantation of skin, in Epstein, E. (ed.): Skin Surgery, ed. 2. Philadelphia, Lea & Febiger, 1962.
17. Converse, J. M., Ballantyne, D. L. Jr., Rogers, B. O., et al.: "Plasmatic circulation" in skin grafts. Transplant. Bull. 4:154, 1957.

---

*Ketaset Plus is available from Bristol Laboratories, a Division of Bristol-Myers Co., Syracuse, NY 13201.

18. Converse, J. M., McCarthy, J. G., Brauer, R. O., et al.: Transplantation of skin: Grafts and flaps, in Converse, J. M. (ed.): Reconstructive Plastic Surgery: Principles and Procedures in Correction, Reconstruction, and Transplantation, ed. 2. Philadelphia, W. B. Saunders Co., 1977, vol. 1.
19. Converse, J. M., Smahel, J., Ballantyne, D. L. Jr., et al.: Inosculation of vessels of skin graft and host bed: A fortuitous encounter. Br. J. Plast. Surg. 28:274, 1975.
20. Converse, J. M., Uhlschmid, G. K., and Ballantyne, D. L. Jr.: "Plasmatic circulation" in skin grafts: The phase of serum imbibition. Plast. Reconstr. Surg. 43:495, 1969.
21. Conway, H.: Skin graft, in Cooper, P. (ed.): The Craft of Surgery, ed. 2. Boston, Little, Brown and Co., 1971, vol. 1.
22. Davis, J. S., and Traut, H. F.: Origin and development of the blood supply of whole thickness skin grafts: An experimental study. Ann. Surg. 82:871, 1925.
23. Davis, L.: The return of sensation to transplanted skin. Surg. Gynecol. Obstet. 59:533, 1934.
24. Divencent, F. C., Curreri, P. W., and Pruitt, B. A.: Use of mesh skin autografts in the burned patient. Plast. Reconstr. Surg. 44:464, 1969.
25. Douglas, B.: The sieve graft: A stable transplant for covering large skin defects. Surg. Gynecol. Obstet. 50:1018, 1930.
26. Dragstedt, L. R., and Wilson, H.: A modified sieve graft: A full thickness skin graft for covering large defects. Surg. Gynecol. Obstet. 65:104, 1937.
27. Elliott, R. A., and Hoehn, J. G.: Use of commercial porcine skin for wound dressings. Plast. Reconstr. Surg. 52:401, 1973.
28. Fackelman, G. E.: A new technique of skin transplantation and preliminary evaluation of the effects of solcoseryl on graft acceptance. Equine Vet. J. 5:105, 1973.
29. Feller, I., and Hill, C. C.: A technique for increasing skin autograft coverage. Arch. Surg. 91:545, 1965.
30. Fitzgerald, M. J. T., Martin, F., and Paletta, F. X.: Innervation of skin grafts. Surg. Gynecol. Obstet. 124:808, 1967.
31. Gingrass, P., Graff, W. C., and Gingrass, R. P.: Skin graft survival on avascular defects. Plast. Reconstr. Surg. 55:65, 1975.
32. Grabb, W. C., and Smith, J. W.: Basic techniques of plastic surgery, in Grabb, W. C., and Smith, J. W. (eds.): Plastic Surgery: A Concise Guide to Clinical Practice, ed. 2. Boston, Little, Brown and Co., 1973.
33. Haller, J. A., and Billingham, R. E.: Studies of the origin of the vasculature in free skin grafts. Ann. Surg. 166:896, 1967.
34. Hanselka, D. V.: Inexpensive mesh grafting technique in the horse. Proc. Ann. Conven. Am. Assoc. Equine Pract. 21:191, 1975.
35. Hanselka, D. V., and Boyd, C. L.: Use of mesh grafts in dogs and horses. J. Am. Anim. Hosp. Assoc. 12:650, 1976.
36. Hoffer, R. E., and Alexander, J. W.: Pinch grafting. J. Am. Anim. Hosp. Assoc. 12:644, 1976.
37. Hogle, R., Kingrey, B. W., and Jensen, E. C.: Skin grafting in the horse. J. Am. Vet. Med. Assoc. 135:165, 1959.
38. Hynes, W.: The early circulation in skin grafts with consideration of methods to encourage their survival. Br. J. Plast. Surg. 6:257, 1954.
39. Jeffery, K. L.: Lyophilized porcine cutaneous dressing used in dogs. J. Am. Anim. Hosp. Assoc. 14:132, 1978.
40. Jensen, E. C.: Canine autogenous skin grafting. Am. J. Vet. Res. 20:898, 1959.
41. Johnston, D. E.: Wound healing and reconstructive surgery. Am. Anim. Hosp. Assoc. Sci. Proc. 2:383, 1975.
42. Kernwein, G. A.: Recovery of sensation in split thickness skin grafts. Arch. Surg. 56:459, 1948.
43. King, M. K.: Immediate skin grafting following injuries. Surg. Gynecol. Obstet. 81:75, 1945.
44. Kountz, S. L.: Autotransplantation, in Sabiston, D. C. (ed.): Davis-Christopher: Textbook of Surgery, ed. 11. Philadelphia, W. B. Saunders Co., 1977.
45. Kredel, F. E., and Evans, J. P.: Recovery of sensation in denervated pedicle and free skin grafts. Arch. Neurol. Psychiatr. 29:1203, 1933.
46. Kredel, F. E., and Phemister, D. B.: Recovery of sympathetic nerve function in skin transplants. Arch. Neurol. Psychiatr. 42:403, 1939.
47. Levin, J. M., and Masters, F. W.: A simple method for applying and changing a bolus dressing. Plast. Reconstr. Surg. 55:500, 1975.
48. Lynch, J. B., and Blocker, T. G.: Thermal burns, in Converse, J. M. (ed.): Reconstructive Plastic Surgery: Principles and Procedures in Correction, Reconstruction, and Transplantation, ed. 2. Philadelphia, W. B. Saunders Co., 1977, vol. 1.
49. Mackay-Smith, M. P., and Marks, D.: A skin grafting technique for horses. J. Am. Vet. Med. Assoc. 152:1633, 1968.
50. MacMillan, B. G.: The use of mesh grafting in treating burns. Surg. Clin. North Am. 50:1347, 1970.
51. McGregor, I. A.: Degloving injuries: Hand. J. Br. Soc. Surg. Hand 2:130, 1970.

52. McGregor, I. A.: Fundamental Techniques of Plastic Surgery, ed. 6. Edinburgh, Churchill Livingstone, 1972.
53. Meagher, D. M., and Adams, O. R.: Skin transplantation in horses. Can. Vet. J. 11:239, 1970.
54. Meagher, D. M., and Adams, O. R.: Split-thickness autologous skin transplantation in horses. J. Am. Vet. Med. Assoc. 159:55, 1971.
55. Merwin, R. M., and Algire, G. H.: The role of graft and host vessels in the vascularization of grafts of normal and neoplastic tissue. J. Natl. Cancer Inst. 17:23, 1956.
56. Miry, M. L.: Biology of the skin graft: New aspects to consider in its revascularization. Plast. Reconstr. Surg. 8:378, 1951.
57. Napier, J. R.: The return of pain sensibility in full thickness grafts. Brain 75:147, 1952.
58. Neal, P. A.: Skin grafting in horses: A report of three cases. Vet. Rec. 70:401, 1958.
59. Neal, P. A.: Skin grafting in the treatment of granulating wounds of the horse's legs. Vet. Rec. 73:1399, 1961.
60. Obel, N.: Tunnelplastik vid behandling av Caro luxurians hos häst. Nord. Vet. Med. 3:869, 1951.
61. O'Donoghue, M. N., and Zarem, H. A.: Stimulation of neovascularization: Comparative efficacy of fresh and preserved skin grafts. Plast. Reconstr. Surg. 48:474, 1971.
62. Padgett, E. C., and Stephenson, K. L.: Plastic and Reconstructive Surgery. Springfield, Ill., Charles C Thomas, Publisher, 1948.
63. Peacock, E. E., and Van Winkle, W.: Wound Repair, ed. 2. Philadelphia, W. B. Saunders Co., 1976, pp. 204–366.
64. Polk, H. C.: Adherence of thin skin grafts. Surg. Forum 17:487, 1966.
65. Psillakis, J. M., DeJorge, F. B., Vilardo, R. A., et al.: Water and electrolyte changes in autogenous skin grafts. Plast. Reconstr. Surg. 43:500, 1969.
66. Pullen, C. M.: Reconstruction of the skin, in Bojrab, M. J. (ed.): Current Techniques in Small Animal Surgery. Philadelphia, Lea & Febiger, 1975.
67. Raynor, A. C., Yoakum, S. T., and Munster, A. M.: A simple technique for obtaining split-thickness skin grafts in small laboratory animals. J. Am. Anim. Hosp. Assoc. 12:648, 1976.
68. Rees, T. D.: Use of rubber bands in tie-over dressings on the chest wall. Plast. Reconstr. Surg. 43:635, 1969.
69. Rees, T. D., Ballantyne, D. L. Jr., Hawthorne, G. A., et al.: Effects of Silastic sheet implants under simultaneous skin autografts in rats. Plast. Reconstr. Surg. 42:339, 1968.
70. Rogers, B. O.: Transplantation of skin, in Peer, L. A. (ed.): Transplantation of Tissue. Baltimore, Williams & Wilkins Co., 1959, vol. 2.
71. Ross, G. E.: Clinical canine skin grafting. J. Am. Vet. Med. Assoc. 153:1759, 1968.
72. Santoni-Rugiu, P.: An experimental study on the reinnervation of free skin grafts and pedicle flaps. Plast. Reconstr. Surg. 38:98, 1966.
73. Schebitz, V. H.: Zur Hauttransplantation nach Braun beim Pferd. Berl. Munch. Tieraerztl. Wochenschr. 68:443, 1955.
74. Self, R. A.: Skin grafting in canine practice J. Am. Vet. Med. Assoc. 84:163, 1934.
75. Shoul, M. I.: Skin grafting under local anesthesia using a new safety razor dermatome. Am. J. Surg. 112:959, 1966.
76. Smahel, J.: Free skin transplantation on a prepared bed. Br. J. Plast. Surg. 24:129, 1971.
77. Smahel, J.: Preparation-phenomenon in a free skin graft. Br. J. Plast. Surg. 24:133, 1971.
78. Snow, J. W.: Safety razor dermatome. Plast. Reconstr. Surg. 41:184, 1968.
79. Spreull, J. S. A.: The principles of transplanting skin in the dog. J. Am. Anim. Hosp. Assoc. 4:71, 1968.
80. Stark, R. B.: Plastic Surgery. New York, Harper & Row, Publishers, Inc., 1962.
81. Tanner, J. C., Shea, P. C., Bradley, W. H., et al.: Large-mesh skin grafts. Plast. Reconstr. Surg. 44:504, 1969.
82. Tanner, J. C., Vandeput, J., and Olley, J. F.: The mesh skin graft. Plast. Reconstr. Surg. 34:287, 1964.
83. Terui, A.: Reinnervation in the free skin graft. Jpn. J. Plast. Reconstr. Surg. 18:392, 1975.
84. Uberreiter, V. O.: Die Hauttransplantation nach Thiersch. Berl. Munch. Tieraerztl. Wochenschr. 69:435, 1956.
85. Wallace, A. B., Spreull, J. S. A., and Hamilton, H. A.: The use of autologous free full thickness skin graft in the treatment of a chronic inflammatory skin lesion in a dog. Vet. Rec. 74:286, 1962.
86. Wexler, M. R., and Neuman, Z.: Use of foam rubber sponge in tie-over dressings for skin grafts. Plast. Reconstr. Surg. 50:301, 1972.
87. Williams, R. G.: Experiments on the growth of blood vessels in thin tissue and in small autografts. Anat. Rec. 133:465, 1959.
88. Woolsey, J. H., and Schaffer, M. H.: Treatment of granulating wounds in horses by means of skin grafting. J. Am. Vet. Med. Assoc. 121:173, 1952.
89. Zarem, H. A., Zweifach, B. W., and McGhee, J. M.: Development of microcirculation in full thickness autogenous skin grafts in mice. Am. J. Physiol. 212:1081, 1967.

11

BLEPHAROPLASTY

Stephen Bistner, D.V.M.;
George Batik, M.S., and
Michael Schenk, M.S., Medical Illustrators

BASIC TECHNIQUES IN OPHTHALMIC PLASTIC SURGERY*

INSTRUMENTATION

A large number of highly sophisticated instruments are not necessary to perform good ocular plastic surgery. A basic set of ophthalmic instruments for plastic surgery should include the following: a knife handle, such as Bard-Parker No. 9 handle with a No. 15 knife blade, Elschnig's fixation forceps, Bishop-Harmon tissue forceps, small blunt-pointed scissors such as Stevens tenotomy scissors, Barraquer's wire lid speculums (small and large), a Castroviejo needle holder, standard jaws with a lock, a Bishop-Harmon anterior chamber irrigating cannula and bulb, assorted hemostats, and a standard needle holder (Fig. 11–1).

In addition to having the appropriate set of instruments, certain procedures must be followed for good results in ophthalmic plastic surgery. The plastic surgical techniques that are used on the eye differ from those that are used on other areas of the body.

PREPARATION

The skin around the eye must be surgically prepared, as must any other external body area that is being readied for surgery. The hair should be carefully clipped, being careful not to excoriate the skin with the clipper blades. The eyelashes of the upper lid are clipped with scissors, the blades of which have been coated with a thin layer of petroleum jelly. The cut hairs will then stick to the blades of the scissors and will not enter the surgical field. The use of a plastic scleral shell to cover the cornea (Smith Corneal Protection Shield) while the skin around the eye is being clipped and washed is helpful (Fig. 11–2). The skin about the eye, including a wide margin around the

---

*Portions of this chapter have been adapted from Bistner, S. I., Aguirre, G., and Batik, G.: Atlas of Veterinary Ophthalmic Surgery. Philadelphia, W. B. Saunders Co., 1977, pages 22 through 26, 34, 71 through 88, and 92 through 94.

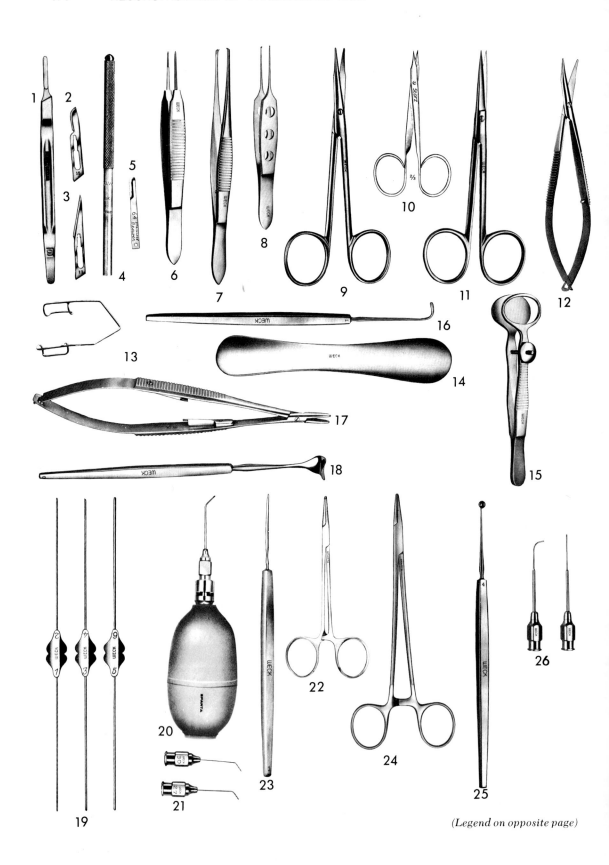

(Legend on opposite page)

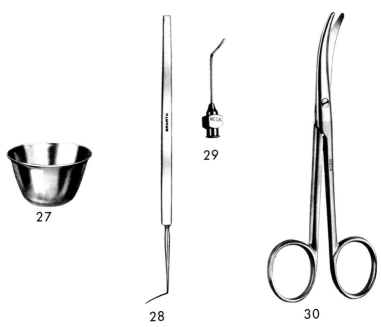

Figure 11–1: Basic and emergency ocular instrument set: *1*, Bard-Parker knife handle No. 9; *2*, Bard-Parker knife blade No. 15; *3*, Bard-Parker knife blade No. 11; *4*, Beaver knife handle No. 3K, round; *5*, Beaver blade No. 64 (Courtesy of Rudolph Beaver, Inc., Belmont, MA); *6*, Castroviejo suturing forceps; *7*, Elschnig fixation forceps, one- and two-angled teeth; *8*, Bishop-Harmon tissue forceps; *9*, Stevens tenotomy scissors, standard straight; *10*, suture scissors; *11*, eye scissors, standard straight; *12*, Westcott tenotomy scissors; *13*, Barraquer wire lid speculum, small, large; *14*, Jaeger lid plate; *15*, Desmarres chalazion forceps; *16*, Graefe muscle hook; *17*, Castroviejo holder, standard jaws with lock; *18*, Desmarres lid retractor, size 2; *19*, Bowman's lacrimal probes; *20*, Bishop-Harmon anterior chamber irrigating cannula and bulb; *21*, air injection cannulas; *22*, Halsted mosquito forceps, 5 inches; *23*, iris spatula; *24*, Crile Wood needle holder, 5 inches; *25*, Meyerhoefer chalazion curette; *26*, lacrimal cannula, curved and straight; *27*, small stainless steel iodine cup; *28*, cyclodialysis spatula; *29*, anterior chamber and cyclodialysis irrigating needle; and *30*, medium-curved enucleation scissors. (Most of these instruments can be obtained from the following manufacturers: Sparta Instrument Corp., 305 Fairfield Ave., Fairfield, N.J. 07006; Storz Instrument Co., 3365 Tree Court Industrial Blvd., St. Louis, MO. 63122; Rudolph Beaver, Inc., 480 Trapelo Rd., Belmont, MA 02178; Alcon Surgical Products Division, Alcon Laboratories, Inc., P.O. Box 1959, Fort Worth, TX 76101; Edward Weck and Co., Inc., 49–33 31st Pl., Long Island City, N.Y. 11101; and Katena Products, Inc., 10 Great Meadow Lane, East Hanover, N.J. 07936.) (From Bistner, S. I., Aguirre, G., and Batik, G.: Atlas of Veterinary Ophthalmic Surgery. Philadelphia, W. B. Saunders Co., 1977, pp. 2 and 3.)

surgical field, is carefully scrubbed with a mild antiseptic soap solution containing povidone-iodine.* Sterile cotton swabs moistened in this solution are used to "scrub" the lid margins.[14] Following this, the skin, the lid margin, and the conjunctival cul-de-sac are irrigated with sterile saline solution and the surgical field is dried with sterile sponges. Sterile cotton swabs that are impregnated with povidone-iodine solution (full strength, 1 per cent iodine) are used to paint the lid margins and the surgical field. One-half strength povidone-iodine solution can be used to topically irrigate the conjunctival

---

*Betadine Surgical Scrub is manufactured by The Purdue Frederick Co., Norwalk, CT 06856.

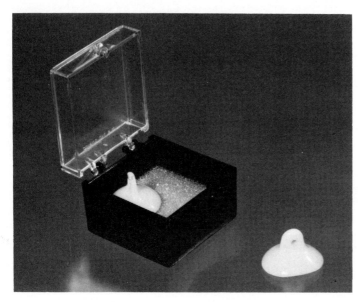

Figure 11–2: Smith's corneal protection shield. This shield, designed by Byron Smith, M.D., is made in either transparent or opaque acrylic and is used to cover the globe during surgical procedures in the lid area. A thin handle at the center area enables easy placement and removal. Three sizes are available: 18 mm., 21 mm., and 25 mm. (Mager and Cougelman, Inc., 30 N. Michigan Ave., Chicago, IL 60602). These scleral shells should not be steam autoclaved but sterilized with ethylene oxide gas. Other types of scleral shells are also available, including those manufactured by Sparta Instrument Co., Fairfield, N. J. (shells—catalog No. 18-300). (From Bistner, S. I., Aguirre, G., and Batik, G.: Atlas of Veterinary Ophthalmic Surgery. Philadelphia, W. B. Saunders Co., 1977, p. 21.)

cul-de-sac. Finally, the surgical site is dried with sterile gauze sponges prior to draping.

DRAPING THE PATIENT

After the hair has been clipped and the operative site has been cleaned and prepared, the patient is draped. The author utilizes disposable Steri-Drapes and finds that the small aperture drape (16 × 16 in.), the large aperture drape (32 × 50 in.), and the special incise drape (48 × 50 in.) all work well (Fig. 11–3). The small aperture drape has an opening at 2.5 in. in diameter that

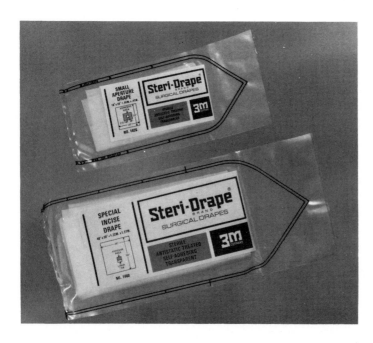

Figure 11–3: Steri-Drapes are available in either small aperture (16 × 16 in.) or large aperture (32 × 50 in.; not shown). In addition, a special incise drape is available. (From Bistner, S. I., Aguirre, G., and Batik, G.: Atlas of Veterinary Ophthalmic Surgery. Philadelphia, W. B. Saunders Co., 1977, p. 21.)

is surrounded by an adhesive area. The large aperture drape contains a more oval and slightly larger aperture. The special incise drape has a central area that is coated with adhesive. After the drape has been placed over the surgical site, a portion of the drape may be incised and removed, exposing the surgical field.

In performing intraocular, corneal, or conjunctival surgery, the author utilizes a piece of sterile medium-weight rubber dental dam material in which has been cut a small incision that is the size of the lid aperture. The dental dam is placed over the lids, the lid speculum is positioned, and the Steri-Drape is placed over the rubber dental dam, to which it adheres.

SETTING UP THE OPERATING ROOM

The proper organization of equipment is extremely important in ophthalmic surgery. The position of the patient, the availability of instrumentation, and the comfort of the surgeon are all important factors. The animal should be positioned so that the head rests on towels, sandbags, or Vac-Pacs,* and the eye should be well exposed and positioned for surgery. The surgeon should be seated while operating so that his arms are steadied, and the small ophthalmic instruments should be manipulated by finger and wrist motion. A chair that can be moved easily (preferably on casters) in helpful (Fig. 11–4).

---

*Vac-Pacs are available from Olympic Medical Corp. 4400 Seventh South, Seattle, WA 98108.

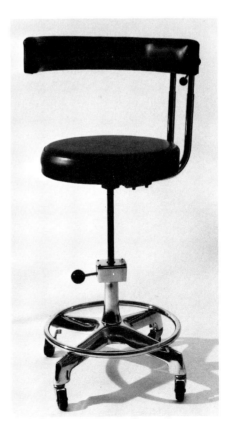

Figure 11–4: The Reliance adjustable stool, model 456, provides parallelogram movement of the support arm, allowing use of the arm as chest support or arm rest. The seat height is adjustable and the chair is on casters (Reliance, F. and F. Koenigkramer Co., 96 Caldwell Dr., Cincinnati, OH 45216). (From Bistner, S. I., Aguirre, G., and Batik, G.: Atlas of Veterinary Ophthalmic Surgery. Philadelphia, W. B. Saunders Co., 1977, p. 15.)

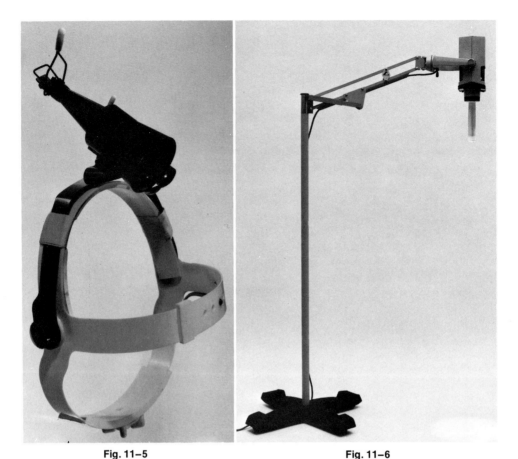

Fig. 11–5   Fig. 11–6

Figure 11–5: The Hallpike operating headlamp (Keeler Optical Products, Inc., Broomall, PA 19008). (From Bistner, S.I., Aguirre, G., and Batik, G.: Atlas of Veterinary Ophthalmic Surgery. Philadelphia, W. B. Saunders Co., 1977, p. 16.)

Figure 11–6: The Burton Polaris/3200 surgical light on floor-mounted stand (Burton, Division of Cavitron Corp., 7922 Haskell Ave., Van Nuys, CA 91406). (From Bistner, S.I., Aguirre, G., and Batik, G.: Atlas of Veterinary Ophthalmic Surgery. Philadelphia, W. B. Saunders Co., 1977, p. 16.)

The small surgical field, the use of delicate instruments and fine suture materials, and the delicate nature of the tissues make it advantageous to utilize some degree of magnification in ocular sugery. Additionally, good focal illumination is very important in ocular surgery. Several sources of high-intensity focal illumination are available: (1) "cold illumination" in which light is provided by halogen illumination that is transmitted via a Lucite rod; (2) an operating headset; (3) fiberoptic lighting; or (4) overhead surgical lighting (Figs. 11–5 and 11–6).

The Opti-Visor loupe, which is the simplest and least expensive type of magnification device, is a binocular magnifier that is worn on the head; it utilizes a continuous dial-type headband. The loupe can fit over regular prescription eyeglasses and can swing up when it is not in use. It has a variety of interchangeable magnifying lenses with variable focal lengths (Fig. 11–7).

Wide-field magnifying spectacles can be very helpful in ocular surgery. The Keeler hinged wide-angle spectacle loupe offers a range of magnifications that provide a wide field of view. The surgeon has a choice of three working distances and two magnifications. The spectacle frame can be select-

Fig. 11–7

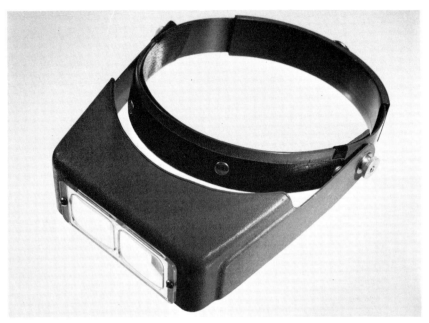

Figure 11–7:   Opti-Visor loupe.

Model	Focal Length	Actual Power
2	20″ (51 cm.)	1.50
3	14″ (35.5 cm.)	1.75
4	10″ (25.5 cm.)	2.0
5	8″ (20.5 cm.)	2.50
7	6″ (15 cm.)	2.75
10	4″ (10 cm.)	3.50

(Donnegan Optical Co., Kansas City, MO; available through most surgical supply companies, including Storz and Sparta). (From Bistner, S.I., Aguirre, G., and Batik, G.: Atlas of Veterinary Ophthalmic Surgery. Philadelphia, W. B. Saunders Co., 1977, p. 18.)

Fig. 11–8

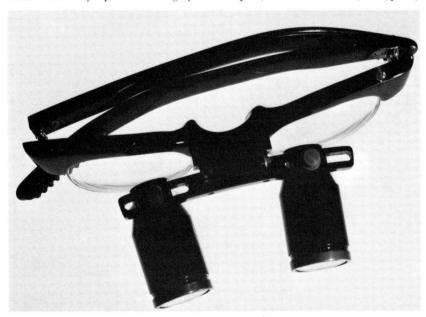

Figure 11–8:   Keeler hinged wide-angle spectacle loupe. Frame No. 1 with 18/20-mm. bridge; frame No. 2 with 20/22-mm. bridge; frame No. 3 with 22/24-mm. bridge (Keeler Optical Products, Inc., 456 Parkway, Broomall, Pa.). (From Bistner, S.I., Aguirre, G., and Batik, G.: Atlas of Veterinary Ophthalmic Surgery. Philadelphia, W. B. Saunders Co., 1977, p. 18.)

ed for approximate size by the surgeon. Different magnification lenses can be screwed into the bar mounts without altering the pupillary distance. Prescription lenses with bifocal reading attachments can be mounted in the frame behind the magnifying lens. The telescope is attached to the spectacle frame by a hinged pin assembly, allowing the telescope to be swung entirely clear of the field of view (Fig. 11–8).

MISCELLANEOUS SURGICAL EQUIPMENT

Small cautery units and electrosurgical units can be very helpful in ophthalmic surgery. Disposable presterilized self-contained battery-operated cautery units are available through several manufacturers. Concept disposable cauteries* can be obtained in large and small sizes. The tip of the regular temperature cautery reaches approximately 1650°F, while the low temperature cautery that is used on more delicate tissues (e.g., the conjunctiva) delivers a temperature of approximately 900°F. The tip heats instantly when the power button is depressed. The tip size of the small cautery unit is satisfactory for ophthalmic surgery (Fig. 11–9).

The Mentor variable temperature cautery unit† must be plugged into an electrical outlet; however, no patient-grounding plate is required. The unit

---

*These cauteries are available from Concept, Inc., 12707 U.S. 19S., Clearwater, FL 33516.

†This unit is manufactured by Codman and Shurtleff, Inc., Randolph, MA 02368.

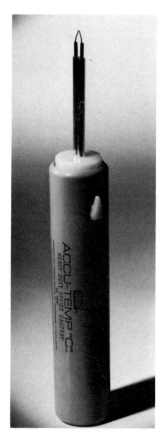

Figure 11–9: The Concept disposable cautery, size C, with a shaft 25 mm. in diameter. This size disposable cautery has a continuous burning time of approximately 20 to 30 minutes. The Concept cautery unit, size AA, is 12.7 mm. in diameter and more suitable for ophthalmic surgery. It is lightweight and permits easy, precise handling. The units may be disposed of after a single use; however, we have found that sterilization with ethylene oxide gas is satisfactory to allow repeated use of these cautery instruments (Concept, Inc., 12707 U. S. 19 South, Clearwater, FL 33516). (From Bistner, S.I., Aguirre, G., and Batik, G.: Atlas of Veterinary Ophthalmic Surgery. Philadelphia, W. B. Saunders Co., 1977, p. 7.)

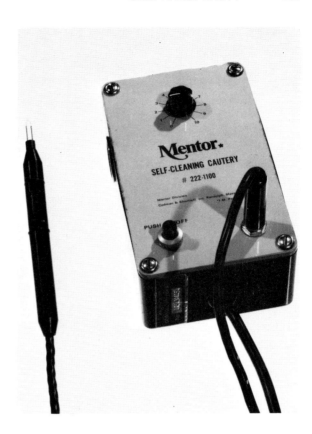

Figure 11–10: The Mentor variable temperature cautery unit (Codman and Shurtleff, Inc., Randolph, MA 02368). (From Bistner, S.I., Aguirre, G., and Batik, G.: Atlas of Veterinary Ophthalmic Surgery. Philadelphia, W. B. Saunders Co., 1977, p. 8.)

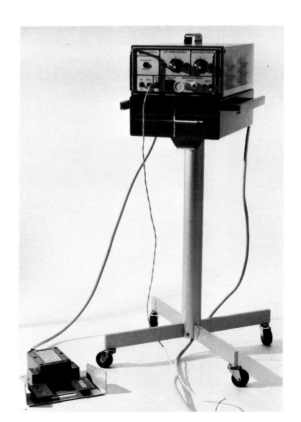

Figure 11–11: The 3M brand model 300 electrosurgical systems unit with stand and foot switch (Medical Products Division, 3M Co., 3M Center, St. Paul, MN 55101). (From Bistner, S.I., Aguirre, G., and Batik, G.: Atlas of Veterinary Ophthalmic Surgery. Philadelphia, W. B. Saunders Co., 1977, p. 8.)

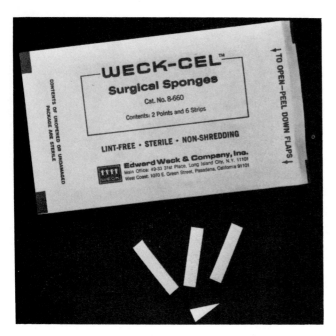

Figure 11–12: Weck-Cel surgical sponges. (From Bistner, S.I., Aguirre, G., and Batik, G.: Atlas of Veterinary Ophthalmic Surgery. Philadelphia, W. B. Saunders Co., 1977, p. 32.)

may be attached to the operating table. The temperature control and fine tip make this a suitable ophthalmic cautery unit. The unit will self-clean when the temperature is raised, thus allowing debris to vaporize (Fig. 11–10).

Electrosurgical units that are capable of cutting and coagulating tissue are frequently used in glaucoma surgery and in surgery involving the uveal tract. A fine spatula tip is frequently used, and the handle should be narrow and lightweight. The 3M model 300 electrosurgical unit* is extremely versatile and reliable. The unit, which is transistorized, may be obtained with a positive hand control attachment (Fig. 11–11). The Cameron-Miller electroscalpel model 26–250† has also been extensively utilized for ocular surgery and may also be used for electroepilation. Prepackaged, sterile disposable cellulose sponges‡ can be used to control hemorrhage effectively in both plastic and intraocular surgery. This material is superior to cotton, which leaves residual fibers in the wound to serve as a nidus for the formation of granuloma (Fig. 11–12).

SELECTION OF SUTURE MATERIALS FOR OPHTHALMIC SURGERY

New developments in suture manufacture have provided excellent ophthalmic sutures that are of very small size, have good tensile strength, and

---

*The Medical Products Division of the 3M Co. is located at 3M Center, St. Paul, MN 55101.

†The Cameron-Miller Co. is located at 329 S. Wood St., Chicago, IL 60612.

‡Weck-Cel sponges are available from Edward Weck and Co., Inc., Long Island City, NY 11101. Merocel sponges are manufactured by Mentor, a Division of Codman & Shurtleff, Inc., Randolph, MA 02368.

produce minimal tissue reaction. Very fine suture materials (8–0 to 10–0 silk or nylon) with fine micropoint or spatula needles have made corneal and conjunctival surgery less traumatic and have greatly minimized scar tissue formation. The use of these very fine suture materials requires adequate magnification.

The minimization of scar tissue formation is a major concern in selecting the appropriate suture material for ocular surgery. Scar tissue can be cosmetically unacceptable in ocular plastic surgery, and if its formation is excessive, it can lead to the abnormal physiological functioning of the eye and the adnexal structures. There are several important factors to consider in minimizing the formation of scar tissue in ophthalmic surgery: (1) maintenance of an aseptic technique; (2) reduction of tissue trauma to a minimum during the course of surgery; (3) choice of the appropriate suture materials; (4) a well thought-out plan and careful execution of the surgical technique; and (5) achievement of complete hemostasis. Of the factors mentioned, the reduction of tissue trauma and the selection of appropriate suture materials are the most important. Throughout the discussion of surgical procedures, emphasis is placed on the utilization of delicate instruments which inflict minimal tissue trauma during surgery. Additionally, the veterinarian who is performing ophthalmic surgery must become familiar with the use of fine suture materials and needles. A brief review of the most commonly used suture materials in ophthalmic surgery will help in the selection of the proper suture materials for the appropriate surgical procedures. Numerous types of these materials are available for ophthalmic surgery. An ideal suture material would meet the following criteria: (1) good tensile strength; (2) good compatibility with tissues; (3) a predictable, uniform rate of absorption; (4) a secure knot-holding ability; and (5) ease in handling and tying.

Nonabsorbable Suture Materials

Silk is a natural material that is principally a polypeptide. Individual silk fibers are relatively short and must be braided to provide adequate length and tensile strength. Braiding imparts a spring-like character to silk. Silk is used in a wide variety of ophthalmic procedures, in both plastic and intraocular surgery. Because of the braided nature of surgical silk, however, organisms and debris penetrate the suture material. When silk is used in the cornea, it has a tendency to produce epithelial proliferation along the suture tract and possible epithelial downgrowth. Although silk tends to loosen after being in tissue for a short period of time, it rarely breaks. The initial tissue reaction to silk is less intense than the reaction to absorbable gut or collagen; however, scar tissue forms earlier than with absorbable sutures. If silk is left in skin incisions for 21 to 28 days or longer, chronic inflammation with the formation of microabscesses frequently occurs.

Because of its excellent pliability and tensile strength, we often use silk in basic plastic procedures of the eyelid and remove the sutures in 14 to 20 days.

Monofilament polypropylene is a synthetic and relatively inert nonabsorbable suture material. It can be used for skin closure in plastic surgery, and it has also been used to cannulate the parotid duct in parotid transplant operations. Its main disadvantage is its lack of pliability, which makes knot tying more difficult. The author's major use of the suture has been in plastic surgery involving the lids, and here the smaller sizes, viz., 5–0 and 6–0, have been used. Care should be used in tying knots, utilizing the same techniques as for tying nylon.

Monofilament nylon is a synthetic suture material of uniform diameter and tensile strength. It has a smooth surface that does not injure tissue as it passes through. This type of suture material is being utilized extensively for anterior segment ocular surgery, especially for microsurgery of the cornea. Nylon suture material is elastic and will hold tissues in exact apposition; it tends to adjust to internal and external stresses. A knot that is tied with nylon suture is secured by the elastic nature of the suture material. This very secure knot permits the surgeon to cut the threads almost flush with the knot. In microsurgery, using 10–0 monofilament nylon, the knot can be moved into the needle tract cut so that it is not exposed on the surface of the cornea or the sclera. Monofilament nylon produces minimal tissue irritation. Ethilon is the trade name for Ethicon's monofilament nylon sutures. Dermalon and Surgilon are the trade names for Davis & Geck's nylon sutures. Ethiflex and Tevdek are Ethicon's and Deknatel's trade names, respectively, for Teflon-coated polyester fiber sutures.

Dacron is the trade name for the polyester fiber that was developed in 1939 and introduced into the United States in 1946 by E. I. DuPont. Mersilene is the trademark adapted by Ethicon, Inc., for their polyester fiber suture, which is a polymer of ethylene glycol and terephthalic acid. The fine Mersilene polyester fiber filaments are tightly braided and the suture material has approximately 30 per cent greater tensile strength than silk and causes less tissue reaction than silk. The author has utilized this material for plastic surgery and finds that it is easy to handle being very pliable. Knots must be tied carefully, and loosening of the knots can occur.

Absorbable Suture Materials

Natural. Catgut is made of twisted collagen strands derived from the submucosal layers of sheep intestine or the serosal layer of beef intestine. Catgut consists of 95 per cent collagen and 5 per cent impurities. Improved processing has provided uniformly strong and smooth surgical gut material. Gut and collagen have little or no elasticity. Both gut and collagen material must be handled carefully to prevent damage to the suture material that could reduce its tensile strength. Absorbable sutures can be moistened in sterile saline solution prior to use but should not be soaked, since this will cause swelling of the suture material and can reduce tensile strength by as much as 30 per cent. In tissue, gut begins to lose tensile strength as early as the fifth postoperative day. The rate of absorption of gut and collagen depends primarily upon the amount of proteolytic enzyme in the tissue. When gut or collagen is placed in close proximity to mucous membrane tissue, rapid absorption can occur. Absorption can be retarded to some degree by adding chromic salts to the suture material; however, this increases the extent of the inflammatory reaction. In using gut or collagen suture material, one should remember that the thread will fracture long before the knot resorbs, and the usefulness of the suture material will be lost.[37]

Synthetic. The development of new synthetic absorbable suture materials has provided the ocular surgeon with two materials that appear to be superior to chromic catgut and chromic collagen. These new suture materials are polyglycolic acid* (P.G.A.) and polyglactin 910.†

Polyglycolic acid suture is a homopolymer of glycolic acid. This material is inert, noncollagenous, nonantigenic, and nonpyrogenic. The material is braided and has a natural beige color; it is of uniform size and tensile strength but is smaller in diameter than other absorbable sutures of equivalent tensile strength. Polyglycolic acid suture has properties of both silk and catgut suture materials. The time of absorption is prolonged: significant absorption begins at 30 days. The author has used this suture material in plastic surgery. It is easy to work with and will become resorbed over a period of time; therefore it does not have to be removed, which is a significant advantage in fractious dogs and cats or in animals that cannot be returned for suture removal.

Polyglactin 910 (Vicryl) is made by the copolymerization of a mixture of lactide and glycoside. The suture material is absorbable and multifilamentous and is designed to lose its strength at a rate closely paralleling that of catgut. Polyglactin 910 suture material possesses several advantages over catgut: the material is nonprotein and nonantigenic, and it has excellent uniformity, improved handling, superior tensile strength retention in the wound, and greater tensile strength with minimal tissue reaction. The suture material is dyed violet and is available in sizes ranging from 4–0 to 7–0, with a needle as small as a GS 14 needle (reverse cutting).

Local tissue hypersensitivity to the naturally occurring tissue proteins of chromic catgut and collagen in eye surgery has always been a problem. The new synthetic absorbable sutures that are described here have several distinct advantages:

1. Good tensile strength when compared with that of chromic catgut and chromic collagen.
2. Good pliability, with handling qualities similar to those of silk.
3. Good knot-holding ability, provided a double loop with a second and a third throw of square knots has been used.
4. Minimal tissue reaction.
5. Good wound healing and the ability to remain for a prolonged time in tissue wounds, allowing adequate healing.

The mechanisms of degradation and of absorption differ for the natural and for the synthetic absorbable sutures. The absorption of both collagen and surgical gut sutures is dependent on cellular enzyme activity. The monocytic cells that are associated with suture absorption in corneal sites do not appear to be macrophages of bone marrow origin. This is indicated by the absence of acid phosphatase in corneal monocytes. There is definite alkaline phosphatase activity, indicating that the transformation of corneal stromal cells is the probable source of monocytes. The time by which the absorption of suture materials has been completed has been estimated according to experimental results:[3, 16, 36]

collagen – 35 to 42 days
polyglactin 910 – 35 days
surgical gut – 42 to 60 days
silk – 42 to 90 days

nylon and polypropylene – encapsulated by 90 days in noncorneal sites

---

*Dexon ophthalmic suture is manufactured by Davis & Geck Co., a Division of American Cyanamid Co., Pearl River, NY 10965.
†Vicryl Suture is available from Ethicon, Inc., Somerville, NY 08876.

TABLE 11-1 COMPARATIVE STUDY OF SWAGED CORNEAL NEEDLES*

Model	Type	Metal	Diameter, in.	Cord Length, mm.	Radius, mm.	Curvature, Degrees	Point Edges	Finish
Ethicon, Inc.								
GS-9	Spatulate	Stainless steel	0.008	5.17	2.78	137	Very sharp	Bright, smooth
GS-8	Spatulate	Stainless steel	0.008	5.95	3.96	97	Very sharp	Bright, smooth
G-7	Reverse cutting	Stainless steel	0.008	5.52	2.78	165	Very sharp	Bright, smooth
G-6	Reverse cutting	Stainless steel	0.008	6.50	3.97	110	Very sharp	Bright, smooth
G-1	Reverse cutting	Stainless steel	0.013	8.80	4.76	135	Very sharp	Bright, smooth
S-14	Spatulate	Stainless steel	0.013	7.24	4.37	112	Very sharp	Bright, smooth
Davis & Geck								
CE-20	Reverse cutting	Carbon steel	0.011	7.14	3.18	130	Sharp	Bright, smooth
CE-30	Reverse cutting	Carbon steel	0.009	5.55	2.78	115	Sharp	Bright, smooth
DO-1	Spatulate	Carbon steel	0.014	7.94	5.16	90	Sharp	Bright, smooth

*Data are taken from the suture material catalogues of Ethicon, Inc., and Davis & Geck.

SURGICAL NEEDLES

Surgical needles are manufactured from high quality steel wire. Either carbon or stainless steel is used. Most manufacturers use stainless steel because it is corrosion resistant and needle points can be made very sharp. In describing needles we can refer to the blade, the point, the body, and the shank or the swage. Needle points are of variable types, depending on what tissues they are to be used in. The types of needle points that are available are (1) flat reverse cutting, (2) reverse cutting, (3) regular cutting, and (4) round or tapered.

Needle curvature refers to the arc or portion of a circle that is formed by a needle and is recorded in degrees, i.e., one-half circle is 180 degrees.

For most surgical problems dealing with plastic surgery, reverse cutting and regular cutting needles are used. Specialized needles that are spatulate have been developed for corneal surgery. Table 11–1 compares several types of needles from major suture material manufacturers, viz., Ethicon, Inc., and Davis & Geck.

BASIC PRINCIPLES OF EYELID RECONSTRUCTION

INTRODUCTION

The field of ocular plastic and reconstructive surgery is very broad and includes reconstructive surgery of the lids, the orbit, the adnexa, and the globe. The types of conditions that may be treated include deformities of the lids, both congenital and acquired, tumors, and trauma-induced abnormalities of all ocular and adnexal structures. The primary goal in ophthalmic plastic surgery is the maintenance of vision by the protection of the globe and by the proper functioning of the orbital adnexa.

In order to maintain the normal physiological function of the lids and of the adnexal structures, a definitive plan of surgical approach should be mapped out prior to beginning any plastic procedure. Included in the plan should be answers to the following questions:
1. How will the eye be protected during surgery?
2. How will the lid tissues be surgically manipulated to retain their normal cosmetic function?
3. Will repair of the lid tissues involve the lacrimal puncta?
4. Will there be any excess skin or deficient lid tissue?

APPLIED ANATOMY OF THE LIDS FOR OCULAR SURGERY

The eyelids of vertebrates have multiple functions. Basically, the lids protect and help to maintain the normal environment of the eye. Protection of the eye involves (1) the tactile action of the cilia; (2) the protective action of the sebaceous glands of the lids; and (3) the movements of the lids, enabling closure of the palpebral fissure.

The lids are covered externally by epidermis and internally by conjunctivae, and between these layers are contained muscular and adnexal structures. In the dog and the cat, cilia are present on the upper eyelid but not on the lower eyelid. The cilia may be present in two or three rows, with each cilium emerging from an individual follicle.

A clearly marked furrow is present in the margin of the upper and of the lower lid. Openings for the meibomian glands are located within this furrow. In the dog, these openings are usually evenly spaced and number 20 to 40 per lid. The meibomian gland orifices lie posterior to the cilia. The glands themselves are situated in a poorly developed tarsal plate. Poor development of this tarsal plate in domestic animals makes manipulation of the lid easier; however, it makes plastic surgery more difficult because adequate support for the normal lid structure is lacking.

Mild pressure over the meibomian glands can produce extrusion of sebum from the openings at the lid margin. The oily layer that is produced by the secretion of these glands forms the most superficial layer of the precorneal tear film.

Besides the meibomian glands, a number of epidermal appendages are present in the lids. The ciliary glands, or glands of Moll, are modified apocrine sweat glands that lie near the palpebral margin and may open directly to the lid margin by tiny ducts or may empty into the follicles of the lashes. The sebaceous glands, or glands of Zeis, are rudimentary glands that are situated at the lid margin.

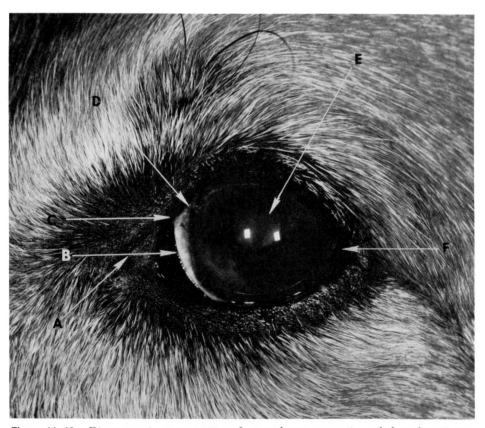

Figure 11–13:   Diagrammatic representation of external canine eye: *A*, medial canthus; *B*, membrana nictitans; *C*, upper nasolacrimal puncta; *D*, limbus (corneoscleral junction); *E*, pupil; and *F*, lateral canthus. (From Bistner, S. I., Aguirre, G., and Batik, G.: Atlas of Veterinary Ophthalmic Surgery. Philadelphia, W. B. Saunders Co., 1977, p. 42.)

The lid aperture in the dog varies widely, depending on age and breed. Horizontal dimensions of the lid aperture may vary from 10 to 35 mm. The two eyelids converge to form medial and lateral angles (Fig. 11–13). The extremities of the palpebral aperture are maintained in their normal position by the two palpebral ligaments. The upper eyelid is more mobile than the lower, and the medial canthus is more obtuse than the lateral.

There are two main patterns of motility of the lids — closure and elevation. The eyelids are closed by the action of the orbicular muscle (orbicularis oculi), which is a flattened muscle that completely surrounds the palpebral fissure. It is attached to the orbital wall by the medial (nasal) palpebral ligament and blends laterally with the retractor muscle of the angle of the eye (retractor anguli oculi). The aponeurotic sheath of the orbicular muscle is fused on its deep face with the palpebral ligament, a portion of the palpebral fascia. The palpebral ligament is formed in the upper lid by the tendon of insertion of the levator muscle (levator palpebrae superioris) and the deep sheath of the orbicular muscle. The orbicular muscle is innervated by the seventh cranial nerve.

The upper lid is elevated mainly by the levator muscle. This muscle arises dorsal to the optic canal between the dorsal rectus (rectus dorsalis) and the dorsal oblique (obliquus dorsalis) muscles and inserts into the upper lid by a wide, flat tendon that passes between fascicles of the orbicular muscle. It is innervated by the oculomotor nerve (third cranial nerve).

In addition to the levator muscle, elevation of the upper lid is aided by the smooth muscle fibers, called Müller's fibers, that arise from this muscle. The lower eyelid is much less mobile than the upper lid and is weakly depressed when the orbicular muscle is relaxed.

The superciliary muscle (superciliaris) is a small muscle that assists in elevating the upper lid, especially the nasal portion. It arises from the medial line on the frontal bone and extends over the orbicular muscle into the medial half of the upper lid.

The retractor muscle of the angle of the eye, a division of the frontal muscle (frontalis), arises from the temporal fascia and extends horizontally to the lateral palpebral angle. This muscle acts as a lateral palpebral ligament and, with its homologue, the medial palpebral ligament, serves to maintain the normal size of the palpebral aperture.

The sensory nerve supply to the palpebral region is via the ophthalmic branch of the trigeminal nerve to the upper lid and via the maxillary branch of the trigeminal nerve to the lower lid. The orbicular and corrugator supercilii muscles are innervated by the palpebral branch of the facial nerve. The levator muscle is innervated by the oculomotor nerve. The blood supply to the eyelids is via the malar and superficial temporal arteries.

The puncta lacrimale are located in the upper and in the lower eyelid, usually 2 to 4 mm. from the medial canthal angle. They are usually present at the mucocutaneous junction of the lid. A small amount of pigment frequently surrounds their opening.

BASIC PLASTY TECHNIQUES

In discussing basic ophthalmic surgical techniques, a knowledge of the basic plasties, or plastic surgical techniques, is extremely important. These techniques permit the surgeon to increase or to reduce tension on areas of the skin, to reconstruct defects on the lids or on the face with flaps or grafts, and to correct excessive scarring or traumatic insults.

The Y-V Plasty

This procedure is used to increase tension on the lid margin in cases of entropion or cicatricial contracture of the conjunctiva. As shown in Figure 11–14, *1,* the initial incision *A–D–B* is made with the arms of the "Y" encompassing the area of the lid or of the skin on which the tension is to be increased. The flap *A–C–B* is thoroughly undermined so that point *C* can be advanced to point *D*. The flap is then sutured into place with simple interrupted fine sutures of 5–0 or 6–0 material. The more acute (longer) the "V" (*A–C–B*), the greater is the chance that the vascular supply will be inadequate at point *C*.

The V-Y Plasty

The V-Y plasty is a tension-relieving procedure that can be used with small areas of cicatricial ectropion. As illustrated in Figure 11–14, *2* the incision *A–D–B* is made, and then the "V"-shaped flap *A–C–B* is thoroughly undermined. Any scar tissue in the subcutaneous area is removed. The incision is then closed with simple interrupted sutures, permitting relaxation of points *A* and *B*.

Blepharoplastic procedures are often indicated in brachycephalic breeds of dogs whose very prominent eyes are prone to injury and irritation. A large

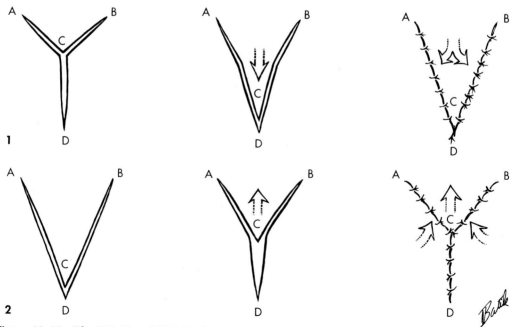

Figure 11–14: The Y-V (*1*) and V-Y (*2*) plasties. See text for further explanation. (From Bistner, S. I., Aguirre, G., and Batik, G.: Atlas of Veterinary Ophthalmic Surgery. Philadelphia, W. B. Saunders Co., 1977, p. 57.)

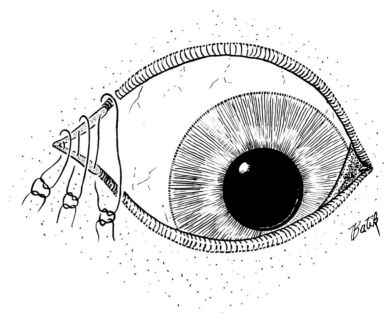

Figure 11–15: Permanent shortening of palpebral fissure. (From Bistner, S. I., Aguirre, G., and Batik, G.: Atlas of Veterinary Ophthalmic Surgery. Philadelphia, W. B. Saunders Co., 1977, p. 51.)

palpebral aperture may predispose to lagophthalmos and chronic exposure of the cornea. Prominent nasal folds may cause corneal irritation. The following procedures may be helpful in the long-term management of some of the chronic problems in these breeds.

Permanent Shortening of the Palpebral Fissure

The palpebral fissure may be easily shortened at the lateral canthus without interfering with the nasolacrimal puncta. This procedure has been helpful in brachycephalic breeds when wide palpebral apertures and very prominent globes prevent the dog from blinking properly (lagophthalmos), which results in chronic superficial keratitis. Numerous procedures can be used to shorten the palpebral fissure permanently, the simplest being to débride and then to suture the upper and the lower lid margins together.

The simple technique of shortening the palpebral fissure, which is depicted in Figure 11–15, involves removing equal-sized pieces of lid margin from the upper and from the lower lid. The amount of tissue that is removed depends on the desired length of the palpebral fissure. The lateral canthus is then carefully recreated with the placement of the first sutures. Sutures of 6–0 silk are recommended, and they are left in place for 14 to 21 days.

INJURIES TO THE LIDS

GENERAL INFORMATION

In assessing injuries to the lids, it is important to determine the extent of any associated injuries to the underlying globe. The globe should be inspected and note should be taken of the following: (1) hemorrhage into the anterior chamber of the vitreous cavity; (2) corneal or scleral lacerations with possible uveal incarceration; (3) luxation of the lens; (4) subconjunctival hemorrhage; and (5) variation in the depth of the anterior chamber.

Trauma to the lids is frequently the result of bites from other animals or of mechanical injury, such as that produced by barbed wire or an automobile accident. Lid tissue is especially prone to posttraumatic edema and hemorrhage. Repair of a traumatized lid should to be accomplished prior to the development of severe edema. Once lid tissue has become swollen and edematous, it is better to wait until the swelling has subsided before attempting primary repair. In cases in which the lids are markedly edematous following trauma, the animal should be anesthetized and the globe should be inspected to assess the extent of injury. The wounds should be irrigated with sterile saline solution, and hair and debris should be removed from the wounds. Systemic and topical antibiotics should be administered, and cold packs may be applied initially to reduce edema and swelling.

The objective in the surgical repair of lid injuries is to perform a primary repair that will maintain the normal physiological function of lid tissue. This can often prove a difficult task. The principles of wound repair of eyelid tissue are basically the same as those for other parts of the body, except that extreme care should be taken not to débride the lid tissue too extensively and fine sutures should be used.

Various types of lacerations of the lids may be present, ranging from multiple extramarginal lacerations and puncture wounds to a large marginal lid avulsion. In suturing extramarginal lesions, the wound edges should be débrided and any devitalized tissues should be removed. The wound edges are sutured together, and all attempts are made not to deform the lid margins. Sutures of 6–0 silk or nylon can be used, and often the wounds are sutured in a "crazy quilt" pattern in order to oppose adjacent tissues.[9, 18, 21, 28, 33]

Marginal lid lacerations are often difficult to treat. The horizontal pull of the orbicularis muscle fibers tends to make a notch in a marginal lid laceration. In repairing lids it should be remembered that the lid margin must be continuous in order to maintain its contour and its normal physiological function. Marginal lid lacerations can be corrected in a number of ways.

SURGICAL TECHNIQUES

Simple Apposition Using Two-Layered Approach

With this technique the tarsoconjunctival layer is closed first with interrupted 6–0 absorbable sutures (Fig. 11–16, 1). The knots are tied on the anterior surface to avoid irritation of the cornea. The muscle layer can then be closed with additional 6–0 or 7–0 interrupted sutures, and the skin layer is closed separately with 7–0 or 8–0 silk or nylon sutures (Fig. 11–16, 2). Care should be taken to close the lid margin so that gapping and notch formation are prevented.

Figure-of-Eight Suture for Repair of Lid Laceration

Defects in the lid margin frequently assume a triangular shape because the lips of the marginal laceration retract with the pull caused by the broken

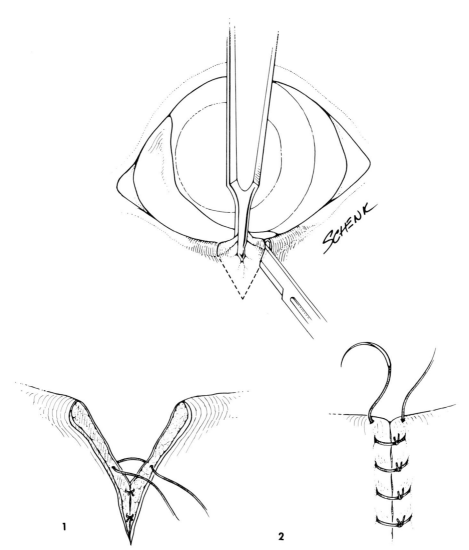

Figure 11–16: Two-layered approach to the repair of marginal lid laceration. See text for explanation of parts *1* and *2*.

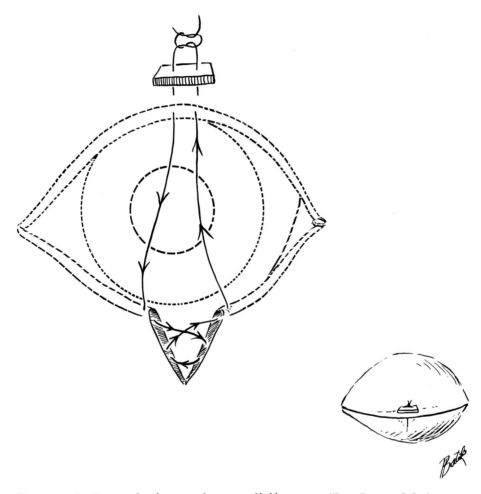

Figure 11–17:   Figure-of-eight suture for repair of lid laceration. (From Bistner, S. I., Aguirre, G., and Batik, G.: Atlas of Veterinary Ophthalmic Surgery. Philadelphia, W. B. Saunders Co., 1977, p. 61.)

orbicular muscle fibers. A figure-of-eight suture will effectively close small marginal incisions or lacerations. The suture may be passed through the opposing lid margin so that the normal lid can be used as a splint in immobilizing the lacerated lid. Using 5–0 or 6–0 ophthalmic silk and rubber, plastic, or cotton pegs to prevent pressure necrosis of the skin, a needle is passed through the middle of the opposing lid margin and then enters the lower lid (the notched portion), emerging about 2 mm. below the lid margin. The suture needle enters the opposite wound margin about midway and emerges about 1 mm. below the point at which it entered. This same procedure is repeated, creating a figure-of-eight suture (Fig. 11–17).

If the suture is carefully placed, the wound margins should be brought into apposition without creating a marginal defect or notching. If a slight notch develops, a single 6–0 silk suture can be placed at the lid margin.

Marginal Lid Wound Repair by Lid Splitting and Two-Layered Closure:

This technique of lid repair involves lid splitting in which the lid is separated into two separate components, viz., the skin and the orbicular muscle portion and the conjunctival portion. This enables the surgeon to close the marginal lid defect (Fig. 11–18, 1) in two layers by mobilizing the skin and sliding the wound defect closed. The lid margin is split to a depth that encompasses the wound (Fig. 11–18, 2). The conjunctival wound is sutured

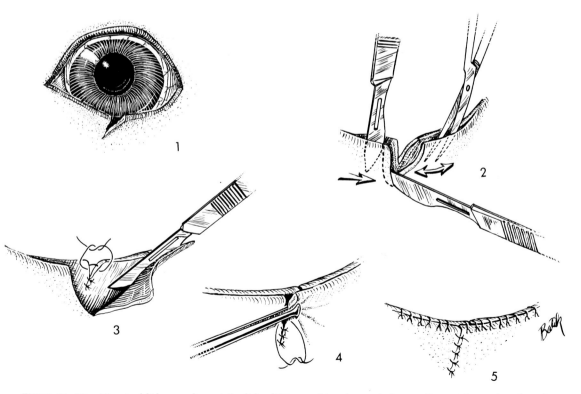

Figure 11–18: Marginal lid wound repair by lid splitting and two-layered closure. See text for explanation of parts *1* through *5*. (From Bistner, S. I., Aguirre, G., and Batik, G.: Atlas of Veterinary Ophthalmic Surgery. Philadelphia, W. B. Saunders Co., 1977, p. 79.)

with 6–0 ophthalmic gut, and the knots are tied between the conjunctiva and the skin (Fig. 11–18, 3). The skin (lid margin) is then closed with simple interrupted 5–0 or 6–0 silk sutures. Care should be taken to avoid notching of the lid margin (Fig. 11–18, 4). The conjunctiva is sutured to the lid margin with 6–0 simple interrupted chromic gut sutures and the knots are tied on the outside of the lid to prevent irritation of the cornea (Fig. 11–18, 5).

Marginal Lid Wound Repair By Lid Splitting and Conjunctival Resection (Indirect Halving Technique)

This technique is especially useful when a tumor involves the epithelial (skin) as well as the conjunctival surface or when a tumor is present near the nasal punctum. This technique permits good mobilization of the skin, avoiding both undue tension on the conjunctiva and distortion of the punctum.

The lower lid in the area of the lower punctum is split into the skin-or-bicular muscle layer and the conjunctival layer. The punctum is not incised. The tumor-containing portions of the epidermal and conjunctival tissues are removed as wedge resections. The edges of the skin and orbicularis portion are undermined. If the skin cannot be adequately mobilized, a lateral canthotomy should be performed. The conjunctiva is closed with 6–0 chromic catgut sutures, the knots of which are tied between the conjunctiva and the skin (Fig. 11–19, 1). The undermined skin and orbicular muscle area is closed with simple interrupted 6–0 silk sutures. The lateral canthotomy permits the lid to be moved nasally to facilitate closure. The split lid margin is closed with 6–0 silk sutures, with the knots tied on the outside of the lid margin. The sutures are removed in ten to 14 days (Fig. 11–19, 2).

POSTOPERATIVE PROTECTION

Following any of the plastic surgical procedures that are performed on the lid margin, adequate protection against self-induced trauma has to be

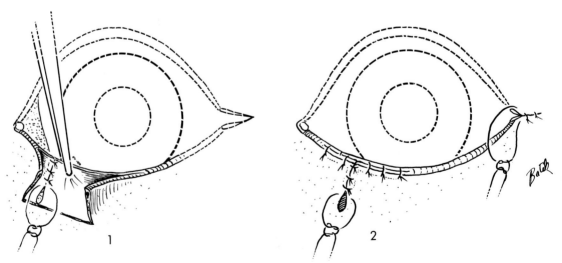

Figure 11–19: Marginal lid wound repair by lid splitting and conjunctival resection. See text for explanation of parts *1* and *2*. (From Bistner, S. I., Aguirre, G., and Batik, G.: Atlas of Veterinary Ophthalmic Surgery. Philadelphia, W. B. Saunders Co., 1977, p. 79.)

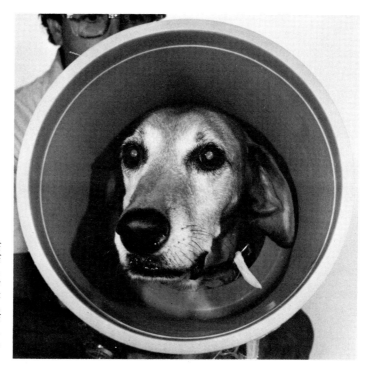

Figure 11-20: Demonstration of plastic bucket used for protection of eye and adnexa following surgery. The bucket is fastened to the collar with gauze passed through holes at the base. (From Bistner, S. I., Aguirre, G., and Batik, G.: Atlas of Veterinary Ophthalmic Surgery. Philadelphia, W. B. Saunders Co., 1977, p. 79.)

provided. The use of plastic buckets works well. Additionally, cardboard collars or polyethylene collars can be used to protect the head area (Fig. 11-20).

The polyethylene collar has proved to be very helpful in restraining animals from irritating surgical wounds and in preventing self-inflicted trauma. It is available in a variety of sizes and has snap-on fasteners (Table 11-2).*

LESIONS OF THE EYELID

Neoplasms

Eyelid neoplasms are not uncommonly seen in domestic animals, particularly in the dog, and occasionally in the cat and in the horse. In small animals,

---

*The polyethylene collar is available from Ejay Veterinary Specialties, Grand Central Box 5101, Glendale, CA 91201.

TABLE 11-2 POLYETHYLENE COLLARS

Size	Shield Diameter, in.	Neck Opening, in.
Tiny	6	0.75–1
Small	12	2–3
Medium	18	3–4
Large	24	4–5
Jumbo	30	4–5.5
Super	36	7.5–9.5

lid tumors may occur at any age but are seen frequently in the middle aged and older dog (8 to 9 years). There appears to be a breed predisposition for eyelid tumors, with the cocker spaniel, boxer, collie, and wire-haired fox terrier predominating. Multiple lid tumors of different types may occur in one dog. In the dog, the epithelium-derived lid tumors predominate by 5 or 6 to 1, and roughly 75 per cent of the tumors are classified histologically as benign. The three most common types of epithelium-derived tumors are adnexal tumors, papillomas, and squamous cell carcinomas. Of those tumors of mesenchymal cell origin, mastocytomas, histiocytomas and fibromas predominate. Melanomas are also frequently found, being more prevalent around the lids than in other areas of the body.[2, 19]

In one study on a large series of dogs with lid tumors, it was found histogenetically that 82.1 per cent of the eyelid tumors were sebaceous gland tumors, melanomas, or papillomas. Sebaceous gland tumors in this study accounted for 44 per cent of the total number of tumors studied.[19]

Papillomas

These benign, epithelial growths are frequently found on the eyelids of older dogs. They may be pedunculated or sessile, and more than one papilloma is frequently found. Since these lesions are benign, they may be left alone unless they interfere with lid movement or cause corneal irritation. Those papillomas that are pedunculated can be removed easily by an electroscalpel. Sessile papillomas that involve the margin of the lid can often be removed most easily by a lid-splitting technique. Papillomas of the eyelid are occasionally seen in young animals from 6 months to 3 years old, and these lesions may closely resemble viral papillomatosis, which is commonly seen on the mucous membranes and skin.

Adenomas

Benign adenomas of the sebaceous glands and of other adnexal tissues are common tumors of the skin in the dog. Sebaceous adenomas are the most frequent tumor encountered on the lid margin of the dog. Adenomas are tumors of advancing age (usually 8 to 9 years) and tend to be multiple. The sebaceous adenoma is found on the lid margin. The lesion is usually small, firm, and hairless, ranges in color from gray to black, and will ulcerate the epithelial surface as the tumor becomes larger. The sebaceous gland adenoma can be seen in many breeds of dogs but is most commonly seen in our practice in the cocker spaniel. The tumor is composed of proliferating, distinctly lobulated masses of cells whose architecture resembles that of the sebaceous gland. There is frequently a low-grade inflammatory response within the surrounding tumor mass. These tumors are benign and may recur locally if they are not completely excised. Although the tumor mass frequently rises above the lid margin, resembling a fibropapilloma, the tumor cannot be removed effectively by cutting it off flush with the lid margin. The tumor tissue arises within the meibomian gland, and therefore removal of the tumor mass usually requires a full-thickness lid resection.

Adenocarcinomas have also been found to involve the lids but are not, in our experience, found frequently.

Squamous Cell Carcinoma

Squamous cell carcinoma affects the lids of dogs, cats, horses, and cattle. Squamous cell carcinoma is more frequently seen in white cats and in white and gray horses. These tumors on the eyelids tend to grow rapidly, to be highly invasive, and to ulcerate early. The tumor can be highly malignant, metastasizing to regional lymph nodes, lungs, and other organs. Our experience has indicated that an early biopsy and complete surgical removal offer the best opportunity for treatment of these lid tumors. The use of radon seed and cobalt implants may be useful in treating some of the more extensive lesions, especially those in the horse.

Basal Cell Carcinomas

Basal cell carcinomas appear to be a common type of malignant tumor around the eyelids of humans, although they are seldom found involving the eyelids of domestic animals. The basal cell tumor is usually more discrete than the squamous cell carcinoma. Basal cell tumors often occur in the shape of a circular nodule involving the lid margin, whose surface ulcerates. The tumor rarely metastasizes, but there may be local invasion. As distinguished from squamous cell carcinomas, basal cell tumors are usually fairly well circumscribed, spread less rapidly, and ulcerate later.

Melanomas

Unfortunately, most veterinarians refer to all pigmented tumors as melanomas, thus implying that most of them are malignant. Most "melanomas" of the lids are benign, whereas melanomas in the mouth and on the feet are usually malignant.

There appears to be some debate about classification among those who have studied canine melanomas. Conroy[6] has, on the basis of examining 100 melanocytic tumors from dogs, classified the benign melanocytic lesions as junctional nevi, canine compound nevi, dermal nevi, and canine dermal melanocytoma. Barron,[2] in his study, found no canine lesion that resembled the classic nevus found in humans; however, he does mention finding two lid tumors that have junctional components, one of which metastasized to the eye.

The benign dermal melanocytoma is frequently seen on the eyelids and periocular skin. These small tumors are usually 0.5 to 2 cm. in diameter, are darkly pigmented, and have smooth surfaces. They may be pedunculated or sessile and are slow growing. There is frequently more than one of this type of tumor on the lid. These tumors are benign, and malignancy from a junctional nevus has rarely been reported in the dog.

Malignant melanomas have been observed occasionally in the lid tissue. They are most frequently seen in heavily pigmented breeds and are more common in male dogs, with an age predilection of between 7 and 14 years. Barron[2] reported four cases of malignant melanoma that arose in the eyelid and spread to the globe. Malignant melanomas in the dog are most common on the gums, lips, and digits. Malignant melanomas may be rapidly enlarging, dome shaped, or flat and vary in color and vascularity. They metastasize by way of the blood and lymphatics to regional lymph nodes and other organs. Canine malignant melanomas can arise from melanocytes in "normal" epidermis and oral epithelium or from junctional and dermal elements in canine pigmented nevi.

Histiocytomas

Histiocytomas are not infrequently seen on the eyelids of young dogs. There is some debate about whether these lesions constitute a true tumor. The lesions are benign and, once removed in their entirety, they do not recur. Histiocytomas appear frequently as raised, solitary, hairless, pink nodules on the head, lips, ears, legs, neck, and abdomen. These tumors grow rapidly but may regress spontaneously.

The aim in treating any tumor surgically is to remove the growth so that it will not recur locally. When dealing with the eyelids, this involves performing surgery so that the physiological and cosmetic functions of the lids are preserved. Small lid lesions can be removed by lid-splitting procedures or by resecting a small full-thickness wedge of lid tissue.

RECONSTRUCTIVE SURGERY OF EXTRAMARGINAL AND MARGINAL EYELID LESIONS

There is a wide variety of plastic surgical procedures that can be used to correct marginal lid defects associated with the removal of neoplasms. All of the procedures attempt to remove the lesions surgically while preserving the physiological integrity of the lid. In surgically correcting any defect of the lid margin, the surgeon must follow a basic plan of wound closure. The techniques that are described in this section allow the surgeon to evaluate and modify several different approaches.

Removal of Extramarginal Lid Lesions

The normal orientation of the orbicular muscle fibers is roughly parallel to that of the lid margins. When removing an extramarginal lid lesion, such as a tumor, or when suturing a laceration, the incision should be made parallel to the lid margin in the direction of the orbicular muscle fibers whenever possible. Incisions should be made cleanly, with no jagged margins, and when removing tumors normal tissue should be present around the mass. Skin closure is accomplished by utilizing fine silk or nylon suture material and carefully approximating the wound edges. Undermining the wound edges and using subcuticular sutures may be required to close the incision without placing undue tension on the suture line.

With larger extramarginal lesions (greater than 1 to 2 cm.), a perpendicular rather than a parallel incision can be made to prevent postsurgical ectropion.

A chalazion forceps may be used to support the lid when removing an extramarginal tumor. An alternative method is to insert a Jaeger's lid plate or a tongue depressor into the inferior fornix of the conjunctiva. An elliptical incision is made parallel to the lid margin and following the orientation of the or-

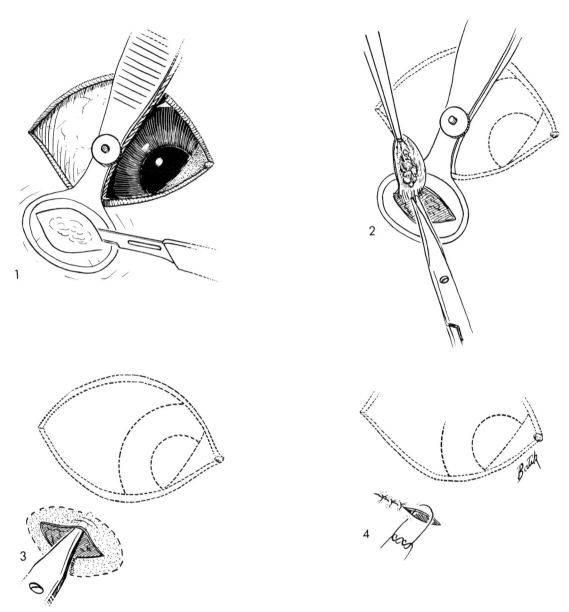

Figure 11–21: Removal of extramarginal lid lesion. See text for explanation of parts *1* through *4*. (From Bistner, S. I., Aguirre, G., and Batik, G.: Atlas of Veterinary Ophthalmic Surgery. Philadelphia, W. B. Saunders Co., 1977, p. 73.)

bicular muscle. The incision should leave a border of healthy tissue around the tumor (Fig. 11–21, *1*). Using Stevens tenotomy scissors, the skin ellipse with the tumor is dissected from the underlying orbicular muscle (Fig. 11–21, *2*). The margins of the incision are undermined with blunt dissection in order to relax the wound edges (Fig. 11–21, *3*). The incision is carefully apposed using simple interrupted sutures of 6–0 silk or nylon (Fig. 11–21, *4*). The sutures are left in place for ten to 14 days.

Vertical Closure of Lid Margin Defects Utilizing a Lid-Splitting Technique

Lesions involving only the anterior half of the lid and not involving the conjunctiva can be removed by a lid-splitting technique. The skin-muscle layer provides adequate mobility so that the lid margin defect can be closed without disturbing the functioning of the lid.

This technique is used with such a lesion as a small broad-based fibro-papilloma that involves the skin on the lower lid. The lid is split into an anterior skin-muscle layer and a posterior tarsoconjunctival layer. The incision is made with a No. 15 blade or a No. 64 Beaver blade to a depth of at least 2 to 3 mm. below and around the border of the lid tumor (Fig. 11–22, *1*). The tumor is removed utilizing a wedge incision in the undermined skin. Stevens tenotomy scissors are utilized to cut the skin (Fig. 11–22, *2*). Hemorrhage is easily controlled and pin-point cautery is used if necessary. The incision is

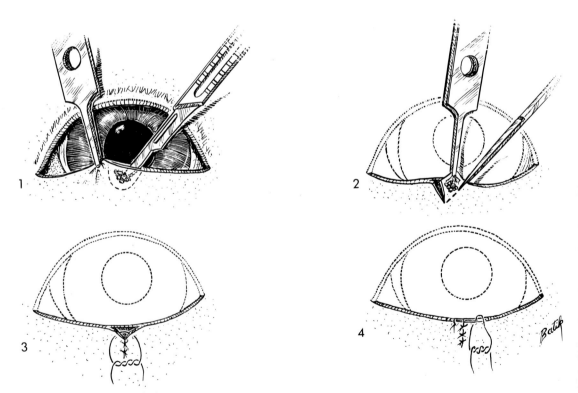

Figure 11–22: Vertical closure of defects of lid margin utilizing a lid-splitting technique. See text for explanation of parts *1* through *4*. (From Bistner, S. I., Aguirre, G., and Batik, G.: Atlas of Veterinary Ophthalmic Surgery. Philadelphia, W. B. Saunders Co., 1977, p. 75.)

closed with sutures of 6–0 silk or P.G.A. after the skin has been adequately mobilized. Care must be taken in suturing the lid margin to prevent the development of any notching (Fig. 11–22, 3). The lid margin at the point of lid splitting is closed with sutures of 6–0 silk or P.G.A., and the knot is tied on the outside of the lid margin to avoid any irritation to the cornea (Fig. 11–22, 4). When working near the medial canthus, the nasolacrimal punctum should be located so that it is not accidentally incised or damaged.

Full-Thickness Wedge Resection

When carefully performed, a full-thickness lid resection can produce good cosmetic results. The danger in performing this type of surgery is that the area that is excised may be too large, thus causing a lid deformity when closure is attempted. Additionally, if the wound margins are not properly aligned or if the lid margin is not sutured tightly closed, notching of the lid margin will occur.

We prefer not to perform a full-thickness lid resection with vertical closure if more than one fourth of the lid tissue must be removed. The technique that is described here permits closure of a lid defect in which more than one fourth of the lid tissue must be removed. When operating near the medial canthus, the lacrimal punctum must be located prior to surgery.

When a full-thickness wedge excision of a lower lid tumor is performed, care must be taken to make the arms of the triangle of equal length, leaving normal appearing tissue around the tumor margins (Fig. 11–23A, 1). Hemorrhage is controlled with pressure and pin-point electrocautery. A lateral canthotomy can be performed, which permits the lid defect to be closed by sliding the lid nasally (Fig. 11–23A, 2). This technique is helpful if excessive tension is to be placed on a vertical lid closure. A new lateral canthus is thus created by suturing the canthal incision. If the lid is advanced too far medially, a slight ectropion could develop. The lid margin should be in its normal position after the vertical marginal sutures are in place (Fig. 11–23A, 3).

The incision can also be closed by (1) a figure-of-eight vertical lid closure (Fig. 11–23B); or (2) a double-layered closure in which the conjunctiva is sutured first with 6–0 chromic catgut, the knots of which are tied on the muscle-mucocutaneous surface. The skin is then closed with simple interrupted sutures of 6–0 silk or P.G.A.

Split-Thickness Vertical Advancement Flap

Marginal and some extramarginal lid lesions involving the skin may be large enough that wedge removal will make closure of the lid defect difficult. Additionally, lid lesions may be over the medial canthal or punctal area. A vertical advancement flap with lid splitting is a method of removing large lesions of the upper and of the lower lid without severely distorting the lid margin. If the lid lesion is sufficiently large that mobilization of a vertical advancement flap creates tension, ectropion will result. A vertical skin-muscle flap (Fig. 11–24) procedure will have to be performed.

The lid margin is split into a skin-orbicular muscle layer and a layer of underlying tarsoconjunctiva. The area of the lower lid that encompasses the tumor is split and undermined (Fig. 11–24, 1). The tumor mass, including a

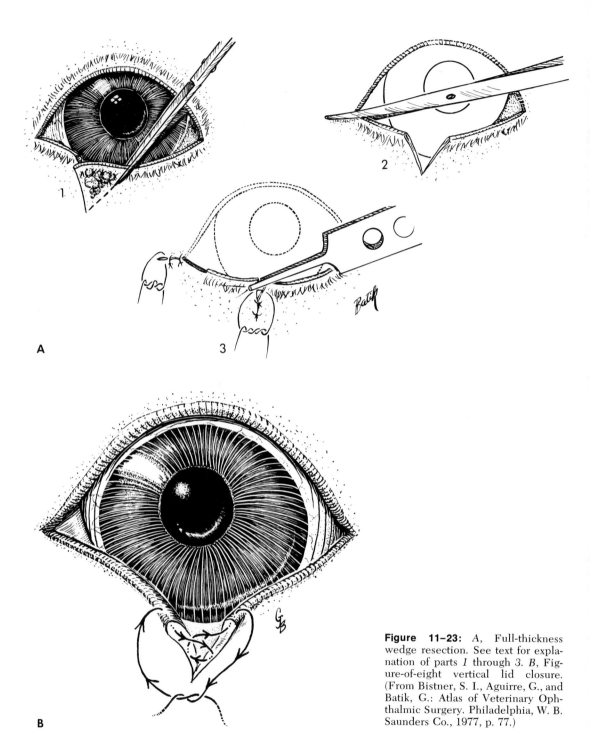

A

B

Figure 11–23: *A,* Full-thickness wedge resection. See text for explanation of parts *1* through *3. B,* Figure-of-eight vertical lid closure. (From Bistner, S. I., Aguirre, G., and Batik, G.: Atlas of Veterinary Ophthalmic Surgery. Philadelphia, W. B. Saunders Co., 1977, p. 77.)

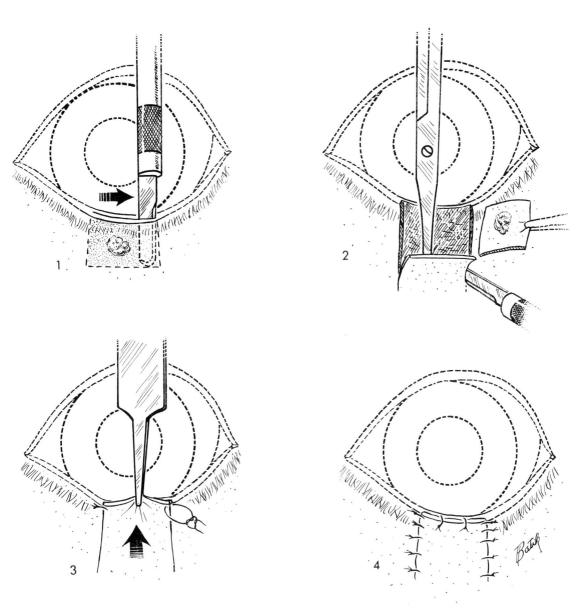

Figure 11–24: Split-thickness vertical advancement. See text for explanation of parts *1* through *4* (From Bistner, S. I., Aguirre, G., and Batik, G.: Atlas of Veterinary Ophthalmic Surgery. Philadelphia, W. B. Saunders Co., 1977, p. 81.)

margin of healthy tissue, is removed. Two parallel vertical incisions are extended through the skin-orbicular muscle layer. The length of these incisions is equal to the amount of skin and orbicular muscle that is removed in the resection. The vertical skin-orbicular muscle flap is undermined and the flap is drawn up and sutured to the tarsal edge, creating a new lid margin (Fig. 11–24, 2 and 3). The lid margin is carefully recreated, and a small amount of the skin-orbicular-muscle layer may be left at the lid margin to allow for wound contracture. The remainder of the flap is sutured with 6–0 silk using a simple interrupted pattern (Fig. 11–24, 4).

Full-Thickness Resection of Eyelid Lesions with Vertical Skin-Muscle Flap

A full-thickness resection, including normal-appearing lid tissue surrounding the lid lesion (tumor), is made. The full thickness of lid tissue is removed, leaving a defect in the palpebral conjunctiva and skin (Fig. 11–25, 1 and 2). The palpebral conjunctiva is mobilized by blunt dissection and undermining of the conjunctival attachments on either side of the lid defect and of the remaining conjunctiva below the lid defect. Enough conjunctiva to line the vertical advancement flap must be mobilized. The vertical incisions that were made to remove the tumor mass are extended through the skin-orbicular muscle layer to twice the length of the original incision. The vertical flap is bluntly dissected and undermined (Fig. 11–25, 3). Two triangles are created at the base of the vertical flap, and the skin-orbicular muscle layer associated with these triangles is bluntly dissected and removed (Fig. 11–25, 4).

The entire vertical flap is undermined by blunt dissection. The palpebral conjunctiva that has been mobilized is elevated until it is even with the existing palpebral margin, and then it is sutured to the lid margin on either side of the defect with 6–0 chromic catgut. The conjunctiva must be sutured to the lid margin in order to line the vertical flap, which is advanced into position. All sutures that are placed in the conjunctiva are tied so that the knots lie between the conjunctiva and the skin-orbicular muscle layer (Fig. 11–25, 5). The vertical flap is advanced to create a new lid margin. The flap is positioned slightly above the existing lid margin, providing for tissue contracture following healing. The flap is sutured into position using 5–0 or 6–0 silk. The sutures are placed in the sequence outlined (Fig. 11–25, 6 and 7). Care must be taken to suture the conjunctiva to the vertical flap in order to create a new conjunctiva-lined lid margin. All sutures on the lid margin should be placed so that they will not irritate the cornea.

Numerous other methods are available for closure of large defects of the lower lid margin; among these is the bridge-flap blepharorrhaphy, which has been described for the cat, the dog, and the horse.[2, 3]

Horizontal Pedicle Flap for Correction of Eyelid Agenesis

Incomplete development of the outer half of one or of both superior eyelids is not uncommon in domestic short-haired and Persian cats. In the involved area, some or all of the lid is missing. Generally there is no trace of the tarsus, the meibomian glands, or the orbicular muscle, and the blink reflex

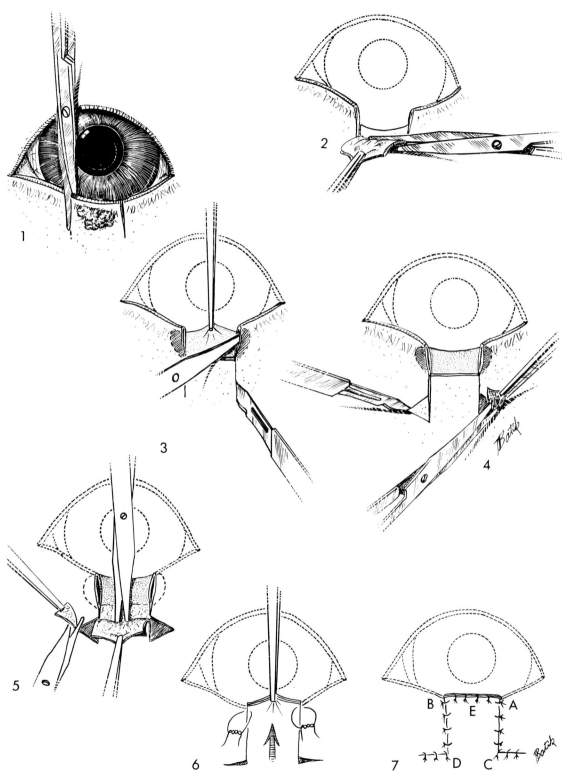

Figure 11–25: Full-thickness resection of an eyelid lesion with vertical skin-muscle flap. See text for explanation of parts *1* through *7*. (From Bistner, S. I., Aguirre, G., and Batik, G.: Atlas of Veterinary Ophthalmic Surgery. Philadelphia. W. B. Saunders Co., 1977, p. 83.)

in the affected portion is absent, although the orbicular muscle is present elsewhere in the lid and is functional.[4]

The defect is bordered by thin, hair-covered skin that is lined by conjunctiva. It may be a small (1 to 3 mm.) notch involving the superior lid at the lateral canthus, although small lesions such as this seldom produce clinical signs. More extensive defects can involve one half to three fourths of the eyelid. Eyelid closure in these cases is not complete, and exposure of the cornea and chronic superficial keratitis or ulceration may develop.

The correction of eyelid agenesis involves a horizontal pedicle flap. The surgical principles that are utilized in performing this procedure may also be used in removing lid tumors or in correcting other large marginal lid defects.

Incomplete development of the temporal aspect of the upper eyelid can result in chronic keratitis (Fig. 11–26, *1*). A recipient bed is prepared in the

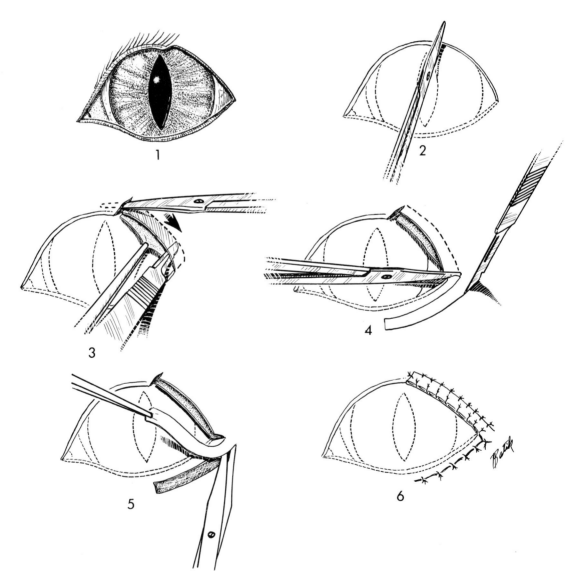

Figure 11–26: Horizontal pedicle flap for correction of eyelid agenesis. See text for explanation of parts *1* through *6*. (From Bistner, S. I., Aguirre, G., and Batik, G.: Atlas of Veterinary Ophthalmic Surgery. Philadelphia, W. B. Saunders Co., 1977, p. 85.)

upper lid to receive the pedicle flap. The nasal end of the lid defect is made square by trimming the defect with Stevens tenotomy scissors (Fig. 11–26, 2). Lid splitting is performed along the length of the upper lid defect, separating the skin-orbicular muscle layer from the underlying conjunctiva. The lid splitting is continued nasally for a distance of 3 mm. into the normal lid (Fig. 11–26, 3).

The horizontal pedicle flap that is to be transposed is prepared by making two incisions through the skin and orbicular muscle of the lower lid. The first incision is made parallel to and 2 mm. from the lid margin; the second incision is made 5 mm. from the lid edge, creating a 3-mm. horizontal flap. The length of the pedicle flap depends on the size of the defect to be filled. The incisions into the lower lid are parallel but diverge slightly to form a broader base as they reach the lateral canthus (Fig. 11–26, 4). The lateral canthus is cut to the uppermost edge of the pedicle, permitting the pedicle to be rotated to its new position in the upper lid. The horizontal skin-orbicular muscle pedicle flap is bluntly dissected free (Fig. 11–26, 5). A thin strip of the skin-orbicular muscle layer in the recipient bed is removed from the upper lid, thereby creating a fresh wound to receive the pedicle flap. The pedicle flap is moved to its new position, where it is sutured into place with interrupted 6–0 silk, nylon, or P.G.A. sutures. The conjunctiva is sutured to the edge of the pedicle flap, creating a new lid margin. All sutures should be placed to avoid corneal irritation. Hair will not grow on the new lid margin, which consists of tarsus that epithelializes and heals with a smooth border. The lower lid defect is closed with simple interrupted sutures (Fig. 11–26, 6). The sutures are removed in 14 to 21 days. Normal hair of the superior lid and of the head is directed temporally. The hair on the horizontal pedicle flap is directed downward. If this hair becomes too long and irritates the cornea, it may be clipped or petroleum jelly may be applied to keep the hair down.

Juxtapunctal Neoplasms of the Medial Canthus

Neoplasms of the lids involving the medial canthus can present difficult surgical problems. The mass must be removed in its entirety, and the nasolacrimal punctum should be salvaged if at all possible. Large tumors may completely destroy the lacrimal puncta, and surgery or radiation therapy may result in the excessive formation of scar tissue, which can destroy the puncta. The nasolacrimal punctum of the lower lid is physiologically more important than the punctum of the upper lid.

In performing any lid surgery around the medial canthus, the lacrimal puncta should be located and marked. A 5–0 silk suture may be placed in the punctum and in the canaliculus. Additionally, the punctum can be located and marked with a lacrimal probe, which can be left in place while the tissue is being dissected. Following surgery in cases in which the lacrimal punctum and the canaliculus are involved, an indwelling polyethylene or Teflon catheter can be left in place to prevent excessive scarring of the canaliculus.

The following procedure is just one method for preserving the lower lacrimal punctum and canaliculus while removing a tumor of the lower lid involving the medial canthus.

To remove a lower lid tumor in a juxtapunctal position, the lacrimal punctum of the lower eyelid is located, and a piece of size PE 90 polyethylene tubing is inserted into the punctum and into the canaliculus. The tubing is threaded as far as possible. A lateral canthotomy is performed to facilitate

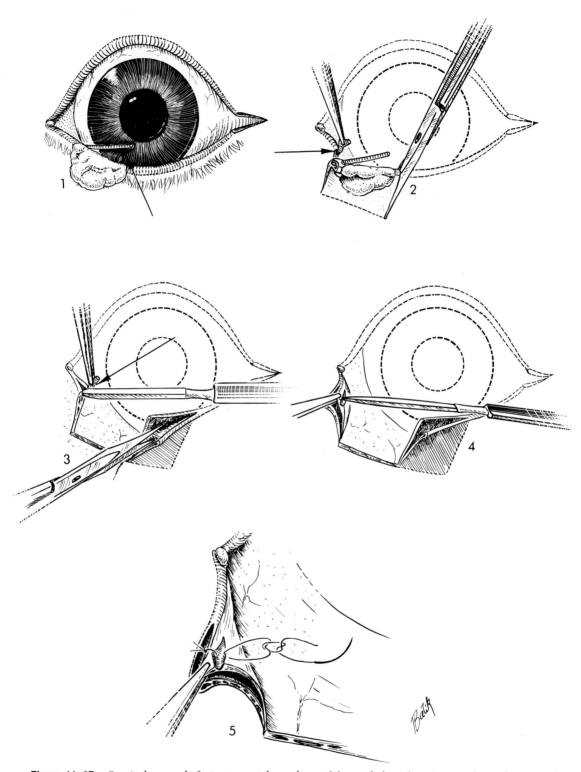

Figure 11–27: Surgical removal of a juxtapunctal neoplasm of the medial canthus. See text for explanation of parts *1* through *5*. (From Bistner, S. I., Aguirre, G., and Batik, G.: Atlas of Veterinary Ophthalmic Surgery. Philadelphia, W. B. Saunders Co., 1977, p. 87.)

exposure of the inner aspect of the lower lid and to permit closure of the lid defect following surgical resection of the tumor (Fig. 11–27, *1*). A full-thickness resection of the tumor of the lower lid is made, and a 2-mm. margin of normal-appearing tissue is left around the tumor. Full-thickness resection of the tumor necessitates removal of a portion of the lacrimal canaliculus. The medial aspect of the remaining canaliculus can be located by finding and by withdrawing slightly the end of the polyethylene catheter (Fig. 11–27, *2*).

A lid-splitting procedure is performed, separating the skin-orbicular muscle layer from the underlying tarsoconjunctival layer. The lacrimal canaliculus of the lower lid in which the polyethylene catheter has been inserted should again be located and isolated so that it will not be cut during the lid-splitting procedure (Fig. 11–27, *3*). The remaining portion of the lower canaliculus is isolated by finding the end of the polyethylene tubing, and, utilizing Graefe's cataract blade or a Bard-Parker No. 11 blade, the canaliculus is incised for a distance of 2 mm. nasally to increase the opening. Two 6–0 silk sutures are used to maintain the enlargement of the canalicular opening (Fig. 11–27, *4* and *5*).

The conjunctival wound margins in the lid-splitting defect are closed with 6–0 catgut sutures, the knots of which are tied and buried between the conjunctival layer and the skin-orbicular muscle layer. The skin-orbicular muscle layer is closed using 6–0 silk sutures. The lateral canthotomy and lid splitting permit closure of the lid defect by sliding. If the skin-orbicular muscle layer defect cannot be closed, a vertical pedicle flap can be created, pulling the flap nasally to close the defect. The skin-orbicular muscle layer is closed with simple interrupted sutures of 5–0 or 6–0 silk that are left in place for 14 to 21 days. The marginal lid split is closed by using several 6–0 catgut simple interrupted sutures, with the knots tied so as to avoid irritating the cornea. A Teflon tube may be left in the nasolacrimal duct for seven to ten days while healing is taking place, although it is not often required.

Repair by Split-Thickness Advancement Flap

This technique can be used to correct defects caused by a neoplastic growth, such as a squamous cell or a basal cell carcinoma. A rectangular resection of this growth is made by incising the skin and the underlying orbicular muscle and by removing the tumor tissue (Fig. 11–28, *1*). A pedicle consisting of skin and orbicular muscle is created. The length of the incision to *create* the pedicle is roughly two times that of the incised tumor tissue. The pedicle is undermined and two triangles are removed from the base (Fig. 11–28, *2*). The pedicle flap is sutured into place with 6–0 nylon, Dermalon, or silk sutures (Fig. 11–28, *3*).

Utilizing an advancement flap from either the medial or the lateral area is very feasible in the dog and in the cat. A problem may be encountered, however, with the medial advancement flap owing to the difficulty of mobilizing the skin from the bridge of the nose.

Repair by Lower Lid Bridge Flap

With this technique a marginal lid tumor is excised along with the involved conjunctiva. The wound that is created in the upper lid resembles a

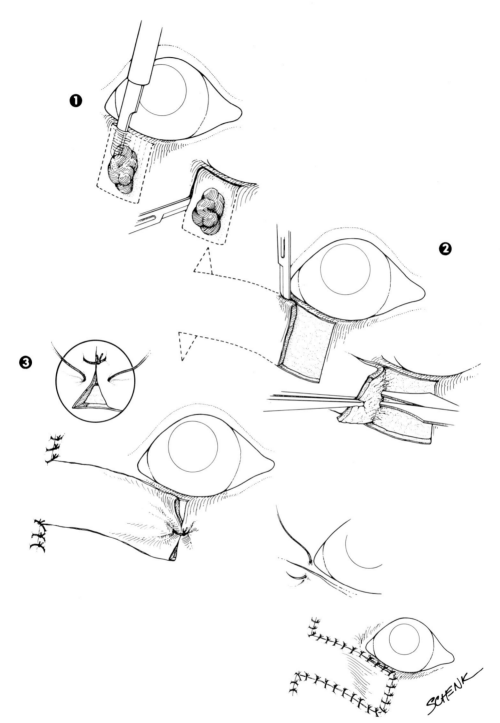

Figure 11–28: Repair by split-thickness advancement flap. See text for explanation of parts *1* through *3*.

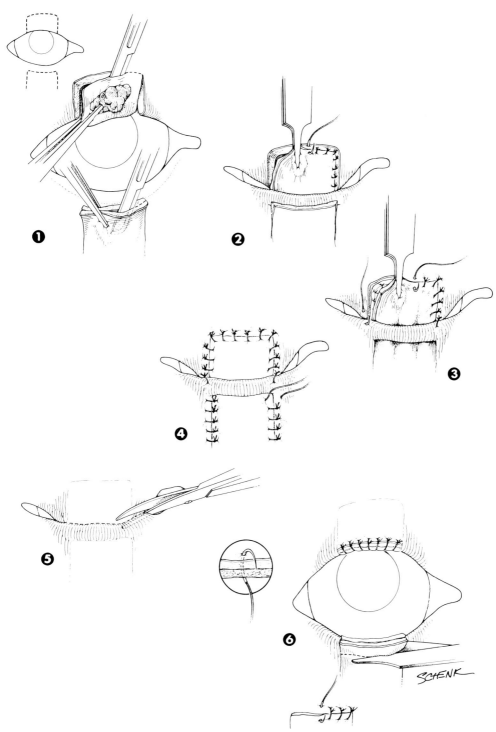

Figure 11–29:   Repair by lower lid bridge flap. See text for explanation of parts *1* through *6*.

rectangle. Hemorrhage is controlled by the use of pin-point electrocautery. A full-thickness horizontal incision is then made in the lower lid just below the lower lid's tarsal border. Two vertical incisions are made to create a full-thickness rectangular advancement flap. Stevens tenotomy scissors are usually used to help incise the conjunctiva to create the advancement flap. The advancement flap is split into two component layers, viz., the skin-orbicular muscle layer and conjunctival layer (Fig. 11–29, *1*).

The conjunctival layer of the bridge flap is brought through the horizontal incision in the lower lid and sutured into place in the upper lid defect. The conjunctiva is sutured with simple interrupted 6–0 ophthalmic chromic gut sutures, and the knots are tied on the temporal side of the conjunctival flap (Fig. 11–29, *2* and *3*).

The skin-muscle flap is then drawn up and sutured to the skin's edges with interrupted sutures of 5–0 or 6–0 silk, nylon, or Dermalon. Two temporary tarsorrhaphy sutures are added at the medial and the lateral aspects of the flap to help stabilize the upper and the lower lid. Sutures are left in place for three weeks, at which time they are removed. The bridge flap is allowed to remain in place for six weeks (Fig. 11–29, *4*).

After six weeks the new margin of the upper lid is marked with a pen, creating a convex line to allow for lid retraction (Fig. 11–29, *5*). The lids are divided with Stevens tenotomy scissors, and the skin of the raw upper lid edge is sutured to the conjunctiva with interrupted sutures of 6–0 silk, the knots of which are tied on the upper lid margin. The lower lid flap is freed from its adhesions, and any extraneous portion of the flap is surgically excised and sutured back into position with 6–0 silk (Fig. 11–29, *6*). All sutures are removed in 14 days.

REFERENCES

1. Arruga, H.: Ocular Surgery. New York, McGraw-Hill Book Co., 1952.
2. Barron, C. N.: The comparative pathology of neoplasms of the eyelids and conjunctiva with special reference to those of epithelial origin. Acta Derm. Venereol. *42 (suppl. 51)*:1, 1962.
3. Blaydes, J. E.: The use of Vicryl (polyglactin 910) suture in muscle surgery. Ophthalmic Surg. 6:39, 1975.
4. Callahan, A.: Reconstructive Surgery of the Eyelids and Ocular Adnexa. Birmingham, Ala., Aesculapius Publishing Co., 1966.
5. Castroviejo, R.: Atlas of Keratectomy and Keratoplasty. Philadelphia, W. B. Saunders Co., 1966.
6. Conroy, J. D.: Melanocytic tumors of domestic animals. Arch. Dermatol. 96:372, 1967.
7. Doherty, M. J.: A bridge-flap blepharorrhaphy method for eyelid reconstruction in the cat. J. Am. Anim. Hosp. Assoc. 9:238, 1973.
8. Fasanella, R. M.: Complications in Eye Surgery, ed. 2. Philadelphia, W. B. Saunders Co., 1965.
9. Fox, S. A.: Ophthalmic Plastic Surgery, ed. 5. New York, Grune & Stratton, 1976.
10. Gelatt, K. N.: Equine ophthalmology, in Proceedings of the 17th Annual Convention of the American Association of Equine Practitioners, 1971, p. 323.
11. Gelatt, K. N.: Recent advances in veterinary and comparative ophthalmology, in Brandly, C. A., and Jungherr, E. L. (eds.): Advances in Veterinary Science and Comparative Medicine. New York, Academic Press, Inc., 1972, pp. 1–33.
12. Gelatt, K. N.: Ocular surgery, in Equine Medicine and Surgery. ed. 2., Santa Barbara, Calif., American Veterinary Publications Inc., 1972.
13. Gelatt, K. N., and Titus, R. S.: The special sense organs — eye and eyelid, in Oehme, F. W., and Prier, J. E. (eds.): Large Animal Surgery. Baltimore, Williams & Wilkins Co., 1974.
14. Hale, M. L.: Povidone-iodine in ophthalmic surgery. Ophthalmic Surg. *1*:9, 1970.
15. Harms, H., and Mackensen, G.: Ocular Surgery Under the Microscope. Chicago, Year Book Medical Publishers, 1967.

16. Helveston, E., and Meyers, S.: Synthetic absorbable suture. Ophthalmic Surg. 5:63, 1974.
17. King, J. H., and Wadsworth, J.: An Atlas of Ophthalmic Surgery, ed 2. Philadelphia, J. B. Lippincott Co., 1970.
18. Mustarde, J. C., Jones, L. T., and Callahan, A.: Ophthalmic Plastic Surgery. Birmingham, Ala., Aesculapius Publishing Co. 1970.
19. Krehbiel, J. D., and Langham, R. F.: Eyelid neoplasms of dogs. Am. J. Vet Res. 36:115, 1975.
20. Partridge, J., Rich, A., Dunlap, W., et al.: Ocular tissue fluids and nylon, virgin silk and collagen sutures. Arch. Ophthalmol. 90:271, 1973.
21. Paton, D., and Goldberg, M. F.: Management of Ocular Injuries. Philadelphia, W. B. Saunders Co., 1976.
22. Paton, R. T., Smith, B., and Katzin, H.: Atlas of Eye Surgery. New York, McGraw-Hill Book Co., 1962.
23. Physicians' Desk Reference for Ophthalmology 1978/1979. Oradell, N.J., Medical Economics Co., 1978.
24. Ragland, W. L., Keown, G. H., and Spencer, G. R.: Equine sarcoid. Equine Vet. J. 2:2, 1970.
25. Smith, B.: Eyelid surgery: Symposium on reconstructive plastic surgery. Surg. Clin. North Am. Vol. 39, 1959.
26. Smith, B., and Cherubini, T. D.: Oculoplastic Surgery. St. Louis, The C. V. Mosby Co., 1970.
27. Smith, B., and Converse, J. M.: Plastic and Reconstructive Surgery of the Eye and Adnexa. St. Louis, The C. V. Mosby Co., 1967.
28. Smith, B., and English, F. P.: Techniques available in reconstructive surgery of the eyelid. Br. J. Ophthalmol. 54:450, 1970.
29. Sparta Ocular Instrument Corp. Catalogue, Fairfield, N.J., 1978.
30. Stallard, H. B.: Eye Surgery, ed 2. Baltimore, Williams & Wilkins Co., 1959.
31. Storz Instrument Co. Catalogue, ed. 12. St.Louis, 1978.
32. The Surgical Armamentarium for Ophthalmology. Chicago, V. Mueller Co., 1979.
33. Troutman, R. C.: Non-penetrating and penetrating injuries of the anterior segment, in Gombos, G. M.: Handbook of Ophthalmologic Emergencies: A Guide for Emergencies in Ophthalmology. Flushing, N.Y., Medical Examination Publishing Co., 1973.
34. Troutman, R. C.: Microsurgery of the Anterior Segment of the Eye: Introduction and Basic Techniques. St. Louis, The C. V. Mosby Co., 1974.
35. Uberreiter, O.: Examination of the eye and eye operations on animals. Adv. Vet. Sci. 5:1, 1959.
36. White, R. H., and Parks, M.: Polyglycolic acid sutures in ophthalmologic surgery. Trans. Am. Acad. Ophthalmol. Otolaryngol. 78:632, 1974.
37. Wille, C. R., and McPherson, S. D.: Evaluation of 8–0 chromic collagen suture material. South. Med. J. 67:54, 1974.
38. Willoughby, R. A.: The eye and its adnexa, in Gibbons, W. D., Catcott, E. J., and Smithcors, J. F.: Bovine Medicine and Surgery. Santa Barbara, Calif., American Veterinary Publications, Inc., 1970.

12

RECONSTRUCTIVE EAR SURGERY

Trauma, Infection, Neoplasia, and Developmental Deformities

Ralph A. Henderson, D.V.M., M.S.

INTRODUCTION

Ear scratching and head shaking in small animals have long been important client complaints for veterinarians. The hospital prevalence of external ear disease in small animals, as seen by 14 teaching hospitals, was 6200/100,000 cases.

The ear is an extension of the central nervous system to the integumentary system. Like those of other body parts, the problems of the ear require a diagnostic protocol in order to establish a diagnosis and to prescribe properly: identification of complaint, history taking, inspection, and clinical examination. The client expects the veterinarian to show concern, to examine the affected part, and to discuss the problem and the solution.

Reconstructive surgery of the ear is often indicated for management of trauma, neoplasia, or developmental anomalies, and as an adjunctive therapy in the management of infection. Although the ear is flexible and resilient, surgical procedures are hampered by the paucity of local tissues with which reconstruction can be performed; this may lead to postoperative ear asymmetry and a cosmetically unacceptable reconstruction. If these complicating factors are taken into account in the initial design of operative reconstruction, the therapeutic and surgical objectives of reconstruction are more likely to be achieved.

ANATOMY AND PHYSIOLOGY

MACROSCOPIC ANATOMY

Anatomical discussions of the ear are generally confusing because the proper anatomical terminology of the external ear is not universally used, and the reference points seem to change between dogs with erect ears and

520

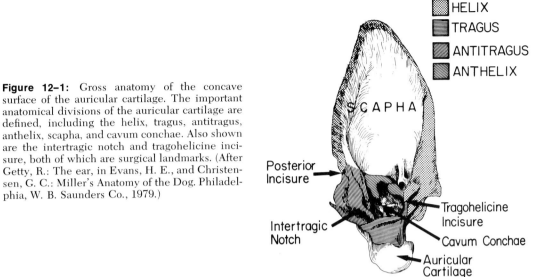

Figure 12-1: Gross anatomy of the concave surface of the auricular cartilage. The important anatomical divisions of the auricular cartilage are defined, including the helix, tragus, antitragus, anthelix, scapha, and cavum conchae. Also shown are the intertragic notch and tragohelicine incisure, both of which are surgical landmarks. (After Getty, R.: The ear, in Evans, H. E., and Christensen, G. C.: Miller's Anatomy of the Dog. Philadelphia, W. B. Saunders Co., 1979.)

dogs with pendulous ears. In order to reduce the confusion, the terms concave and convex will be used to refer to the surfaces of the external ear. These correspond to the hairless rostral and haired caudal surfaces of the aurical (pinna), respectively (Fig. 12–1).[14]

Macroscopically, the external ear is composed of three elastic cartilages: the annular, the scutiform, and the auricular. The annular cartilage is a portion of the horizontal canal and conjoins the osseous meatus of the temporal bone and the auricular cartilage. The annular cartilage is not usually involved in surgery of the external ear. The scutiform cartilage is boot-shaped and lies medial to the auricular cartilage, adjoining its convex surface; it is within the auricular muscles and assists in the attachment of the auricular cartilage to the head. This cartilage is important in correcting ear carriage,[21, 38] but not in reconstructive procedures.

The auricular cartilage is the largest cartilage of the ear and the most complicated anatomically. It is cone shaped from its origin at the annular cartilage and flares distally to form the pinna. It is heavily convoluted, which gives it a more intricate appearance. The six important surgical landmarks of the auricular cartilage are the helix, the anthelix, the tragus, the antitragus, the scapha, and the cavum conchae (Fig. 12–1).

The helix is the free margin of cartilage around the pinna that borders the scapha on three sides. The scapha is bordered on the fourth side by a ridge and a prominent tubercle termed the anthelix, which is on the medial concave aspect of the auricular cartilage at the entrance to the vertical canal. The tragus is a heavy cartilaginous rim that forms the lateral aspect of the vertical canal meatus; it is directly opposite the anthelix. The tragohelicine incisure separates the tragus and the helix. The antitragus is a plate of cartilage that is caudal to the tragus and separated from it by the intertragic notch. Finally, the cavum conchae is the rolled or funnel-shaped portion of the auricular cartilage that forms the vertical canal and a portion of the horizontal canal with the annular cartilage. It also forms the external auditory meatus of the vertical canal with the tragal, antitragal, and anthelicine borders (Fig. 12–1).[25]

The principal arteriovenous system of the external ear is the great auricular arborization of the external carotid artery and the internal maxillary vein. The lateral, intermediate, and medial vascular rami course along the convex surface and wrap around the helicine margins; they also directly penetrate the scapha to supply the concave epithelium.[25] The maxillary artery is closely associated with the rostromedial aspect of the ventral canal as it branches from the external carotid artery. It is therefore a potential surgical hazard.

The second cervical nerve is the principal sensory innervation caudodorsally on the convex surface, while the auriculotemporal branches of the trigeminal nerve are the source of sensory innervation on the concave surface. Motor function is by way of the auricular branch (auriculopalpebral trunk) of the facial nerve.[25] Both the facial and the trigeminal nerves are associated with the ventral and the rostral aspects of the vertical canal, and accidental transection of these is another potential surgical hazard with relatively irreversible consequences.

MICROSCOPIC ANATOMY

The skin is closely adherent to the concave aspect of the perichondrium and thus is difficult to undermine for suturing. The convex surface, in contrast, has subcuticular (areolar) tissue interposed between the skin and perichondrium. Thus, movement of tissue is facilitated on the convex surface because it is easier to undermine the skin, and small defects are easily closed.

PHYSIOLOGY

Cerumen is produced by the sebaceous and tubular glands that are located in the skin of both the cartilaginous and the osseous ear canals. The cerumen acts as a protector against and mechanical binder of detritus or foreign material, thus facilitating its removal.

The ear is normally cleaned by horizontal epithelial migration.[24] Although they are intimately associated, the epithelium and the perichondrium are separate, and the epithelium glides over its connective tissue junction with the perichondrium. This migration originates at the umbo (the attachment of the malleus to the tympanic membrane) and ends at the external auditory meatus as a result of desquamation. It is thought that infection results in vertical proliferation, which exceeds or interrupts the horizontal migration and results in obstructive hyperkeratosis.[24]

The normal microbial flora of the ear is the same as that of the skin and includes *Staphylococcus epidermidis* and several streptococcal and corynebacterial species. Cerumen is the normal substrate of these microorganisms. Depending upon the state of health of the individual, other nonpathogenic opportunists may also be cultured.

The ear canal temperature averages 0.6° C below the rectal temperature, and there is no significant difference in temperature between erect- and pendulous-eared dogs. Changing environmental temperatures have little effect on the temperature of the ear canal.[16]

The mean pH of the external ear canal is between 6.1 and 6.2; however, the pH increases to 6.8 in dogs with chronic otitis. The buffering capacity of the ear is such that a chemically induced pH of 4.6 is raised to a normal value within one hour. This should be considered in cases in which buffering could reduce the effectiveness of a chemotherapeutic agent.[17]

The mean relative humidity of the normal ear canal is 80 per cent, whereas in those dogs with a vertical canal resection it is 70 per cent. The mean relative humidity of an individual animal is not affected by environment. The presence of active otitis externa raises the relative humidity to 89 per cent.[18]

PHYSICAL INJURIES

AURAL HEMATOMA

Aural or auricular hematoma is the most common physical injury of the dog's ear. It is a self-inflicted injury caused by scratching and head shaking. It is seen most commonly in pendulous-eared dogs, but it is also found in the erect-eared breeds. The underlying causes of this condition are reported to be acute or chronic inflammation, parasitic infestation such as with *Otodectes cynotis* or tick species, and the presence of foreign bodies in or near the ear canal.

Hematomas are normally confined to the concave surface of the ear (Fig. 12–2); however, they may be on either or both sides of the auricular cartilage, depending upon the severity and duration of trauma. The hematoma does not, however, extend to the helix.

The great auricular artery is the source of hemorrhage that accumulates between the skin and the perichondrium. When the arterial pressure is equaled by the pressure within the hematoma, the bleeding ceases. Additional pressure on the hematoma during head shaking or scratching causes further separation of the tissues and a secondary decrease in the pressure within the hematoma, which allows the hemorrhage to resume.

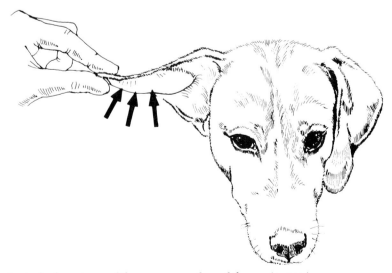

Figure 12–2: Auricular hematoma of the concave surface of the ear (*arrows*).

Fibrin is deposited along the walls of the hematoma, leaving a sanguinous seroma centrally. If this condition is chronic, the ear becomes thickened and deformed. Fibrous reorganization of the ear and secondary contracture result in the convoluted "cauliflower" configuration.[31, 33]

Treatment

The therapeutic objectives in the management of an aural hematoma are to identify the source of irritation, to maintain tissue apposition, to reduce fibrin deposition, and to prevent its recurrence. The management of hematomas is surgically oriented.

Conservative Management. Needle aspiration or cannulation of a hematoma may be effective when the diagnosis is made early in the course of formation, in which case the minimum therapeutic objectives include elimination of the causative irritant and tissue apposition. The serum of the hematoma must be removed to allow tissue apposition, and aseptic precautions are necessary to protect the hematoma from bacterial contamination. Performing needle aspirations frequently is troublesome, and instilling cortisone is dangerous in addition to leaving material to separate the tissues. A pressure bandage should be applied following aspiration.

Longer standing hematomas in which minimum fibrin is present may be treated by inserting a self-retaining disposable teat cannula rather than relying upon multiple needle aspirations. The cannula is aseptically placed through a small stab incision in a dependent portion of the hematoma. The application of continuous pressure for five to seven days decreases the chance of recurrence. Recurrence is, however, fairly common following either conservative method.

Management by Incision. Large, severe, or chronic (thick-walled) hematomas should be treated by surgical incision and suturing. The therapeutic objectives of this mode include the elimination of the inciting irritant, the removal of the clot, and the reapposition of tissues under aseptic conditions. Hematomas may be opened with straight, cruciate, or "S"-shaped incisions, depending upon the surgeon's preference and the size of the hematoma. The "S"-shaped incision may reduce linear contraction of the chronically scarred ear.[30]

It has been advocated that the hematoma be allowed to organize for 10 to 14 days prior to incision.[30] If the surgeon believes that there are advantages in delaying incision, the situation should be fully explained to the client. An uninformed client will often seek help elsewhere if the hematoma worsens in the interim. It is acceptable and effective to incise the hematoma immediately after physical and clinical evaluation of the animal, but the sanguineous drainage is heavier in the early postoperative period than when the incision is delayed.

When a hematoma is incised, the cut should be bold, exposing the cavity of the hematoma from end to end. The clot is thoroughly curetted with a blunt instrument, and the cavity is copiously irrigated. These measures promote better drainage and reduce the formation of scars and the potential for infection. Unless dead space and pockets are obliterated, the hematoma will re-form in these areas.[33] Although a pressure bandage applied in such a way that the ear is pressed over the dorsum of the neck is effective in reducing the recurrence of hematomas, drainage may not be adequate. In-

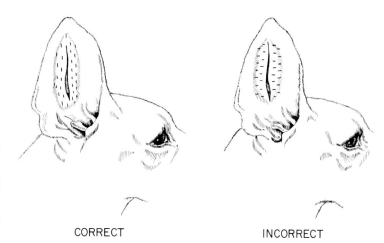

Figure 12–3: Sutures are placed in the auricular hematoma to obliterate dead space. Sutures are correctly placed when parallel to and not including the blood vessels. Incorrectly placed sutures may cause avascular necrosis.

CORRECT   INCORRECT

stead it is recommended that mattress sutures be placed through the ear. These sutures should be placed parallel to the auricular cartilage's long axis and to the vasculature. The three main great auricular branches are visible on the convex surface and should be avoided. The placement of mattress sutures perpendicular to the incision (and to vessels) increases the risk of vascular damage and necrosis (Fig. 12–3). The incisional edges are not apposed or sutured, as drainage must pass through this area. If it is desired, a reinforcing stent, such as radiographic film, may be used on the convex surface, but this is not usually necessary if the sutures are not greater than 0.5 cm. in width and if they are not tied too tightly.

A light protective bandage may be applied to immobilize the ear against the dorsum of the neck. The bandage is changed after three days, and sutures are removed between seven and ten days. As an alternative, a sterile leather punch can be used to make holes in the epithelium; the holes are between 0.3 and 0.4 cm. in size and are spaced 0.75 cm. apart. It is necessary to insert a tongue depressor through a small incision in the skin to protect the cartilage. A pressure bandage is applied to the ear for five days, and then the ear is cleaned and bandaged for another five days. Healing of the punched epithelium is by contracture and reepithelialization.[7]

WOUNDS OF THE PINNA

Therapeutic Objectives and General Management

The dog's ear is commonly injured during fights because it protrudes in an unprotected position, especially in pendulous-eared breeds. The wounds range from abrasions to serious avulsion injuries in which major portions of the pinna are lost. Regardless of the severity of the wound, the therapeutic objectives are similar and include cleansing, débridement, apposition of tissues, protection, and prevention of secondary infection.

Following an initial rinse, the wound is packed with a sterile water soluble ointment or lubricant, and a razor blade or clippers are used to remove the hair from the area. Loose hair clippings are entrapped in the lubricant rather than in the wound and are thus more easily washed away.

While the lubricant is still protecting the wound, clean gauze, a balanced pH soap, and saline solution or tap water are used to wash the periphery of the wound and the matted hair, freeing them of dried blood and serum. The cleansing is then continued to the margins and finally to the depths of the wound, during which time the gauze is changed and the wound is irrigated frequently. Topical agents are then applied to disinfect the wound before surgery or to débride the wound prior to bandaging. Wound management is more thoroughly described in Chapter 4.

The tissues may require sutures for apposition, or healing by second intention (contraction and epithelialization) may be adequate. The margins of fresh wounds with minimal contamination may be apposed following cleansing, while more contaminated or infected wounds should be bandaged and débrided chemically for 24 hours before closing. Small wounds, wounds in which the tissues remain in good apposition, and grossly infected wounds may be treated openly; however, generalizations are not good substitutes for sound clinical judgement.

Ear Lacerations

Three types of lacerations of the ear may be distinguished on the basis of wound depth or the structures involved. A laceration may involve the skin only, the skin and the underlying cartilage, or the skin, the contralateral skin, and the interposed cartilage (a through-and-through wound) (Fig. 12–4).

Ear Lacerations Involving the Skin Surfaces Only.   Linear lacerations involving the skin only (Fig. 12–5) usually heal adequately by second intention because of the rigid cartilaginous template that underlies the wound and maintains tissue apposition. Although it is not necessary, careful suturing may improve the cosmetic appearance.

Suturing is mandatory, however, when a two- or three-sided pedicle flap has been traumatically raised (Fig. 12–6). If the flap is not sutured, contracture during the healing process usually creates a defect that either cannot epithelialize or does so without a covering of hair. These wounds must be sutured at the margin as well as through the center of the flap as is done with aural hematomas, to obliterate the dead space (Fig. 12–7). Dead space allows

A   B

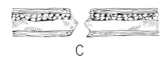

C

Figure 12–4:   Lacerations of the ear flaps may include, *A*, the skin only (convex surface), *B*, the skin and cartilage, or *C*, cartilage and both skin surfaces.

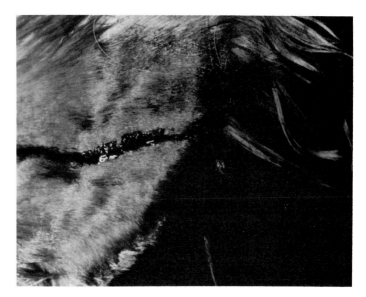

Figure 12–5: Laceration of the concave ear skin superficial to the scapha and helix. The cartilage is intact, and the tissue apposition is excellent because of the skin's adherence to the cartilage template.

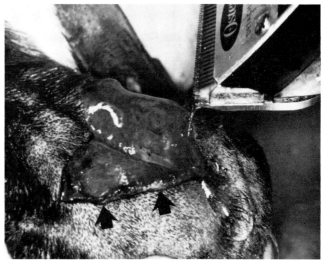

Figure 12–6: A traumatically raised pedicle flap (*arrows*) on the convex surface of an ear. This wound must be sutured to prevent contracture and a hairless scar. (Sterile lubricant is applied to protect the wound during clipping.)

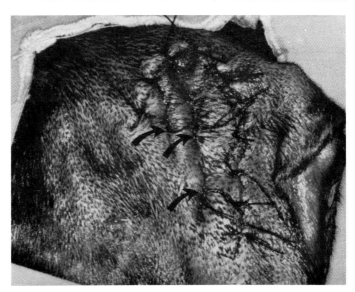

Figure 12–7: Sutured pedicle flap from Figure 12–6. The dead space has been obliterated with three through-and-through mattress sutures (*arrows*), as was done with the aural hematoma.

A 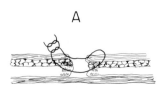   B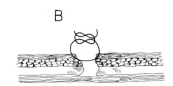

Figure 12–8: Suturing partial ear lacerations. *A*, Vertical mattress sutures may be used to align and stabilize the cartilage and skin. *B*, If the cartilage is stable, the wound may be closed with sutures in the skin's surface only.

the formation of hematomas, and disfiguring contractures may occur or sepsis may arise from this area, causing dehiscence.

Lacerations of One Skin Surface and the Cartilage.   Unsutured lacerations that extend through one skin surface into the cartilage respond similarly to wounds of the skin only, except that in longer wounds the cartilage template effect is lost and healing is delayed until the tissues acquire an adequate fibrous union. In this instance, healing by second intention may result in malalignment of the margins of the cartilage and disfigurement of the ear. Cosmetically, it is best to suture the skin at least, and if the cartilage is unstable at its margin, a vertical mattress suture is placed, with the deeper sutures aligning the cartilage and the superficial sutures aligning the skin (Fig. 12–8).

Lacerations That Extend Through Both Skin Surfaces and Cartilage.   The lacerations that extend through the pinna but not through the helical border, e.g., punctures or tears, heal adequately with conservative treatment (Fig. 12–9). Long tears may benefit cosmetically by suturing (Fig. 12–10), as do lacerations of one skin surface and the cartilage.

The most serious lacerations are those in which the full thickness of the ear is lacerated through a helical border (Fig. 12–11). When left untreated, the margin of such wounds epithelialize to form a permanent defect. Wound contraction during healing causes the defect to gap, resulting in a defect that is larger than the initial wound; consequently, these lacerations must be sutured soon after injury. A line of simple interrupted sutures engaging the skin is placed on each surface, beginning at the helical margin, or one row of simple interrupted sutures is placed on one side while vertical mattress sutures align both skin and cartilage from the other side (Fig. 12–10).

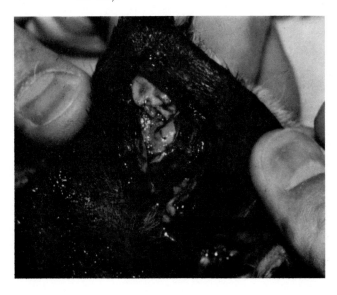

Figure 12–9: Contaminated wound penetrates the entire ear but does not extend through the helical border. This wound may be adequately managed with chemical débridement and healing by second intention. Pendulous-eared dogs may have a greater tendency toward contractural deformity.

Figure 12–10: Suturing full-thickness ear lacerations. *A,* A vertical mattress suture may be used to align and stabilize the cartilage and the skin on one side of the ear. Simple interrupted sutures are placed in the skin on the remaining side of the ear. *B,* The wound may also be closed by simple interrupted sutures that are placed only through the skin on both ear surfaces.

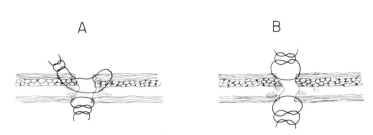

A   B

Avulsions of a Portion of the Pinna

The manner of healing for the margins of untreated avulsed wounds of the pinna is the same as that for through-and-through lacerations, i.e., by contracture and epithelialization. These injuries also widen as a result of chronic wound contracture. Rarely, if ever, will the avulsed portion be narrow enough to suture without causing excessive cupping or folding; thus, these wounds must be managed by other means.

The primary therapeutic objectives for treating the ear after a portion has been avulsed are to control hemorrhage, to prevent infection, and to allow wound epithelialization. These objectives can be achieved, simply, but the result of such conservative treatment is an ear with a defect, which may not be readily accepted by the owner. Other methods of therapy will result in a more cosmetic appearance.

Correction of Auricular Defects by Partial Amputation. Ears that have shallow auricular avulsions may be made cosmetically acceptable by partial amputation of the auricle. The amputation need not include the apex of the avulsion, and the amount of tissue that is excised should be minimal. Partial amputation is more completely discussed in the section on ear fissures.

Reconstruction of Small Auricular Defects With Pedicle Flaps. A defect of the auricular margin may be reconstructed by transposing a pedicle flap from the lateral cervicobuccal region. If a pedicle transposition is considered, preparation of the recipient site (the area of the auricular defect) is initiated early in the wound management, and it must be remembered that

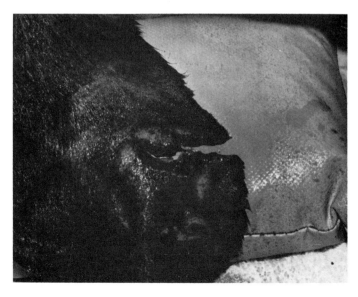

Figure 12–11: Auricular full-thickness lacerations through the helical border must be sutured.

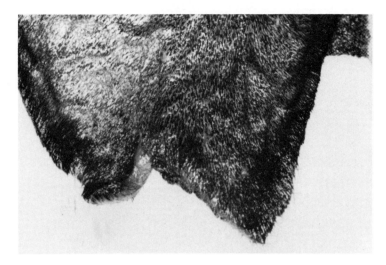

Figure 12–12: Marginal auricular defect to be corrected with a pedicle flap.

it is necessary to reconstruct both the concave and the convex epithelial surfaces. In this technique, no cartilage will be interposed.

After clipping the hair and cleansing the area around the auricular defect, sharp scissors are used to débride and reshape the margins of the defect, transforming them from ragged to straight edges while removing as little tissue as possible. A bactericidal ointment is applied and the ear is bandaged. The bandage is changed after three days. By seven days after the site has been prepared, the epithelium of the ear is more vascular and thicker, which facilitates the acceptance of a pedicle.

The best area from which to obtain skin for reconstructing an auricular defect is the cervicobuccal region. The skin of this area is loose and vascular and can be easily transferred. It will also provide a hair covering on the convex surface of the ear. The direction of hair growth in this area is generally similar to that on the convex surface of the ear, except near the ventral midline where the hair grows away from the midline and caudally. However, the pattern of hair growth in this area will vary with different dogs.

The hair from the donor (cervicobuccal) area and from the recipient

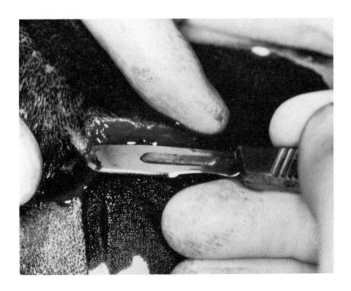

Figure 12–13: Splitting the margin of the defect and débriding the edges.

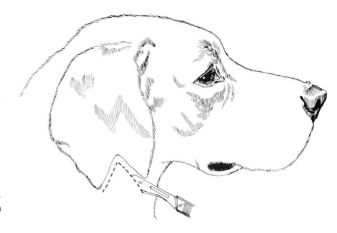

Figure 12–14: Ear in position over cervicobuccal area, with defect outlined on the skin.

(ear) area is clipped, and the sites are scrubbed 24 hours before surgery. The auricular defect is evaluated and measured (Fig. 12–12). The margins of the defect are split and sharply, but sparingly, débrided (Fig. 12–13). The ear is then placed over the cervicobuccal area in a comfortable position, and a skin marker or a light incision is used to outline the shape of the auricular defect on the cervicobuccal skin (Fig. 12–14). Full-thickness incisions are made along these lines but extend for 5 mm. past the lines. This produces the flap that will fill the auricular defect (Fig. 12–15). The flap is sutured into the defect beginning at the wound angle or centrum. Simple interrupted sutures of 4–0 polypropylene are placed from 3 to 5 mm. apart (Fig. 12–16).

The ear is protected under bandages for two weeks postoperatively. A bactericidal ointment is applied topically prior to the initial bandaging. Ideally, this bandage should suffice for the first week. More frequent bandage changes could disrupt the epithelial union and endanger the blood supply. After the flap has healed into the defect (two weeks), the area is ready for final transfer of the flap (Fig. 12–17).

Transfer of the pedicle flap may be completed by several methods: (1) the flap may be severed from the donor site at its base, and a pedicle flap

Figure 12–15: Pedicle flap formation. The pedicle flap shape is inscribed on the donor site by direct superimposition of the recipient site defect. The incisional lengths are 0.5 cm. longer than those of the recipient's margin.

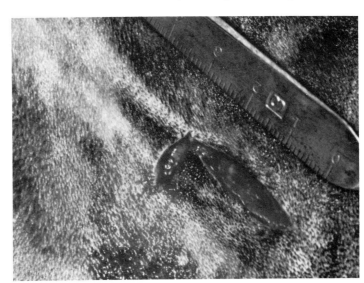

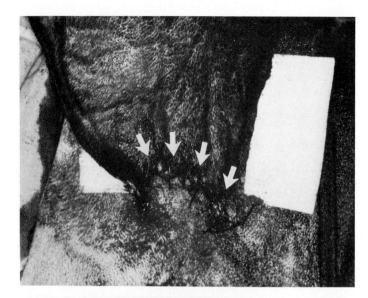

Figure 12–16: The pedicle is sutured into the defect with simple interrupted sutures (*arrows*).

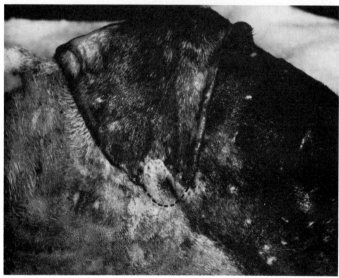

Figure 12–17: Two weeks after pedicle transposition the healed flap is ready for transfer. Note the proposed line of excision (*dotted line*).

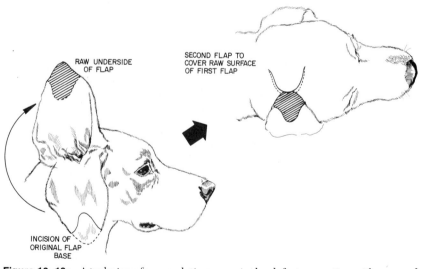

RAW UNDERSIDE
OF FLAP

SECOND FLAP TO
COVER RAW SURFACE
OF FIRST FLAP

INCISION OF
ORIGINAL FLAP
BASE

Figure 12–18: A technique for completing an auricular defect correction with a second flap.

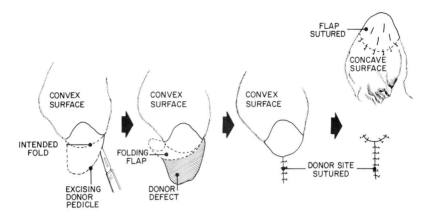

Figure 12–19: A second technique for completing an auricular defect correction with a folded pedicle. Vascular kinking and necrosis are more likely to occur with this technique.

from another site may be used to cover the concave auricular surface (Fig. 12–18). (2) After the flap has been severed, the concave surface may be left to heal by contraction and epithelialization if the area is not too large. (3) The site of pedicle origin may be incised in the shape of the contralateral defect, folded upon itself, and sutured. Avascular necrosis may result from crimping the blood vessels in the patch of skin when it is folded over (Fig. 12–19).

The transferred pedicle flap should be protected by applying antibiotic ointment and bandaging the ear over the dorsal cervical area. Bandages are changed twice or as often as necessary during healing, and the sutures are removed in ten days.

Ear Fissures and Ear Tip Dermatitis

Ear fissure wounds begin along the distal helical border and extend for differing lengths toward or into the scapha of the auricle (Fig. 12–21). They are most common in pendulous-eared dogs. These wounds are caused by continuous abrasion and ear margin seborrhea, which is especially prevalent

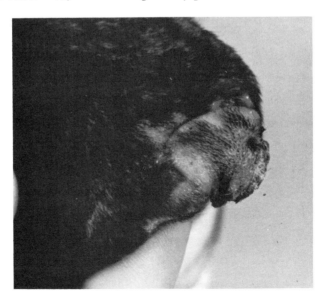

Figure 12–20: Completed pedicle flap after two weeks (convex surface).

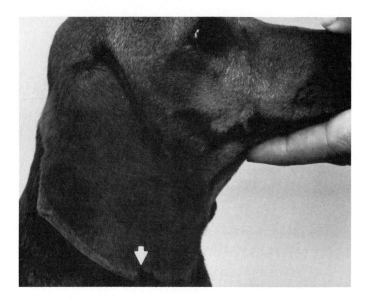

Figure 12–21: Ear fissure (*arrow*).

in dachshunds.[28] Fissures are aggravated by the shearing forces that are exerted on the ear during head shaking. They differ from lacerations in that they are chronic, suffer from repetitive trauma, and exhibit several stages of healing simultaneously.[28] Although they are dissimilar in onset, the ear tip dermatitis of erect-eared dogs that is caused by biting flies may be similar to ear fissures in effect.

The primary therapeutic objective in treating these two conditions is to interrupt the head shaking by treating the cause. Protecting the animal from insects by physical barriers or by repellents usually resolves the ear tip dermatitis, but the cause of ear fissures often seems to be related to some aspect of the fissure itself or to chronic irritation of the pinna. The secondary objectives of therapy are directed toward the fissure. Small fissures may be débrided, trimmed, and sutured, as may long fissures of short duration that have little tissue loss. Long fissures are normally chronic, however, and tissue contracture usually makes apposition of the wound edges by suturing impossible. These fissures are generally removed by partial amputation.

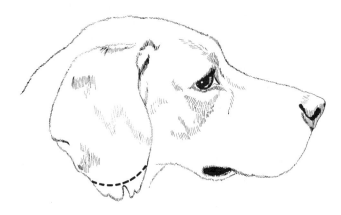

Figure 12–22: Partial amputation of the auricle. As little tissue as possible is removed when amputating a portion of the auricle, except when neoplasias are present, in which case wide amputation is suggested.

Partial Amputation of the Auricle. The amputation is performed in normal ear tissue as distally as possible on the auricle. The excisional amputation is made with scissors, and the wound is smoothed and curved to approximate the previous ear shape (Fig. 12–22). If significant hemorrhage is encountered, it is managed, when possible, by crushing and twisting vessels rather than by applying ligatures. The skin edges are apposed with a simple continuous suture of size 3–0 or smaller. The shortened ear may be cosmetically acceptable to the owner, or the owner may wish the contralateral ear to be shortened to match. As an alternative, single deep fissures may be managed by pedicle flaps that are taken from the neck and head, as is done with avulsed wounds of the auricle.

Regardless of the therapy, ears with these conditions must be protected from trauma until they are completely healed, and even then recurrence is common.

SOLAR, THERMAL, AND PRESSURE TRAUMA

SOLAR DERMATITIS OF WHITE EARS OF CATS

The white ears of cats are apparently more sensitive to the sun, which predisposes them to auricular solar dermatitis. The skin of the ear tip is exposed to more direct sunlight owing to the direction and quantity of hair growth. This condition is seen most often in warm, sunny climates.[28]

The initial lesion appears as a mild sunburn and results in alopecia. Because fewer hairs are protecting the lesion, its exposure to sunlight is increased and it burns. Over a period of years, the cartilage and overlying skin begin to deform. Ulceration of the skin over the helix is not uncommon. It is believed that solar dermatitis predisposes the ear to squamous cell carcinomas (Figs. 12–23 and 12–24).[4, 28]

The therapeutic objectives are to decrease the ear's exposure to direct sunlight by keeping the animal indoors during the afternoon or by applying sunscreening ointment to protect the ear margins and to amputate progres-

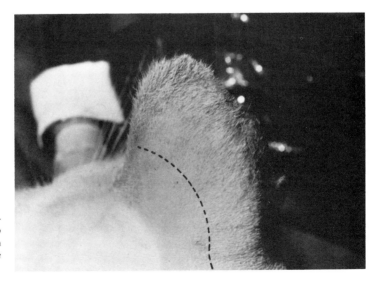

Figure 12–23: Feline solar dermatitis. Solar changes (*distal to dotted line*) are most common on the white ears of cats and are caused by chronic sunburn.

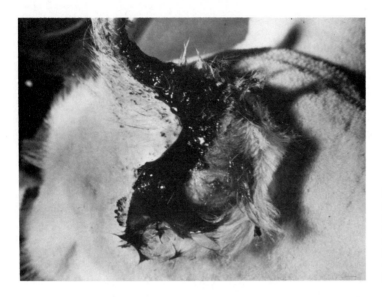

Figure 12–24: Squamous cell carcinoma. The contralateral ear of the cat in Figure 12–23 is shown with a squamous cell carcinoma. The lesion, which is crateriform and appears as a chronic wound, resulted from chronic solar exposure.

sive ulcerative lesions. Partial amputation of the auricle has been discussed in the section on ear fissures. Postoperative therapy is identical to preventive therapy.[28] (See also the section on neoplasia of the external ear in this chapter.)

COLD INJURIES OF THE AURICLE

Although the temperature of the ear canal is about the same as, and remains in a relatively constant relationship with, the temperature of the body core, the auricle is subjected to more radical variations in temperature because of its thinness and dependent position.

Cold injuries may occur when the environmental temperature is well above freezing owing to wind chill or exposure to water. The dog ear with a covering of hair is well insulated against this type of exposure. Cold injury of the dog's auricle is most likely to result from exposure to extreme cold in dogs with less refined preservational instincts. Cold injury resulting in tissue loss is fairly common in the northern regions of the United States and in Canada.[40]

In acute cold injury, the auricle may feel hard and there may be no response to painful stimuli. The most severe cases have clinical signs of avascular necrosis.[33] Systemic manifestations are rarely seen, and the frozen portion forms a dry eschar and desquamates. White hair regrows on the margin, and the cosmetic appearance is generally acceptable.[40]

Pathophysiologically, cold injuries progress to the point of dry gangrene and pass through three stages. Initially, cold induces severe arteriospasm and prevents capillary flow. Second, the vessels dilate, with a marked increase of capillary perfusion and permeability. The skin becomes reddish, warm, and painful. Third, red cells form aggregates and thrombi because of endothelial damage and plasma loss. Without treatment, the aggregates will organize within 72 hours to form an irreversible occlusive thrombus, and dry gangrene results.[33]

Current therapeutic recommendations for cold injury include rapid warming by placing the animal in a warm environment and by applying

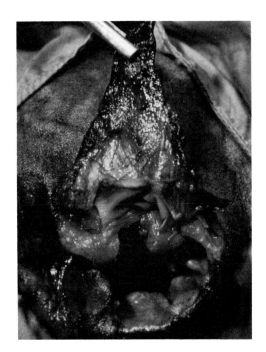

Figure 12–25:   Avascular necrosis of the auricle resulting from a bandage that was applied too tightly following cosmetic auriculoplasty.

warm (not hot) compresses to the affected part.[40] If gangrene occurs, amputation· at the line of demarcation is contraindicated because less tissue will generally slough than is suspected. The gangrenous area should be protected with sterile dressings. Additionally, it should be noted that healed tissues are more susceptible to subsequent exposure to cold[28] and may be predisposed to neoplasia.[23]

PRESSURE NECROSIS

Bandages that are applied too tightly to ears can impair auricular circulation. The result can be avascular necrosis of the auricle (Fig. 12–25). This should be kept in mind when bandages are applied following cosmetic auriculoplasty.

INFECTION

ETIOLOGY

There are several theories on the etiology of otitis externa. The possible causes include parasitism, fungal or bacterial infection, allergy,[16, 30] and endocrine alterations of substrates that allow opportunists to proliferate.[29] Under experimental conditions ear mites have been shown to play a more important role in causing otitis externa than do pure cultures of *Pseudomonas aeruginosa* (obtained from active otitis infections) or controlled trauma to the external ear canal.[15] The early histological changes that are associated with ear mite infestation include hyperemia, hyperplasia of the sebaceous and ceruminous glands, and infiltration of the tissues with macrophages and lymphocytes. Chronically, a crusty dried serum layer, ceruminous secretion, mites, mite detritus, and exfoliated epithelium are seen.[39]

Hypersecretion results in the exhaustion of the sebaceous glands, which become epithelial cords. The primary secretion-producing glands then become the apocrine ceruminous glands, which secrete a more watery substance; thus, the ear humidity increases.[8, 10]

Both *Candida albicans* and *Pityrosporon pachydermatitis* infections are common in dogs, but the importance of Pityrosporon as a primary pathogen has been questioned, and it has been called a nonpathogenic commensal instead.[2]

The common primary bacterial invaders are *Staphylococcus* and *Streptococcus* species.[28] The prevalence of these species is lower overall than that of other species, probably because of the resistance of the secondary invaders, such as *Pseudomonas, Proteus,* and coliform species, which are more common in chronic otitis.[11, 12] It is interesting to note that the 65 per cent prevalence of *Staphylococcus aureus, Pseudomonas aeruginosa,* and *Proteus* species has remained unchanged over the past 20 years; however, these organisms are currently more likely to be resistant to antibiotics.[3] Clostridial organisms may also be considered frequent pathogens.[29]

Otitis may also occur secondary to other skin diseases, such as seborrhea or allergic dermatitis.[11] Seborrhea causes hypersecretory ceruminous otitis in which the increased amount of cerumen obstructs the vertical canal and acts as a substrate for bacterial growth. Owners complain of foul odors around the head, and the condition does not respond to therapy, as do most cases of otitis. Remission is temporary, with a very high recurrence rate. Intradermal sensitivity testing and desensitization have not proved otitis to be initiated by inhalation or by atopic or contact dermatitis.

DIAGNOSIS

Certain minimum diagnostic methods are required for a thorough evaluation of an infected ear. The ear should be inspected grossly and with an otoscope to determine the extent of changes, the canal size, the condition of the epithelium, and the integrity of the eardrum and to look for the presence of foreign material or parasites. A microscopic examination of the exudate may be necessary to identify parasites or exfoliated cells.

In chronic cases a bacterial culture and sensitivity testing are mandatory. The exudate of the ear should ideally be cultured initially, and the exudate should be recultured after 48 to 72 hours, during which time the ear has been thoroughly cleaned with ceruminolytics or alcohol. By the time of the second culture, the number of opportunists will have been reduced, and the organisms in the deep tissue can then be identified. Sensitivity examinations will often reveal the resistant strains of organisms. It is unfortunate that sensitivity to individual antibiotics cannot be predicted;[4, 30] therefore laboratory assistance is necessary in cases of chronic otitis.

THERAPY

Conservative Therapy

Medical therapy is advocated in the presence of acute inflammation, suppuration, and evidence of systemic involvement and in milder infections in which the vertical and horizontal canals are adequately patent. Such therapy includes cleaning, drying, and specific chemotherapy.

Prior to cleansing, it may be necessary to sedate the animal. Cleansing methods include soap and water irrigation and curettage with a wire loop, as well as the application of ceruminolytic oils or alcohol. Following cleansing, drying is necessary and may be accomplished mechanically or by evaporation. The selection of antibiotics, antiparasitics, and antifungals should be based upon the identification of an organism and its sensitivity. The manufacturer's precautions should be heeded if ototoxic antibiotics are used concomitantly. Corticosteroids may be indicated topically and appear to be effective in reducing hyperkeratosis. Radiation and electric desiccation are also effective in controlling hyperkeratosis.[36]

Surgical Therapy

Surgical resection of the lateral vertical canal wall is advocated in cases in which three exacerbations of otitis have occurred in less than a year. The same operation is indicated when the vertical canal is obstructed but the horizontal canal is patent, when it becomes necessary to provide drainage laterally for the middle ear, or when curettage of a bulla of the middle ear is necessary.[32]

Resection of the Lateral Ear Canal.   Removal of the lateral aspect of the vertical canal has been called lateral wall resection, resection of the vertical canal and the Lacroix procedure. This procedure has been modified to include the relocation of a portion of the canal, as a ventral pedicle flap, this modification has been termed a lateral wall resection with a ventral graft and a Lacroix-Zepp or a Zepp procedure.[6, 41] Both the procedure and its modification provide adequate drainage, but the modification has gained greater acceptance because it reduces the likelihood of obstruction by hair around the cutaneous canal opening. Resection of the entire vertical canal to eliminate the source of proliferative otitis while maintaining the horizontal canal will be discussed in the section on management of neoplasia. Only the lateral wall resection with a ventral pedicle flap will be described here.

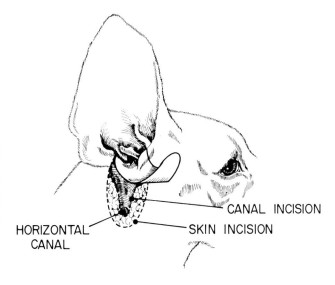

Figure 12–26: Incisions are made for resection of the lateral ear canal to form a ventral pedicle flap. Skin incisions from the tragohelicine incisure and intertragic notch are joined below the plane of the horizontal canal. The vertical canal is dissected clean. Here dotted lines show the proposed incision of the vertical canal cartilage. Although it is not actually seen at this point, the horizontal canal is shown for reference.

HORIZONTAL CANAL

CANAL INCISION

SKIN INCISION

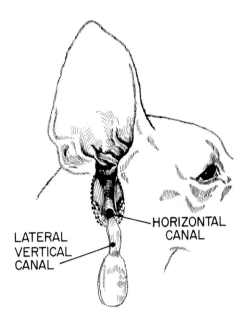

LATERAL VERTICAL CANAL

HORIZONTAL CANAL

Figure 12–27: Preparation for ventral pedicle flap placement. Following its incision, the vertical canal is pulled ventrally and used as a pedicle flap. Unnecessary skin and portions of the vertical canal are excised.

A vertical skin incision from the tragohelicine incisure and one from the intertragic notch are joined from 1 to 2 cm. ventral to the long axis of the horizontal canal. The skin flap thus formed is undermined and retracted dorsally. The lateral cartilage wall is then carefully dissected, and the parotid salivary gland is retracted ventrally. The lateral canal wall (cartilage) is incised from the skin incision's origins to the long axis of the horizontal canal (Fig. 12–26). In some instances, chronic inflammation induces osseous metaplasia of the canal cartilage,[8] and an osteotome or oscillating saw is required to incise the canal. A pedicle flap that is continuous with the floor of the ventral horizontal canal is maintained. This flap is folded ventrally after the cartilage

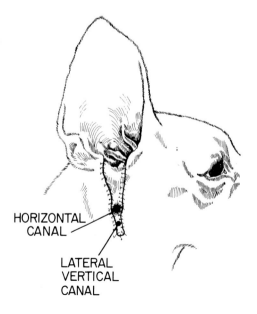

HORIZONTAL CANAL

LATERAL VERTICAL CANAL

Figure 12–28: Suturing the lateral canal resection and ventral pedicle flap formation. Sutures are placed in the flap, and enough tension is applied to open the horizontal canal and tilt it ventrally. The remaining vertical canal and skin are apposed with sutures that are placed 3 to 5 mm. apart.

(or bone) has been grooved, if necessary (Fig. 12–27). All but 1 cm. of the pedicle flap is excised and discarded.

The pedicle flap is anchored rostroventrally and caudoventrally to the skin with 4–0 monofilament sutures, placing moderate tension on the pedicle to open the horizontal canal and to tilt it ventrally. These and other sutures may penetrate the cartilage, if necessary, to provide security.[26] Additional sutures are placed to appose the skin and the epithelium of the cavum conchae (Fig. 12–28). Redundant hyperkeratotic epithelium may be removed by sharp resection or by electrosurgery from both the medial vertical and horizontal canals.

Partial Resection of the Horizontal Canal. Although it is infrequent, the horizontal canal may be compressed dorsoventrally as a result of fibrosis or of calcification and hypertrophy of the horizontal cartilages. The lumen may be enlarged by resecting the caudodorsal perimeter of the horizontal cartilages in lieu of total ablation. The site can be approached only after a lateral wall resection has been performed.

The epithelium of the cavum conchae is incised in the shape of an inverted "Y," with the arms extending cranially and caudally to the opening of the horizontal canal. The flap is undermined to expose the cartilage of the horizontal canal, and the obstructing cartilage is carefully rongeured away. This resection may be carried to the dorsal nuchal line of the squamous temporal bone. Finally, the inverted flap of the "Y" is advanced to an inverted "V" to pull the canal epithelium dorsally and to open the meatus (Fig. 12–29).

Ablation of the Ear Canal. Although it is possible, it is unlikely that otitis will progress to a state that requires ablation of the cavum conchae and the annular cartilage. These operations are more commonly associated with resections of neoplasia and are dealt with in that section.

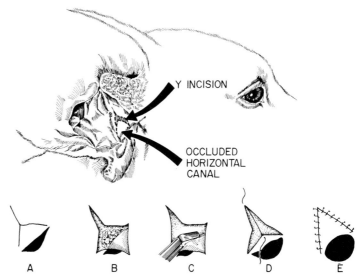

Figure 12–29: Partial resection of the horizontal canal. The vertical canal was previously resected. *A,* The skin is incised in an inverted "Y" in the caudodorsal region of the horizontal canal opening. The arms extend to the cranial and caudal aspects of the horizontal canal. *B,* The skin flaps of the "Y" are undermined to reveal the horizontal cartilage, *C,* which is rongeured away. *D,* Sutures are placed to reconstruct the inverted "Y" to an inverted "V" (*E*), thus opening the horozintal canal.

Aftercare

Although most animals tolerate the operation and the sutures with no evidence of irritation or discomfort, a sufficient number of animals mutilate the operative site to necessitate close observation at least. One episode of scratching can destroy the entire reconstruction. The ear needs to be allowed to dry and drain, but if the dog cannot be observed, protective measures must be taken. Sedation is not very effective in controlling self-mutilation because 5 per cent of the dogs will continue to traumatize the ear.[6] The better course is to use Elizabethan collars or plastic buckets with the bottom cut to fit the neck; if other means are not available, the ear may be covered by bandages.[12] Bandages must be changed daily, beginning immediately after the operation until about the third to the fifth day, when the drainage begins to cease. At this time dressings should be applied every third day until the time when the animal does not attempt to scratch the ear.

Systemic antibiotics are indicated because of the chronic and resistant nature of the associated organisms. The incidence of postoperative soft tissue infection is low. Topical agents should be applied to help dry the ear for the first three to five days. Medical aftercare is identical to conservative therapy.

Sutures are not usually removed before ten days. If topical corticosteroids have been used, the sutures are left for 14 days or until the wound is adequately healed.

NEOPLASIA OF THE EXTERNAL EAR

Neoplasia arising within the external ear canal must originate from the skin, the adnexa, or the cartilage; however, neoplasia arising outside the ear canal may develop from nearly any cell type of the body. The common neoplastic cell types that are associated with the ear canal are ceruminous gland adenomas (adenocarcinomas), papillomas, squamous cell carcinomas, histiocytomas, mastocytomas (sarcomas), sebaceous adenomas (carcinomas), basal cell tumors (carcinomas), and melanomas (sarcomas).

The management of neoplasia of the ear is identical to that of neoplasia of any other body part. Neoplasia must initially be diagnosed and the treatment must be prescribed accordingly. Diagnosis is based upon signalment (that portion of a patient's record that provides vital statistics), the biological activity of the neoplasia, and cytological and histopathological findings. Currently, the successful modes of therapy for ear neoplasia that are useful to the veterinarian include chemotherapy, radiation, and surgery, but the condition must be properly diagnosed before sensible therapeutic decisions can be made.

DIAGNOSIS

Signalment may help the veterinarian to decide which tumors are most likely to occur in an individual. For instance, an ulcerating neoplasia on the white ear of a cat would likely be a squamous cell carcinoma, or a raised tumor on the ear of a young dog would more likely be a histiocytoma than another similar-appearing neoplasia. Definite breed and sex predispositions are gradually being documented in the veterinary literature.[9, 19]

CHARACTERISTICS OF NEOPLASIA

Individual neoplasias of the same cell type are generally similar in site, origin, appearance, growth rate, growth pattern, and metastatic pattern, all of which may be summated as the biological activity of that particular neoplasia. It is this biological activity, along with the sex, age, breed, and color of the animal, that enables the veterinarian to make an educated guess regarding the tumor type and the therapeutic methods that may be required. The eight previously mentioned common cell types are briefly discussed here from the standpoint of biological activity.

TYPES OF NEOPLASIA

Ceruminous Gland Adenomas and Carcinomas. The ceruminous gland tumors arise from the apocrine glands of the ear canal at any point within the ear. They are small, rounded, nodular, or pedunculated lesions with a smooth surface and a pinkish coloration (Fig. 12–30). They remain small but recur readily after incomplete excision. The carcinomas may metastasize to the regional lymph nodes and the lungs.[22, 27]

Sebaceous Adenomas and Carcinomas. Sebaceous adenomas are very common in the external portion of the ear of older dogs. They are usually small, firm, smooth, and pedunculated. Their usual color is grayish white. Although it is unlikely, sebaceous carcinoma, which is rare, may metastasize, and surgical resection usually results in a cure.[4]

Papillomas. Papillomas may arise from any skin surface and appear as small (2 to 20 mm.), horny projections that may be pedunculated or may arise from a broad, flat base. The surface is irregular and cauliflower-like in appearance. Papillomas are usually singular in the ear canal. They do not metastasize and are not locally invasive.[4, 20, 27] Surgical excision is indicated.

Squamous Cell Carcinomas. Papillomas have a malignant counterpart in squamous cell carcinomas. When they are associated with the ear they are most often seen on the white auricle of the cat, but they may arise from

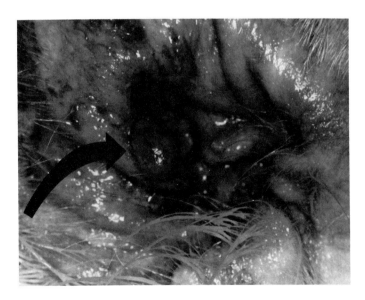

Figure 12–30: Ceruminous gland adenoma (*arrow*). Small tumors such as this one, as well as hyperkeratotic epithelium, may be surgically removed with very little hemorrhage.

any epidermal tissue on the ear. Their appearance is one of a chronic, granulating, infected wound with a crateriform center and proliferative margins Fig. 12–24). These tumors may be slow to metastasize systemically, but locally they are determinedly invasive.[4, 27] They may respond to radiation therapy.

Histiocytomas and Mastocytomas.   These two tumors are impossible to differentiate on gross examination. When they arise from the ear, they are usually located on the convex surface of the pinna, where they develop from the thin hypodermal or dermal tissues. They are reddish, raised, round, and dome-shaped as they displace the epidermis and become noticeable. Histiocytomas may regress spontaneously, whereas mastocytomas may become invasive and metastasize to regional lymph nodes. The surgical resection of single nodules is usually curative. Mastocytomas are sensitive to radiation and can be forced into temporary regression with the administration of prednisone.[4, 27]

Basal Cell Tumors.   Basal cell tumors arise from the stratum basale of the epidermis and are common on the head. They are usually raised, hard plaques but may ulcerate and become infected. These tumors may recur after incomplete surgical excision, but they do not metastasize.[4] Carcinomas are often responsive to radiation.

Melanomas.   Melanomas are round, raised, dome-shaped neoplasias that are common on the head. Depending upon the degree of malignancy, the growth rate may be slow or rapid and the tumor may be invasive. The color varies from black to pink, with the more anaplastic tumors being less pigmented. Heavily pigmented basal cell tumors may be confused clinically with melanomas.

Nonneoplastic New Growth

Nonneoplastic inflammatory polyps and papillary verrucose hyperkeratosis[14] are commonly confused with neoplastic processes. Verrucose lesions are epithelial exuberances that are possibly related to infection or local metabolic changes. Ultimately, the vertical canal becomes obstructed, and the functional changes in the canal liken the condition to a benign neoplasia.

Inflammatory polyps are more commonly seen in the cat than in the dog, and they arise from a thin pedicle that is usually attached to the tympanic area. They lie in the external auditory canal or communicate by way of their pedicle and the eustachian tube to the nasopharynx. Polyps are composed of richly cellular connective tissue, blood vessels, and leukocytes. The recommended therapy is surgical excision, although they may recur.[34]

Morphological Identification

Cytology and histopathology are the only reliable determinants of clinical impressions. Cytological specimens can be obtained by aspirating tumor cells with a fine needle and expelling them on a slide or by touching a slide to the open lesion in an attempt to isolate a few exfoliating cells. Conventional stain preparations may allow accurate diagnosis or at least further categorization of the cell as to type (i.e., round cells vs. spindle cells and so on.) These methods, along with textbook morphological descriptions of tumors, allow practitioners to train themselves to some aspects of cytodiagnostics.

Whether or not cytological findings confirm preoperative clinical suspicions, every tumor should ideally be subjected to histopathological examination following removal. Since histopathological methods can establish most neoplastic types and confirm or deny the previous clinical diagnosis, the practitioner gains experience in recognizing neoplastic types. Even the strongest suspicion should not preclude the use of histopathological confirmation.

Histopathological specimens may be harvested by biopsy needle or by total or partial excision. If cartilage is included in a biopsy specimen, the cartilaginous defect should be made triangular so as not to weaken the cartilage in any one plane and to prevent a deforming contracture. All tissues that are removed should be routinely submitted for histopathological study, but the cost to the client is occasionally of concern; thus, all excised tumors that are potentially neoplastic should, at the very least, be retained in 10 per cent formalin until the veterinarian believes that recurrence is not probable. If a tumor does recur, the specimen may be submitted for examination with very little time lost or insult added to the patient.

Regional lymph nodes should be palpated and surgically removed for histopathological examination when they are enlarged. This technique occasionally interrupts the metastatic process.

TREATMENT BY EXCISION

It is unfortunate that excisional surgery of or around the ear is usually avoided because of the fear of disfigurement and the misconception that the surgery is difficult or dangerous. Exposing the area for optimum manipulation can be difficult, but either resecting the lateral canal or simply incising and opening the vertical canal temporarily facilitates exposure. Surgical considerations may be divided between the two areas of occurrence, the auricle and the canal.

Neoplasia of the Auricle

Surgical Management. Neoplasias that arise in the centralmost portions of the auricle seem to occur more commonly on the convex surface. Small tumors on this surface are excised easily because the skin is mobile and a defect can be closed after undermining. Here the tumor should be adequately marginated based upon clinical suspicions. When undermining for closure, the dissection should remain close to the cartilage to avoid contact with vessels. It is usually necessary to suture the skin only. If a tumor has been removed from the concave ear surface and there is inadequate tissue for closure, the result of healing by second intention under a light bandage is usually cosmetically acceptable.

Management of neoplasia of the ear margin is the same as that of ear fissures, i.e., by partial amputation. Since it is better to have no auricle than an auricle with neoplasia, a wide excision is indicated. Reconstruction of the auricle with pedicle flaps, as described in a previous section, may also be considered.

Neoplasia of the External Canal

Surgical Management. Small neoplasms may be excised with scissors if they are near the surface or through an operating otoscope if small instru-

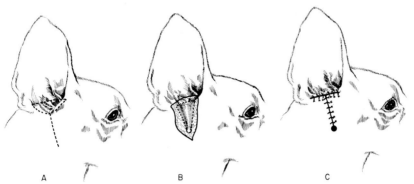

Figure 12–31: Excision of the vertical canal. *A*, The skin is elliptically incised around the cavum conchae's opening and down to the level of the horizontal canal. *B*, The soft tissues are undermined and the vertical canal is exposed. *C*, The vertical canal is excised, and the skin is sutured to the edges of the horizontal canal.

ments are available. Generally, though, a lateral resection or single incision of the vertical canal facilitates exposure. The single incision is conveniently and routinely closed.

Resection of the Entire Vertical Canal. Larger, more aggressive neoplasms or verrucose lesions may be removed along with the entire vertical canal while sparing the horizontal canal.[13] An elliptical skin incision is made from the anterior helix across the anthelix to the antitragus and around the proximal lateral aspect of the cavum conchae. Another skin incision is made down to the long axis of the horizontal canal. The vertical canal is dissected from the lateral to the medial aspect. The horizontal canal is transected, and the vertical canal is excised by completing the incision in the cartilage around the medial aspect of the cavum conchae near the anthelix. The skin flaps are advanced and sutured in the form of a "T," and the base of the "T" is sutured around the horizontal canal (Fig. 12–31).[13]

Ablation of the Ear Canal. Neoplasia that is confined to the limits of the external canal and below the opening of the external meatus may be excised by ablation of the cavum conchae and the annular cartilage. The skin is incised in the basic form of a "T," as in the resection of the entire vertical canal, but the dissection of the canal is carried to the squamous temporal bone. Dead space is obliterated with sutures, and the skin is sutured in a "T"-shaped closure (Fig. 12–32).[36]

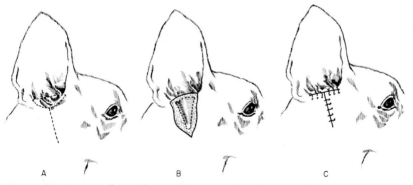

Figure 12–32: *A* and *B*, Ablation of the vertical and horizontal canals. Incisions are made and the canals are exposed, as with the vertical canal excision. *C*, The entire external ear canal is resected and the skin is closed as a "T," obliterating external communication of the ear.

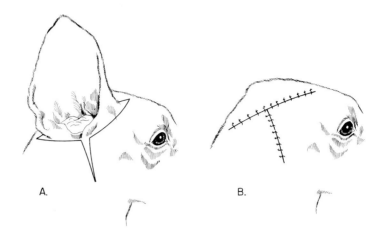

Figure 12–33: Amputation of the external ear. *A*, The skin is elliptically incised around the ear base, and an incision is made exposing the vertical canal. *B*, Alternate sharp and blunt dissection, which is performed close to the cartilage and extends to the squamous temporal bone, completes the dissection, and the skin is closed as a "T."

A.   B.

Auricular Ablation. Ablation of the entire ear is indicated when neoplasia involves the cavum conchae and the pinna. The skin is initially incised around the base of the ear and vertically over the vertical canal. The dissection is carried through the auricular muscles and vessels, which are ligated where appropriate. The dissection is again carried close to the cartilage and ends at the squamous temporal bone. Dead space is closed with sutures, and the skin is closed in the shape of a "T." (Fig. 12–33).[30]

When ablation is performed, care must be taken to avoid the parotid salivary gland, the internal maxillary artery, and the facial and trigeminal nerves.

MANAGEMENT OF DEVELOPMENTAL DEFORMITIES

Developmental deformities are not uncommon, but because they are symmetrical when associated with the pinna or hidden when associated with the canal, they are usually undetected except upon careful examination.[31] Several deformities of both the auricle and the canal will be discussed briefly.

AURICULAR DEFORMITIES

Owners frequently request euthanasia for a young puppy with auricular deformities, such as excessively small (microtia) or excessively large (macrotia) auricles, especially since these deformities are associated with other congenital abnormalities.[30] If the condition is asymmetrical and the owner desires, a portion of the larger ear can be excised to match the smaller ear (reduction auriculoplasty). Enlarging (augmenting) auriculoplasties have been reported in humans[26] but none have been reported in the dog.

CANAL DEFORMITIES

The ear canal is normally nonluminal until the 14th to the 21st day of life. The presence of an occluding membrane has been suggested but has not been determined definitely.[5, 30] It is possible for the canal lumen to form improperly (atresia or hypoplasia) and thereby prevent the normal expulsion of desquamated cells and sebum. The clinical signs of canal atresia resemble those of an abscess in a young dog — swelling of the canal, pain, and heat. The diagnosis of canal atresia is confirmed by the inability to detect a normal conchae. The condition is corrected by a lateral resection of the horizontal canal or ablation of the mass.[5]

Inflammation may also be present in conjunction with a dentigerous cyst (temporal odontoma). A fistula is usually present and, if it is dissected, an ectopic, incompletely developed tooth is found. Excision is usually curative.[30]

REFERENCES

1. Austin, V. H.: Selected case reports in small animal dermatology: Atypical feline cutaneous papillomatosis. Mod. Vet. Prac. 56:31, 1975.
2. Baxter, M.: *Pityrosporum pachydermatitis* in pendulous and erect ears of dogs. N. Z. Vet. J. 24:69, 1976.
3. Blue, J. L., and Wooley, R. E.: Antibacterial sensitivity patterns of bacteria isolated from dogs with otitis externa. J. Am. Vet. Med. Assoc., 171:362, 1977.
4. Bostock, D. E., and Owens, L. N.: Neoplasia in the Cat, Dog and Horse. Chicago, Year Book Medical Publishers, 1975.
5. Brodey, R. S.: Atresia of the vertical ear canal in a dog. J. Am. Vet. Med. Assoc. 155:1457, 1969.
6. Coffey, D. J.: Observations on the surgical treatment of otitis externa in the dog. J. Small Anim. Pract. 11:265, 1970.
7. Cowley, F.: Treatment of hematoma of the canine ear. Vet. Med Small Anim. Clin. 71:283, 1976.
8. Daniels-McQueen, S., Directo, A. C., and Garcia, J. P.: Ossification of the ear canal in an American cocker spaniel. Vet. Med. Small Anim. Clin. 69:747, 1974.
9. Dorn, C. R.: Epidemiology of canine and feline tumors. J. Am. Anim. Hosp. Assoc., 12:307, 1976.
10. Fernando, S. D. A.: Certain histopathologic features of the external auditory meatus of the cat and dog with otitis externa. Am. J. Vet. Res. 28:278, 1967.
11. Fraser, G.: Etiology of otitis external. J. Small Anim. Pract. 6:445, 1965.
12. Frazer, G., Gregor, W. W., McKenzie, C. P., et al.: Canine ear disease. J. Small Anim. Prac. 10:725, 1970.
13. Fraser, G., Withers, A. R., and Spreull, J. S. A.: Otitis externa in the dog. J. Small Anim. Pract. 2:32, 1961.
14. Getty, R., Foust, H. L., Presley, E. T., et al.: The macroscopic anatomy of the ear of the dog. Am. J. Vet. Res., 17:364, 1956.
15. Grono, L. R.: Etiology of otitis externa. Vet. Rec. 85:34, 1969.
16. Grono, L. R.: Studies of the microclimate of the external auditory canal in the dog. I. Aural temperature. Res. Vet. Sci. 11:307, 1970.
17. Grono, L. R.: Studies of the microclimate of the external auditory canal in the dog: II. Hydrogen ion concentration of the epithelial surface of the external auditory meatus. Res. Vet. Sci. 11:312, 1970.
18. Grono, L. R.: Studies of the microclimate of the external auditory canal in the dog: III. Relative humidity within the external auditory meatus. Res. Vet. Sci. 11:316, 1970.
19. Hardy, W. D., Jr.: General concepts of canine and feline tumors. J. Am. Anim. Hosp. Assoc. 12:295, 1976.
20. Hayden, D. W.: Squamous carcinoma in a cat with intraocular and orbital metastases. Vet. Pathol. 13:332, 1976.
21. Horne, R. D.: Personal communication, 1977. School of Veterinary Medicine, Dept. of Small Animal Surgery and Medicine, Auburn University, Auburn, AL 36830.
22. Jabara, A. G.: A mixed tumor and an adenoma both of ceruminous gland origin in a dog. Aust. Vet. J. 52:590, 1976.
23. Katsas, A., Agnantis, J., Smyrnis, S., et al.: Carcinomas of old frostbite. Am. J. Surg. 133:377, 1976.
24. Litton, W. B.: Epidermal migration in the ear: The location and characteristics of the generatii center revealed by utilizing a radioactive deoxyribose nucleic acid precursor. Acta Otolaryngol. Suppl. 240:5, 1968.

25. Miller, M. E., Christensen, G. C., and Evans, H. E. (eds.): The sense organs and integument, in Anatomy of the Dog. Philadelphia, W. B. Saunders Co., 1964; Evans, H. E., and Christensen, G. C.: Miller's Anatomy of the Dog. Philadelphia, W. B. Saunders Co., 1979.
26. Milton, J. L.: Personal communication, 1977. School of Veterinary Medicine, Dept. of Small Animal Surgery and Medicine, Auburn University, Auburn, AL 36830.
27. Moulton, J. E.: Tumors of the skin and subcutis, In Tumors in Domestic Animals. Berkeley, University of California Press, 1961, pp. 21–63.
28. Muller, G. H., and Kirk, R. W.: Feline solar dermatitis, in Small Animal Dermatology, ed. 2. Philadelphia, W. B. Saunders Co., 1976, p. 518.
29. Nesbit, G. H.: Chronic bacteria otitis and dermatitis: 195 cases. J. Am. Anim. Hosp. Assoc. 13:442, 1977.
30. Ott, R. L.: Ears, in Archibald, J. (ed.): Canine Surgery. Santa Barbara, Calif., American Veterinary Publications, Inc., 1965, pp. 243–281.
31. Pandy, A. N. J.: Experimental production of "cauliflower ear" in rabbits. Plast. Reconstr. Surg. 53:534, 1973.
32. Parker, A. J.: Bulla curettage for chronic otitis media and interna in dogs. J. Am. Vet. Med. Assoc. 168:931, 1976.
33. Shambaugh, G. E.: Surgery of the Ear. ed. 2. Philadelphia, W. B. Saunders Co., 1967.
34. Smith, H. M., and Jones, T. C.: Organs of special sense, in Veterinary Pathology, ed. 3. Philadelphia, Lea & Febiger, 1966, p. 1146.
35. Snow, J. B.: Surgical disorders of the ears, nose, paranasal sinuses, pharynx, and larynx, in Sabiston, D. C. (ed.): Davis-Christopher Textbook of Surgery, ed. II. Philadelphia, W. B. Saunders Co., 1977, pp. 1204–1215.
36. Spreull, J. S. A.: Ablation of the ear canal, in Borjrab, M. J.: (ed.): Current Techniques in Small Animal Surgery. Philadelphia, Lea & Febiger, 1975, pp. 68–70.
37. Tanzer, R. C., Bellucci, R. J., Converse, J. M., et al.: Deformities of the auricle, in Converse, J. M. (ed.): Reconstructive and Plastic Surgery: Principles and Procedures in Correction, Reconstruction and Transplantation, ed. 2. Philadelphia, W. B. Saunders Co., 1977, vol. 3.
38. Vine, L. L.: Corrective ear surgery. Vet Med. Small Anim. Clin. 69:1015, 1974.
39. Weisbroth, S. H., Powell, M. B., Roth, L., et al.: Immunopathology of naturally occurring otodectic otoacariasis in the domestic cat. J. Am. Vet. Med. Assoc. 165:1088, 1974.
40. Withrow, S. J.: Personal communication, 1978. School of Veterinary Medicine, Colorado State University, Fort Collins, Colo.
41. Zepp, C. P.: Surgical correction of diseases of the ear in the dog and cat. Vet. Rec. 61:643, 1949.

13

CORRECTION OF SPECIFIC SKIN DISEASES

D. J. Krahwinkel, Jr., D.V.M., M.S.

INTRODUCTION

Many skin problems that are encountered in veterinary practice are best treated surgically. Some of these conditions involve skin folds that lead to specific diseases; others are related to certain breeds of animals and their etiology is unknown. These problems will be dealt with in this chapter.

Skin folds in the dog and the cat cause a variety of problems, but most common is a moist pyoderma. Facial (nasal), tail (screw tail), and vulvar folds are the skin folds that cause the majority of problems. The statement that "the only satisfactory treatment of any skin fold pyoderma is surgical elimination of the fold"[20] is very apropos. Owners of animals that are to undergo surgery that will alter their appearance must be made fully aware of the consequences and must consent to the procedure, since skin folds are a desirable characteristic in some breeds and may affect the animal's future for show purposes.

FACIAL FOLDS

These skin folds across the nose have also been described as nasal folds[18] and lip folds.[8] The terms facial and nasal are more appropriate, since these skin folds are located across the bridge of the nose in brachycephalic breeds (Fig. 13–1). The problems arising from these folds are pyoderma[11, 20] and pigmentary keratitis.[1, 8, 18] The affected breeds are the Pekingese, the pug, the Boston terrier, and the English bulldog.[12] The long-haired breeds tend to have more problems with pigmentary keratitis because their hair lies against the cornea and causes irritation. The Pekingese can be severely affected, and the disease is more prevalent in highly inbred dogs.[8] The chronic irritation that is caused by the hair from the folds brushing against the cornea produces inflammation and vascularization, resulting in superficial pigment deposits on the cornea.[1]

The more common problem in short-haired dogs is the presence of pyoderma in the recesses of the folds. The accumulation in the folds of ocular discharges, sebum, and sweat secreted by the apocrine glands creates a

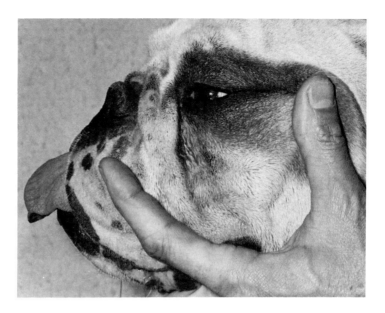

Figure 13–1: An English bull-dog with facial folds resulting in pyoderma.

favorable environment for a moist pyoderma.[20] This problem can be temporarily resolved by cutting the hair from the folds and treating the pyoderma topically. Permanent cure requires resection of the folds.

SURGICAL EXCISION

Any active infection in the folds should be treated with topical drying agents and antibiotics before surgery is performed. Anesthesia is induced with a barbiturate that produces an effect of ultrashort duration and is maintained with an inhalant anesthetic. It is essential to perform endotracheal intubation immediately owing to the potential obstruction in the upper airway

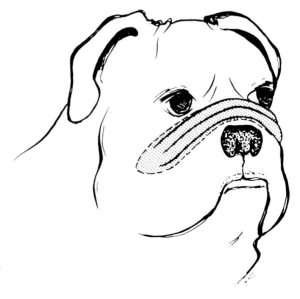

Figure 13–2: Paired skin incisions are made to remove facial folds.

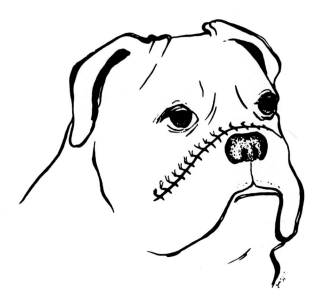

Figure 13–3: The resulting skin closure following excision of facial folds.

of the brachycephalic breeds. A protective ophthalmic ointment is applied to prevent injury to the eye during the surgical scrub. Hair is clipped from the folds, and a surgical preparation is applied. The procedure should be done as aseptically as possible.

Paired elliptical incisions are made from the ends of the folds on one side of the cheek, across the bridge of the nose, to the ends of the folds on the opposite cheek (Fig. 13–2). The incisions should be made far enough apart to remove all of the folds but not so far apart as to put tension on the resulting suture line. The skin between the incisions is bluntly separated from the subcutaneous tissue and removed. Deep dissection is not performed in order to avoid injury to the facial muscles and nerves.[12] The folds can be elevated and excised close to the face with scissors;[18] however, healing occurs more readily when the incisions are made with a scalpel. In some dogs, especially in Boston terriers, the folds do not extend across the bridge of the nose and therefore the incision should not cross the nose. The folds are removed by making paired incisions on each cheek. In chronic cases, hemorrhage may be profuse and should be controlled with electrocoagulation or ligation. If too much skin is removed, ectropion may result. Subcutaneous tissues are closed with 3–0 polyglycolic acid (P.G.A.) sutures, and the skin is closed with 4–0 monofilament nylon in a simple interrupted pattern (Fig. 13–3). If hemorrhage is profuse, a 0.25–in. Penrose drain may be left in the wound for 48 hours to prevent hematoma or seroma formation.

Postoperative care includes the administration of broad-spectrum antibiotics for five days as a prophylaxis against infection; they may also be administered to treat infection that is already present in the folds. An Elizabethan collar or tape applied to the front dewclaws is used to prevent scratching at the suture line. Sutures should be left in for 14 days, since healing may be retarded in these chronically inflamed areas.

INGROWN TAILS

In many dogs and cats with naturally short tails, the coccygeal vertebrae deviate ventrally and may ankylose in a corkscrew fashion. This has been

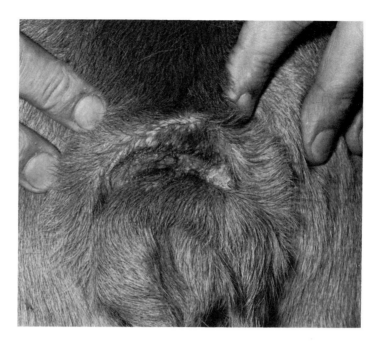

Figure 13-4: Ingrown tail on an
English bulldog resulting in tail
folds and pyoderma.

termed screw tail[20] and corkscrew tail[12] and has been reported to occur in the
Boston terrier, the English bulldog, the Schipperke, the pug, and the Manx
cat.[20] The ingrowth results in the deep skin folds that are lateral and ventral to
the tail (Fig. 13-4). Sebum, sweat from the apocrine glands, and fecal material
accumulate in the folds, resulting in a moist pyoderma. The pressure exerted
on the perineum by the ingrown tail and the itching of the pyoderma cause
the animal to scoot and to lick. Medical treatment of this problem is of no
value.[20]

EXCISION OF TAIL FOLDS

Some authors recommend excising only the skin folds, but most feel that
excision of the ingrown coccygeal vertebrae is necessary.[12, 20] The dog is
anesthetized and a purse-string suture is placed in the anus to include the anal
sac openings. Hair is clipped from the surgical site, and the area is prepared
for aseptic surgery. With the dog in a position of ventral recumbency, paired
elliptical incisions are made beginning at the level of the sacrum, continuing
lateral to the tail, and ending above the anus (Fig. 13-5). The incision is
carried through the subcutaneous tissue until the tail can be identified digitally. The coccygeal and levator ani muscles are severed close to their attachment to the coccygeal vertebrae (Fig. 13-6). The loose fascial attachment of
the rectum to the ventral side of the vertebrae is separated by blunt dissection. Bone cutters are used to transect the vertebrae where they deviate
ventrally. The coccygeal vessels are ligated, and any hemorrhage from the cut
bone is controlled with sterile bone wax. Penrose tubing is placed into the
depths of the wound for postoperative drainage and exits ventral to the
primary incision. The roof of the pelvic canal is reformed by apposing the
severed muscles and the deep fascia. The subcutaneous tissue and the skin
are closed in a routine fashion (Fig. 13-7).

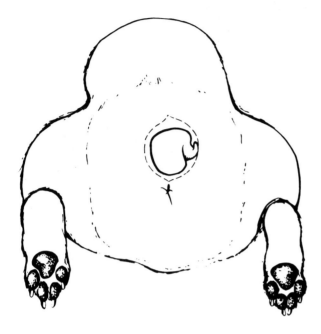

Figure 13–5: The skin incisions that are to be made for removal of ingrown screw tail.

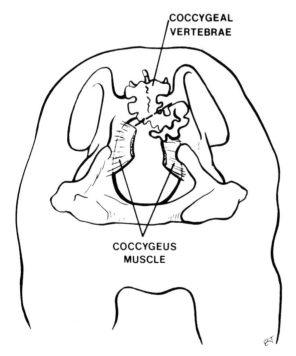

Figure 13–6: Pelvic area showing incision of coccygeus muscle and coccygeal vertebrae.

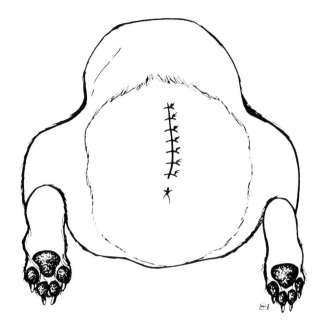

Figure 13–7: Skin is closed following excision of ingrown tail and associated skin folds.

The drainage tube is removed on the second or the third postoperative day. Parenterally administered antibiotics are continued for five days after removal of the tube. An Elizabethan collar is used if necessary to prevent the animal from traumatizing the wound. Skin sutures are removed in ten days.

VULVAR FOLDS

In the older, obese bitch with an immature vulva, skin folds tend to develop dorsal and lateral to the vulva (Fig. 13–8). There is no breed predilection, but the condition is reported to be worse in bitches that have been spayed at an early age.[20] The accumulation of moisture and urine results in an

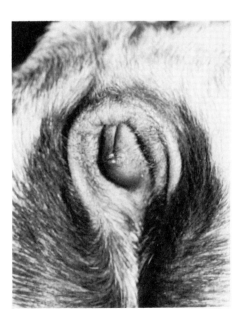

Figure 13–8: Dog with recessed vulva and perivulvar skin folds.

intertriginous irritation and a perivulvar pyoderma. A reduction in body weight helps to reduce the severity of the disease. Topical therapy that consists of cleansing, drying, and applying protective lotions and powders is helpful in the palliative treatment or preoperative preparation of the patient.[1, 20, 27] The bitch usually exhibits symptoms of scooting, licking, and discomfort, and the owner may complain of a bad odor from the vulvar area.

EPISIOPLASTY

The treatment of choice is to excise the redundant folds and to reconstruct the perineum in order to lift the vulva from its recessed position. Surgery is performed with the animal under general anesthesia and in a position of ventral recumbency. A purse-string suture is placed in the anus to prevent fecal contamination of the surgical site. An approximation is made of the amount of skin that must be removed to eliminate the folds.[6] A pair of crescent-shaped incisions is made in the perivulvar skin. The incisions extend dorsally from the 8-o'clock position to the 4-o'clock position (Fig. 13–9). The inner incision is made approximately 5 to 10 mm. away from the vulva, and the outer incision is made at a sufficient distance to eliminate the folds.[6, 27] The skin between the folds is elevated and excised, with close attention being given to hemostasis. Enough subcutaneous fat should be removed to insure that the vulva does not rest in a recessed position.[27] Simple interrupted skin sutures of monofilament nylon are placed at the 9-, 12-, and 3-o'clock positions to ascertain if a sufficient amount of skin and fat has been removed (Fig. 13–10). If it has not, these sutures are removed and additional tissues are excised. If the excision is adequate, interrupted subcutaneous sutures of 3–0 P.G.A. are placed to help relieve tension on the skin and the skin is closed with additional monofilament sutures that are placed alternately between the previous three sutures (Fig. 13–11).

Possible postoperative complications include seroma, wound dehiscence

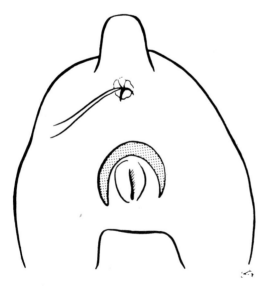

Figure 13–9: The skin that is to be removed in eliminating vulvar folds. (After Cawley, A. J., and Archibald, J.: Plastic surgery, in Archibald, J. (ed.): Canine Surgery. Santa Barbara, Calif., American Veterinary Publications, Inc., 1974, p. 168.)

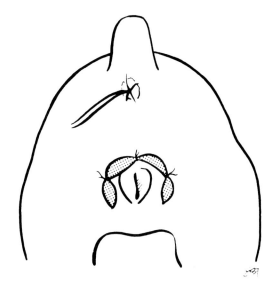

Figure 13–10: Placement of sutures at the 9-, 12-, and 3-o'clock positions to determine if sufficient skin has been removed. (After Cawley, A.J., and Archibald, J.: Plastic surgery, in Archibald, J. (ed.): Canine Surgery. Santa Barbara, Calif., American Veterinary Publications, Inc., 1974, p. 168.)

that is attributable to swelling or mutilation, and infection.[6] An Elizabethan collar may be used to prevent the dog from licking at the wound, and antibiotics may be administered parenterally for five days to control infection. Sutures are removed in ten days.

ACROPRURITIC GRANULOMA

These thickened, firm plaques on the dorsal surfaces of the front and hind limbs of the dog are also termed lick granuloma or acral pruritic nodules.[20] The lesions develop as a result of the dog's persistent licking of the affected area (Fig. 13–12). Even though the exact cause is unknown, nervousness or

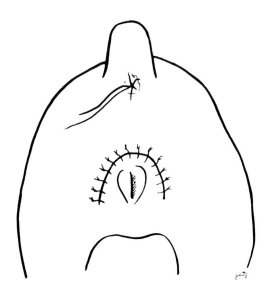

Figure 13–11: Completed suture line following excision of vulvar folds. (After Cawley, A. J., and Archibald, J.: Plastic surgery, in Archibald, J. (ed.): Canine Surgery. Santa Barbara, Calif., American Veterinary Publications, Inc., 1974, p. 168.)

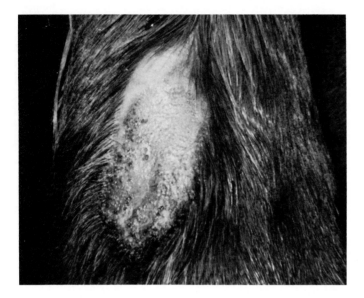

Figure 13–12: Acropruritc granuloma on the front foot of an Irish setter.

boredom may contribute to the behavior.[25] The lesions sometimes occur following an injury or surgical incision. The large breed dog over 5 years of age is most often affected.[20] In most cases the lesion is single, but multiple lesions may occur. The carpus and metacarpus are the common sites for this insidious yet persistent lesion.[20]

TREATMENT

When they are discovered and treated early, the lesions may respond to conservative therapy consisting of the intralesional injection of long-acting corticosteroids.[25] The area must be protected from further mutilation by the dog with the use of bandages, Elizabethan collars, and sedatives. Radiation therapy has produced favorable results in approximately 50 per cent of the cases.[3]

The intralesional and perilesional injection of cobra venom* has been successful in a high percentage of cases of lick granulomas.[20, 25] Up to 50 mouse units mixed with a 1:1000 solution of epinephrine results in six to eight months of remission and, in some cases, a permanent cure. Weekly treatments for two to three weeks are usually required. Intralesional and intramuscular injections of orgotein† have been highly successful in the treatment of canine lick granuloma.[21] The injection of 5 mg. of orgotein followed by a second injection one week later caused regression of the lesions that had failed to respond to other modalities.

If a small lesion can be removed surgically and its resulting wound can be closed without excessive tension, it should respond favorably. Careful suturing of the defect, using stent sutures when needed, is imperative for good results. The wound must be protected during the healing process by ban-

---

*Cobroxin is manufactured by Hynson, Westcott, & Dunning, a Division of Becton, Dickinson and Co., Baltimore, MD 21201.

†Palosein is available from Diagnostic Data, Mountain View, CA 94043.

dages, casts, or protective collars. Otherwise the dog may mutilate the wound, resulting in a second lick granuloma that is more extensive than the first. Even after healing is complete, the animal should be watched carefully, since boredom or compulsion to lick the area may cause a recurrence at the same site or at a different location. Skin grafts may be used to cover a defect that is too large for primary closure. Postoperative protection of the grafted site is essential, lest the animal destroy the graft and further aggravate the lesion.

Cryosurgery has been advocated recently as a treatment of lick granuloma.[11, 28] Liquid nitrogen applied by a probe or in a spray in a double freeze-thaw pattern to a minus 20° C results in the regression of some lesions. The cryonecrosis causes a slough of the lesion and healing occurs by contracture and epithelial migration. The resulting analgesia of the frozen area most likely accounts for the success in these instances. Some cases that respond initially and heal may recur within four to eight months. This phenomenon of recurrence is noted regardless of the mode of treatment.

ELBOW HYGROMA

Elbow hygromas occur in large and giant breed dogs as a result of trauma to the soft tissues overlying the olecranon (Fig. 13–13). The trauma is usually attributed to the animal's lying on hard surfaces. In mature dogs, this repeated trauma produces a protective skin callus over the caudolateral aspect of the elbow that helps to prevent the formation of hygromas. If no callus is present, the trauma produces an inflammatory response that results in a dense-walled, fluid-filled cavity. The fluid is characteristic of a serum transudate, ranging from yellow to red and being less viscid than synovial fluid.[22] The hygroma is a false bursa and is not associated with the synovial bursa that lies under the tendon of the triceps muscle.[9] One or both elbows may be affected.

Early in the course of the disease, a painless, fluctuant swelling is present over the olecranon process. As inflammation becomes more severe and ulceration occurs, the area becomes infected and fistulas develop.[20] The condition

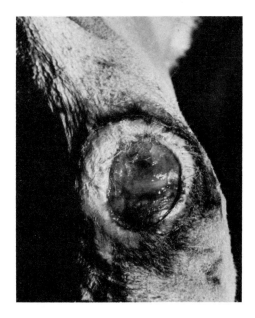

Figure 13–13: Ulcerated elbow hygroma on a giant-breed dog. (Courtesy of Dr. A. S. Dorn, University of Tennessee.)

becomes very painful, and the dog resists getting up and lying down. Occasionally the skin may show localized areas of calcification.[24]

If the condition is diagnosed and treatment is begun when the hygromas are small, surgical intervention is unnecessary. It is imperative to provide soft bedding in order to prevent further trauma. Padded "breeches" can be fitted to the dog to arrest the disease process.[20] Aseptic needle drainage of the fluid from small hygromas and the elimination of the cause of the elbow trauma are successful methods of treatment early in the course of the disease.[19] The injection of steroids into the hygroma is controversial. Some authors recommend their use,[1] while others are opposed.[8, 22] Small hygromas whose development can be arrested by eliminating the cause of trauma do not require treatment.

SURGICAL TREATMENT

When conservative medical therapy does not arrest the disease process or when ulceration has occurred, surgery is the treatment of choice. Large nonulcerated hygromas are treated by surgical drainage.[8] Early reports advocated the dissection and removal of the sac "in toto,"[1, 24] but this extensive and difficult dissection is probably not necessary. Following aseptic surgical preparation, stab wounds are made into the hygroma at the most proximal and distal boundaries. Fibrin masses and loculi are digitally removed through the stab wounds. A Penrose drain (0.25 in.) is placed through the hygroma and exits dorsally and ventrally at the stab wounds. The drain is sutured at both exits and left in place for two to three weeks. A bulky, well-padded bandage (e.g., Robert Jones' bandage) is placed over the elbow and changed at weekly intervals until the skin has adhered down and the pocket is obliterated (usually between three and four weeks). This technique does not excise any skin and saves any protective callus that may have developed over the olecranon. Other techniques involve incising the hygroma and removing the redundant skin.[22] When this procedure is performed, the resulting wound may break down, resulting in a large dehiscence and a more severe problem than the original one.

Advanced cases of hygroma may have large ulcerations and granulating wounds over the olecranon. These ulcerated wounds occur as a result of wound dehiscence, necrosis secondary to repeated trauma, or infection that is due to repeated needle aspirations. Complete resection of the ulcerated area is the treatment of choice.[9] An antibiotic dressing should be applied to the wound for one week to clear up any infection before surgery. The elbow is surgically prepared, and elliptical incisions are made around the area of ulceration (Fig. 13–14). Healthy skin should be preserved to prevent undue tension on the wound closure. The entire ulcerated area is excised, and the surrounding skin is undermined. Hemorrhage will be profuse because of the chronic nature of the disease. The skin closure is positioned so that the suture line lies either medial or lateral to the point of the elbow, which promotes healing. Stent sutures of monofilament material are placed through tubing to relieve tension on the primary suture line (Fig. 13–15). The skin is closed with simple interrupted sutures of monofilament material. When a large ulceration is excised and simple undermining fails to provide adequate closure, an advancement pedicle flap[10] can be constructed to cover the defect (Fig. 13–16A and B). This moves the suture line to one side of the elbow. Penrose

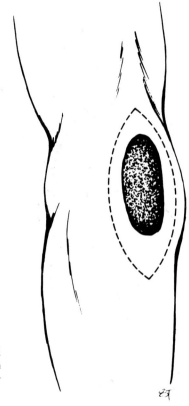

Figure 13–14: An ulcerated elbow hygroma illustrating the proposed skin incisions. (After Johnston, D. E.: Hygroma of the elbow in dogs, in Bojrab, M. J. (ed.): Current Technics in Small Animal Surgery. Philadelphia, Lea and Febiger, 1975, p. 294.)

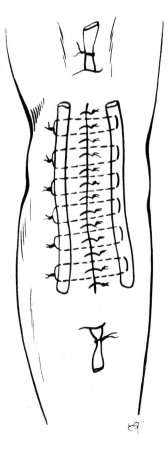

Figure 13–15: A drain tube is placed through the wound, and stent sutures are used to relieve tension on the skin sutures.

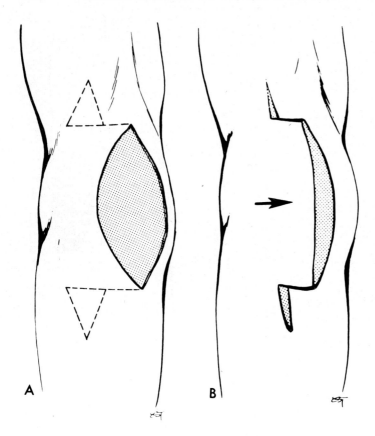

Figure 13–16: *A*, An advancement flap is fashioned by excising two triangular pieces of skin at the proximal and distal extents of the defect. *B*, The skin is moved by undermining the pedicle flap and advancing it (*arrow*) across the defect, thereby closing the triangles.

drains are used to prevent the development of postoperative hematomas or seromas. The wound is covered with a padded bandage and the elbow is immobilized with a Schroeder-Thomas splint or Robert Jones' bandage. Drains are taken out within three to five days, and the stent sutures are removed within five to seven days. The skin sutures and splint are removed in two weeks. The elbow should remain bandaged for an additional two weeks.

The inciting cause must be corrected postoperatively to prevent recurrence. The dog must be kept off hard surfaces, or elbow pads can be used to prevent further trauma.

PERIANAL FISTULA

Perianal fistula (also known as perianal sinus, perianal fissures, and furunculosis) is a progressive, necrotizing disease of the perineal region of the dog. It occurs most commonly in the adult German shepherd between the ages of 3 and 8 years.[5] Other breeds that are affected include the English setter, the Irish setter, the Labrador retriever, the cocker spaniel, and crossbreds.[4, 14] The condition appears to be equally distributed between males and females.

The cause is uncertain but is usually attributed to the accumulation of fecaliths in the anal sinuses (or crypts). These lead to necrosis, with resulting abscess formation and fistulas that erode into the ducts of the circumanal or hepatoid glands.[2, 4] The fistulas progress along the ducts of the glands and erupt through the skin around the anus. The broad, tight tail carriage of the German

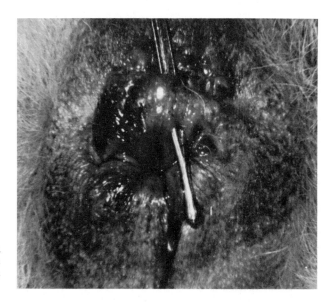

Figure 13-17: A German shepherd with a mild case of perianal fistulas. A probe has been inserted through one of the fistulous tracts.

shepherd may contribute to the disease by maintaining a fecal film over the anus and preventing adequate ventilation of the perineal region.[7, 23] The anal sacs may be secondarily involved but do not appear to contribute to the cause of fistulas.[2]

The clinical signs include tenesmus, dyschezia (painful defecation), perianal licking, odoriferous anal discharge with bleeding, weight loss, personality change, and pain on examination. Examination of the perianal region reveals fistulous tracts radiating from the anus into the surrounding tissue. In mild cases only a few tracts may be evident (Fig. 13-17) while in severe cases the tracts may coalesce and be so extensive that the anal opening is nearly obliterated.

TREATMENT

Medical therapy may help to control the problem, but it is seldom curative.[2] This treatment involves cleansing, cauterization, antibiotics, topically applied enzymes, hormones, and laxatives.[2, 23] Small isolated fistulas may be treated by opening the tract, dissecting away the lining, and permitting the area to heal by granulation.[17] Opening the tract followed by cauterizing the involved area may be effective in mild cases,[15] but this method does not produce results in advanced cases of the disease.

Surgical treatment has a high cure rate if it is performed in the early stages of the disease.[20] The surgical procedure involves excision of all diseased perianal tissue, including the anal sacs and the external anal sphincter when it is involved.[2, 4, 5] The dog is fasted for 24 hours preoperatively after which a warm water enema is administered to evacuate the colon. The oral administration of neomycin for 48 hours before surgery helps to reduce the intestinal flora and to prevent wound infection. Anesthesia is induced and then maintained with inhalant agents. Intravenous fluids are administered, since blood loss may be extensive. The cranial portion of the rectum is packed with gauze to prevent fecal contamination, and the hair from the perineal area is clipped liberally, including that from the base of the tail. Anal sacs are

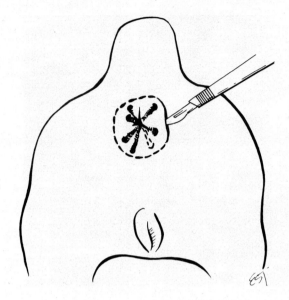

Figure 13–18: The initial skin incision is made to excise perianal fistulas. (After Christie, T. R.: Perianal fistula in a dog. Vet. Clin. North Am. 5: 353, 1975.)

flushed with antiseptic, and the perineum and anal canal are surgically prepared. The dog is placed in a perineal position with the tail retracted cranially.

If possible, the tracts are dissected individually, and the anal mucosa is sutured to the skin. In most cases this is impossible, and a 360° resection is required. The initial incision is made outside the fistulous openings in normal skin (Fig. 13–18). It is imperative that all diseased tissue be removed. Blunt dissection is directed toward the anus and separates the healthy deep tissues

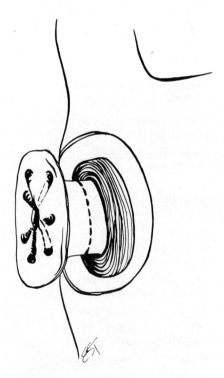

Figure 13–19: The diseased skin and anal canal are dissected free and excised. An attempt is made to preserve the external anal sphincter. (After Christie, T. R.: Perianal fistula in a dog. Vet. Clin. North Am. 5:353, 1975.)

from the superficial necrotic tissues. The anal sacs are removed as they are encountered in the dissection. The external anal sphincter is preserved if possible; however, if it is diseased, the affected portion is resected. When the rectal canal is reached in the dissection, it is transected cranial to the fistulous tracts (Fig. 13–19). The cranial and caudal rectal arteries, which lie on the dorsal and ventral aspects of the rectum, and the caudal rectal nerves to the sphincter should be preserved.[4] The anal canal and its associated fistulous tissues are removed. The surgical site is irrigated with antibacterial solution, and a rectocutaneous anastomosis is made. An absorbable suture is used to close the subcutaneous and perirectal tissue. Interrupted monofilament sutures are placed through the rectal wall and the skin to complete the anastomosis (Fig. 13–20).

Postoperative care consists of the systemic administration of antibiotics for one week. A low-residue diet and fecal softeners help to prevent straining and to minimize bowel movements. An Elizabethan collar is used if the dog licks at the surgical wound. Excessive handling of the tail should be avoided, since tension on the suture line may cause it to break down. Hot soaks can be used if swelling and inflammation are present. Sutures are removed in 14 days.

Complications, such as wound dehiscence, fecal incontinence, anal stenosis, flatulence, and diarrhea, are not uncommon.[5] A wound that has broken down can be resutured or left to granulate if the area is small. Fecal continence can be enhanced by preserving the caudal one quarter of the rectal wall[4] or by sparing the anal sphincter. Partial continence is achieved by the action of the pelvic diaphragm.[15] Anal strictures are best handled by incising the stenotic ring in four to six places, dilating the ring, and resuturing the mucosa to the skin.[4] If the entire anal canal is not excised, recurrence is possible. If this happens, a second surgical procedure is required.

A ventral coccygeal myotomy to set the tail has been reported to be successful in treating perianal fistulas.[26] The tail is placed in a vertical position and held by a brace during the healing period.

Cryosurgery has recently become a popular mode of therapy for perianal fistula. It has been advocated to "attempt cryosurgical treatment of perianal

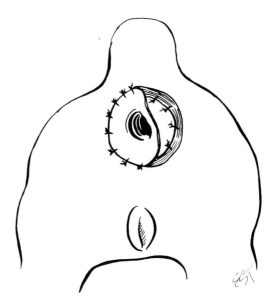

Figure 13–20: A rectocutaneous anastomosis is made by closing the deep tissues and suturing the rectum to the skin. (After Christie, T. R.: Perianal fistula in a dog. Vet. Clin. North Am. 5:353, 1975.)

pyoderma regardless of the appearance of the lesion."[20] Success has been reported with this method, the techniques of which are discussed in the literature.[13, 14, 16] The fistulous lesions are frozen with liquid nitrogen or nitrous oxide. Sinuses are opened and frozen using a repeated freeze-thaw cycle. The anal sacs are excised simultaneously. Frozen tissues are permitted to slough and healing takes place by granulation. Repeated treatments may be required at two- to four-week intervals until all diseased tissue has disappeared and has been replaced by healthy granulation tissue. Healing may require several weeks.

Postoperative complications of cryosurgical treatment are anal stenosis, odor and discharge, fecal incontinence, scrotal edema, and recurrence. The incidence of complications with this method appears to be no higher than that which occurs with conventional scalpel excision. Advantages of cryosurgery include the ease and the speed of treatment, the lack of hemorrhage, and low recurrence and incontinence rates.

REFERENCES

1. Cawley, A.J., and Archibald, J.: Plastic surgery, in Archibald, J. (ed.): Canine Surgery. Santa Barbara, Calif., American Veterinary Publications, Inc., 1974.
2. Christie, T.R.: Perianal fistula in the dog. Vet. Clin. North Am. 5:353, 1975.
3. Gillette, E.L.: Radiation therapy, in Carlson (ed.): Veterinary Radiology. Philadelphia, Lea & Febiger, 1977.
4. Greiner, T.P., and Betts, C.W.: Diseases of the rectum and anus, in Ettinger (ed.): Textbook of Veterinary Internal Medicine: Diseases of the Dog and Cat. Philadelphia, W. B. Saunders Co., 1975.
5. Harvey, C.E.: Perianal fistula in the dog. Vet. Rec. 91:25, 1974.
6. Hoffer, R.E.: Atlas of small animal surgery, ed. 2. St. Louis, The C. V. Mosby Co., 1977.
7. Horney, F.D., and Archibald, J.: Colon, rectum and anus, in Archibald, J. (ed.): Canine Surgery, Santa Barbara, Calif. American Veterinary Publications, Inc., 1974.
8. Jensen, H.E.: Ophthalmic Surgery of Domestic Animals. St. Louis, The C. V. Mosby Co., 1973.
9. Johnston, D.E.: Hygroma of the elbow in dogs. J. Am. Vet. Med. Assoc., 167:213, 1975.
10. Krahwinkel, D.J. Jr.: Reconstruction of skin defects by the use of pedicle grafts. J. Am. Anim. Hosp. Assoc. 12:844, 1976.
11. Krahwinkel, D.J. Jr., and Howard, D.R.: Reconstructive surgery. Proceedings of the American Animal Hospital Association, 1975.
12. Krahwinkel, D.J. Jr., and Merkley, D.F.: Surgical correction of facial folds and ingrown tails in brachycephalic dogs. J. Am. Anim. Hosp. Assoc. 12:654, 1976.
13. Krahwinkel, D.J. Jr., Merkley, D.F., and Howard, D.R.: Cryosurgical treatment of cancerous and noncancerous diseases of dogs, horses, and cats. J. Am. Vet. Med. Assoc. 169:201, 1976.
14. Lane, J.G., and Burch, D.G.S.: The cryosurgical treatment of canine anal furunculosis. J. Small Anim. Pract. 16:387, 1975.
15. Lewis, D.G.: Symposium on canine recto-anal disorders: III. Clinical management. J. Small Anim. Pract. 9:329, 1968.
16. Liska, W.D., Greiner, T.P., and Withrow, S.J.: Cryosurgery in the treatment of perianal fistulae. Vet. Clin. North Am. 5:449, 1975.
17. Lowry, E.C.: The perianal and anovaginal region, in Bojrab, M.J. (ed.): Current Techniques in Small Animal Surgery. Philadelphia, Lea & Febiger, 1975.
18. Magrane, W.C.: Canine Ophthalmology, ed. 2. Philadelphia, Lea & Febiger, 1976.
19. McCurnin, D.M.: Surgery of the canine elbow joint. Vet. Med. Small Anim. Clin. 71:909, 1976.
20. Muller, G.H., and Kirk, R.W.: Small Animal Dermatology. Philadelphia, W. B. Saunders Co., 1976.
21. Neibert, H.C.: Orgotein treatment of canine lick granuloma. Mod. Vet. Pract. 56:529, 1975.
22. Newton, C.D., Wilson, G.P., Allen, H.L., et al.: Surgical closure of elbow hygroma in the dog. J. Am. Vet. Med. Assoc. 164:147, 1974.
23. Palminteri, A.: Anorectal disease, in Kirk, R.W. (ed.): Current Veterinary Therapy: IV. Philadelphia, W. B. Saunders Co., 1971.

24. Piermattei, D.L.: Surgery of the skin and adnexa: Hygroma of the elbow. Proceedings of the American Animal Hospital Association, 1973.

25. Reid, J.S.: Acropruritic granuloma, in Kirk R.W. (ed.): Current Veterinary Therapy: V. Philadelphia, W. B. Saunders Co., 1974.

26. Smith, K.: Ventral coccygeal myotomy in the treatment of perianal pyoderma, in Proceedings of the 47th Annual Western States Veterinary Conference of the Intermountain Veterinary Medical Association, 1975.

27. Welser, J.R.: Episioplasty, in Bojrab, M.J. (ed.): Current Techniques in Small Animal Surgery: I. Philadelphia, Lea & Febiger, 1975.

28. Withrow, S.J., Greiner, T.R., and Liska, W.D.: Cryosurgery: Veterinary considerations. J. Am. Anim. Hosp. Assoc. *11*:271, 1975.

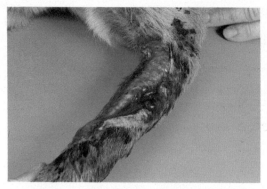

I-A: See Figure 2–2 (p. 42) for legend.

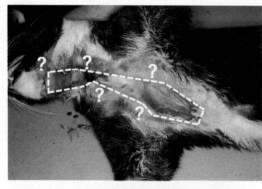

I-B: See Figure 2–4 (p. 44) for legend.

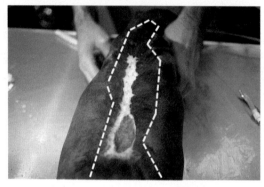

I-C: See Figure 2–5 (p. 47) for legend.

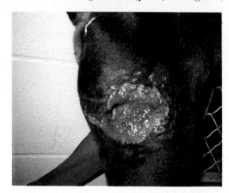

I-D: See Figure 2–11 (p. 58) for legend.

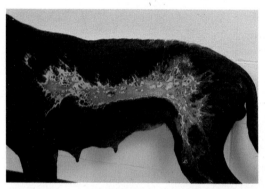

I-E: See Figure 2–15 (p. 63) for legend.

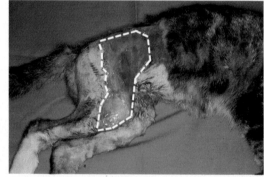

I-F: See Figure 2–16 (p. 64) for legend.

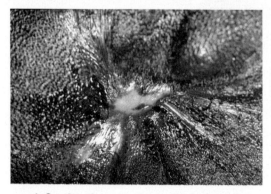

I-G: See Figure 3–20*B* (p. 95) for legend.

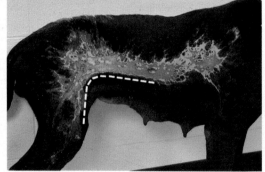

I-H: See Figure 3–21 (p. 96) for legend.

PLATE I

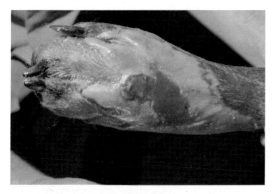

II–A: See Figure 3–22 (p. 97) for legend.

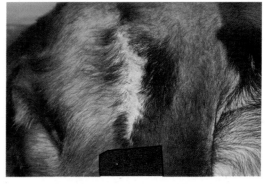

II–B: See Figure 3–24 (p. 99) for legend.

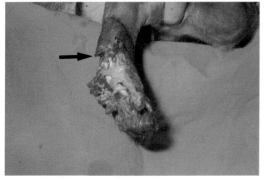

II–C: See Figure 4–10 (p. 168) for legend.

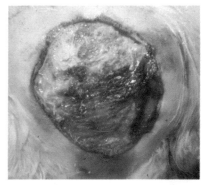

II–D: See Figure 4–15 (p. 175) for legend.

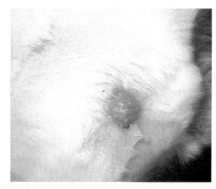

II–E: See Figure 4–16 (p. 176) for legend.

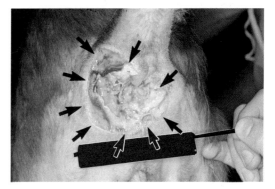

II–F: See Figure 4–27 (p. 203) for legend.

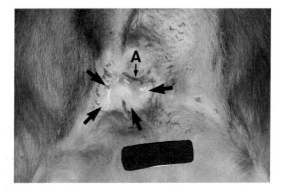

II–G: See Figure 4–28 (p. 204) for legend.

PLATE II

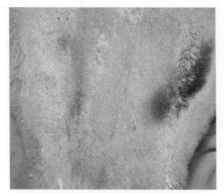

III–A: See Figure 5–1 (p. 216) for legend.

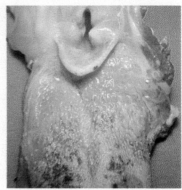

III–B: See Figure 5–2 (p. 217) for legend.

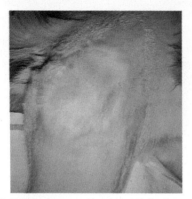

III–C: See Figure 5–4 (p. 223) for legend.

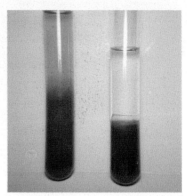

III–D: See Figure 5–5 (p. 225) for legend.

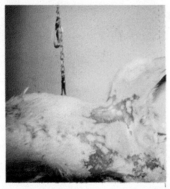

III–E: Left, See Figure 5–6A (p. 228) for legend.

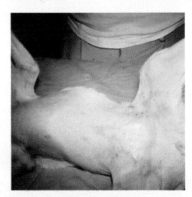

III–E: Right, See Figure 5–6B (p. 228) for legend.

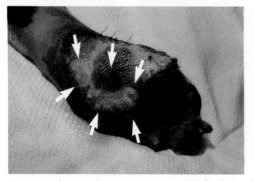

III–F: Left, See Figure 10–3A (p. 426) for legend.

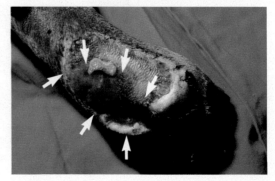

III–F: Right, See Figure 10–3B (p. 426) for legend.

PLATE III

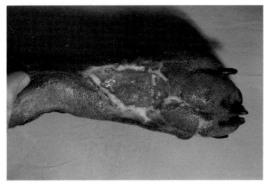

IV–A: Left, See Figure 10–9A (p. 436) for legend.

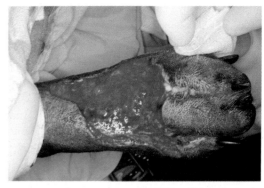

IV–A: Right, See Figure 10–9B (p. 436) for legend.

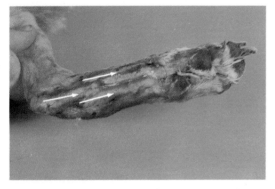

IV–B: See Figure 10–49 (p. 462) for legend.

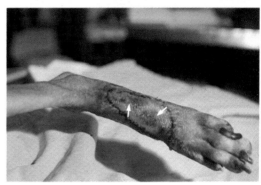

IV–C: See Figure 10–52 (p. 468) for legend.

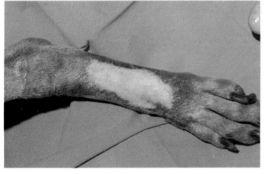

IV–D: See Figure 10–53 (p. 469) for legend.

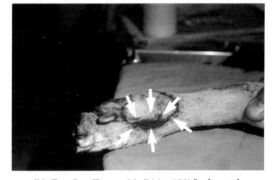

IV–E: See Figure 10–54 (p. 469) for legend.

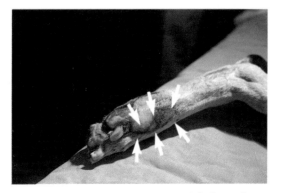

IV–F: See Figure 10–55 (p. 469) for legend.

PLATE IV

INDEX

Note: Page numbers in *italics* refer to illustrations. Page numbers followed by the letter "t" refer to tables.

Abrasion(s), epidermal, 90
Abscess(es)
  management of, 182–183
    antibiotics in, 155
Acetic acid, in wound lavage, 142–143
Acral granuloma, 65, *65*
Acropruritic granuloma, 557–559, *558*
Adenocarcinoma, feline, 52
Adenoma
  hepatoid, 49
  of ceruminous gland, 543, *543*
  of eyelids, 502
  perianal, 49
  sebaceous, of external ear, 543
Adhesive, liquid, for wound closure, 261
Adhesive tape, surgical, for wound closure, 260–261
Adipose tissue, 13–14
Advancement skin flaps, 358–362, 365–366, 368
  bipedicle, 365–366, *366–368*, 368
  single pedicle, 358–359, *359–363*, 361–362
Age, effect of, on wound healing, 100
Agenesis, eyelid, horizontal pedicle graft for, 510, *512*, 512–513
Aging
  hair changes in, 6–7, 19
  skin changes in, 6
Allografts, 463
Alopecia, epithelialized wounds and, 87, *88*
Anagen, 21, *22*
Anal sacs, 26
  removal of, in perianal reconstruction, 354, 357, 563 to 566, *565*
Anemia
  effect of, on wound healing, 100–101
  in burn patients, 220, 230
  induced, in skin flaps, 339
Anesthesia
  in skin flaps, 390–391
  in wound débridement, 128–129
Antibiotic(s)
  for dog bite wounds, 186
  for snakebite wounds, 191
  in wound lavage, 138
  in wound therapy, 101, 149–157
    history of, 149–150
    systemic, 154–156
    systemic and topical, 156–157

Antibiotic(s) *(Continued)*
  in wound therapy, topical, 150–154
    cytotoxicity of, 150
    scrubbing with, 153
    time factor in, 152–153
Antihistamines, for snakebite, 191
Antiseptics, in wound lavage, *140*, 140–143
Antivenins, for snakebite, 190–191
Anuria, in burn patients, 226
Anus
  fistula of, 562–566, *563–565*
  reconstruction of, transposition skin flaps in, 354, *357*
Apocrine glands, 24–25
Arrector pili muscle, 29
Artery(ies), of skin, *30–31*, 30–32, *33*
Asepsis, in wound débridement, 131
Aspirin, in wound healing, 101
Atrophy, of hair follicles, 17
Atropine absorption test, for skin flap circulation, 337
Aural hematoma, *523*, 523–525, *525*
Auricle. See *Ear(s)*.

Bacitracin, in wound therapy, 151
Bacterium(a), in wounds. See also *infections.*
  burn, 194–195, 230
  infection with, 63–65, 120–122
  quantitative analysis of, 160–161
  skin loss in, 64, *64, 568*
Balsam of Peru, in wound débridement, 148
Bandage(s)
  and injury, 62
  application of, 292–293
  changing of, 293–294
  for open wounds, 177–182
  for tubed pedicle skin flaps, 382, 383, *383*
  for skin grafts, 464–466
  in wound healing, 103
  pressure, 293
    and hemostasis, 243–244
    for open wounds, 178
    for skin grafts, 464
  tie-over, for skin grafts, 464–466, *465*
  waterproofing of, 293
Basal lamina, epidermal, 8–9

Basal layer, epidermal, 9
Basophil(s), 13
Bed(s), skin graft, 424–425, *426–427,*
    433–434, *436, 571*
Bee stings, 47–48
Bite(s), dog, *43,* 43–44, 184–186, *185*
    insect, 46–48, *47, 568*
    snake. See *Snakebite(s)*
Blepharoplasty, 477–519. See also *Eyelid(s).*
    corneal protection shield in, 477, *480*
    draping of patient for, *480,* 480–481
    instruments for, 477, *478–479*
    minimizing scar tissue in, 487
    operating room in, 481–482, 484
    preparation for, 477, 479–480
    principles of, 491–495
    surgical equipment for, 481–482, 484, 486,
        481–486
    surgical needles for, 490(t), 491
    suture materials for, 486–489
    techniques basic to, 493–495
        for shortening palpebral fissure, 495,
            495
        V–Y–plasty, *494,* 494–495
        Y–V–plasty, 494, *494*
Blood clot formation, in wound healing,
    72–73
Blood pressure
    control of, by skin, 4
    in burn patients, 218
    in skin flaps, 333
Blood supply, in skin flaps. See *Flaps, skin,
    blood supply in.*
    in wound healing, 100–101
    to skin, *30–31,* 30–32, *33*
Blood vessel(s)
    in degloving injury, 41–42
    in tubed pedicle skin flaps, 371–373, 376
    injury to, wound débridement in, 133–134
    of skin, *30,* 30–32, *33*
Bone, injury to, 183
    wound débridement in, 131–132
Bridging phenomenon, in skin grafts, 425,
    425
Brown dermatome(s), 445–446, *447*
Bunnell method, in tubed pedicle skin
    flaps, 371, *372*
Burns
    contamination of, bacterial, 194–195
    electrical, 215–216
    eschar of, removal of, 198–199
    mechanical therapy for, 198–199
    systemic therapy for, problem with, 195
    thermal, 62–63, *63,* 214–233, *568*
        and anemia, 220, 230
        and anuria, 226
        and cardiovascular changes, 218
        and Curling's ulcer, 217
        and electrolyte shifts, 218–220
        and fluid shifts, 218–220
        and hematological changes, 220, *221,*
            225
        and liver damage, 216
        and metabolic disturbances, 220–221
        and organic damage, 217–218
        and protein shifts, 218–220
        and renal damage, 216
        and respiratory tract damage, *217,*
            217–218, *570*

Burns *(Continued)*
    thermal, and shock 226
        classification of, 214–215
        depth of, 223–224
        effect of, on blood pressure, 218
        full-thickness, 215, *216, 570*
        surgical treatment of, 230
        management of, 222–230
        partial-thickness, 215, *223, 228, 570*
        pathological physiology of, 218–222
        severity of, determination of, 222(t),
            222–224, 225
        superficial, 215
    topical therapy for, 195–198, 227–229
Burn patient
    convalescent care of, 229–230
    dietary needs of, 229–230
Burn therapy
    corticosteroids in, 226
    enzymatic, 228–229
    exposure method of, 227–228, *228*
    fluid replacement in, 225–226
    local, 227–229
    steroids in, 230
Burn wound(s), reconstruction of, skin grafts
    in, 230, 473–474
Burow's triangle(s), in skin flaps *345,* 346
    single pedicle advancement, *361, 361*

Canthus, medial, neoplasms of, 513, *514,*
    515
Capillary infiltration, in wound healing,
    81–83
Carcinoma
    basal cell, of eyelid, 503
    of ceruminous gland, 543
    sebaceous, of external ear, 543
    squamous cell, 49
        of ear, 535, *536,* 543–544
        of eyelid, 503
Cardiovascular system, effect of thermal
    burns on, 218
Cartilage, in wound healing, 103
Castor oil, in wound débridement, 148
Cast(s), 62, 293, 466
Catagen, 21, *22*
Caterpillaring technique, in tubed pedicle
    skin flaps, 373, *373–375*
Catgut sutures, 164–165, 250–252, 488–489
Cautery units, in blepharoplasty, 484,
    484–485, 486
Ceruminous gland
    adenoma of, 543, *543*
    carcinoma of, 543
    secretions of, 522
    tumors of, 49
"Chalone," in epithelialization, 84
Chemicals
    cauterizing, and hemostasis, 243
    in wound débridement, 143–144
Chlorhexidine
    in burn therapy, 197–198
    in wound lavage, 142, 185
Chymotrypsin, in wound débridement,
    145–146
Circumanal glands, 24
Clear cell layer, epidermal, 10

Clips, metal, in wound closure, 260, *260*
Clostridium, infection with, 201–202
Closure, of wounds. See *Wound(s), closure of.*
Cold injury, to auricle, 66, 536–537
Collagen, in wound healing, 79–81, 98–99
Collagen fibers, in dermis, 11–12
Collagen sutures, extruded, 253
Collagenase, in wound débridement, 147
Contact guidance, in epithelialization, 86
Contact inhibition, in epithelialization, 86
Contamination
    fecal, antibiotics for, 152, 155–156
    wound, management of, 119–213
Continuous sutures
    cross sutures, 283–284, *283*
    horizontal mattress, 282, *282*
    intradermal, 275–278, *276–278*
    lock sutures, 282–283, *283*
    simple, 279–280, *279*
Contraction
    of skin grafts, 470–471
    wound. See *Wound, contraction of.*
Corium. See *Dermis.*
Cornea, protection of, in blepharoplasty, 477, *480*
Cortex, of hair shaft, 18
Corticosteroids, for thermal burns, 226
Cotton sutures, 255–256
Cross sutures, 283, 283–284
Cryosurgery, 203–208
    advantages of, 207
    cryoprobe in, *206,* 206–207
    disadvantages of, 208
    guidelines for, 205
    in perianal fistula, *203,* 204, *204,* 565–566
    indications for, 204
    media in, 204–205
        application of, 205–206
    protection of tissue in, 205, *206*
    techniques of, 204–207, *205, 206*
    thermocouples in, 205, *205*
Cryotherapy, for snakebite wounds, 189–190
Curling's ulcer, thermal burns and, 217
Cutaneous trunci muscle, 29–30
Cuticle, of hair shaft, 18
Cyanosis, in skin flaps, 339
Cytotoxic drugs, and wound healing, 108–109

Dacron sutures, 256–257
Débridement, 127–149
    and hematomas, 134
    and seromas, 134
    anesthesia in, 128–129
    asepsis in, 131
    blood vessel damage with, 133–134
    chemical, 143–144
    dressings in, synthetic biological, 180, *180*
    en bloc, 129–130, *130*
    enzymatic, 144–149, 145(t)
        castor oil in, 148
        collagenase in, 147
        dextran polymer in, 149
        fibrinolysin-desoxyribonuclease in, 146–147

Débridement *(Continued)*
    enzymatic, indications for, 14
        streptokinase-streptodornase in, 148–149
        sutilains in, 147–148
        trypsin-chymotrypsin in, 145–146
    history of, 127–128
    joint damage with, 131–132
    layered, *129*
    muscle damage with, 132–133
    nerve damage with, 133
    of dog bite wounds, 184–185
    of fascia, 134
    of fat, 134
    principles of, 129–131
    skin edges in, 135, *172*
    skin flaps in, 134–135
    tendon damage with, 132
    vs. excision, 128
Débridement stage of wound healing, 74–77, *75*
    monocytes in, 75–76
    neutrophils in, 74
    phagocytosis in, 75–76, *76*
Decubital ulcers, 60–62, *61–62,* 199–200, *199–201*
    transposition skin flap in, 348, *348–349*
Defect(s), of skin. See *Skin defects.*
Deformity(ies), developmental, of ear, 547–548
Degloving injury(ies), 41–43, *42,* 183–184, *568*
Dehiscence, wound, 168–169
Dehydration, in wound healing, 104
Denervation, in wound healing, 104
Dermatitis
    ear tip, 533–535
    solar, feline, 66, *66,* 535, *535*–536
Dermatome(s), 445–446, *446–447*
Dermis, 7, 10–13, *12*
    innervation of, 32, *33,* 34
Detergents, in wound lavage, 139–140
Dextran, in skin flaps, 339
Dextran polymer, in wound débridement, 149
Diethylstilbestrol, in skin tumors, 49
Dimethyl sulfoxide
    in skin flaps, 339
    in wound therapy, 152
Disease, systemic, skin as indicator for, 5
Dog bite wounds, *43,* 43–44, 184–186, *185*
Dog-ears
    correction of, 308–309, *309–310,* 311
    in transposition skin flaps, 351–352, *353, 354, 354–355*
Drains, in wound management, 157–160, *158–159*
Dressings,
    biological, 179, 463
        synthetic, 179–180, *180*
    for open wounds, 178–182
    for skin grafts, 464–467, *465*
Drugs,
    antibiotic. See *Antibiotic(s).*
    anti-inflammatory, in wound healing, 101–103
    cytotoxic, in wound healing, 108–109
    steroid
        in burn therapy, 226, 230

Drugs (*Continued*)
   steroid, in snakebite, 191
      in wound healing, 100, 101–103

Ear(s), 520–549
   anatomy of, 520–522, *521*
   avulsions of, 529–531, *530–533*, 533
   carcinoma of, squamous cell, 535, *536*
   cerumen production of, 522
   cold injury to, 66, 536–537
   deformities of, developmental, 547–548
   epithelial migration in, horizontal, 522
   external, neoplasia of, 542–547
      excision of, 545–547, *546–547*
   feline, solar dermatitis of, 66, *66*, 535, 535–536
   fissures of, 533–535, *534*
   hematoma of, *523*, 523–525, *525*
   infection in, 537–542
      diagnosis of, 538
      etiology of, 537–538
      medical therapy for, 538–539
      surgical therapy for, 539–541, *539–541*
   injury to, physical, 523–535
   lacerations of
      full-thickness, 528, *528–529*
      partial-thickness, 528, *528*
      superficial, 526, *527*, 528
   physiology of, 522–523
   pressure necrosis of, 537, *537*
   tip of, dermatitis of, 533–534
Ear canal
   ablation of, 541, 546, *546*
   deformities of, developmental, 547–548
   horizontal, resection of, 541, *541*
   lateral, resection of, *539*, *540*, 539–541
   neoplasia of, 545–546, *546*
Echelon sutures, in surface defect closure, 301, *302*
Edema
   in skin flaps, 337–338
   in wound closure, 167–168
   in wound healing, 104
Elastic fibers, 11–12, 81
Elbow, hygroma of, 287, *559*, 559–560, *561*, 562
Electrical burns, 215–216
Electrolyte(s), shifts of, in thermal burns, 218–220
Electrosurgery, and hemostasis, 243
Electrosurgical unit, in blepharoplasty, 484, *485*, 486
Enzymes
   in wound débridement, 144–149
   proteolytic, in burn therapy, 198
Epidermis
   abrasions of, 90
   anatomy of, 7–10
   layers of, *8*, 8–10
   reaction of, in wound healing, 85
   thickness of, 6(t), 8
Episioplasty, *556*, 556–557, *557*
Epithelial migration, horizontal, in ear, 522
Epithelialization in wound healing, 83–90, *84*
   "chalone" in, 84
   contact guidance in, 86

Epithelialization (*Continued*)
   contact inhibition in, 86
   hair follicles in, *85*, 85–86
   macroscopic appearance of, 87–89
   of incised wounds, 89–90, *90*
   of sutured wounds, 89, 89–90
Epithelium, changes in, after wound coverage, 86–87
Eschar, removal of, 198
Excretion, skin function in, 4
Eyelid(s), See also *Blepharoplasty*.
   agenesis of, 510, *512*, 512–513
   anatomy of, 491–493, *492*
   extramarginal lesions of, removal of, 504, *505*, 506
   histiocytoma of, 504
   injury to, 495–496
   lesions of, 501–504
      resection of
         full-thickness wedge, 507, *508*
         with vertical skin-muscle flap, 510, *511*
      skin flap for
         lower lid bridge, 515, *517–518*
         split-thickness advancement, 515, *516*
         split-thickness vertical advancement, 507, *509*, 510
   marginal
      lacerations of, repair of, 496, *497–500*, 499–500
      lesions of, vertical closure of, *506*, 506–507
      postoperative protection of, 500–501, *501*
   medial canthus of, neoplasms of, 513, *514*, 515
   melanoma of, 503–504
   motility of, 493
   neoplasms of, 501–502
   palpebral fissure of, shortening of, 495, *495*
   V-Y-plasty in, *494*, 494–495
   Y-V-plasty in, *494*, 494

Face
   folds of, 550–552, *551–552*
   wounds on, closure of, 355, *357*
Far-far-near-near sutures, 287–288, *288*
Far-near-near-far sutures, 287, *288*
Fascia, débridement of, 134
Fat
   débridement of, 134
   subcuticular, 13–14
Feces, contamination by, antibiotics in, 152, 155–156
Fibers
   dermal, 11–12
   wound, orientation of, 78–79
Fibrin
   in adherence of skin grafts, 427
   in blood clotting, 73
   in hemostasis, 243
   in wound healing, 73, 77–78
Fibrinolysin-desoxyribonuclease, in wound débridement, 146–147
Fibroblasts, 12
   in wound healing, 77–81

Figure-of-eight suture technique, in eyelid
    lacerations, 496, *498*, 499
Fissure(s), of ear, 533–535, *534*
palpebral, shortening of, 495, *495*
Fistula, perianal, 562–566, *563*
    complications of, 565
    cryosurgery in, 565–566
    surgical treatment of, 563–566, *564–565*
Flaps, skin, 321–393
    adaptation of, to recipient bed, 389–390
    advancement
        bipedicle, 365–366, *366–368*, 368
        single pedicle, 358–359, *359–363*,
            361–362
    anesthesia in, 390–391
    blood pressure in, 333
    blood supply in, 332–334, 337–340, 343
        axial, 340, *342*, 343
        impaired, 337–340
        random, 340, *341*
        tests for, 332–334, *335–336*, 337
    color of, 333–334
    cyanotic, surgery in, 339
    débridement of, 134–135
    delay of, 327–332
        advantages of, 331
        disadvantages of, 329–330
        physiological, 330, *330–331*, *331*
        techniques for, 327–329, *328–330*
    delayed, circulatory efficiency in,
        331–332, *332*
    dermal bleeding in, 333
    design of, 322–327
        length to width ratio in, 324–326
        "planning in reverse" in, 323–324,
            325
    distant, 322, 323(t), 368–389
        direct, 384–386, *385–389* 388–389
        indirect, 368–384
    edema in, 337–338
    effect of, on wound contraction, 97
    for eyelid lesions, 507, *509*, 510,
        511–512, *512–513*, 515, *516–517*, 518
    French, 358–362, *359–363*
    hair growth on, 333, 384–385, *385*
    hemostasis in, 326
    hyperbaric oxygen in, 339–340
    hypothermia in, 340
    indications for, 321
    infection in, 327, 338
    interpolation, 358, *358*
    island, axial, *342*, 384
    kinking of, 337–338, *338*
    local, 322, 323(t), 343–368
        nonpivotal, 358–368
        pivotal, 343–358
    long, delay of, *329–330*
    necrosis of, 337
    on limbs, 321, *322–324*, 384–389,
        385–389
    pattern for, 323, *324*
    pedicle
        horizontal, in eyelid agenesis, *510*,
            512, 512–513
        in auricular defects, 529–533,
            530–533
        single, 389, *389*
        subcutaneous, 362–365, *364–365*
    pouch, 384–386, *385–388*, 388

Flaps (*Continued*)
    skin, pressure on, 338
        radioisotope test of circulation in, 333
        reinnervation of, 390
        revascularization of, 389–390
        rotation, 343–347, *344–347*
        suturing of, *326*, 326–327
        temperature in, 333
        transposition, 347–358
            angle of, 351, *351–353*, 356
            areas where indicated, *348*
            bilobed, 354–355, *357–358*
                in facial wounds, 355, *357*
                tension on, 355, *357*, 358
            design of, 348, *350–353*
            dog-ears in, 351–352, *353*, 354,
                354–355
            double, 354, *357*
            in decubital ulcers, 348, *348–349*
            in perianal reconstruction, 354, *357*
            rotation of, *347*, 347–348
            sutures in, 353
            tension on, 350–352, *350–353*, 356
        tubed pedicle, 368–384
            advantages of, 382
            aftercare of, 382–384
            bandaging of, 382–383
            Bunnell method in, 371, *372*
            caterpillaring of, 373, *373–375*
            creation of, 369–371, *370*
            design of, 369
            disadvantages of, 382
            lengthening of, 381–382, *382*
            modifications of, 371, *372*
            on limbs, 368–369, *369*
            "pancake" technique in, *379*, 381
            recipient site of, covering of, 376–378.
                376–380, 381
            revascularization in, 376
            scar tissue in, excision of, 378, *379*,
                381
            sloughing in, 382, *383*
            sutures in, 370–371, *371*
            transfer of, 373–374, *373–378*, 376
            trap-door technique in, 374, *375*, 376
            tumbling of, 338, *373*, 373–374
            vasculature of, 371–373
            waltzing of, 373–374, *375*
        vascular insufficiency in, 337–340
        viability of, 134–135
Fluid(s)
    replacement of, in burn therapy, 224–226
    shifts of, in burn patients, 218–220
Fluorescein test, of skin flap circulation,
    334, *335*, *336*
Folds
    facial, 550–552, *551–552*
    vulvar, 555–557, *555–557*
Follicles, hair, *14–16*, *14–17*
    in wound epithelialization, 85, *85–86*
    terminal nerve receptors in, 32, 34
Foot pad, 34–36, *35–36*
    immobilization of following surgery,
        181–182
Foreign bodies, in wounds, 104, 135–136
French skin flaps, 358–362, *359–363*
Frostbite, 66, 536–537
Full-thickness skin grafts. See *Grafts, skin,
    full-thickness.*

Fungal infections, 65
Furunculosis, 562–566, 563

Gangrene, gas, 201–202
Gelatin foam, in hemostasis, 243
Gentamicin
  in burn therapy, 198
  in wound therapy, 151, 152, 155
Glands, 22–29
Graft(s), skin, 423–476
  adherence of, to bed, 427
  areas capable of supporting, 424–425
  areas not capable of supporting, 425
  bandaging of, 464–466
  bridging phenomenon in, 425, 425
  casts for, 466
  contraction of, 470–471
  degenerative changes in, 467–468
  delayed, 429
  donor site for, closure of, 441, 449, 459,
    459–460
  dressings for, 464, 466–467
  effect of, on wound contraction, 97
  fat in, dissection of, 13, 437, 438, 439
  full-thickness, 434–435, 437, 439, 441
    advantages of, 441
    application of, 439–441, 439, 441
    cutting of, 437, 437–438, 439
    disadvantages of, 441
    donor sites for, 435
    elevation of, 437, 438, 439
    indications for, 434–435
    patterns for, 435, 436, 437, 437
    sutures in, 439, 439–440
  growth of, 473
  hair coat of, 20–21, 441, 450, 450
  hematomas in, 430–431, 430–431
  immobilization of, 433, 464
  in burn wounds, 473–474
  indications for, 423
  infection in, 431–432
  loss of, 429–433
  mesh, 451, 453–455
    application of, 452, 453–454, 454
    cutting of, 451, 452–453, 453
    dressings for, 467
    healing of, 455, 455
    sutures in, 454, 454
  metaplasia in, 473
  plasmatic imbibition in, 427–428, 428
  postoperative appearance of, 468, 470,
    468–469, 571
  preparation phenomena of, 429
  pressure bandage on, 464
  reinnervation of, 471–473
  revascularization of, 428, 428–429
  sebaceous secretions in, 473
  seed-type, 456–461, 467
    application of, 457–459, 458–459
    cobblestone appearance of, 460, 461
    cutting of, 457, 457–458
    donor sites for, 457
      closure of, 459, 459–460
    granulation tissue bed of, 458, 459
    growth of, 460, 460
    placement of, 457–458, 458–459
  sensation in, return of, 472

Graft(s) (Continued)
  skin, sieve, 456, 456
    splints for, 466
    split-thickness, 423, 424, 442–451
      application of, 446, 447–448, 448–449
      capillary network in, 450, 450
      dermatomes in, 445–446, 446–447
      disadvantages of, 450–451
      donor sites for, 442
        healing of, 449, 449
      freehand cutting of, 442–445, 443–445
      hair growth on, 450, 450
      indications for, 442
      overlapped edges in, 446–447,
        447–448
    stamp, 461
    storage of, 434
    strip, 461–462, 462, 571
    success of, 427–429
    sweat secretions in, 473
    tie-over bandage for, 464–466, 465
    tie-over sutures in, 464–466, 465
    tunnel, 462
    Wolfe's. See Graft(s), skin,
      full-thickness.
Graft bed(s), skin, 424–425, 426–427,
  433–434, 436, 571
Granny knot, 272, 272–273
Granulation tissue, in wound healing, 82,
  82–83, 171–172, 172
Granular cell layer, epidermal, 10
Granuloma(s), 65, 65–66, 557–559, 558
Ground substance, 11
Gunshot wounds, 55–59, 56, 58, 192,
  192–194, 568

Hair, 5–7, 17–22
  anatomy of, 17–18
  pigmentation of, 19–20
  types of, 18
Hair bulb, 15
Hair bundles, 17
Hair coat
  age-related changes in, 6–7, 19
  density of, 6
Hair follicle(s), 14–15, 14–16, 17
  in wound epithelialization, 85, 85–86
  terminal nerve receptors in, 32, 33, 34
Hair growth, 7, 20, 20–22, 22
  cycle of, 21–22, 22
  on healing wounds, 88
  on skin flaps, 20–21, 333, 384–385, 385
  on skin grafts, 20–21, 450, 450
Hair root, 14, 17
Hair shaft, 14, 17–18
"Half-Z" Z-plasty, 403, 403
Halothane, in skin flaps, 390
Healing, wound. See Wound healing.
Heat loss, skin function in, 3–4
Hematoma(s)
  aural, 523, 523–525, 525
  débridement and, 134
  in skin grafts, 430–431, 430–431
  in wound healing, 109–110
Hemorrhage, in wound excision, 242–244
Hemostasis
  in dog bite wounds, 185

Hemostasis (Continued)
  in skin flaps, 326
  in Z-plasty, 408
  ligation and, 242–243
  techniques of, in wound excision,
    242–244
Heparin, mast cells and, 13
Heterografts, 463
Histamine, mast cells and, 13
Histamine wheal test, of skin flap
  circulation, 334
Histiocytes, 12
Histiocytoma(s), 49
  of external ear, 544
  of eyelids, 504
Homografts, 463
Hormone(s), in wound healing, 105
Horny layer, epidermal, 10
Hydrogen peroxide, in wound lavage,
  140–141
Hygroma, elbow, 559, 559–560, 561–562,
  562
Hypoproteinemia, in wound healing,
  105–106
Hypothermia, in skin flaps, 340

Immobilization, of open wounds, 180–182,
  181
Incision lines, relationship of, to tension
  lines, 300, 301
Indomethacin, in wound healing, 101
Infection
  abscesses, 182–183
  and wound scarring, 290
  bacterial, 63–65, 120–122
  clostridial, 201–202, 202
  fungal, 65
  in burn patients, during convalescence,
    230
  in decubital ulcers, 61
  in dog bite wounds, 43–44
  in ear, 537–542
  in gunshot wounds, 58–59
  in skin flaps, 327, 338
  in skin grafts, 431–432
  in wasp stings, 48
  in wounds, 106–107, 120–125, 135–136
    effect of sutures on, 165–166
    foreign bodies in, 135–136
    leukocytes in, 123–124
    lymph in, 123–124
    management of, 119–213
    resistance to, 124–125
    snakebite, 45
    soil and, 123
    Streptococcus in, β-hemolytic, 161
Inflammatory stage, of wound healing, 72,
  72–74, 74
Ingrown tails, 552–553, 553–555, 555
Injury(ies)
  bandage, 62
  cast, 62
  degloving, 41–43, 42, 183–184, 568
  missile, 55–59, 56, 58, 192–194, 192, 568
  physical, to ear, 523–535
  radiation, 59, 59–60
  to eyelids, 495–496

Inosculation, in skin grafts, 428, 428–429
Insect bites, 46–48, 47, 568
Insulin, in wound healing, 105, 175–177,
  176
Interpolation skin flap, 358, 358
Interrupted sutures, simple, 278, 279
Interrupted tension sutures, simple, 285,
  285
Intradermal knot, 277, 277–278
Intradermal sutures, 167, 274–278, 276–278
Intradermal tension sutures, 289
Irritants, and skin trauma, 63
Ischemia, 60–61

Joint(s), injury to, wound débridement in,
  131–132

Kanamycin, in wound therapy, 152
Keratinization, 8
Keratinocytes, 9
Ketamine, in skin flaps, 391
Kidney(s), damage to, and thermal burns,
  216
Knots, suture, 269–274
  granny, 272, 272–273
  intradermal, 277, 277–278
  square, 271, 271–272, 273, 273–274
  surgeon's, 272, 273
  tension of, 270–271, 270–271

Laceration(s)
  management of, 182
  of ear, 526–528, 526–529
  of eyelid, 496, 497–500, 499–500
  of skin, dog bite and, 43–44, 43, 184–186,
    185
  simple, 41
Lacroix-Zepp procedure, in ear canal
  surgery, 539
Langerhans' cells, 9
Lavage, wound, 136–143
  acetic acid in, 142–143
  antiseptics in, 140, 140–143
  chlorhexidine in, 142
  detergents in, 139–140
  high pressure, 137–138
  hydrogen peroxide in, 140–141
  moderate pressure, 137
  of dog bites, 185
  povidone-iodine in, 141
  saline solution in, 138
  water in, 138
Lesions, of eyelid. See Eyelid(s), lesions of.
Leukocytes
  in débridement stage of wound healing,
    74–76
  in infected wounds, 123–124
Lick granuloma, 65–66, 65, 557–559, 558
Ligation, and hemostasis, 242–243
Ligatures, sizes of, 250(t)
Limbs
  Z-plasties on, 411–412, 412
Lipomas, 50

Liver, damage to, and thermal burns, 216
Lock sutures, continuous, 282–283, 283
Lymph, in infected wounds, 123–124
Lymphatic(s), 32
    mammary, drainage of, 28

Mafenide, in burn therapy, 196, 227
Mammary glands, 26–29, 27
    innervation of, 27
    lymphatics of, 28
    neoplasms of, 28–29
    vasculature of, 28
Mammary tumors, 52–55
    growth of, 52–53
    incidence of, 52
    inguinal, 52
    malignant, 53
    metastasis of, 53
    surgical removal of, 53–55, 54
Mast cells, 13
Mast cell tumors, 50–51, 50–52
Massage, in skin flap circulation, 339
Mastectomy, 28–29, 53–54, 54
Mastocytomas, 50
    of external ear, 544
Mattress sutures
    horizontal
        adjustable, 285–286, 286
        continuous, 282, 282
        interrupted, 281, 281–282
        tension, 285–286, 286
    vertical, 280, 280–281
        tension, 286–287, 287
Maturation stage, of wound healing, 88,
    98–100
Medulla, of hair shaft, 18
Melanocytes, 9, 19
Melanoma(s)
    malignant, 49
    of external ear, 544
    of eyelids, 503–504
Merocrine glands, 25–26, 26
Mesh skin grafts. See Graft(s), skin, mesh.
Metabolism, disturbances of, thermal burns
    and, 220–221
Metal clips, for wound closure, 260, 260
Metaplasia, in skin grafts, 473
Metastasis, of mammary tumors, 53
Methy 2-cyanocrylate, for wound closure,
    261
Migration, epithelial, horizontal, in ear, 522
Migratory phase, in wound healing, 78
Missile injury(ies), 55–59, 56, 58, 192,
    192–194, 568
Monocytes, in wound healing, 75–76
Muscle(s), 29–30
    in axial island skin flaps, 384
    injury to, débridement in, 132–133
Mycosis, 65
Myofibroblast(s), in wound contraction, 92
Myositis, clostridial, 201–202

Nasal skin, 37, 37–38
Necrosis
    in open wounds, 175
    in Z-plasty, 407–408

Necrosis (Continued)
    of skin flaps, 337
    pressure, of auricle, 537
Needle(s), suture, 261–264, 262–264
        and tissue trauma, 263, 264
        in blepharoplasty, 490(t), 491
        passage of, 265–267, 266
Neomycin, in wound therapy, 151
Neoplasia
    in wound healing, 107
    of auricle, 546
    of ear canal, 545–546
    of external ear, 542–547
Neoplasm(s)
    mammary, 28–29
    of eyelids, 501–504
    of medial canthus, 513, 514, 515
Nerves
    in skin flaps, 390
    in skin grafts, 471–473
    injury to, wound débridement in, 133
    of mammary glands, 27
    of skin, 32, 33, 34
Neutrophils, in wound healing, 74
Nocardiosis, 65
Nodules, acral pruritic, 557–559, 558
Nutrition, in burn therapy, 229–230
Nylon sutures, 258, 488

Obesity, effect of, on wound healing, 100
Ophthalmic plastic surgery. See
    Blepharoplasty and Eyelid(s).
Otitis externa. See Ear, infection in.
Ovariohysterectomy, 55
Oxygen
    hyperbaric, in skin flaps, 339–340
    in wound healing, 81–82, 108

Padgett-Hood dermatome, 445, 446
Palpebral fissure, shortening of, 495, 495
"Pancake" technique, in tubed pedicle skin
    flaps, 376, 379–381, 381
Papilla
    dermal, 11
    epidermal, 8
Papilloma
    of external ear, 543
    of eyelid, 502
Pedicle skin flaps
    single, 389, 389
    subcutaneous, 362–365, 364–365
Perianal glands, 24
Perianal reconstruction, transposition skin
    flaps in, 354, 357
Phagocytosis, in wound healing, 75–76, 76
Phenylbutazone, in wound healing, 101
Pigmentation
    of hair, 19–20
    of skin, 5, 9
Pinna. See Ear(s).
Planum nasale, 37, 37–38
Plasmatic imbibition, in skin grafts,
    427–428, 428
Plastic surgery, ophthalmic. See
    Blepharoplasty and Eyelid(s).
Plasty(ies). See V-Y-plasty, W-plasty, Y-V
    plasty, and Z-plasty(ies).

Plexuses, arterial, 31–32
Polyamide sutures, 258–259
Polyester sutures, 256–257
Polyglactin 910 sutures, 254, 489
Polyglycolic acid sutures, 165, 253–254, 489
Polymyxin B, in wound therapy, 151
Polyolefin sutures, 257–258
Pouch skin flaps, 384–386, 385–388, 388
Poulard's technique, in fusiform defects, 307–308
Povidone-iodine
  in blepharoplasty, 479
  in burn therapy, 197
  in granulation tissue bed preparation, 434
  in wound lavage, 141
  in wound preparation, 126
Precollagen, 12
Pressure bandages, 293
  and hemostasis, 243–244
  for open wounds, 178
  for skin grafts, 464
Prickle cell layer, epidermal, 9–10
Proliferative phase, in wound healing, 80
Protein(s)
  recognition of, by skin, 5
  shifts of, thermal burns and, 218–220
Proteolytic enzymes, in burn therapy, 198, 228–229
"Pseudohealing," 168, 168
Pulley sutures, 287, 288
Pyoderma, 64–65
  in facial folds, 550–551, 551
  in ingrown tails, 552–553, 553
  in vulvar folds, 555, 555–556

Quantitative analysis, of bacteria, 160–161

Radiation, and wound healing, 108–109
Radiation injury, 59, 59–60
Radioisotope test, of skin flap circulation, 333
Rapid-slide technique, in quantitative analysis of bacteria, 161
Reese dermatome(s), 445
Reinnervation
  of skin flaps, 390
  of skin grafts, 471–473
Repair, of skin, 5
Repair stage, of wound healing. See Wound healing, repair stage of.
Respiratory tract, damage to, thermal burns and, 217–218, 217
Rete ridges, 8
Reticulin fibers, 11–12
Revascularization
  of skin flaps, 376, 389–390
  of skin grafts, 428, 428–429
Root sheaths, of hair follicles, 14–15
Rotation skin flaps, 343–347, 344–347

Sacrum, skin flaps over, 359, 359, 360
Sacs, anal, 26
  removal of, in perianal reconstruction, 354, 357, 563–566, 565
Saline solution, in wound lavage, 138

Saline wheal test, of skin flap circulation, 334
Scab formation, in wound healing, 72–73
Scar(s)
  infection and, 290
  tension and, 289, 289–290
  widened, 99, 99–100, 569
    W-plasty in, 417–418, 416–418
    Z-plasty in, 408–409, 408–409
Scar tissue, excision of, from tubed pedicle skin flaps, 378, 379, 381
Scrotum, 36
Sebaceous glands, 23, 23–24
Sebaceous secretions, in skin grafts, 473
Sebum, 23–24
Secretion, skin function in, 4
Seed-type skin grafts. See Grafts, skin, seed-type.
Sensory perception, skin function in, 4
Seroma(s)
  débridement and, 134
  in wound healing, 109–110
  under skin grafts, 430–431
Shock, thermal burns and, 226
Sieve skin grafts, 456, 456
Silk sutures, 254–255
Silver nitrate solution, in burn therapy, 195–196
Silver sulfadiazine, in burn therapy, 196–197, 227
Skin
  age-related change in, 6
  anatomy of, 3–39, 7
  blood supply to, 30–32, 30–31, 33
  breakdown of, in decubital ulcers, 61
  degloving of, 41–43, 42, 183–184, 568
  denervation of, 104
  diseases of, 550–567
  functions of, 3–5
  innervation of, 32, 33, 34
  nasal, 37, 37–38
  physiology of, 3–39
  pigmentation of, 5, 9
  reparation properties of, 5
  thickness of, 6, 6(t)
  trauma to, 40–69. See also specific types of trauma, e.g., Burns, Snakebite(s), etc.
    in wound healing, 110–111
    injection of irritants and, 63
    miscellaneous sources of, 67
    suture needle and, 263, 264
  undermining of, in wound closure, 240–242, 241
Skin defects, 297–320
  chevron-shaped, 314, 315, 317
  circular, 317, 318, 319
  crescent-shaped, 316, 317
  fusiform, 305–308, 305–306, 308
  oval, 316, 317
  parallel, 316, 317
  rectangular, 311, 311
  reorientation of, by Z-plasty, 396–397, 408–411, 409
  square, 310, 311
  triangular, 312, 312–314
  wedge-shaped, 312–314, 312–314
Skin edge(s)
  débridement of, 172
  excision of, 135
Skin flaps. See Flaps, skin.

Skin folds, 17, *17*
  of face, 550–552, *551–552*
  of tail, 553–555, *553–555*
  of vulva, 555–557, *555–557*
Skin grafts. See *Graft(s), skin.*
Skin tumors, 48–52
Snakebite(s), 44–46, 186–192
  cryotherapy for, 189–190
  drugs in, 190–191
  lethal, 44
  reaction to, 45
  venom of, *44*, 44–45, *568*
Soaps, in wound lavage, 139–140
Soil, and wound infection, 123
Solar dermatitis, 66, *66*
Spider bites, 46–47
Spinous cell layer, epidermal, 9
Splints, 293, 466
Split-thickness skin grafts. See *Graft(s), skin, split-thickness.*
Square knots, *271*, 271–272, *273*, 273–274
Stainless steel sutures, 256
Stamp skin graft, 461
Stent sutures, *288*, 288–289
Steroids
  in burn therapy, 230
  in snakebite, 191
  in wound healing, 100, 101–103
Stings, insect, 46–48
Stratum basale, 9
Stratum corneum, 10
Stratum cylindricum, 9
Stratum granulosum, 10
Stratum lucidum, 10
Stratum malpighii, 9
Stratum spinosum, 9
Streptococcus, β-hemolytic, in wound infection, 161
Streptokinase-streptodornase, in wound débridement, 148–149
Strip skin graft, 461–462, *462*, *571*
Subcutis, 13–14
Sugar, in wound healing, 174–175
Surface defects, of skin. See *Skin defects.*
Surgeon's knot, *272*, *273*
Surgery, reconstructive, 395–422.
Sutilains, in wound débridement, 147–148
Suture(s), 247–260
  history of, 247–248
  in closure of dead space, 246–247, *247*
  in closure of skin defects, 301–305
  in closure of wounds, 164–168, 245–246, *245*
  in skin flaps, *326*, 326–327
    pouch, *386*, *387*
    transposition, 353
    tubed pedicle, 370–371, *370–371*
  placement of, 264–274
    knots in. See *Knots, suture.*
    passage of needle in, 265–267, *266*
    wound edges in, 264–265, *265*, 267, *268*, 269, *269*
  removal of, 290–292, *291–292*
  selection of, 248–250
  sizes of, 249–250, 250(t)
  tension of, 270–271, *270–271*
  tension on, 249, *249*

Suture materials, 248, 250–260
  catgut, 164–165, 250–252, 488–489
  collagen, extruded, 253, 488–489
  cotton, 255–256, 259
  handling of, 269
  in blepharoplasty, 486–489
  natural, absorbable, 250–253, 488
  nonabsorbable, 254–256, 487
  polyamides, 258–259
  polyester, 256–257
  polyglactin 910, 254, 489
  polyglycolic acid, 165, 253–254, 489
  polyolefin, 257–258
  silk, 254–255, 487–489
  stainless steel, 256
  synthetic, absorbable, 253–254, 488–489
    nonabsorbable, 256–259, 487–488
Suture needles, 261–264, *262–263*
  and tissue trauma, 263, *264*
  in blepharoplasty, 491, 492(t)
  passage of, 265–267, *266*
Suture patterns, 274–289
  continuous, simple, *279*, 279–280
  cross suture, *283*, 283–284
  echelon, 301, *302*
  figure-of-eight, 496, *498*, 499
  horizonital mattress,
    continuous, *282*, *282*
    interrupted, *281*, 281–282
  interrupted, simple, *278*, 279
  intradermal, 167, 274–278, *275–278*
  lock, continuous, 282–283, *283*
  mattress
    vertical, *280–281*, 280–281
    X, 284, *284*
  tension, 285–289
    echelon, 301, *302*
    far-far-near-near, 287–288, *288*
    far-near-near-far, 287, *288*
    interrupted, simple, 285, *285*
    intradermal, 289
    mattress
      horizontal, 285–286, *286*
      vertical, 286–287, *287*
    pulley, 287, *288*
    stent, *288*, 288–289
    walking, 289, 302–304, *303–304*
Sweat glands, *23*, 24–26, *26*
Sweat secretions, in skin grafts, 473
Swelling, in wound closure, 167–168

Tail, amputation of, in skin flap construction, 354, *357*
  ingrown, 552–553, *553*, 553–555, *555*
Tail glands, 24
Tape, surgical adhesive, in wound closure, 260–261
Telogen, 21
Temperature and wound healing, 110
  in skin flaps, 333
Tendon, injury to, débridement in, 131–132, 183, 188–189
Tension
  diffusion of, Z-plasties and, 397–398, 411, 413, *413*

Tension *(Continued)*
  of sutures, 270–271, *270–271*
    and wound scarring, 289, 289–290
    on skin flaps, 344, *345*, 346, 350–352,
      350–353, 355, *356–357*, 358
    on sutures, 249, *249*
Tension lines, in wound healing, 298–299,
  299–300, 301, 418
Tension sutures. See *Suture patterns,
  tension.*
Tetanus, 202, *202*
Thermal burns. See *Burns, thermal.*
Thermoregulation, skin function in, 3–4
Tie-over bandage, for skin grafts, 464–466,
  465
Tissue
  adipose, 13–14
  destruction of
    in gunshot wounds, 57–58, *58*, 568
    in snakebite, 45–46
  granulation, in wound healing, *82*,
    82–83, 164, 171–172, *172*
  protection of, in cryosurgery, 205–206,
    206
  trauma to, 119
    suture needles and, 263, *264*
Tonofibrils, 9
Tourniquets, for snakebite, *187*, 187–188,
Tranquilizer(s), for snakebite, 191
Transposition skin flaps. See *Flaps, skin,
  transposition.*
Trap-door technique, in tubed pedicle skin
  flaps, 374, *375*, 376
Trauma
  in wound healing, 110–111
  thermal. See *Burns, thermal.*
  to skin, 40–69. See also specific types of
    trauma, e.g., *Burns, Snakebite(s),* etc.
  irritants and, 63
  miscellaneous sources of, 67
  to tissue, 119
    suture needles and, 263, *264*
  weather and, 66, *66*, 536–537
Trypsin, in wound débridement, 145–146,
  148
Tubed pedicle skin flaps. See *Flaps, skin,
  tubed pedicle.*
Tumbling technique, in tubed pedicle skin
  flaps, *338*, *373*, 373–374
Tumor(s)
  basal, of external ear, 544
  mammary, 28–29, 52–55
  mast cell, 50–52, *50–51*
  of eyelids, 501–504
  of skin, 48–52
Tunnel skin grafts, 462

Ulcer(s)
  Curling's, thermal burns and, 217
  decubital, 60–62, *61–62*, 199–201, *199–200*
    transposition skin flap in, 348, *348–349*
  in radiation injury, 59–60

Vascular insufficiency, in skin flaps,
  337–340

Vasculature
  in classification of flaps, 340, *341–342*, 343
  of flaps in Z-plasty, 407, *407*
  of mammary glands, 28
  of skin, 30–32, *30–31*, 33
  of tubed pedicle skin flaps, 371–373
Vasoconstrictors, and hemostasis, 243
Vasodilators, in skin flaps, 338–339
Veins, of skin, 30–32, *30–31*, 33
Venom, snake, *44*, 44–45
Vessels, lymphatic, 32
Vitamin(s), in wound healing, 111–112
Vitamin A, in wound healing, 102–103
Vitamin D, synthesis of, by skin, 4
Vulva, folds of, 555–557, *555–556*
V-Y-plasty, 415, *416*, 417
  in eyelids, *494*, 494–495

Walking sutures, 289, 302–305, *303–304*
Walking tension sutures, 289
Waltzing techniques, in tubed pedicle skin
  flaps, *373*, 373–374, *375*
Wasp stings, 47–48
Water, in wound lavage, 138
Weather trauma, 66, *66*, 536–537
Wolfe's skin grafts. See *Graft(s), skin,
  full-thickness.*
Wound(s)
  bacterial analysis in, 160–161
  classification of, 119–120
  closure of, 162–168
    adhesives for, 260–261
    dead space in, 246–247, *247*
    delayed, 237–240
      primary, *163*, 163–164
    edema with, 167–168
    in dog bites, 185
    in structure damage, 246–247
    metal clips for, 260, *260*
    primary, 162–164
    secondary, *163*, 164
    surgical instruments for, *244*, 244–246
    sutures for, 164–168
    swelling in, 167–168
    undermining of skin in, 240–242, *241*
  contaminated, management of, 119–213
  contraction of, 91–98
    benefits of, 94, 96
    cessation of, *93*, 93–94
    disadvantages of, *96*, 96–97, *97*, 568,
      569
    myofibroblasts in, 92
    skin flaps in 97
    skin grafts in, 97
    skin reaction in, 92–93
    wound shape and, 94, *95*, 568
  débridement of. See *Débridement.*
Wound(s), dehiscence of, 168–169
  disrupted, healing of, 169
  dog bite, *43*, 43–44, 184–186, *185*
  early management of, 125
  epithelialized, 87–89
  excised, following reconstructive surgery,
    239
  foreign bodies in, 104–105, 135–136
  gunshot, 55–59, *56*, *58*, *192*, 192–194, *568*
  incised, epithelialization in, 89–90, *90*

Wound(s) *(Continued)*
　infection in. See *Infection, in wounds.*
　management of, drains in, 157–160,
　　158–159
　nonhealing, 168–169, *169*
　open, 169–182, *297*
　　bandaging of, 177–182
　　granulation tissue in, 171–172
　　immobilization of, 180–182, *181*
　　insulin in, 175–177, *176*
　　mobilization of, 180–182
　　necrotic tissue in, *175*
　　pH in, 173, 173(t)
　　sugar in, 174–175
　　vital structures in, exposed, *172,*
　　　172–173
　protection of, 125–127, *126*
　puncture. See *Bite(s), dog.*
　shape of, and contraction, 94, *95, 568*
　snakebite. See *Snakebite(s).*
　sutured, epithelialization in, *89,* 89–90
Wound edges, in suture placement,
　264–265, *265–267*
Wound fibers, orientation of, 78–79, *79*
Wound healing, 70–115
　age in, 100
　anemia in, 100–101
　bandaging in, 103
　blood supply in, 100–101
　by second intention, *163,* 170, *170, 298*
　cartilage in, 103
　capillary infiltration in, 81–83
　collagen in, 79–81, 98–99
　condition of patient in, 105
　contact guidance in, 86
　contact inhibition in, 86
　cytotoxic drugs in, 108–109
　débridement stage of, 74–77, *75*
　　monocytes in, 75–76
　　neutrophils in, 74
　　phagocytosis in, 75–76, *76*
　dehydration in, 104
　denervation in, 104
　disruption of, *169*
　drugs in, 101
　edema in, 104
　effect of movement on, 107
　epithelialization in. *See Epithelialization*
　　in wound healing.
　factors affecting, 100–113
　foreign bodies in, 104–105, 135–136
　granulation tissue in, 82, *82–83,* 171–172,
　　172
　hematomas in, 109–110
　hormones in, 105
　hypoproteinemia in, 105–106
　infection in, 106–107
　inflammatory stage of, *72,* 72–74, *74*
　insulin in, 105, 174–177, *176*
　maturation stage of, *88,* 98–100
　neoplasia in, 107
　obesity in, 100
　oxygen in, 81–82, 108
　patterns of, 71, *71*
　pH in, 173(t), 173–174
　radiation and, 108–109

Wound healing *(Continued)*
　repair stage of, 77–97
　　capillary infiltration in, 81–83
　　epidermal changes in, 85
　　epithelialization in, 83–90, *84–85, 89–90*
　　fibroblasts in, 77–81
　　migratory phase in, *78*
　　proliferative phase in, *80*
　　wound contraction in, 91–98
　scab formation in, 72–73
　secondary, 109
　seromas in, 109–110
　steroids in, 100, 102–103
　sugar in, 174–175
　temperature in, 110, 173(t), *173–174*
　trauma in, 110–111
　vitamin A in, 102–103
　vitamins and, 111–112
　zinc and, 112–113
Wound lavage. See *Lavage, wound.*
Wound scarring. See *Scar(s).*
Wound scrubbing, 143
Wound strength, 79–81, 98–100
Wound therapy, antibiotics in. See
　Antibiotic(s), in wound therapy.
W-plasty, 417–421
　contraindications for, 418
　design of, 418–419, *419*
　in hypertrophic scars, 417, *416–418*
　indications for, 417–418
　surgical technique for, *416–418,* 419–420,
　　420
　tension reorientation with, *420,* 420–421

Xenografts, 463

Y-V-plasty, in eyelids, 494, *494*
　in resection of horizontal canal, 541, *541*

Zepp procedure, 539
Zinc, and wound healing, 112–113
Z-plasty(ies), 395–415
　"half-Z," 403, *403*
　modified, in skin flaps, 362, *362*
　multiple, *399,* 411–415, *412–415*
　　design of, 412–413
　　in crescent-shaped wounds, 415, *415*
　　in lengthening contractures, 414
　　indications for, 411–412
　　on limbs, *399,* 411–412, *412*
　　relief of constriction by, *400,* 414, *414*
　single, 395–411
　　angles of, 395, *395, 402,* 402–405, *404*
　　arms of, 395, *395,* 403–406, *404–405*
　　changes produced by, 398, 400, *400*
　　components, of, *395*
　　design of, 404–406
　　　without protractor, *410,* 410–411

Z-plasty(ies) (*Continued*)
    diagonals of, 401, *401*
    dynamics of, *396*
    flaps in, vasculature of, 407, *407*
    four-flap, 402, *403*
    hemostasis in, 408
    in hypertrophic scars, 408–409, *408–409*
    in reorientation of defects, 396–397,
      408–411
    in structure realignment, 399, 411

Z-plasty(ies) (*Continued*)
    in tension relief, 397–398, 411, 413, *413*
    indications for, 395, 396–400, 398, 400
    length gain with, 396, 400–404,
      400–402, 404
    necrosis in, 407–408
    scar tissue excision in, 406, *406–407*
    surgical technique for, 406–407
    tension on, prevention of, 408